D1082750

Practical Gastroenterology and Hepatology:
Esophagus and Stomach

Companion website

This book has a companion website:

practicalgastrohep.com

with:

- Videos demonstrating procedures

- The videos are all referenced in the text where you see this symbol:

Practical Gastroenterology and Hepatology

Esophagus and Stomach

EDITOR-IN-CHIEF

Nicholas J. Talley, MD, PhD

Pro Vice Chancellor and Professor of Medicine Faculty of Health
University of Newcastle, NSW, Australia;
Adjunct Professor of Medicine
College of Medicine
Mayo Clinic
Rochester, MN, and Jacksonville, FL, USA;
Foreign Adjunct Professor of Gastroenterology
Karolinska Institute
Stockholm, Sweden;
Adjunct Professor
University of North Carolina
USA

EDITORS

Kenneth R. DeVault, MD

Professor and Chair, Department of Medicine
College of Medicine, Mayo Clinic
Consultant, Division of Gastroenterology and Hepatology
Mayo Clinic
Jacksonville, FL, USA

David E. Fleischer, MD

Professor of Medicine
College of Medicine, Mayo Clinic
Consultant, Divisions of Gastroenterology and Hepatology
Mayo Clinic
Scottsdale, AZ, USA

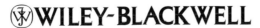

A John Wiley & Sons, Ltd., Publication

This edition first published 2010, © 2010 by Blackwell Publishing Ltd

Blackwell Publishing was acquired by John Wiley & Sons in February 2007. Blackwell's publishing program has been merged with Wiley's global Scientific, Technical and Medical business to form Wiley-Blackwell.

Registered office: John Wiley & Sons Ltd, The Atrium, Southern Gate, Chichester, West Sussex, PO19 8SQ, UK

Editorial offices: 9600 Garsington Road, Oxford, OX4 2DQ, UK
 The Atrium, Southern Gate, Chichester, West Sussex, PO19 8SQ, UK
 111 River Street, Hoboken, NJ 07030-5774, USA

For details of our global editorial offices, for customer services and for information about how to apply for permission to reuse the copyright material in this book please see our website at www.wiley.com/wiley-blackwell

The right of the author to be identified as the author of this work has been asserted in accordance with the Copyright, Designs and Patents Act 1988.

All rights reserved. No part of this publication may be reproduced, stored in a retrieval system, or transmitted, in any form or by any means, electronic, mechanical, photocopying, recording or otherwise, except as permitted by the UK Copyright, Designs and Patents Act 1988, without the prior permission of the publisher.

Wiley also publishes its books in a variety of electronic formats. Some content that appears in print may not be available in electronic books.

Designations used by companies to distinguish their products are often claimed as trademarks. All brand names and product names used in this book are trade names, service marks, trademarks or registered trademarks of their respective owners. The publisher is not associated with any product or vendor mentioned in this book. This publication is designed to provide accurate and authoritative information in regard to the subject matter covered. It is sold on the understanding that the publisher is not engaged in rendering professional services. If professional advice or other expert assistance is required, the services of a competent professional should be sought.

The contents of this work are intended to further general scientific research, understanding, and discussion only and are not intended and should not be relied upon as recommending or promoting a specific method, diagnosis, or treatment by physicians for any particular patient. The publisher and the author make no representations or warranties with respect to the accuracy or completeness of the contents of this work and specifically disclaim all warranties, including without limitation any implied warranties of fitness for a particular purpose. In view of ongoing research, equipment modifications, changes in governmental regulations, and the constant flow of information relating to the use of medicines, equipment, and devices, the reader is urged to review and evaluate the information provided in the package insert or instructions for each medicine, equipment, or device for, among other things, any changes in the instructions or indication of usage and for added warnings and precautions. Readers should consult with a specialist where appropriate. The fact that an organization or Website is referred to in this work as a citation and/or a potential source of further information does not mean that the author or the publisher endorses the information the organization or Website may provide or recommendations it may make. Further, readers should be aware that Internet Websites listed in this work may have changed or disappeared between when this work was written and when it is read. No warranty may be created or extended by any promotional statements for this work. Neither the publisher nor the author shall be liable for any damages arising herefrom.

ISBN: 9781405182737

A catalogue record for this book is available from the British Library and the Library of Congress.

Set in 9/12 pt Minion by Toppan Best-set Premedia Limited
Printed and bound in Singapore by Fabulous Printers Pte Ltd

1 2010

Contents

A companion website for this book is available at:
practicalgastrohep.com

Contributors

Sami R. Achem, MD
Professor of Medicine
Gastroenterology Consultant
Division of Gastroenterology and Hepatology
Mayo Clinic
Jacksonville, FL, USA

Deepak Agrawal, MD
Director of Endoscopy
Parkland Hospital
Assistant Professor Digestive and Liver Diseases
University Texas Southwestern Medical Center
Dallas, TX, USA

Jeffrey A. Alexander, MD
Assistant Professor of Medicine
Department of Gastroenterology and Hepatology
Division of Internal Medicine
Mayo Clinic
Rochester, MN, USA

Yasser M. Bhat, MD
Director, Interventional Endoscopy
Assistant Clinical Professor of Medicine
Division of Digestive Diseases
David Geffen School of Medicine at UCLA
Los Angeles, CA, USA

Ernest P. Bouras, MD
Assistant Professor of Medicine
Division of Gastroenterology and Hepatology
Mayo Clinic
Jacksonville, FL, USA

Eugene M. Bozymski, MD
Professor of Medicine
Department of Medicine
University of North Carolina Medical Center
Chapel Hill, NC, USA
Adjunct Professor of Medicine
Department of Medicine
Division of Gastroenterology and Hepatology
Duke University Medical Center
Durham, NC, USA

Colin Brown, MD
Fellow in Gastroenterology and Hepatology
Division of Gastroenterology and Hepatology
University of Alabama, Birmingham
Birmingham, AL, USA

Peter Bytzer, MD, PhD
Professor of Medicine
Copenhagen University
Department of Medicine
Køge University Hospital
Køge, Denmark

Matthew D. Callister, MD
Assistant Professor of Oncology
Department of Radiation Oncology
Mayo Clinic
Scottsdale, AZ, USA

Rebecca R. Cannom, MD, MS
General Surgery Resident
Division of Thoracic Foregut Surgery
Department of Surgery, Keck School of Medicine
University of Southern California
Los Angeles, CA, USA

Donald O. Castell, MD
Professor of Medicine
Division of Gastroenterology and Hepatology
Medical University of South Carolina
Charleston, SC, USA

Amitabh Chak, MD
Professor of Medicine and Oncology
Division of Gastroenterology
Case Western Reserve University School of Medicine
Cleveland, OH, USA

Francis K.L. Chan, MD
Professor of Medicine
Chief of Gastroenterology & Hepatology
Assistant Dean (General Affairs)
Department of Medicine and Therapeutics
The Chinese University of Hong Kong
Shatin, NT, Hong Kong SAR, China

Joseph Y. Chang, MD, MPH
Instructor in Medicine
Division of Gastroenterology and Hepatology
Mayo Clinic
Rochester, MN, USA

Jonathan Cohen, MD
Clinical Professor of Medicine
Division of Gastroenterology
Department of Internal Medicine
New York University School of Medicine
New York, NY, USA

Roberto de Franchis, MD
Department of Medical Sciences
University of Milan
Head, Gastroenterology Unit
IRCCS Ca' Granda Ospedale
Maggiore Policlinico Foundation
Milan, Italy

Evan S. Dellon, MD, MPH
Assistant Professor of Medicine
Division of Gastroenterology and Hepatology
Department of Medicine
University of North Carolina School of Medicine
Chapel Hill, NC, USA

Tom R. DeMeester, MD
Professor, General and Thoracic Surgery
Department of Surgery
Keck School of Medicine
University of Southern California
Los Angeles, CA, USA

Neelendu Dey, MD
Fellow in Gastroenterology
University of California San Francisco
San Francisco, CA, USA

John K. DiBaise, MD
Professor of Medicine
Divisions of Gastroenterology and Hepatology
Mayo Clinic
Scottsdale, AZ, USA

Guy D. Eslick, PhD, MMedSc (Clin Epi), MMedStat
Associate Professor of Epidemiology
Discipline of Surgery
The University of Sydney
Nepean Hospital
Penrith, NSW, Australia

Ronnie Fass, MD
Professor of Medicine
Department of Medicine
Section of Gastroenterology
University of Arizona
Head, Neuroenteric Clinical Research Group;
Chief of Gastroenterology
Section of Gastroenterology
Southern Arizona VA Health Care System
Tucson, AZ, USA

Dawn L. Francis, MD, MHS
Assistant Professor of Medicine
Associate Chair
Division of Gastroenterology and Hepatology
Mayo Clinic
Rochester, MN, USA

Gregory G. Ginsberg, MD
Professor of Medicine
Department of Medicine
Division of Gastroenterology
University of Pennsylvania School of Medicine
Executive Director of Endoscopic Services
University of Pennsylvania Health Systems
Philadelphia, PA, USA

Stuart Gordon, MD
Associate Professor of Medicine
Department of Medicine
Dartmouth Medical School
Director of Endoscopy
Section of Gastroenterology and Hepatology
Dartmouth Hitchcock Medical Center
Lebanon, NH, USA

David Y. Graham, MD
Professor of Medicine, Molecular Virology and Microbiology
Michael E. DeBakey Veterans Affairs Medical Center and
Baylor College of Medicine
Houston, TX, USA

David Greenwald, MD
Associate Professor of Clinical Medicine
Albert Einstein College of Medicine
Associate Director
Division of Gastroenterology
Montefiore Medical Center
New York, NY, USA

Gerald Holtmann, MD, PhD
Professor of Medicine
University Hospital Essen
Essen, Germany;
Faculty of Health Sciences
University of Adelaide
Adelaide, SA, Australia

James E. Huprich, MD
Division of Radiology
Mayo Clinic
Rochester, MN, USA

Dennis M. Jensen, MD
Professor of Medicine
Department of Medicine
David Geffen School of Medicine at UCLA
Los Angeles, CA, USA

David A. Johnson, MD
Professor of Medicine
Chief of Gastroenterology
Division of Gastroenterology
Eastern VA Medical School
Norfolk, VA, USA

Daniel B. Jones, MD, MS
Professor
Harvard Medical School
Chief, Section Minimally Invasive Surgery
Beth Israel Deaconess Medical Center
Boston, MA, USA

Kee Wook Jung, MD
Advanced Fellow, Diseases of the Esophagus
Division of Gastroenterology and Hepatology
Department of Medicine
Mayo Clinic
Rochester, MN, USA

Philip O. Katz, MD
Chairman, Division of Gastroenterology
Albert Einstein Medical Center
Clinical Professor of Medicine
Jefferson Medical College
Philadelphia, PA, USA

David A. Katzka
Professor of Medicine
Division of Gastroenterology and Hepatology
Mayo Clinic
Rochester, MN, USA

H. Jae Kim, MD, MSc
Assistant Professor of Medicine
Divisions of Gastroenterology and Hepatology
Mayo Clinic
Scottsdale, AZ, USA

Kazufumi Kimura, MD, PhD
Research Fellow
Microbiology and Immunology
School of Biomedical, Biomolecular and Chemical Sciences
University of Western Australia
Perth, WA, Australia

Christen Klochan, MD
Resident, Department of Internal Medicine
Vanderbilt University Medical Center
Nashville, TN, USA

Michael L. Kochman, MD
Wilmott Family Professor of Medicine
Professor of Medicine in Surgery
Division of Gastroenterology
University of Pennsylvania Health System
Philadelphia, PA, USA

Thomas O.G. Kovacs, MD
Professor of Medicine
CURE/Digestive Diseases Research Center
Department of Medicine
David Geffen School of Medicine at UCLA
Los Angeles, CA, USA

Benjamin E. Levitzky, MD
Digestive Disease Institute
Cleveland Clinic Foundation
Cleveland, OH, USA

James H. Lewis, MD
Professor of Medicine
Division of Gastroenterology
Georgetown University Medical Center
Washington, DC, USA

Charles J. Lightdale, MD
Professor of Clinical Medicine
Division of Digestive and Liver Diseases
Columbia University Medical Center
New York, NY, USA

Henry Lin, MD
Head of Bariatrics
National Naval Medical Center and Walter Reed
Army Medical Center
Bethesda, MD, USA

Hendrik Manner, MD
Internal Medicine Specialist
Department of Gastroenterology and Hepatology
Horst Schmidt Klinik (HSK)
Wiesbaden, Germany

Barry J. Marshall, MD
Clinical Professor
Microbiology and Immunology
School of Biomedical, Biomolecular and Chemical Sciences
University of Western Australia
Perth, WA, Australia

Rodney J. Mason, MD, PhD
Associate Professor of Surgery
Division of General and Laparoscopic Surgery
University of Southern California Los Angeles
Los Angeles, CA, USA

Stephen A. McClave, MD
Professor of Medicine
Division of Gastroenterology/Hepatology
University of Louisville School of Medicine
Louisville, KY, USA

Kenneth McQuaid, MD
Professor of Clinical Medicine
University of California San Francisco
Chief, GI Section
San Francisco VA Medical Center
San Francisco, CA, USA

David C. Metz, MD
Professor of Medicine
Division of Gastroenterology
University of Pennsylvania School of Medicine
Philadelphia, PA, USA

Vikneswaran Namasivayam, MB, BS
Advanced Fellow, Diseases of the Esophagus
Division of Gastroenterology and Hepatology
Department of Medicine
Mayo Clinic
Rochester, MN, USA

Lori A. Orlando, MD, MHS
Assistant Professor of Medicine
Division of General Internal Medicine
Duke University Medical Center
Durham, NC, USA

Roy C. Orlando, MD
Mary Kay and Eugene Bozymski and Linda and William
Heizer Distinguished Professor of Gastroenterology
Adjunct Professor of Cell and Molecular Physiology
Division of Gastroenterology and Hepatology
University of North Carolina School of Medicine
Chapel Hill, NC, USA

Henry P. Parkman, MD
Professor of Medicine
Director of GI Motility Laboratory
Temple University School of Medicine
Philadelphia, PA, USA

Oliver Pech, MD, PhD
Associate Professor
Gastroenterology Attending Physician
Department of Gastroenterology and Hepatology
Horst Schmidt Klinik (HSK)
Wiesbaden, Germany

Carlos A. Pellegrini, MD
The Henry N. Harkins Professor and Chair
Department of Surgery
University of Washington
Seattle, WA, USA

Heiko Pohl, MD
Assistant Professor of Medicine
Section of Gastroenterology
Dartmouth Medical School
VAMC White River Junction, VT;
Section of Gastroenterology and Hepatology
Dartmouth Hitchcock Medical Center
Lebanon, NH, USA

Joel E. Richter, MD
Professor of Medicine
The Richard L. Evans Chair
Department of Medicine
Temple University School of Medicine
Philadelphia, PA, USA

Jason R. Roberts, MD
Fellow
Division of Gastroenterology and Hepatology
Medical University of South Carolina
Charleston, SC, USA

Yvonne Romero, MD
Assistant Professor of Medicine
GI Epidemiology/Outcomes Unit
Division of Gastroenterology and Hepatology
Department of Medicine
Mayo Clinic
Rochester, MN, USA

Richard I. Rothstein, MD
Professor of Medicine and of Surgery
Dartmouth Medical School
Chief, Section of Gastroenterology and Hepatology
Dartmouth Hitchcock Medical Center
Lebanon, NH, USA

Massimo Rugge, MD
Professor of Pathology
Department of Diagnostic Medical Sciences and
Special Therapies
Pathology Unit
University of Padova
Padova, Italy

Thomas J. Savides, MD
Professor of Clinical Medicine
Division of Gastroenterology
University of California, San Diego
San Diego, CA, USA

Virender K. Sharma, MD
Director
Arizona Center for Digestive Health
Phoenix, AZ, USA

Peter D. Siersema, MD, PhD
Professor of Gastroenterology
Department of Gastroenterology and Hepatology
University Medical Center Utrecht
Utrecht, The Netherlands

C. Daniel Smith, MD
Professor and Chair
Department of Surgery
Mayo Clinic
Jacksonville, FL, USA

Michael S. Smith, MD, MBA
Assistant Professor of Medicine
Associate Director, Esophageal Program
Gastroenterology Section
Department of Medicine
Temple University School of Medicine
Philadelphia, PA, USA

Geoffrey Spencer, MD, MSCE
Instructor of Medicine
Division of Gastroenterology
Hospital of the University of Pennsylvania
Philadelphia, PA, USA

Mark E. Stark, MD
Consultant in Gastroenterology
Associate Professor of Medicine
Division of Gastroenterology and Hepatology
Mayo Clinic
Jacksonville, FL, USA

Ellen Stein, MD
Fellow in Gastroenterology
Division of Gastroenterology
Albert Einstein Medical Center
Philadelphia, PA, USA

Kazuki Sumiyama, MD, PhD
Clinical Associate, Consultant Endoscopist
Department of Endoscopy
The Jikei University School of Medicine
Minato-ku, Tokyo, Japan

Jan Tack, MD, PhD
Professor of Medicine
Department of Pathophysiology
Gastroenterology Section
University of Leuven
Leuven, Belgium

Hisao Tajiri, MD, PhD
Chairman and Professor
Division of Gastroenterology and Hepatology
Department of Internal Medicine
The Jikei University School of Medicine
Minato-ku, Tokyo, Japan

Roger P. Tatum, MD
Assistant Professor
Department of Surgery
University of Washington
Seattle, WA, USA

Stephen W. Trenkner, MD
Associate Professor
Division of Radiology
Mayo Clinic
Rochester, MN, USA

Michael F. Vaezi, MD, PhD, MSc(Epi)
Professor of Medicine
Director, Clinical Research and Center for Swallowing and
Esophageal Disorders
Clinical Director, Division of Gastroenterology, Hepatology
and Nutrition
Vanderbilt University Medical Center
Nashville, TN, USA

John J. Vargo, II, MD, MPH
Associate Professor of Medicine
Cleveland Clinic Lerner College of Medicine of Case Western
Reserve University
Head, Section of Therapeutic and Hepatobiliary Endoscopy
Digestive Disease Institute
Cleveland Clinic Foundation
Cleveland, OH, USA

Ganesh R. Veerappan, MD
Senior Fellow in Gastroenterology
Gastroenterology Service
Walter Reed Army Medical Center
Washington, DC, USA

C. Mel Wilcox, MD
Professor of Medicine
Division of Gastroenterology and Hepatology
University of Alabama at Birmingham
Birmingham, AL, USA

Helen M. Windsor, PhD
Research Fellow
Microbiology and Immunology
School of Biomedical, Biomolecular and Chemical Sciences
University of Western Australia
Perth, WA, Australia

John M. Wo, MD
Professor of Medicine
Director of Swallowing and Motility Center
Division of Gastroenterology/Hepatology
University of Louisville School of Medicine
Louisville, KY, USA

Herbert C. Wolfsen, MD
Professor of Medicine
Mayo Clinic
Rochester, MN, USA
Consultant, Division of Gastroenterology and Hepatology
Mayo Clinic
Jacksonville, FL, USA

Vincent W.S. Wong, MD, MRCP
Associate Professor
Department of Medicine and Therapeutics
The Chinese University of Hong Kong
Shatin, NT, Hong Kong SAR, China

Preface

Welcome to *Practical Gastroenterology and Hepatology*, a new comprehensive three volume resource for everyone training in gastroenterology and for those certifying (or re-certifying) in the subspecialty. We have aimed to create three modern, easy to read and digest stand-alone textbooks. The entire set covers the waterfront, from clinical evaluation to advanced endoscopy to common and rare diseases every gastroenterologist must know.

Volume one specifically deals with disorders of the upper GI tract including mainly the stomach and esophagus. Each chapter highlights, where appropriate, a clinical case which demonstrates a common clinical situation, its approach, and management. Simple easy to follow clinical algorithms are demonstrated throughout the relevant chapters. Endoscopy chapters provide excellent video examples, all available electronically.

Each chapter has been written by the best of the best in the field, and carefully peer reviewed and edited for accuracy and relevance. We have guided the writing of this textbook to help ensure experienced gastroenterologists, fellows, residents, medical students, internists, primary care physicians, as well as surgeons all will find something of interest and relevance.

Each volume and every chapter has followed a standard template structure. All chapters focus on key knowledge, and the most important clinical facts are highlighted in an introductory abstract and as take home points at the end; irrelevant or unimportant information is omitted. The chapters are deliberately brief and readable; we want our readers to retain the material, and immediately be able to apply what they learn in practice. The chapters are illustrated in color, enhanced by a very pleasant layout. A Web based version has been created to complement the textbook including endoscopy images and movies.

In this volume, section one addresses the pathobiology of the esophagus and stomach, providing a scientific basis for disease. The emphasis here is, as in all volumes, on the practical and clinically relevant, as opposed to the esoteric. Section two deals with endoscopy issues including preparation, endoscopic anatomy and both routine and advanced (EMR, ablation of neoplasia, NOTES and other) procedures. Section three covers the other "non-endoscopic" approaches to the upper gastrointestinal tract including radiologic, motility, reflux and capsule testing and physiologic testing. Section four approaches disorders from a problem or symptom based standpoint with a simple, clear guide to diagnosis and management strategies. Section five covers important diseases of the esophagus including GERD and its complications, motility disorders, other mucosal diseases, esophageal cancer and others. Section six addresses diseases of the stomach including peptic ulcer disease, gastritis, gastroparesis, cancer, other mucosal diseases and surgical issues. Section eight covers functional gastrointestinal disorders of the upper gastrointestinal tract.

We have been thrilled to work with a terrific team in the creation of this work, and very much hope you will enjoy reading this volume as much as we have enjoyed developing it for you.

Nicholas J. Talley
David E. Fleischer
Kenneth R. DeVault

Foreword

Dr. Talley and colleagues are to be congratulated for providing a very informative and thorough review of diseases affecting the upper portion of the gastrointestinal tract, including the clinical presentations, diagnostic testing and management. In this first volume of their complete treatise, they have assembled experts from around the world to succinctly discuss individual aspects of upper gastrointestinal disorders. They have identified the right individuals to share their knowledge in each one of the individual chapters. What a delight it was for me to have my personal knowledge and awareness of the various conditions and their management expanded by reviewing this collection. I can easily promise that the reader will find their personal knowledge enhanced and gain a greater awareness to the clinical aspects of esophageal and gastric disorders. I applaud Dr. Talley and his associates for their conscientious effort and I thank them for providing this exceptional work to the GI community. I believe it will find a place in the active personal library of clinicians worldwide.

Donald O. Castell, MD, AGAF, MACG
Professor of Medicine
Director, Esophageal Disorders Program
Medical University of South Carolina

PART 1

Pathobiology of the Esophagus and Stomach

1

CHAPTER 1

Anatomy, Embryology, and Congenital Malformations of the Esophagus and Stomach

Lori A. Orlando[1] and Roy C. Orlando[2]

[1] Division of General Internal Medicine, Duke University Medical Center, Durham, NC, USA
[2] Division of Gastroenterology and Hepatology, University of North Carolina School of Medicine, Chapel Hill, NC, USA

Summary

Understanding the anatomy and embryology of the esophagus and stomach is necessary for dealing with clinically important congenital malformations. The esophagus acts as a conduit for the transport of food from the oral cavity to the stomach which, as a J-shaped dilation of the alimentary canal, connects with the duodenum distally. Sphincters at the upper esophagus, distal esophagus/proximal stomach, and distal stomach have strategic functions. Formation of the esophagus (primitive foregut) begins at 6 weeks and the stomach is recognizable in the fourth week of gestation as a dilation of the distal foregut. Congenital abnormalities of the esophagus are common and of the stomach are rare.

Case

A 7-year-old male developed dysphagia while attending a birthday party. A hot dog did not pass despite retching and giving the boy carbonated beverages. He was seen in the emergency room where an esophagram was performed. A contrast radiograph outlined a 1-cm length of hot dog above a 10-cm stricture in the mid-esophagus. There was no associated tracheal–esophageal fistula. With anesthesia, an endoscopy was performed and the hot dog was removed. The patient was seen in follow-up evaluation and causes for mid-esophageal stricture were explored. No etiology was found and the clinical findings were attributed to congenital esophageal stenosis. At a later time, endoscopy was repeated and dilation was carried out with bougies. Further dilations were undertaken and surgery was being discussed.

Practical Gastroenterology and Hepatology: Esophagus and Stomach, 1st edition. Edited by Nicholas J. Talley, Kenneth R. DeVault and David E. Fleischer. © 2010 Blackwell Publishing Ltd.

Anatomy

The esophagus is a conduit for the transport of food from the oral cavity to the stomach. It is an 18 to 22-cm long, hollow, muscular tube with an inner "skin-like" lining of stratified squamous epithelium. The esophagus is collapsed and airless at rest but, during swallowing, is distended by the food bolus. When the bolus is delivered to the stomach, it is stored in the gastric fundus, then mixed with acid and ground in the gastric body and antrum. Finally, it is propulsed through the pylorus and into the duodenum.

Structurally, the esophageal wall is composed of four layers: innermost mucosa, submucosa, muscularis propria, and outermost adventitia; unlike the remainder of the gastrointestinal tract, the esophagus has no serosa [1,2]. The esophageal musculature is comprised of skeletal muscle in the upper third and smooth muscle in the lower two-thirds. Both skeletal and smooth muscle are innervated by the Vagus nerve with nuclei located within the central medullary swallowing center. The stomach is also innervated by the Vagus nerve, which splits into two branches—the left which innervates the dorsal wall (greater curvature) and the right which innervates the ventral wall (lesser curvature).

Upper Esophageal Sphincter

Proximally, the esophagus begins where the inferior pharyngeal constrictor merges with the cricopharyngeus, an area of skeletal muscle known as the upper esophageal sphincter (UES). The UES is contracted at rest, creating a high-pressure zone that prevents inspired air from entering the esophagus. UES contraction is mediated by intrinsic muscle tone and vagal acetycholine release, while relaxation is mediated by inhibition of acetylcholine release [3].

Esophageal Body

The esophageal body lies within the posterior mediastinum behind the trachea and left mainstem bronchus [1]. At the T10 vertebral level the esophageal body leaves the thorax through a hiatus within the right crus of the diaphragm. Within the hiatus the esophageal body ends in a 2 to 4-cm asymmetrically thickened, circular smooth muscle known as the lower esophageal sphincter [4]. Pain within the esophagus is mediated by stimulation of chemoreceptors in the esophageal mucosa or submucosa and mechanoreceptors in the esophageal musculature [5].

Lower Esophageal Sphincter (LES)

The LES is contracted at rest due to intrinsic smooth muscle tone and vagal acetylcholine release. This contraction creates a high-pressure zone that prevents gastric contents from entering the esophagus. The high-pressure zone is also aided by contraction of the diaphragm and weakened in the presence of a hiatal hernia. During swallowing, LES relaxation occurs by vagal release of nitric oxide (and vasoactive intestinal peptide), enabling peristalsis to push the bolus from the esophagus into the stomach [4]. The same mechanism initiates receptive relaxation of the gastric fundus to accommodate a meal without a concomitant increase in intragastric pressure.

Mucosa

On endoscopy, the esophageal stratified squamous-lined mucosa appears smooth and pink while the stomach's simple columnar mucosa is red. Their junction is recognized by an irregular, white, "Z-shaped" line (ora serrata). Squamous cells have no secretory capacity while gastric cells can secrete both into the lumen (acid, pepsin, and a variety of other products) and the blood (gastrin). Below the epithelium is the lamina propria, a loose network of connective tissue with blood vessels and scattered white cells. A thin layer of smooth muscle, the muscularis mucosae, separates the lamina propria from the submucosa, a network of dense connective tissue comprised of blood vessels, lymphatic channels, Meissner neuronal plexus and, in the esophagus, submucosal glands. The esophageal glands secrete mucus and bicarbonate into collecting ducts that deliver the fluid to the esophageal lumen. Between the inner circular and outer longitudinal layers of the muscularis propria is Auerbach neuronal plexus.

Embryology

In the developing fetus, the gastrointestinal tract and the respiratory tract develop from a common tube of endoderm. Between weeks 7 and 10, a ventral diverticulum is formed, which subsequently develops into the respiratory tract; the remaining dorsal part of the tube becomes the primitive foregut. The foregut is initially lined by ciliated columnar epithelium, but begins to transform into stratified squamous epithelium by week 16. This epithelial transition is complete by birth. At embryonic week 4, the stomach is discernable as a dilation of the distal foregut. As the stomach grows, it rotates 90° around its longitudinal axis so that the greater curvature is located dorsally and the lesser curvature ventrally.

Congenital Malformations of the Esophagus and Stomach

Congenital anomalies of the esophagus are relatively common (1 in 3000 to 1 in 4500 live births) and are due to either transmission of genetic defects or intrauterine stress that impedes fetal maturation [6–8]. A clinical overview is presented in Table 1.1. In premature infants about 50% of esophageal anomalies are also associated with anomalies at other sites; this has given rise to the term VACTERL. The letters in VACTERL represent a mnemonic depicting these anomalies which include:

Table 1.1 Clinical aspects of esophageal developments anomalies. (Reproduced with permission from Long JD, Orlando RC. Anatomy, histology, embryology, and developmental anomalies of the esophagus. In: Feldman M, Friedman LS, Sleisenger MH, eds. *Sleisenger and Fordtran's Gastrointestinal and Liver Disease; Pathophysiology/Diagnosis/Management,* 7th edn. Philadelphia: Saunders (an imprint of Elsevier Science): 2002: 556.)

Anomaly	Age at presentation	Predominant symptoms	Diagnosis	Treatment
Atresia alone	Newborns	Regurgitation of feedings Aspiration	Esophagogram* Radiograph—gasless abdomen	Surgery
Atresia + distal fistula	Newborns	Regurgitation of feedings Aspiration	Esophagogram* Radiograph—gasless abdomen	Surgery
H-type fistula	Infants to adults	Recurrent aspiration pneumonia Bronchiectasis	Esophagogram* Bronchoscopy	Surgery
Esophageal stenosis	Infants to adults	Dysphagia Food impaction	Esophagogram* Endoscopy†	Bougienage‡ Surgery§
Duplication cysts	Infants to adults	Dyspnea, stridor, cough (infants) Dysphagia, chest pain (adults)	EUS* MRI/CT† Esophagogram	Surgery
Vascular anomalies	Infants to adults	Dyspnea, stridor, cough (infants) Dysphagia (adults)	Esophagogram* Angiography† MRI/CT/EUS	Diet modification‡ Surgery§
Esophageal rings	Children to adults	Dysphagia Food impaction	Esophagogram* Endoscopy†	Bougienage
Esophageal webs	Children to adults	Dysphagia	Esophagogram* Endoscopy†	Bougienage

*Diagnostic test of choice.
†Confirmatory test.
‡Primary therapeutic approach.
§Secondary therapeutic approach.
CT, computed tomography, EUS; endoscopic ultrasonography; MRI, magnetic resonance imaging.

Vertebral, Anal, Cardiac, Tracheal, Esophageal, Renal, and Limb systems. Specific defects within this group are the patent ductus arteriosus, cardiac septal deformity, and imperforate anus.

Esophageal Atresia and Tracheoesophageal (TE) Fistula

Esophageal atresia, a failure of the primitive foregut to re-canalize, occurs as an isolated anomaly in 7% and in conjunction with a TE fistula in 93%. In the isolated type of esophageal atresia the upper esophagus ends in a blind pouch and the lower esophagus connects to the stomach. The condition is suspected at birth by the occurrence of choking, coughing, and regurgitation on first feeding in combination with a scaphoid gasless abdomen. The diag-

nosis can be confirmed by failure to pass a nasogastric tube into the stomach and air in the upper esophagus on chest radiograph following air insufflation via a naso-esophageal tube.

When esophageal atresia is associated with a TE fistula, the majority of the cases are accompanied by the distal type in which the upper esophagus ends in a blind pouch and the distal esophagus connects to the trachea. The clinical presentation of the distal type is similar to isolated esophageal atresia, with the addition of recurrent aspiration pneumonia and increased abdominal air. Both of these are attributed to the communication between the esophagus and trachea, permitting reflux of gastric contents into the trachea and air into the esophagus and stomach (which can be seen on plain radiographs) [7].

There are three less common types of TE fistula. The first is when both upper and lower segments of the atretic esophagus communicate with the trachea; the second is when just the upper segment communicates with the trachea; and the third or "H-type fistula" is when the esophagus is *not* atretic, but still communicates with the trachea. All TE fistula types present with recurrent aspiration pneumonia due to the communication between the esophagus and trachea; however, they can be differentiated by other clinical features. The first two types present in infancy and are distinguished from each other by the presence or absence of bowel gas on a plain radiograph (gas present when there is an accompanying distal TE fistula). In contrast, diagnosis of the H-type TE fistula may be delayed until childhood or young adult-hood [8]. The diagnosis of an H-type fistula is usually made either on bronchoscopy after ingestion of methy-lene blue to stain the fistula site or on esophagography.

The treatment of almost all esophageal anomalies is surgical. Success rates depend upon the type and severity of accompanying genetic abnormalities. For isolated atresias, surgical success is about 90%; however, there is an increased risk of gastroesophageal reflux disease after correction due to abnormalities of both esophageal motility and luminal acid clearance.

Congenital Stenosis

Esophageal stenosis, which varies in length from 2 to 20 cm is rare and typically occurs in males [9]. The precise cause is unknown and most present with solid-food dysphagia and regurgitation in infancy or child-hood. Diagnosis is made by either esophagography or endoscopy. Treatment is by endoscopic-guided bougie-nage, which has variable efficacy depending upon the length and the complexity of the stricture. It is possible that some, perhaps many, of the cases once considered congenital stenosis actually are involved with eosino-philic esophagitis (see Chapter 34).

Esophageal Duplications

Congenital duplications of the esophagus are rare and arise as epithelial-lined outpouchings off the primitive foregut. There are two types: cystic and tubular. Cysts account for 80% of the duplications and are usually single, fluid-filled structures. They do not communicate with the lumen and when large are often associated with compression of the adjacent tracheobronchial tree,

resulting in cough, stridor, wheezing, cyanosis, or chest pain. When asymptomatic they may be detected as medi-astinal masses on chest radiography or submucosal lesions on esophagogram. The diagnosis is confirmed by computed tomography (CT), magnetic resonance imaging (MRI) or endoscopic ultrasonography (EUS). Surgical excision is usually required to exclude a cystic neoplasm [10].

Tubular esophageal duplications are less common and, unlike the cystic type, *do* communicate with the true lumen [10]. They usually cause chest pain, dysphagia, or regurgitation in infancy, and the diagnosis is established by esophagography or endoscopy. Reconstructive surgery is indicated for those patients who are symptomatic [10–12].

Vascular Anomalies

Intrathoracic vascular anomalies are present in 2–3% of the population. Most are asymptomatic, however some may develop symptoms from esophageal compression (dysphagia and regurgitation) in childhood or adult-hood. Dysphagia lusoria, the most common vascular compression of the esophagus, is due to an aberrant right subclavian artery, arising off the left side of the aortic arch [13]. Diagnosis is made by a pencil-like extrinsic esophageal compression at the level of the third to fourth thoracic vertebrae on barium esophagogram [13]. Con-firmation is made by CT, MRI or EUS [13,14]. Initial treatment is dietary modification (mechanical soft diet) for symptom control with surgery reserved for refractory cases.

Esophageal Rings

The distal esophagus may contain up to two "rings", the muscular A ring and the mucosal B or Schatzki ring. The A ring is 4–5 mm thick and represents an enlargement of the upper end of the LES [15,16]. It is both uncommon and rarely symptomatic. The B ring, which is 2 mm thick, represents the squamocolumnar junction [15,16]. It is common and usually asymptomatic, unless the lumen size is compressed to less than 15 mm, at which point intermittent solid-food dysphagia or acute impaction may occur [15,16].

Esophageal Webs

Esophageal webs are thin mucosal protrusions extending from the anterior wall of the esophagus in the cervical region. They are thus best visualized on a lateral view of an esophagram. Unlike rings, webs rarely encircle the lumen [17]. Nonetheless, cervical webs can cause solid-food dysphagia. The triad of cervical webs, dysphagia, and iron-deficiency anemia is referred to as the Plummer–Vinson or Paterson–Brown-Kelly syndrome [17]. The syndrome is significant as it increases the risk of squamous cell carcinoma of the pharynx and esophagus and may also be associated with celiac sprue [17,18]. Treatment with iron has been reported to not only correct the iron deficiency but to also induce resolution of the web. Isolated cervical webs are treated by esophageal bougienage.

Heterotopic Gastric Mucosa

Heterotopic gastric mucosa is also known as the "inlet patch". It is seen on 10% of endoscopies as a small, red island of mucosa just below the UES. Typically, inlet patches are asymptomatic though rarely they secrete acid and cause strictures or ulcers [19] and even more rarely evolve into adenocarcinoma [20].

Congenital Malformations of the Stomach

Congenital malformations of the stomach are very uncommon and include: gastric atresia, microgastria, gastric volvulus, gastric diverticulum, and gastric duplications. When symptomatic, these lesions typically present with epigastric pain, nausea, and vomiting, reflecting the degree of gastric outlet obstruction. Gastric atresia may be associated with both Down syndrome and epidermolysis bullosa. Unlike esophageal duplications, gastric duplications rarely communicate with the lumen and therefore develop into masses within the stomach wall. Congenital laxity of ligaments attaching stomach to duodenum, spleen, liver, and diaphragm are contributing causes of gastric volvulus, which are either mesenteroaxial or organoaxial in type based on the axis of rotation. Mesenteroaxial gastric volvulus may be asymptomatic or symptomatic with chronic, intermittent, upper gastrointestinal symptoms [21]. Organoaxial gastric volvulus is typically acute, presenting with abdominal pain, retching, and inability to pass a nasogastric tube (Borchardt triad). It is commonly associated with a diaphragmatic hernia and a gas-filled viscus in the thorax may be seen on chest radiography. Diagnosis is confirmed by upper gastrointestinal series.

Take-home points

Anatomy:
- The upper esophageal sphincter (UES) is a skeletal-muscled structure that prevents inhaled air from entering the esophagus. The lower esophageal sphincter (LES) is a smooth-muscled structure that prevents gastric contents from refluxing into the esophagus.
- The distal end of the LES demarcates the anatomic gastroesophageal junction. This muscular junction on endoscopy is approximated by the proximal (orad) end of the gastric folds.
- The squamocolumnar junction on endoscopy is denoted by a white, irregular, "Z-shaped" line that is the transition between esophageal and gastric epithelia.
- The stomach is comprised of a cardia, fundus, body, antrum, and pylorus and is completely invested by peritoneum except at the gastroesophageal junction.

Embryology:
- The formation of the esophagus (primitive forgut) begins at 6 weeks in the embryo; it is initially lined by a ciliated columnar epithelium but this is completely replaced by stratified squamous epithelium by birth.
- The stomach is identifiable by week 4 in the embryo as a dilation of the distal foregut. As it grows it rotates 90° around its longitudinal axis so that the greater curvature lies to the left and lesser curvature to the right.

Congenital malformations of the esophagus and stomach:
- Congenital anomalies of the esophagus are common and gastric anomalies are rare.
- Most esophageal atresias are accompanied by a distal-type TE fistula.
- The only TE fistula that may go undetected until adulthood is known as the H type.
- The inlet patch is usually an incidental finding on endoscopy, appearing as a small island of red-appearing gastric mucosa just below the UES.
- The B or Schatzki ring is a 2-mm thick mucosal indentation located at the squamocolumnar junction. When reducing the esophageal lumen to <15mm, it commonly causes intermittent solid-food dysphagia or acute solid-food impaction.
- Cervical webs, dysphagia, and iron-deficiency anemia are a triad known as the Plummer–Vinson or Paterson–Brown-Kelly syndrome.
- Gastric volvulus can be mesenteroaxial or organoaxial in type, the latter typically an acute event producing abdominal pain, retching an inability to pass a nasogastric tube (Borchardt triad).

References

1 Skandalakis JE, Ellis H. Embryologic and anatomic basis of esophageal surgery. *Surg Clin North Am* 2000; **80**: 85–155.

2 Ergun GA, Kahrilas PJ. Esophageal muscular anatomy and physiology. In: *Atlas of Esophageal Diseases*, 2nd edn. Philadelphia: Current Medicine, Inc., 2002: 2–18.

3 Mittal RK, Balaban DH. The esophagogastric junction. *N Engl J Med* 1997; **336**: 924–32.

4 Hornby PJ, Abrahams TP. Central control of lower esophageal sphincter relaxation. *Am J Med* 2000; **108** (Supp. 4A): 90S.

5 Orlando RC. Esophageal perception and noncardiac chest pain. *Gastroenterol Clin N Am* 2004; **33**: 25–33.

6 Spitz L, Kiely EM, Morecroft JA, *et al.* Oesophageal atresia: At-risk groups for the 1990s. *J Pediatr Surg* 1994; **29**: 723–5.

7 Deurloo JA, Ekkelkamp S, Schoorl M, *et al.* Esophageal atresia: Historical evolution of management and results in 371 patients. *Ann Thorac Surg* 2002; **73**: 267–72.

8 Danton MHD, McMahon J, McGiugan J, *et al.* Congenital oesophageal respiratory tract fistula presenting in adult life. *Eur Respir J* 1993; **6**: 1412.

9 Amae S, Nio M, Kamiyama T, *et al.* Clinical characteristics and management of congenital esophageal stenosis: A report of 14 cases. *J Pediatr Surg* 2003; **38**: 565–70.

10 Geller A, Wang KK, DiMagno EP. Diagnosis of foregut duplication cysts by endoscopic ultrasonography. *Gastroenterology* 1995; **109**: 838–42.

11 Cioffi U, Bonavina L, De Simone M, *et al.* Presentation and surgical management of bronchogenic and esophageal duplication cysts in adults. *Chest* 1998; **113**: 1492–6.

12 Ratan ML, Anand R, Mittal SK, *et al.* Communicating oesophageal duplication: A report of two cases. *Gut* 1988; **29**: 254–6.

13 Janssen M, Baggen MGA, Veen HF, *et al.* Dysphagia lusoria: Clinical aspects, manometric findings, diagnosis, and therapy. *Am J Gastroenterol* 2000; **95**: 1411–16.

14 De Luca L, Bergman JGHM, Tytgat GNJ, *et al.* EUS imaging of the arteria lusoria: Case series and review. *Gastrointest Endosc* 2000; **52**: 670–3.

15 Tobin RW. Esophageal rings, webs, and diverticula. *J Clin Gastroenterol* 1998; **27**: 285–95.

16 Hirano I, Gilliam J, Goyal RK. Clinical and manometric features of the lower esophageal muscular ring. *Am J Gastroenterol* 2000; **95**: 43–9.

17 Dickey W, McConnell B. Celiac disease presenting as the Paterson–Brown-Kelly (Plummer–Vinson) syndrome. *Am J Gastroenterol* 1999; **94**: 527–9.

18 Jessner W, Vogelsang H, Puspok A, *et al.* Plummer–Vinson syndrome associated with celiac disease and complicated by postcricoid carcinoma and carcinoma of the tongue. *Am J Gastroenterol* 2003; **98**: 1208–9.

19 Von Rahden BHA, Stein HJ, Becker K, *et al.* Heterotopic gastric mucosa of the esophagus: Literature-review and proposal of a clinicopathologic classification. *Am J Gastroenterol* 2004; **99**: 543–51.

20 Galan AR, Katzka DA, Castell DO. Acid secretion from an esophageal inlet patch demonstrated by ambulatory pH monitoring. *Gastroenterology* 1998; **115**: 1574–6.

21 Godshall D, Mossallam U, Rosenbaum R. Gastric volvulus: Case report and review of the literature. *J Emerg Med* 1999; **17**: 837–40.

2

CHAPTER 2
Esophageal and Gastric Motor Function

Kenneth R. DeVault[1], Ernest P. Bouras[1], and Nicholas J. Talley[2]

[1]Division of Gastroenterology and Hepatology, Mayo Clinic, Jacksonville, FL, USA
[2]Faculty of Health, University of Newcastle, NSW, Australia

Summary

The esophagus and stomach have specific motor functions that propel ingested material through the upper gastrointestinal tract, while the stomach also helps to grind the food into a more digestible form. The proximal, striated muscle portion of the esophagus quickly moves the bolus into the distal esophagus where smooth muscle contractions propel it through the lower esophageal sphincter into the stomach. In addition to allowing the bolus to pass, the lower esophageal sphincter is tonically contracted in its resting state, which prevents gastroesophageal reflux. The proximal stomach receptively relaxes to accommodate the swallowed bolus, while the distal stomach has functions to grind the food into smaller sizes to facilitate digestion. The antrum and pylorus have an additional function as a "sieve" to prevent emptying of particles until they have been reduced to an appropriate size. The stomach has a specific region that coordinates the motor activity of the stomach and to a degree the entire upper gastrointestinal tract (pacemaker region). This region initiates the periodic contraction profile that pushes both digested and undigested material through the gastrointestinal tract (phase III of the migrating motor complex). This complicated physiology is affected by both hormones and extrinsic innervation, but the pacemaker resides in the specialized nervous system of the gastrointestinal tract, most likely in the interstitial Cajal cells.

Esophageal Motor Function

The esophagus is a tubular structure of approximately 18–25 cm in length (somewhat dependent on body height) with two major functions: propulsion of swallowed material to the stomach and prevention of the reflux gastric content back toward the mouth. At rest, the smooth muscle of the esophagus is relaxed, with the exception of the sphincters located on either end; the striated muscle upper esophageal sphincter and the smooth muscle lower esophageal sphincter. Those sphincters are very important since the pressure of the thoracic cavity is lower than either the external environment or the stomach (without the sphincters, air and gastric content would be pulled into the esophagus).

Innervation of Esophageal Muscle

The proximal portion of the esophagus is composed of striated muscle that is not under voluntary control, but is directly innervated by cholinergic nerves that have their cell bodies in the brainstem (predominantly the nucleus ambiguous). Vagal nerves going to the smooth muscle have their cell bodies in the dorsal motor complex and do not directly synapse on the muscle, but alternatively synapse on myenteric neurons. Cholinergic innervation excites both the longitudinal and circular muscle, while the non-adrenergic, non-cholinergic transmitter mainly inhibits activity in the circular muscle [1]. The final mediator of this relaxation is most likely nitric oxide (NO) or a similar compound [2]. Peristalsis can occur in a deinnervated esophagus through intramural enteric neurological activity.

Practical Gastroenterology and Hepatology: Esophagus and Stomach, 1st edition. Edited by Nicholas J. Talley, Kenneth R. DeVault and David E. Fleischer. © 2010 Blackwell Publishing Ltd.

This motor activity and much of the motor activity of the gastrointestinal tract in general seems to be localized in specialized neurons within the myenteric plexus in the wall of the organ, which are labeled the interstitial Cajal cells (ICCs) [3]. These cells are found between most nerves and smooth muscle and are major moderators of the nerve–smooth muscle interaction. They may have a role in modulating muscle activity independent of central stimulation, have been shown to pay a key role in the relaxation of the lower esophageal sphincter [4], and are abnormal in diseases such as achalasia [5].

Oral, Pharyngeal, and Upper Esophageal Sphincter Function

Coordinated activity in the mouth and pharynx is required in order to process a bolus, to avoid aspiration of that bolus, and to transfer that bolus to the esophagus in order to initiate peristalsis. Chewing and swallowing is a complicated process under control of multiple cranial nerves. The process begins with mastication of the bolus, which is under voluntary control and involves the brainstem and cranial nerves V, VII, and XII. Once the decision is made to initiate the swallow a very rapid process (involving CN V, X, XI, and XII) begins, but quickly (in less than 0.5 second) becomes automatic, involving those nerves and brainstem coordination. The phase begins with the tongue preparing the bolus then forcing it posteriorly and continues with the palate and posterior pharynx closing to prevent nasal regurgitation. The next event is protection of the airway as the pharynx is lifted proximally and anteriorly which results in the closure of the airway by the epiglottis. Sequential contractions of pharyngeal muscle then move the bolus toward the entrance to the esophagus.

The upper esophageal "sphincter" (UES) is not a true smooth muscle sphincter, but is, in fact, a functional closure between the pharynx and the esophagus that is composed of several different muscles and is slit-like rather than round (unlike the other GI tract sphincters). At rest, UES muscle is tonically contracted and closed due to neural excitation. Within 0.3 seconds after a swallow begins, neural stimulation to the UES ceases and the thyrohyoid and other muscles contract, which pull the larynx upward and forward to open the sphincter [6]. This entire process takes 0.5–1 second in most individuals. Assuming the pharynx contracts as the UES opens, the bolus is cleared into the esophageal body by postrelaxation contractions of muscles in the UES region. The UES is also affected by what occurs more distally, in that fluid or acid in the esophagus tends to result in an increase in UES pressure, presumptively to prevent the aspiration of refluxed material. In addition, the UES relaxes to allow air to escape during a belch. The mechanism that distinguishes between air and fluid is not clear (just as the same mechanism is not clear on the other end of the gastrointestinal tract!)

Motor Function of the Esophageal Body

Once a bolus enters the esophagus, it quickly transits the striated muscle portion of the esophagus (which varies from a minimal segment to up to one-third of the length of the esophagus, with a segment of "transition" or mixed muscle). Once the bolus reaches the smooth muscle, the process becomes automated and essentially outside conscious control. The esophageal smooth muscle consists of two layers: an outer longitudinal layer and an inner circular layer. It appears that contraction of the longitudinal muscle allows the circular muscle to have a firmer substrate upon which to act. It has been suggested that the circular muscle contraction would have to increase up to 90% without longitudinal muscle contraction [7].

The circular muscle distal to the bolus relaxes (receptive relaxation) and the muscle proximal to the bolus contracts. Both receptive relaxation and esophageal contraction is at least partially controlled by the vagus nerve, with relaxation moderated by vasoactive intestinal polypeptide (VIP) and NO, and contraction by cholinergic innervation. The smooth muscle of the esophagus actually relaxes and remains relaxed until the bolus arrives and, interestingly, if multiple swallows occur (as in gulping water) the esophagus remains relaxed until the last swallow, at which time peristalsis moves down the organ. This response is termed "deglutitive inhibition" and can result in abnormal motility testing in normal patients who repetitively swallow during esophageal manometry [8]. It takes between 6 and 8 seconds for a bolus to move from the mouth to the stomach with a velocity of 3–4 cm/second. Normal esophageal contraction should last less than 7 seconds and have a bolus pressure between 35 and 180 mmHg [9]. Although air (with belching) and gastric content (with vomiting or regurgitation) can move retrograde through the esophagus, this is due to gastric contraction and normal esophageal muscle cannot produce coordinated retrograde activity. In fact, when isolated muscle from the distal and proximal smooth muscle is electrically stimulation, contraction occurs at different rates, suggesting that peristalsis is programmed into the smooth muscle itself.

The process of transfer of a swallowed bolus through the esophagus is often termed primary peristalsis. Peristalsis can also be initiated independent of swallowing, usually after esophageal distension, and has been termed secondary peristalsis. This response is independent of central nervous system control and is preserved in an isolated organ preparation. Secondary peristalsis is important in the clearance of material left behind after primary peristalsis and material refluxed from the stomach. In addition to primary and secondary contractions of the esophagus, the esophagus at times may activate and produce peristalsis independent of swallowing or intraluminal distension (tertiary peristalsis). This must be distinguished from uncoordinated contractions that radiologists often observe with barium testing and describe as "tertiary" contractions, or from the simultaneous contractions seen at manometry that define diffuse esophageal spasm [10].

Lower Esophageal Sphincter

The muscle of the lower esophageal sphincter (LES) is different from the smooth muscle of the non-sphincteric portions of the gastrointestinal tract in that it is contracted in the resting state and relaxes with stimulation. In a resting state, the majority of the LES pressure is provided by the tonic contraction of smooth muscle, but some additional "pressure" is provide by diaphragmatic contraction. The resting pressure of that sphincter needs to be more than 10 mmHg in order to prevent the spontaneous reflux of gastric material into the esophagus and must relax in order to allow the bolus to pass. Interestingly, the LES relaxes within 1–2 seconds of swallowing and remains relaxed until the bolus arrives and passes (6–8 seconds). This relaxation occurs even with "dry" swallows and the LES can remain relaxed for very long periods of time during repetitive swallowing. Central control appears to enter well proximal to the LES, since surgical vagotomy in the lower esophagus has minimal to no affect on LES pressure or relaxation [11]. LES tone is dependent on the influx of extracellular calcium and can be attenuated with calcium channel blockers [12]. NO plays an important role in LES relaxation. Nitrates and phosphodiesterase inhibitors such as sildenafil also lower LES pressure in health and disease [13].

Gastroesophageal reflux is common when the resting LESP pressure is very low, especially in the presence of a hiatal hernia, but the more common reflux-associated event at the LES is what has been termed transient LES relaxation (TLESR) [14]. TLESR are evoked by gastric

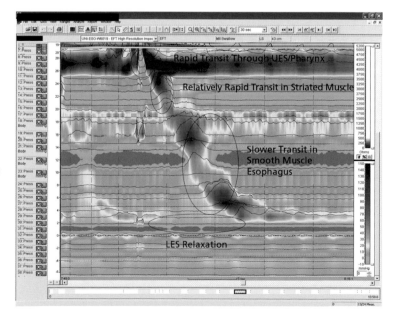

Figure 2.1 Esophageal motility: This figure is an example of high-resolution motility tracing to demonstrate the progression of a bolus through the esophagus. With swallowing there is rapid transit through the UES/pharyngeal region. The bolus then continues to move relatively rapidly through the striated muscle and then transitions into slower transit in the smooth muscle. The LES actually relaxes with the initiation of swallowing and remains relaxed until the bolus passes into the stomach.

distension and by stimulation of gastric vagal afferent neurons. They are also increased by cholecystokinin, acetylcholine and NO, while they are decreased by gamma aminobutyric acid (GABA-B receptor) and opioids [15]. Preventing TLESR is a major target for several ongoing research programs and may eventually represent a more physiologic way to treat some patients with gastric esophageal reflux disease (GERD).

Figure 2.1 illustrates typical esophageal peristalsis as demonstrated with high resolution manometry.

Gastric Motor Function

Motor activity has several major functions in the stomach. In response to eating, the proximal stomach normally relaxes (accommodation). The distal stomach begins to contract in a coordinated fashion to begin to mix (trituration) and eventually empty. In addition, emptying of the stomach helps to coordinate the motility of the rest of the upper gastrointestinal tract.

Electrophysiology of Gastric Motility

Much of the motor activity of the stomach is controlled by an innate, cyclical electrical activity. This activity is felt to originate at a site along the greater curvature of the stomach that has been described as a gastric pacemaker [16]. From this point, electrical activity is transmitted throughout the stomach in the form of an activity occurring at a frequency of about three cycles per minute (CPM) that is known as the slow wave [17]. When this activity is occurring at a low level, no motor activity occurs, but when the amplitude of the cycles are sufficient, calcium channels open, spikes of activity produce action potentials, and motor activity ensues. This electrical activity has different affects on different areas of the stomach due to innate difference in the excitability of muscles in those areas [18]. It is important to understand that the frequency of gastric contractions cannot exceed 3 CPM.

ICCs play a key role in the stomach just as in the esophagus [19]. The ICCs are directly coupled to smooth muscle cells and result in their excitation when 3 CPM activity reaches threshold amplitude. In fact, the

slow wave itself is most likely a function of the ICCs [20]. In contrast to the small bowel and colon, it appears that almost all gastric ICCs receive direct vagal innervation [21]. The ICCs play a role in the relaxation of the pylorus and appear to be lost in infantile pyloric stenosis [22].

The stomach, unlike the esophagus, receives innervation from both the vagus nerve (cell bodies in the dorsal motor nucleus) and from the splanchnic nerves (cell bodies in the prevertebral celiac ganglia). While these nerves certainly affect motility, they contain a predominance of efferent, sensory fibers.

Proximal Stomach

The muscle in the proximal stomach has a degree of tonic contraction at rest and does not usually exhibit 3 CPM activity. With a meal, it relaxes to allow the stomach to distend (up to threefold) and provide a reservoir for the swallowed material. The muscle then contracts and pushes that bolus toward the distal stomach. In the past, this was thought to be due to an overall pressure gradient, but modern studies have found that the activity of even the proximal stomach is pulsatile and under the control of the gastric pacemaker. This relaxation is under vagal control, is diminished or lost with vagotomy or significant vagal neuropathy, and appears to mediated by NO and VIP-releasing nerves [23]. Poor gastric accommodation has also been suggested to play a role in some patients with dyspepsia and may cause early satiation (inability to finish a normal-sized meal) [24]. Other factors that decrease fundic tone (and increase accommodation) include: antral distension (a full stomach) [25], duodenal acidification and distension [26], and intraluminal fat or protein and nutrients in the ileum [27]. The fundus also relaxes with swallowing [28] and during nausea and vomiting. Surgical fundoplication obliterates part of the fundus and seems to impair relaxation, usually due to mechanical means, but some patients also undoubtedly suffer vagus nerve damage during their surgery [29].

Distal Stomach

The muscle from the distal stomach initially contracts at 3 CPM to mix the bolus with secreted acid and enzymes in order to break the food down into smaller particles prior to emptying. When food is sufficiently digested, peristaltic contractions (again at 3 CPM) force the bolus toward the pylorus [30]. The pylorus is the sphincter between the stomach and duodenum, has greater muscular bulk than the remainder of the stomach, and has unique myogenic activity. During trituration, the pylorus is contracted and closed, which keeps the bolus in the stomach or allows only the better-digested (i.e., smaller) portions of the gastric content to empty. Later, when the bolus is more completely digested, the pylorus relaxes in coordination with antral contractions to allow more of the bolus to exit the stomach. In fact, ultrasound-based studies suggest that most flow through the pylorus occurs during relatively prolonged periods of opening when the gastric antrum and duodenal bulb become essentially a common cavity [31].

Gastric emptying of solids classically occurs in two phases. The first phase (lag phase) is characterized by minimal solid emptying and may last up to 60 min. The majority of emptying occurs during the second (linear) phase [32]. The linear phase is felt to begin after the meal has been titurated into particles of 1 mm or less in diameter. Emptying of fats presents an additional challenge in that fats are liquid at body temperature, do not mix well with the aqueous solutions in the stomach, and tend to float on the top of the liquid layer, all of which results in slow emptying of this food component [33].

During fasting, there are periodic "house keeper contractions" which are also known as phase III of the migrating motor complex. Particles that were not broken down sufficiently during tituration are then emptied by these phase III contractions. This event appears to be initiated in the duodenum, but also affects gastric muscle [34]. When a phase III is initiated, the LES contracts, tone increases in the proximal stomach, and 1 CPM high amplitude waves develop in the body of the stomach. The 3 CPM contractions in the antrum become more pronounced and as the activity reaches the distal stomach, the pylorus relaxes, allowing material to move into the duodenum. In the GI tract distal to the stomach, phase III activity is peristaltic, while in the stomach it tends to occur in all areas relatively simultaneously. Motilin is a peptide hormone that appears to induce this activity and offers a therapeutic target for patients with disturbed gastric motility [35].

Gastric Emptying: A Coordinated Activity?

Given the above-described physiology, how does the stomach process and transport an ingested meal? There is no one answer to this question. The stomach (assuming it is intact with intact innervation) handles low or no-calorie liquids in a very simple fashion. The stomach distends, liquids are distributed throughout the stomach and then empty at a steady rate until most have exited the stomach. If there are substantial calories or even osmols in the liquid, emptying is slowed, most likely due to feedback from receptors in the duodenum [36] (Table 2.1). Solids are handled differently, initially dependent on the size of particles in the ingested and later the digested meals. Digestible solids (defined in general as particles that can be broken down to 1 mm or smaller by the stomach), empty more like liquids (after they are digested to that size), while indigestible solids remain in the stomach longer, some of which are not emptied until phase III of the migrating motor complex occurs. The complicated nature of this activity is compounded by the fact that most ingested meals are a combination of liquids and both digestible and indigestible solids, as is illustrated in Figure 2.2.

Table 2.1 Factors that slow gastric emptying.

Meal factors
Volume
Acidity
Osmolarity
Nutrient density
Carbonation
Certain amino acids
L-tryptophan
Medications
Narcotics
Anticholinergics
Calcium channel blockers
Other factors
Rectal or colonic distension
Pregnancy
Female sex
Blood glucose
Circular motion
Cold-induced pain

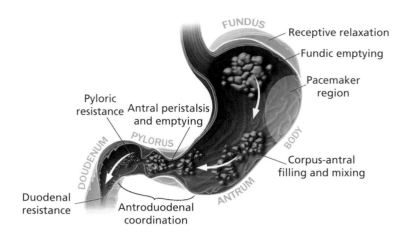

Figure 2.2 Gastric motility: See text for details, but in brief gastric function can be divided into what happens in the proximal stomach (receptive relaxation and fundic empting) and into what happens in the corpus and distal stomach (mixing, peristalsis, and emptying). In addition, there is a gastric pacemaker that helps to coordinate not only gastric motility, but the motility of the upper small intestine. The pylorus provides resistance to emptying that aids mixing and opens to allow the bolus to pass into the duodenum.

Take-home points

- The esophagus and stomach have innate muscle activity with an intramural "nervous" system. This activity is affected and, in some cases, control by extrinsic nervous input (primary via the Vagus nerve).

- The esophagus has striated muscle in the proximal portion, smooth muscle in the distal portion, and a sphincter at either end (upper esophageal and lower esophageal sphincters).

- After swallowing, the bolus enters the esophagus and is passed to the stomach in 5–10 seconds.

- The lower esophageal sphincter is tonically closed (to prevent reflux) and opens with the initiation of swallowing, then closes when the bolus passes into the stomach.

- With eating, the proximal stomach relaxes (receptive relaxation) allowing the bolus to be easily accommodated. This function is under control of the vagus nerve.

- The distal stomach and pylorus are involved in the grinding food into small pieces and in the control of gastric emptying.

- The stomach has an intramural "pacemaker region" that controls specific aspects of both gastric and small bowel motility.

References

1 Crist J, Gidda JS, Goyal RK. Intramural mechanism of esophageal peristalsis: Roles of cholinergic and noncholinergic nerves. *Proc Natl Acad Sci USA* 1984; **81**: 3595–9.

2 Yamato S, Spechler SJ, Goyal RK. Role of nitric oxide in esophageal peristalsis in the opossum. *Gastroenterology* 1992; **103**: 197–204.

3 Daniel EE, Posey-Daniel V. Neuromuscular structures in opossum esophagus: Role of interstitial cells of Cajal. *Am J Physiol* 1984; **246**: G305–15.

4 Morris G, Reese L, Wang X-Y, Sanders KM. Interstitial cells of Cajal mediate enteric inhibitory neurotransmission in the lower esophageal and pyloric sphincters. *Gastroenterology* 1998; **115**: 314–29.

5 Mearin F, Mourelle M, Guarner F, *et al.* Patients with achalasia lack nitric oxide synthase in the gastro-oesophageal junction. *Eur J Clin Invest* 1993; **23**: 724–8.

6 Jacob P, Kahrilas PJ, Logemann JA, *et al.* Upper esophageal sphincter opening and modulation during swallowing. *Gastroenterology* 1989; **97**: 1469–78.

7 Brasseur JG, Nicosia MA, Pal A, Miller LS. Function of longitudinal vs circular muscle fibers in esophageal peristalsis, deduced with mathematical modeling. *World J Gastroenterol* 2007; **13**: 1335–46.

8 Meyer GW, Gerhardt DC, Castell DO. Human esophageal response to rapid swallowing: Muscle refractory period or neural inhibition? *Am J Physiol* 1981; **241**: G129–36.

9 Richter JE, Wu WC, Johns DN, *et al.* Esophageal manometry in 95 healthy adult volunteers. Variability of pressures with age and frequency of "abnormal" contractions. *Dig Dis Sci* 1987; **32**: 583–92.

10 Meyer GW, Castell DO. Anatomy and physiology of the esophageal body. In: Castell DO, Johnson LF, ed. *Esophageal Function in Health and Disease.* New York: Elsevier Biomedical, 1983: 1–29.

11 Higgs RH, Castell DO. The effect of truncal vagotomy on lower esophageal sphincter pressure and response to cholinergic stimulation. *Proc Soc Exp Biol Med* 1976; **153**: 379–82.

12 Biancani P, Hillemeier C, Bitar KN, Makhlouf GM. Contraction mediated by Ca^{2+} influx in esophageal muscle and by Ca^{2+} release in the LES. *Am J Physiol* 1987; **253**: G760–6.

13 Lee JI, Park H, Kim JH, *et al.* The effect of sildenafil on oesophageal motor function in healthy subjects and patients with nutcracker oesophagus. *Neurogastroenterol Motil* 2003; **15**: 617–23.

14 Dodds WJ, Dent J, Hogan WJ, *et al.* Mechanisms of gastroesophageal reflux in patients with reflux esophagitis. *N Engl J Med* 1982; **307**: 1547–52.

15 Hirsch DP, Tytgat GN, Boeckxstaens GE. Transient lower oesophageal sphincter relaxations—a pharmacological target for gastro-oesophageal reflux disease? *Aliment Pharmacol Ther* 2002; **16**: 17–26.

16 Szurszewski JH. Electrophysiological basis of gastrointestinal motility. In: Johnson LR, ed. *Physiology of the Gastrointestinal Tract*, 2nd edn. New York: Raven Press, 1986: 383–42.

17 Wilson P, Perdikis G, Redmond EJ, *et al.* Prolonged ambulatory antroduodenal manometry in humans. *Am J Gastroenterol* 1994; **89**: 1489–95.

18 Hinder RA, Kelly KA. Human gastric pacesetter potential. Site of origin, spread, and response to gastric transection and proximal gastric vagotomy. *Am J Surg* 1977; **133**: 29–33.

19 Horowitz B, Ward SM, Sanders KM. Cellular and molecular basis for electrical rhythmicity in gastrointestinal muscles. *Annu Rev Physiol* 1999; **61**: 19–43.

20 Huizinga JD. Physiology and pathophysiology of the intestinal cell of Cajal: From bench to bedside. II Gastric motility: Lessons from mutant mice on slow waves and innervation. *Am J Physiol* 2001; **281**: G1129–34.

21 Powley T. Vagal input to the enteric nervous system. *Gut* 2000; **47** (Suppl. 4): iv30–32.

22 Vanderwinden J-M, Liu H, De Laet M-H, Vanderhaegen J-J. Study of the interstitial cells of Cajal in infantile hypertrophic pyloric stenosis. *Gastroenterology* 1996; **111**: 279–88.

23 Jansson G. Extrinsic nervous control of gastric motility. An experimental study in the cat. *Acta Physiol Scand* 1969; **326**: 1–42.

24 Tack J, Piessevaux H, Coulie B, *et al.* Role of impaired gastric accommodation to a meal in functional dyspepsia. *Gastroenterology* 1998; **115**: 1346–52.

25 De Ponti F, Azpiroz F. Malagelada JR. Reflex gastric relaxation in response to distention of the duodenum. *Am J Physiol* 1987; **252**: G595–601.

26 Kelly KA, Code CF. Effect of transthoracic vagotomy on canine gastric electrical activity. *Gastroenterology* 1969; **57**: 51–8.

27 Azpiroz F, Malagelada JR. Physiological variations in canine gastric tone measured by an electronic barostat. *Am J Physiol* 185; **248**: G229–37.

28 Jansson G. Extrinsic nervous control of gastric motility: an experimental study in the cat. *Acta Physiol Scand* 1969; **326** (Suppl.): 1–42.

29 DeVault KR, Swain JM, Wentling GK, *et al.* Evaluation of vagus nerve function before and after antireflux surgery. *J Gastrointest Surg* 2004; **8**: 883–8; discussion 888–9.

30 Ehrlein HJ, Heisinger E. Computer analysis of mechanical activity of gastroduodenal junction in unanesthetized dogs. *Q J Exp Phyisol* 1982; **67**: 17–29.

31 Pallotta N, Cicala M, Frandina C, Corazziara E. Antropyloric contractile patterns and transpyloric flow after meal ingestion in humans. *Am J Gastroenterol* 1998; **93**: 2513–22.

32 Siegel JA, Urbain JL, Adler LP, *et al.* Biphasic nature of gastric emptying. *Gut* 1988; **29**: 85–9.

33 Meyer JH, Mayer EA, Jehn D, *et al.* Gastric processing and emptying of fat. *Gastroenterology* 1986; **90**: 1176–87.

34 Kellow JE, Borody TJ, Phillips SF, *et al.* Human interdigestive motility: Variations in patterns from esophagus to colon. *Gastroenterology* 1986; **91**: 386–95.

35 Peeters T, Matthijs G, Depoortere I, *et al.* Erythromycin is a motilin receptor agonist. *Am J Physiol* 1989; **257**: G470–4.

36 Hunt JN, Spurrell WR. The pattern of emptying of the human stomach. *J Physiol (Lond)* 1951; **115**: 157–68.

CHAPTER 3

Gastric Acid Secretion and Hormones

Geoffrey Spencer[1] and David C. Metz[2]

[1] Division of Gastroenterology, Hospital of the University of Pennsylvania, Philadelphia, PA, USA
[2] Division of Gastroenterology, University of Pennsylvania School of Medicine, Philadelphia, PA, USA

Summary

Gastric acid secretion is crucial to initiate digestion and absorption of ingested nutrients. An intricate neurohormonal system regulates hydrogen secretion from the proton pump (H^+, K^+-ATPase enzyme) located on the apical membrane of the parietal cell. Gastrin is released from G cells located in the gastric antrum and stimulates enterochromaffin-like (ECL) cells to release histamine, which in turn directly activates acid secretion from the nearby parietal cell. Acetylcholine release from vagal stimulation also results in stimulation of the parietal cell and hydrogen secretion. This system is kept in balance by the inhibitory influence of somatostatin.

Case

A 45-year-old man presents with fatigue and anemia. He reports a 3-day history of melena and on the day of presentation one episode of hematemesis. His medical history is significant for a duodenal ulcer several years ago treated with a course of antisecretory therapy. He is admitted, started on an intravenous proton pump inhibitor, and transfused 2 units of packed red blood cells. Emergent endoscopy reveals a recurrent duodenal ulcer with a visible vessel that is cauterized. Serologic testing reveals a positive *Helicobacter pylori* (*H. pylori*) antibody. *H. pylori* infection can lead to a hypersecretory state that is associated with duodenal ulcer formation. The pathophysiologic basis of this is described further below.

Introduction

The stomach functions both as a secretory and a digestive organ. It carries out these roles by storing, processing,

Practical Gastroenterology and Hepatology: Esophagus and Stomach, 1st edition. Edited by Nicholas J. Talley, Kenneth R. DeVault and David E. Fleischer. © 2010 Blackwell Publishing Ltd.

and emptying ingested nutrients into the small intestine. The processing of food is dependent on both the secretory and motor function of the stomach. The stomach secretes water and electrolytes at low pH, as well as enzymes and glycoproteins to initiate digestion and absorption and to provide protection of the gastrointestinal tract. Digestion begins in the stomach. This principle was first confirmed in 1833 by William Beaumont, an American army surgeon, studying human digestion via a gastrocutaneous fistula in a young fur trapper (though at the time he was unable to obtain a chemical analysis of the contents of gastric juice) [1]. Since then, the role of gastric acid secretion has been elucidated in both health and disease. Under physiologic conditions, hydrochloric acid provides the optimal pH for pepsin and gastric lipase function, assists in duodenal absorption of inorganic cations, provides negative feedback for gastrin release, stimulates pancreatic bicarbonate release, and plays a role in suppression of ingested microorganisms [2]. Gastric acid secretion must be precisely regulated to carry out these physiologic functions without overwhelming the protective mechanisms of the digestive tract and leading to organ damage. When this balance is disturbed, gastric acid can lead to mucosal disease such as peptic ulcers as well as malabsorption via intestinal damage and inactivation of digestive enzymes.

Functional Anatomy

The stomach is a J-shaped dilation of the alimentary canal that can be divided into four regions defined by anatomic and histologic landmarks (cardia, fundus, corpus, and antrum) [3]. The secretory role of the stomach can be divided into two functional regions, the oxyntic and pyloric gland areas. The oxyntic (*oxys*, Greek for acid) gland area is responsible for acid secretion (Figure 3.1). It comprises 80% of the stomach and is found in the corpus and fundus [4]. The oxyntic glands are fairly straight, tubular glands subdivided into three areas: the isthmus containing predominately mucous cells, the neck containing parietal and mucous cells, and the base containing predominately chief cells but also some parietal and mucous cells. The oxyntic mucosa also contains scattered D cells and enterochromaffin-like cells [2].

Gastric Acid Secretion

The parietal cell of the oxyntic gland is responsible for the secretion of 3×10 hydrogen ions per second at a final HCl concentration of about 160 mmol/L or pH 0.8 [5].

The proton pump (H^+, K^+-ATPase enzyme) is synthesized in the parietal cell cytoplasm, stored in intracellular vesicles and inserted into the apical microvillus membrane of the parietal cell when the cell is stimulated. It is responsible for extruding hydrogen ions into the gastric lumen and is recycled into the cytoplasm when stimulation ceases. During parietal cell stimulation, the apical membrane elongates and long apical microvilli develop as cytoplasmic vesicles fuse with the apical membrane to form channels (cannaliculi) that drain to the apical lumen [6]. With stimulation, potassium–chloride co-transport becomes active, allowing hydrogen–potassium exchange to occur to maintain electrical neutrality. The proton pumps then actively secrete hydrogen ions in an active, energy-dependent process against a large concentration gradient (cytoplasm pH 7.4, acid secreted at pH 0.8).

Mediators of Gastric Acid Secretion

Gastric acid secretion reflects an intricate balance of overlapping paracrine, endocrine, and neural input to the parietal cell. The principal secretagogues are histamine (paracrine), gastrin (endocrine), and acetylcholine (neural). These ligands bind to receptors coupled to two major intracellular signaling pathways leading to activation of the parietal cell (Figure 3.2). Histamine activates adenylate cyclase whereas gastrin and acetylcholine acti-

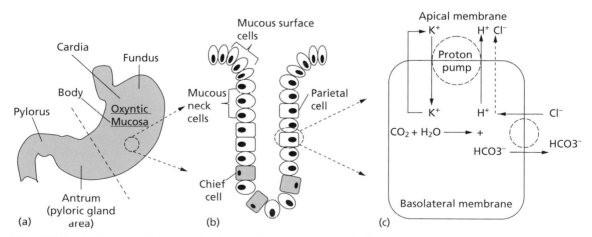

Figure 3.1 Functional anatomy of the stomach. (a) Anatomic regions of the stomach. (b) Oxyntic gland area. (c) Parietal cell and proton pump physiology.

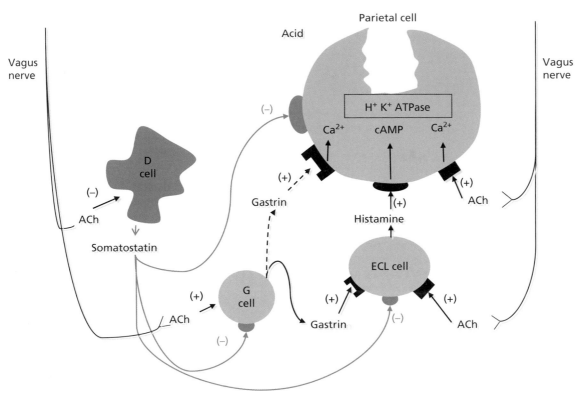

Figure 3.2 Simplified diagram of the physiology of gastric acid secretion and its feedback control.

vate inositol trisphosphate to raise intracellular calcium. In turn, release of these secretagogues is controlled by a feedback mechanism in response to lowering of the gastric luminal pH (Figure 3.2).

Histamine

Histamine is the major paracrine stimulus of acid secretion. It is released from enterochromaffin-like (ECL) cells localized in direct proximity to the parietal cells in the oxyntic mucosa. Histamine binds to H_2 receptors on the parietal cell which are coupled to activation of adenylate cyclase and the generation of the intracellular messenger adenosine 3′,5′-cyclic monophosphate (cAMP) [7]. Histamine also indirectly stimulates acid secretion by binding to H_3 receptors on D cells, inhibiting somatostatin release [8]. Gastrin is the primary stimulus for histamine release. Pituitary adenylate cyclase-activating polypeptide (PACAP), vasoactive intestinal peptide (VIP), and ghrelin also stimulate histamine release whereas somatostatin, calcitonin gene-related peptide (CGRP), prostaglandins, peptide YY, and galanin inhibit its secretion [9].

Gastrin

Gastrin is the major endocrine stimulator of acid secretion. It is the main stimulant of acid secretion during meals and is released from gastrin-expressing cells (G cells) localized to the antrum. Gastrin binds to cholecystokinin B (CCK_2) receptors, which have equal affinity for both CCK and gastrin. These receptors are present on ECL and parietal cells and are coupled to activation of phospholipase C and release of intracellular calcium from inositol trisphosphate. Gastrin stimulates parietal cells, leading to gastric acid secretion largely indirectly through the release of histamine from ECL cells [10]. A lesser, direct action of gastrin on the parietal cell may be to sensitize it to other secretory mediators. It also has a trophic action on parietal and ECL cells and is the best identified regulator of parietal cell mass in humans.

Regulation of gastrin secretion involves a complex interaction among various mediators. As the main stimulant of acid secretion during meals, gastrin is released in response to gastric distension and amino acids. Low-grade distension leads to somatostatin release, inhibiting gastrin, whereas higher grades of distension causes cholinergic activation and increased gastrin release [11]. Amino acids from a meal stimulate G cells both directly and through activation of cholinergic and bombesin (gastrin releasing peptide, GRP) releasing neurons [12]. Other stimulants of gastrin secretion include secretin, $\beta2/\beta3$ adrenergic agonists and calcium. The primary inhibitor of gastrin secretion is somatostatin. Other inhibitors include galanin and adenosine.

Acetylcholine

The stomach is innervated by both the sympathetic and parasympathetic nervous system. The parasympathetic innervation is via the vagal nerves. The preganglionic neurons of the vagus synapse on postganglionic neurons of the enteric nervous system within the stomach, which contain neurotransmitters including acetylcholine (ACh) as well as GRP, VIP, PACAP, nitric oxide, and substance P. ACh is the major neural stimulatory mediator of gastric acid secretion. It binds to muscarinic receptors on parietal cells leading to activation of phospholipase C and intracellular calcium release [13]. ACh also inhibits somatostatin release, thereby indirectly stimulating gastric acid secretion by promoting gastrin and histamine secretion. In the antrum, ACh stimulates gastrin release directly and indirectly through inhibition of somatostatin.

Somatostatin

Somatostatin is the main inhibitor of acid secretion. It is released from D cells found throughout the gastric mucosa in close proximity to target cells, including parietal, ECL, and G cells. The main effect of somatostatin is the inhibition of histamine release from the ECL cell and to a lesser extent inhibition of gastrin release. Luminal acidity and gastrin itself increase secretion of somatostatin acting as a negative feedback on acid production [14]. Other stimulants of somatostatin secretion include GRP, VIP, PACAP, $\beta2/\beta3$ adrenergic agonists, secretin, adrenomedullin, amylin, adenosine, and CGRP. Cholinergic activation suppresses somatostatin release via ACh and leads to an increase in gastric acid secretion.

Regulation of Acid Secretion in Health and Disease

Phases of Acid Secretion

During the fasted state, continuous inhibition by somatostatin leads to low levels of gastric acid production. The physiologic stimulation of gastric acid production by a meal has classically been divided into three phases: the cephalic, gastric, and intestinal phases [15]. During the cephalic phase, anticipation of a meal leads to cholinergic activation via the vagus nerve. ACh stimulates the parietal cell directly, increases gastrin and inhibits somatostatin, thereby increasing histamine release from ECL cells and, in sum, promoting gastric acid secretion. During the gastric phase, distension leads to further cholinergic activation and amino acids stimulate cholinergic and GRP neurons, promoting gastrin release to increase acid secretion. As the meal empties from the stomach, inhibition of acid secretion via somatostatin is restored through several pathways. Gastrin functions as a negative feedback to increase somatostatin release. There is decreased distension leading to reduced activation of cholinergic neural inhibition of somatostatin as well as VIP neural stimulation of somatostatin release. Further, with reduced buffering capacity of the meal and diminished amino acids, gastrin release is reduced. In total, the balance of mediators returns to the fasted state, favoring somatostatin release with less gastrin and histamine production leading to lower basal acid secretion.

Disorders of Acid Secretion

When the balance of gastric acid secretion and protective mechanisms is disturbed ulcers can develop. Understanding these conditions elucidates the mechanisms reviewed above. Gastric acid hypersecretion occurs in several uncommon conditions (Table 3.1). The most recognized, Zollinger–Ellison syndrome (or gastrinoma), results from gastrin over production and loss of its feedback control. Gastrin stimulates histamine release from ECL cells and parietal cells to induce acid secretion and cellular proliferation. Despite an active feedback control of gastrin release from antral G cells, gastrinoma G cells located in the duodenum, pancreas or elsewhere fail to respond to the local paracrine effects of somatostatin in the stomach. Systemic mastocystosis results in elevated levels of histamine produced from increased numbers of mast cells, resulting in stimulation of parietal cells and

Table 3.1 Gastric acid hyper- and hyposecretory conditions.

Hypersecretory states	Hyposecretory states
Zollinger–Ellison syndrome	Chronic atrophic gastritis (autoimmune/*H. pylori*)
H. pylori (antral predominant infection)	Chronic active gastritis (*H. pylori*)
Systemic mastocytosis	Medications (proton pump inhibitor/H_2 receptor antagonists)
Hypercalcemia	Vagotomy
Massive small bowel resection	Hypocalcemia
Retained gastric antrum	Somatostatinoma/VIPoma
	HIV (AIDS)

VIPoma, vasoactive intestinal polypeptide secreting tumor.

acid production. Feedback control fails in this condition for similar reasons. Massive resection of the small bowel may remove negative feedback on gastric acid secretion and lead to hypersecretion. Hypergastrinemia and increased acid secretion may also result from retention of a portion of gastric antrum in the afferent limb of a Billroth II after antrectomy. This portion of antrum is not exposed to acid and loses this negative feedback stimulus on gastrin secretion. Distension during gastric outlet obstruction leads to cholinergic-mediated hypergastrinemia and increased acid secretion. Hypercalcemia can also result in acid hypersecretion by directly stimulating gastrin release and acid secretion from parietal cells. Antral predominant (*H. pylori*) infection can also lead to gastric acid hypersecretion. Under these circumstances, somatostatin release is suppressed, leading to low-level, inappropriate gastric acid hypersecretion sufficient to lead to duodenal ulceration.

On the other hand, there are also numerous causes of gastric acid hyposecretion (Table 3.1). Most important of these are drug-induced hyposecretion (primarily proton pump inhibitor therapy but high-dose H_2 antagonist therapy also leads to gastric acid hyposecretion) and atrophic gastritis (due either to autoimmune pernicious anemia or chronic *H. pylori* pangastritis). Under these circumstances, the infection causes local inflammation in the gastric body with loss of parietal cell function, appropriate hypergastrinemia and a reduction in gastric acid secretion. During the acute phase of *H. pylori* infection,

pangastritis also results in inhibition of the parietal cell mass leading to outbreaks of so-called epidemic achlorhydria.

Take-home points

- Gastric acid secretion is regulated by a complex neurohormonal mechanism.
- Gastrin is the major hormonal mediator of acid secretion. It stimulates histamine release from ECL cells.
- Histamine is the major paracrine mediator of acid secretion. It directly stimulates parietal cells, leading to activation of the proton pumps.
- Acetylcholine release from vagal innervation activates parietal cells directly and through stimulation of G cells and ECL cells. It also inhibits somatostatin release.
- Somatostatin is the primary inhibitory influence on gastric acid secretion. It inhibits gastrin and histamine release and has direct inhibitory effects on the parietal cell.

References

1 Osler W. William Beaumont. A pioneer American physiologist. *JAMA* 1902; **39**: 1223–31.

2 Feldman M, Friedman LS, Brandt LJ. *Sleisenger and Fordtran's Gastrointestinal and Liver Disease*, 8th edn. Philadelphia: W.B. Saunders, 2006.

3 Johnson L. *Gastrointestinal Physiology*, 6th edn. St Louis: CV Mosby, 2001.

4 Joseph IM, *et al.* A model for integrative study of human gastric acid secretion. *J Appl Physiol* 2003; **94**: 1602–18.

5 Schubert ML, Peura DA. Control of gastric acid secretion in health and disease. *Gastroenterology* 2008; **134**: 1842–60.

6 Yao X, Forte JG. Cell biology of acid secretion by the parietal cell. *Annu Rev Physiol* 2003; **65**: 103–31.

7 Soll AH, Wollin A. Histamine and cyclic AMP in isolated canine parietal cells. *Am J Physiol* 1979; **237**: E444–50.

8 Vuyyuru L, *et al.* Reciprocal inhibitory paracrine pathways link histamine and somatostatin secretion in the fundus of the stomach. *Am J Physiol* 1997; **273**: G106–11.

9 Prinz C, Zanner R, Gratzl M. Physiology of gastric enterochromaffin-like cells. *Annu Rev Physiol* 2003; **65**: 371–82.

10 Lindstrom E, *et al.* Control of gastric acid secretion:the gastrin-ECL cell-parietal cell axis. *Comp Biochem Physiol A* 2001; **128**: 505–14.

11 Schubert ML, Makhlouf GM. Gastrin secretion induced by distention is mediated by gastric cholinergic and vasoactive intestinal peptide neurons in rats. *Gastroenterology* 1993; **104**: 834–9.

12 Schubert ML, Makhlouf GM. Neural, hormonal, and paracrine regulation of gastrin and acid secretion. *Yale J Biol Med* 1992; **65**: 553–60, discussion 621–3.

13 Kajimura M, Reuben MA, Sachs G. The muscarinic receptor gene expressed in rabbit parietal cells is the m3 subtype. *Gastroenterology* 1992; **103**: 870–5.

14 Shulkes A, Read M. Regulation of somatostatin secretion by gastrin- and acid-dependent mechanisms. *Endocrinology* 1991; **129**: 2329–34.

15 Lloyd KCK, Debas HT. Peripheral regulation of gastric acid secretion. In: Johnson LR, Christensen J, Jackson MJ, Jacobson ED, Walsh JH, eds. *Physiology of the Gastrointestinal Tract*, 4th edn. New York: Raven Press, 1994.

PART 2

Esophago-gastroduodenoscopy

CHAPTER 4
Preparation and Sedation

Benjamin E. Levitzky and John J. Vargo, II

Digestive Disease Institute, Cleveland Clinic Foundation, Cleveland, OH, USA

Summary

Sedation plays a central role in the practice of endoscopy. It affects the exam quality, patient satisfaction, and compliance. There are a variety of guidelines for training and most follow those by the American Society for Gastrointestinal Endoscopy, who have developed guidelines in association with the American Society of Anesthesiology. In addition to guidelines for training, there are recommendations for preprocedural assessment, the administration of analgesia and sedation, and a wide variety of information about the agents used for sedation and reversal. The endoscopist should also be familiar with postprocedural monitoring.

Case

A 59-year-old male lawyer who recently had a myocardial infarction with attendant congestive heart failure was scheduled to undergo an endoscopy and colonoscopy to evaluate anemia and dark stools following the institution of aspirin and Plavix®, which was begun soon after the infarction. His primary care physician wishes him to have the procedure with sedation given by an anesthesiologist. The gastroenterologist says he is now stable and since he cannot start cases "on time" when anesthesiologists are involved and that it increased the cost of the procedure, he believes it can be done safely with conscious sedation alone. Since there is a difference of opinion, the two physicians contact the Chairman of Anesthesiology who believes that an anesthesiologist should be present to administer the sedation. The gastroenterologist says that that is a predictable response since the Chairman of Anesthesiology would be biased in his opinion. The primary care physician is uncertain about what should be the next step.

Introduction

Sedation plays a central role in the practice of endoscopy. It affects exam quality, patient satisfaction, and compli-

Practical Gastroenterology and Hepatology: Esophagus and Stomach, 1st edition. Edited by Nicholas J. Talley, Kenneth R. DeVault and David E. Fleischer. © 2010 Blackwell Publishing Ltd.

ance with surveillance guidelines. The goals of sedation are to make patients comfortable and to facilitate a successful endoscopic exam. Careful attention must be made to choose the optimal regimen for a particular patient and to adequately assess the patient during and after the procedure. This chapter will address standards of care for sedation and monitoring of patients undergoing endoscopic procedures.

Guidelines for Training

Safe administration of endoscopic sedation mandates the following [1,2]:

• Endoscopists should have current Basic Life Support (BLS) and Advanced Cardiac Life Support (ACLS) certification.

• Endoscopists should be able to provide respiratory support if apnea ensues. This includes working knowledge of jaw-thrust chin-lift maneuvers, use of oropharyngeal and nasopharyngeal airway devices, laryngeal mask airways, and bag mask ventilation.

• Endoscopists and nurses should understand the pharmacologic profiles of all drugs being used for sedation.

• Nursing personnel should be adept at monitoring sedated patients and recognizing signs of oversedation.

• Equipment and personnel to manage complications of sedation must be readily available.

Gastroenterologists targeting moderate sedation must be able to rescue patients who enter deep sedation. Gastroenterologists targeting deep sedation require additional training in advanced airway management to rescue from general anesthesia.

Preprocedural Assessment

A preprocedural patient evaluation, including a targeted history and physical examination, is required prior to performing endoscopy. This assessment helps to identify factors that may increase risks associated with sedation. Patient characteristics to consider include age, health, degree of anxiety, and current medication use. Procedural factors include the anticipated level of sedation, duration of examination, and the potential degree of discomfort experienced by the patient [1–3].

Patient History

All patients should participate in a concise history. Key elements of the medical history include documentation of the following:

• Cardiopulmonary disease
• Neurologic or seizure disorder
• Obstructive airway disease or sleep apnea
• Prior adverse reaction to sedation
• Current medications and known food and drug allergies
• Alcohol or substance abuse
• The time of last oral intake.

A patient's overall co-morbid disease status should be classified by the American Society for Anesthesiology (ASA) status classification (Table 4.1). ASA class I, II, and III patients are appropriate candidates for gastroenterologist-administered sedation. The ASA classification has been shown to be an independent risk factor for cardiopulmonary events [1,4].

Consideration of anesthesiologist support should be given in the following situations:

• ASA class IV or V patient
• History of adverse reaction to sedation
• Alcohol or substance abuse
• Prior inadequate response to moderate sedation
• Patient undergoing endoscopic retrograde cholangio-

Table 4.1 American Society of Anesthesiologists physical classification.

	Definition
Class 1	Healthy patient without medical problems
Class 2	Mild systemic disease that does not limit activity
Class 3	Moderate to severe systemic disease which limits activity
Class 4	Severe systemic disease that is a constant potential threat to life
Class 5	Moribund and at substantial risk of death within 24 hours

pancreatography (ERCP), upper GI stent placement, endoscopic ultrasonography (EUS), or another complex therapeutic procedure.

Preprocedural Physical Exam

The preprocedural physical exam should include the following:

• Vital signs and weight
• Heart and lung auscultation
• Baseline level of consciousness
• Airway assessment

Analgesia and Sedation

"Moderate sedation" is targeted for the majority of endoscopic procedures. A moderately sedated patient remains able to respond purposefully to verbal and gentle tactile stimuli while maintaining ventilatory and cardiovascular function (Table 4.2).

The targeted depth of sedation is dependent on the procedure being performed. Sedation remains optional during flexible sigmoidoscopy and rectal EUS as many patients will tolerate these procedures unsedated. Diagnostic and therapeutic colonoscopy and esophagogastroduodenoscopy (EGD) typically require moderate sedation. For advanced procedures such as EUS and ERCP, deeper levels of sedation are often required.

Lengthy procedures may necessitate deeper levels of sedation that correlate with a greater rate of sedation-related adverse events. Depth of sedation is a continuum and patients may move rapidly between depths of sedation. In light of this, gastroenterologists administering sedatives and analgesics must be able to rescue patients from deeper-than-intended degrees of sedation.

All subjects should be monitored with pulse oximetry and an automated blood pressure cuff. Electrocardiography should be used in those patients over 55 years of age and those with significant cardiopulmonary disease. A crucial but often overlooked part of patient monitoring

is periodic visual inspection for the level of sedation and respiratory activity [1,3].

In patients in whom deep sedation is targeted, the use of extended monitoring with capnography should be considered [1,5] (Figures 4.1 and 4.2). Bispectral index monitoring has been shown to be of limited value in determining the depth of sedation [6].

Table 4.2 Levels of sedation.

Minimal sedation	Patient responds normally to verbal commands. Ventilatory and cardiovascular functions are unaffected.
Moderate sedation	Patient is able to respond purposeful to verbal and light tactile stimuli. Ventilatory and cardiovascular functions are maintained.
Deep sedation	Patient cannot easily be aroused but responds purposefully to repeated or painful stimuli. Airway support may be required. Spontaneous ventilation may be inadequate.
General anesthesia	The patient is not arousable, even after painful stimuli. The ability to independently maintain ventilatory function may be impaired. Cardiovascular function may also be impaired.

Standard Agents for Sedation and Analgesia

Benzodiazepines and opiates are the most commonly used agents for gastroenterologist-administered sedation prior to endoscopic procedures. Premedication may involve either a benzodiazepine alone or a synergistic combination of a benzodiazepine with an opiate. Combination sedation may increase risk of hypoxia, hemodynamic instability, and oversedation and underscores the need for close monitoring. Benzodiazepines provide anxiolysis, sedation, and amnesia while opioids provide additional analgesia and sedation. The use of small, incremental doses with allowance of sufficient time between doses allows the gastroenterologist to titrate to a desired level of sedation. Doses and pharmacodynamic

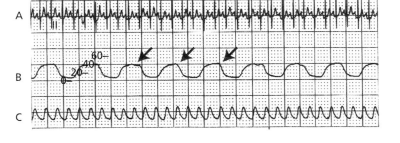

Figure 4.1 Tracing A shows an electrocardiogram (lead II). Tracing B is a normal capnograph. The peaks (arrows) represent expiration and the troughs are inspiration. Tracing C is a pulse oximetry plethysmograph.

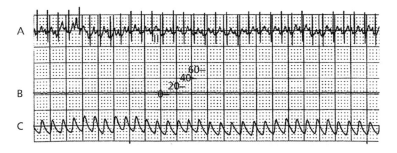

Figure 4.2 Tracing B shows an example of apnea. There is no evidence of respiratory activity. The pulse oximetry value at the time was 94%. Tracing A is the electrocardiogram and C is the pulse oximetry plethysmograph.

Table 4.3 Pharmacologic profile of drugs used for endoscopic sedation.

Drug	Onset of action (min)	Peak effect (min)	Duration of effect (min)	Initial dose	Maximum dose	FDA pregnancy category	Pharmacologic antagonist	Significant adverse effects
Diazepam (mg)	2–3	3–5	360	5–10	20	D	Flumazenil	Respiratory depression, chemical phlebitis
Fentanyl (µg)	1–2	3–5	30–60	50–100	200	C	Naloxone	Respiratory depression, vomiting
Flumazenil (mg)	1–2	3	60	0.1–0.3	>5	C		Agitation, withdrawal symptoms
Meperidine (mg)	3–6	5–7	60–180	25–50	150	C	Naloxone	Respiratory depression, pruritus, vomiting, interaction with monoamine oxidase inhibitor
Midazolam (mg)	1–2	3–4	15–80	1–2	6	D	Flumazenil	Respiratory depression, disinhibition,
Naloxone (mg)	1–2	5	30–45	0.2–0.4	>2	B		Narcotic withdrawal
Propofol (mg)	<1	1–2	4–8	10–40	400	B	None	Respiratory depression, cardiovascular instability

profiles for commonly employed drugs are found in Table 4.3.

Benzodiazepines

Benzodiazepines function by binding intracerebral $GABA_A$ receptors, thereby increasing inhibitory GABA activity. Midazolam (Versed®) and diazepam (Valium®) are the most widely used agents in this class. Many gastroenterologists prefer midazolam over diazepam due to its shorter half-life, lack of active metabolites, and excellent amnestic profile. The longer half-life of diazepam may be of particular concern in elderly patients and other individuals particularly sensitive to sedative effects. The most prominent dose-related side effect of benzodiazepines is respiratory depression.

Opiates

Both meperidine (Demerol®) and fentanyl (Sublimaze®) are widely utilized agents for sedation. Meperidine is a highly cost-effective option and remains the most commonly used opiate for sedation. While fentanyl incurs greater cost, it has been gaining in popularity due to its more rapid onset of action, shorter half-life, the lack of

a pharmacologically active metabolite, and a lower incidence of postprocedural nausea. Morphine may cause smooth muscle and sphincter of Oddi contraction and is not recommended for endoscopic sedation.

The major adverse effects of meperidine and fentanyl are respiratory depression and cardiovascular instability. Opiates may lower the threshold for seizure activity and caution should be exercised in this setting. Meperidine is contraindicated in patients taking monoamine oxidase inhibitors due to significant drug–drug interactions.

Topical Anesthetics

Topical anesthetic agents such as benzocaine, cetacaine, tetracaine, and lidocaine are commonly used to suppress the gag reflex prior to EGD. Efficacy data on topical agents has been mixed. Given their excellent safety profile and possible benefit in facilitating endoscopy, it is reasonable to use topical agents prior to EGD, particularly in patients under minimal to moderate sedation. The major risk of these agents is aspiration from inhibition of gag reflex. Remote risks include methemoglobinemia, arrhythmia, and seizures from systemic absorption.

Propofol

Propofol (Diprivan®) is a rapidly-acting, central GABA-agonist that may be administered alone or in tandem with other sedative-analgesics. It is a pure sedative-hypnotic with no analgesic effects. Administration may be performed with bolus dosing or continuous intravenous infusion. Advantages of this agent include rapid postprocedural recovery times and excellent patient and physician satisfaction. Disadvantages include the lack of reversal agents and potential higher risk for deeper-than-intended levels of sedation. Currently, the FDA does not support non-anesthesiologist administration of propofol and its role for routine endoscopic procedures remains controversial.

Other Agents

Other agents such as ketamine, nitrous oxide, dexmedetomidine, diphenhydramine, and droperidol are occasionally used for endoscopic sedation. Prospective data on the use of these is quite limited and may require specialized training (dexmedetomidine) or special precautions due potential side effects (droperidol).

Reversal Agents

When using benzodiazepines and opiates for sedation, it is imperative to have reversal agents easily accessible to rescue patients from deeper-than-intended levels of sedation. Use of these agents should be considered when patients develop signs of oversedation. Signs of oversedation include:
• Hypoxemia despite supplemental oxygen
• Lack of response to gentle stimulation
• Respiratory depression.

Naloxone

Naloxone (Narcan®) is an opiate antagonist that will rapidly reverse the respiratory depression and CNS depression due to opiate administration. Repeat dosing may be required in patients dosed with long-acting opiates such as meperidine. Naloxone alone may not be sufficient to stabilize a patient with significant hemodynamic compromise from opiate overdosage. In this setting, intravenous fluids or vasopressors may also be required.

Flumazenil

Flumazenil (Romazicon®) may be used to partially reverse the central effects of benzodiazepines by competitively binding the GABA$_A$ receptor. This agent is more effective in reversing sedation and amnesia than in reversing respiratory depression.

It should be emphasized that the use of these agents to hasten recovery from uncomplicated sedation is not warranted. Additionally, due to the risk of resedation, subjects receiving naloxone and/or flumazenil should be observed in the recovery room setting for an extended period of time.

Documentation

Careful documentation should include the following:
• Preprocedure and postprocedure assessments
• Informed consent
• A "time out," which should include identification of the patient, type of procedure, patient positioning, type of sedation, and identification of any type of specialized equipment or personnel that is to be utilized.
• Intraprocedural monitoring should be performed every 5 min at baseline and more frequently should the clinical situation change rapidly
• Recovery time and discharge.

Complications

The most common complications of procedural sedation include hypoxia, hypotension, aspiration, apnea, and allergic reaction to medication administration.

Hypoxemia

Causes of overt hypoxia include central respiratory depression, upper airway obstruction, or a reduction in functional residual capacity leading to ventilation–perfusion mismatches. Initial management should include supplemental oxygen administration and upper airway management with maneuvers such as a head tilt, chin lift, jaw thrust, or placement of an oral or nasal airway device. Administration of naloxone and flumazenil is warranted to counteract effects of benzodiazepines and opiates. Manual bag mask ventilation and/or endotracheal intubation may be required for cases of refractory hypoxemia.

Postprocedural Monitoring

Due to ongoing risk of cardiopulmonary complications following endoscopic sedation, patients should be monitored in a dedicated recovery area until the level of consciousness returns to baseline. This includes ongoing monitoring of vital signs, degree of discomfort, level of consciousness, oxygenation, and respiratory activity. Patients requiring reversal agents during a procedure warrant extended observation. Discharge criteria includes the documentation of baseline vital signs and some measure of recovery of the ability of the patient to perform baseline activities such as ambulating independently and able to tolerate fluid intake. A responsible individual should escort the patient home.

In summary, the evaluation, planning, administration, and recovery from procedural sedation is often overlooked but is crucial to the success of the procedure and paramount to the safety of the patient. It is incumbent on the endoscopist to have a thorough knowledge of the pharmacology of the medications and to utilize the personnel and monitoring equipment to deliver a safe and appropriate level of sedation.

Take-home points

- Endoscopists should have current Basic Life Support and Advanced Cardiac Life Support certification.
- Endoscopists and nurses should understand the pharmacologic profiles of all drugs being used for sedation.
- Equipment and personnel to manage complications and sedation must be readily available.

- The preprocedural assessment should include patient history and a preprocedural physical examination.
- The most common sedative agents used are benzodiazepines, of which midazolam is the most common; opiates of which meperidine and fentanyl are the most common; topical anesthetics and propofol. There is a wide variance of opinion about the role of propofol for "routine endoscopy."
- Reversal agents such as naloxone and flumazenil should be readily available.
- Documenting the events of the sedation is both medically and legally important.
- Postprocedural monitoring and discharge planning is part of the spectrum of preparation and sedation.

References

1 American Society of Anesthesiologists Task Force on Sedation and Analgesia by Non-anesthesiologists. Practice guidelines for sedation and analgesia by non-anesthesiologists. *Anesthesiology* 2002; **96**: 1004–17.

2 Lichtenstein D, Jagannath S, Baron TH, *et al.* Sedation and analgesia in GI Endoscopy. *Gastrointest Endosc* 2008; **68**: 815–26.

3 Vargo JJ, Ahmad A, Aslanian H, *et al.* Training in patient monitoring and sedation and analgesia. *Gastrointest Endosc* 2007; **66**: 7–10.

4 Sharma VK, Nguyen CC, Crowell MD, *et al.* A national study of cardiopulmonary unplanned events after GI endoscopy. *Gastrointest Endosc* 2007; **66**: 27–34.

5 Qadeer M, Vargo JJ, Dumot JA, *et al.* Capnographic monitoring of respiratory activity improves safety of sedation for endoscopic cholangiopancreatography and ultrasonography. *Gastroenterology* 2009; **136**: 1568–76.

6 Qadeer MA, Vargo JJ, Patel S, *et al.* Bispectral index monitoring of conscious sedation with the combination of meperidine and midazolam during endoscopy. *Clin Gastroenterol Hepatol* 2008; **6**: 102–8.

CHAPTER 5
Endoscopic Anatomy and Postsurgical Anatomy

Mark E. Stark

Division of Gastroenterology and Hepatology, Mayo Clinic, Jacksonville, FL, USA

Summary

The endoscopic appearance of the normal esophagus and stomach is described. The typical postsurgical endoscopic appearance of the esophagus and stomach is explained, including surgery performed for esophageal cancer or motility disorders, fundoplication for control of gastroesophageal reflux, gastrectomy for gastric cancer or ulcer disease, and surgery for weight reduction (bariatric surgery).

Case

A 56-year-old man had a laparoscopic Nissen fundoplication 3 years ago. At that time, symptoms of heartburn and regurgitation were judged to result from gastroesophageal reflux disease, and he had incomplete relief with a proton pump inhibitor (PPI). After the surgery, his symptoms improved, and he was able to stop the PPI. However, during the last year he has had a return of heartburn and regurgitation. He has restarted a PPI, but has incomplete relief of symptoms. He has also developed intermittent dysphagia for solid food. His surgeon has referred him to you, to sort out the cause of his symptoms and the status of the fundoplication. You are considering endoscopy to determine the status of the fundoplication.

Normal Endoscopic Anatomy of the Esophagus and Stomach

The esophagus extends from cricopharyngeus (18–20 cm from the incisors) to the gastroesophageal junction (GEJ) (35–45 cm from the incisors). With the patient in the left lateral decubitus position, the endoscope handle buttons toward the patient, and a straight insertion tube, the right esophageal wall is seen at the "12 o'clock" position, the posterior wall at "3 o'clock", the left at "6 o'clock", and the anterior wall at "9 o'clock". The lumen diameter is 1.5–2 cm, and varies in shape from circular to slit like depending on respirations, position in the esophagus, and peristalsis. Longitudinal mucosal columns become flat with air distension. The mucosa is smooth, glistening, and pale pink. Small, red, longitudinal mucosal blood vessels are visible [1].

At the GEJ, the pale-pink mucosa of the esophagus abuts the orange–red gastric mucosa. This mucosal junction appears serrated, and is called the "Z-line" (for "zig-zag"). Approximately 2 cm proximal to the GEJ, a variable ring-like narrowing ("A" ring) marks the proximal extent of the lower esophageal sphincter (LES). An indentation that moves with respiration is seen where the esophagus crosses the diaphragm. The diaphragm usually lies at or below the GEJ, the relationship varying with respiration and gastric distension. If the Z-line remains more than 2 cm above the GE junction, a hiatus hernia is present. The endoscope normally crosses the GEJ with little resistance.

In the stomach, with the lesser curvature positioned at "12 o'clock", the posterior wall is at "3 o'clock", greater curvature at "6 o'clock", and anterior wall at "9 o'clock". At the cardia, the tubular esophageal lumen flares into the wider stomach. With distension, the fundus is a wide

Practical Gastroenterology and Hepatology: Esophagus and Stomach, 1st edition. Edited by Nicholas J. Talley, Kenneth R. DeVault and David E. Fleischer. © 2010 Blackwell Publishing Ltd.

rounded area, with flat, smooth mucosa. The longitudinal axis of the stomach has a "J-shape". At the inside curve of the "J" is the angulus or incisura, a crescentic fold along the lesser curvature marking the junction of the gastric body and antrum. In the body, rugal mucosal folds extend along the longitudinal axis, and flatten with distension. Distal to the angulus, the cone-shaped antrum tapers to the ring-like pylorus. Rugal folds are less prominent or absent in the antrum. Submucosal vessels may be seen in the cardia, fundus, and antrum, but not usually in the body. Peristaltic waves may pass through the antrum.

Endoscopic Appearance of Surgical Anastomoses

When surgery joins organs with different mucosal types, the anastomosis is recognized by the mucosal transition and change in luminal shape. Gathered folds may create a nodular appearance and small outpouchings. Staples or sutures may be visible below the mucosal surface or protrude into the lumen, and superficial ulcerations are common. The diameter varies with the type of surgery, but normal anastomoses are over 10 mm in diameter and allow passage of standard gastroscopes [2].

Endoscopic Appearance after Esophageal Surgery

Surgery for Cancer

With subtotal esophagectomy and gastric pull-up, the stomach is formed into a tube by removal of the fundus and some of the lesser curve, and pulled up through the diaphragm. The gastroesophageal anastomosis is usually 20–30 cm from the incisors. A colonic segment may be interposed in the place of the esophagus. The colonic interposition has typical colonic mucosa and haustra, and can become distended and tortuous, as well as developing the usual problems of colon mucosal including polyps and carcinomas.

Surgery for Motility Disorders and Diverticuli

Esophagomyotomy for achalasia is usually combined with fundoplication. The myotomy site is not typically apparent, except for the absence of the spastic LES.

Esophageal diverticulectomy may create a linear mucosal deformity. Myotomy for esophageal spasm may create a longitudinal defect of the muscle wall and in some cases a diverticulum.

Endoscopic Appearance after Antireflux Surgery

With a Nissen fundoplication, the fundus is pulled around the back of the GEJ, and then sutured anteriorly, creating a 360° wrap (Figure 5.1). The wrap constricts the lumen of the distal esophagus, but the endoscope will pass with slight pressure. The fundoplication is assessed with the endoscope retroflexed in the gastric body, and oriented in front of the lesser curvature (Figure 5.1). There should be a shallow anterior groove, a deep posterior groove, and a nipple valve (2–3 cm long) of stacked mucosal folds oriented parallel to the diaphragm (see Video 1). The mucosa of the nipple valve adheres to the endoscope in all phases of respiration. If the anterior groove is absent, the posterior groove is shallow, or the valve does not adhere to the endoscope, the fundoplication has loosened or become disrupted [3].

If there is a pouch of gastric mucosa above the wrap, the stomach has slipped up through the wrap, or the wrap was improperly constructed around the proximal stomach. A tight fundoplication is suggested by puckering of the distal esophagus, and the need for excess pressure to advance the endoscope. If the wrap remains in position at the GEJ but has herniated above the diaphragm, the fundoplication will appear intact, but the fundoplication and proximal stomach will be above the diaphragmatic pinch across the stomach.

The Toupet fundoplication is a 270° posterior partial fundoplication, which creates a looser constriction at the GEJ. This partial posterior wrap creates an "omega"-shaped valve, with shallow anterior and posterior grooves, and a valve of stacked folds that is loosely adherent to the endoscope.

Endoscopic Appearance after Gastric Surgery for Cancer or Ulcers

With Billroth I surgery (antrectomy and gastroduodenal anastomosis), the antrum and pylorus are absent, and the

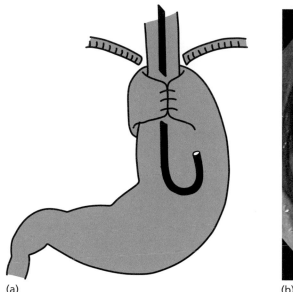

(a)

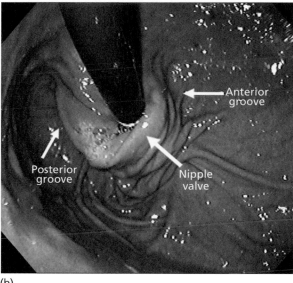

(b)

Figure 5.1 (a) Diagram and (b) endoscopic and photograph of normal Nissen fundoplication. The endoscope is retroflexed and positioned along the lesser curve. There is a shallow anterior groove, deep posterior groove, and nipple valve of stacked mucosal folds.

rugal folds end at a stoma that connects the gastric body to the duodenum. Billroth II surgery is an antrectomy with gastrojejunal anastomosis along the greater curve. A jejunal loop is connected to the stomach side to side, so that two limbs of jejunum can be entered from the stoma. The "afferent" limb comes from the duodenum and is identified by the presence of bile and the ampulla; the "efferent" limb leads downstream. Another variation is a Roux-en-Y esophagojejunostomy; a single limb of small intestine exits the gastrojejunal stoma, and an end-to-side jejunojenostomy is found 30–50 cm downstream. A simple gastrojejunostomy may be used to bypass an obstructed duodenum, and may have the appearance of a typical Billroth II loop anastomosis, or of a Roux-en-Y gastrojejunostomy [1,2].

Wedge resections may create a linear deformity of the gastric mucosa, or a decrease in the usual volume of a portion of the stomach. With total gastrectomy, an end-to-side esophagojejunostomy is formed, usually with a Roux-en-Y jejunal limb. The end of the jejunum may have a J-shape, with a short blind pouch. Sometimes a loop of jejunum is connected as a side-to-side gastrojejunostomy; there may be a side-to-side jejunojejunostomy connecting the afferent and efferent limbs

of the loop several centimeters distal to the esophagojejunostomy.

Endoscopic Appearance after Bariatric Surgery

Roux-en-Y Gastric Bypass

A 15–30 mL pouch of the proximal stomach is separated from the distal stomach, and a Roux-en-Y gastrojejunostomy is formed at the pouch (Figure 5.2). The GEJ is not altered. A normal gastrojejunal anastomosis has a diameter of 10–12 mm, and easily allows a standard gastroscope to pass. The Roux-en-Y jejunojejunostomy may be 50–150 cm downstream, so it may not be within reach of a standard gastroscope. The distal or excluded stomach cannot be seen with a standard gastroscope [4].

Laparoscopic Adjustable Gastric Band

The proximal stomach has been formed into a 15–30 mL pouch, by placing an adjustable silicone band around the stomach. The band gathers the gastric folds to a central point. Moderate resistance is sensed as the endoscope is advanced through the band, and the normal distal

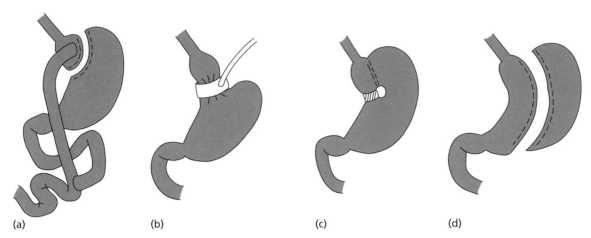

(a)   (b)   (c)   (d)

Figure 5.2 Common bariatric operations: (a) Roux-en-Y gastric bypass; (b) laparoscopic adjustable gastric band; (c) vertical banded gastroplasty; and (d) sleeve gastrectomy.

stomach is entered. There is no anastomosis or stapling, so the visible mucosa of the stomach will be normal. The silicone material of the band should not be visible.

Vertical Banded Gastroplasty

The proximal stomach is stapled into a linear pouch (<50 mL) along the lesser curvature. A band of prosthetic material is placed around the stoma that connects the pouch to the distal stomach, through a donut-shaped hole formed near the lesser curvature, to prevent dilation of the stoma over time. The internal diameter of the stoma is 10–12 mm. The stomach distal to the band has a normal appearance. Although staples or suture material may be visible, the prosthetic material of the band should not be seen.

Sleeve Gastrectomy

The fundus and a portion of the gastric body along the greater curve are removed after stapling, creating a long tubular stomach. The distal antrum and pylorus are normal.

Take-home points

- The esophagus is a 20- to 30-cm tube that has a contracted sphincter at either end.
- The esophagogastric junction is identified (in a normal patient) by the transition from squamous to columnar mucosa.

- The stomach is a long "J-shaped" organ with five endoscopically identifiable regions: cardia, fundus, body, antrum, and pylorus.
- Many operations are performed on the esophagus and stomach, each with a relatively distinct endoscopic appearance, although endoscopy cannot replace a careful review of surgical notes and can be supplemented with appropriately performed radiologic studies.
- Understanding of both the normal and the abnormal endoscopic appearance of the most common of these operations (reflux surgery, gastric resection, and bariatric surgery) is a key part of modern endoscopic practice (described in detail in the text).

References

1 Blackstone MO. *Endoscopic Interpretation*. New York: Raven Press, 1984.
2 Allen JI, Allen MO. Endoscopy in the postoperative upper gastrointestinal tract. In: Sivak MV (ed.), *Gastrointestinal Endoscopy*, 2nd edn. Philadelphia: WB Saunders, 2000: 752–82.
3 Jobe BA, Kahrilas PJ, Vernon AH, *et al.* Endoscopic appraisal of the gastroesophageal valve after antireflux surgery. *Am J Gastroenterol* 2004; **99**: 233–43.
4 ASGE Standards of Practice Committee. Role of endoscopy in the bariatric surgery patient. *Gastrointest Endosc* 2008; **68**: 1–10.

CHAPTER 6

Technique of Esophagogastroduodenoscopy

David Greenwald[1] and Jonathan Cohen[2]

[1] Division of Gastroenterology, Montefiore Medical Center, New York, NY, USA
[2] Division of Gastroenterology, Department of Internal Medicine, New York University School of Medicine, New York, NY, USA

Summary

Esophagogastroduodenoscopy (EGD) is a procedure that allows for visualization of the esophagus, stomach, and proximal small bowel. There are a variety of technical and cognitive aspects that must be mastered in order to perform a high-quality examination. The aim of this chapter is to describe the elements of a complete and thorough EGD, and to review the key elements of the procedure, including tissue sampling

Case

A first-year GI fellow doing his first Endoscopy rotation in August was performing his second endoscopy with a "seasoned veteran faculty member." He reported that the patient was being evaluated for dyspepsia. He wanted to know if it was his responsibility to obtain the informed consent or whether that could be done by a nurse. He asked how does one decide whether to utilize fentanyl or meperidine with midazolam. He asked whether or not the aspirin and clopidogrel would be a problem if biopsies were required; and he asked whether antibiotics should be administered since patient had cirrhosis and ascites. Dr S. Veteran commended him for thinking of these key questions and referred him to national society guidelines on these matters.

with real-time assessment and interpretation of the findings encountered. Mastering the technical and cognitive aspects of this procedure, the operator is able to collect a wide array of diagnostic information. The basic technical components of EGD described in this chapter also serve as the requisite skill set and platform on which many therapeutic interventions depend. The aim of this chapter will be to define and describe all the elements that are required to perform high-quality EGD. The discussion focuses on the key components of *diagnostic* EGD and includes basic tissue sampling, which is considered an essential aspect of standard EGD competency. Therapeutic maneuvers performed during EGD will be covered in other chapters in this textbook.

Introduction

A complete esophagogastroduodenoscopy (EGD) encompasses adequate visualization of the oropharynx, esophagus, stomach, and proximal duodenum, along

Indications for Esophagogastroduodenoscopy

EGD is indicated in the evaluation of signs and symptoms of a wide variety of gastrointestinal disorders. Endoscopy should only be performed for indicated reasons. An American Society for Gastrointestinal Endoscopy guidance document outlines appropriate indications for EGD [1] (Table 6.1).

Practical Gastroenterology and Hepatology: Esophagus and Stomach, 1st edition. Edited by Nicholas J. Talley, Kenneth R. DeVault and David E. Fleischer. © 2010 Blackwell Publishing Ltd.

Table 6.1 Indications for esophagogastroduodenoscopy.

Dyspepsia unresponsive to empiric therapy

Dyspepsia with alarm symptoms

New dyspepsia in a patient age >55

Dysphagia

Odynophagia

Persistent or chronic gastroesophageal reflux disease

Persistent vomiting of unknown cause

Familial adenomatous polyposis syndrome (FAP)

Abnormal upper gastrointestinal tract X-ray

Gastrointestinal bleeding

Iron-deficiency anemia (after unremarkable colonoscopy)

Sampling of small bowel fluid

Foreign body

Portal hypertension: document or treat

Esophageal varices

Following caustic ingestion

A complete EGD must also be high quality. Elements of high-quality performance in endoscopy have been elucidated, and include the following [2,3]:
• Correct indications
• Adherence to guidelines
• Suitable environment
• Adequate support team
• Strategies to minimize risk, including patient preparation and monitoring (see Chapter 4)
• Well prepared and informed patients, consented for the procedure
• Correct selection of equipment
• Appropriate use of sedation/analgesia
• Comfortable intubation
• Complete assessment of target organ(s)
• Recognition and documentation of all abnormalities
• Proper tissue sampling
• Use of appropriate therapy where indicated
• Avoiding, recognizing, and managing complications
• Reasonable duration
• Smooth recovery
• Explanation of procedure and appropriate discharge
• Integrated pathology results
• Clear recommendations and follow-up plan.

Patient Preparation and Informed Consent

The crux of the "Doctrine of Informed Consent" is disclosure, a clear and complete explanation of all portions of the procedure. It is crucial to remember that informed consent is a process, not merely a form, and is really the sum total of all the interactions between a health-care provider and a patient. Full disclosure strengthens the patient–caregiver relationship. Five essential elements to discuss in preparation for EGD include [4,5]:
• Nature of the procedure
• Benefits
• Risks
• Alternatives
• Limitations of procedure.

Consent should be completed using clear and simple language. For example, EGD might be explained as "an EGD is a procedure in which I will pass a flexible tube with a light and a camera though your mouth and esophagus into your stomach and the upper part of your small intestine…" A discussion of the possible risks of EGD, including bleeding, perforation, and missed lesions must occur, while at the same time placing the risks and benefits of the proposed procedure in balance and in a framework the patient can understand. There are very few exceptions where obtaining consent may be waived. Written documentation of the discussion of consent is mandatory. The use of translators and written material in a language in which the patient is fluent is also important when applicable.

Preparation of patients for EGD typically includes taking nothing by mouth for 4–8 h, and longer if there are gastric emptying issues [6]. Most medications can be continued up to the time of endoscopy, usually taken with a small sip of water. Some patients require special consideration prior to EGD; these might include diabetics, who may need their regimens modified in light of decreased oral intake around the time of the procedure. Patients on antiplatelet agents or anticoagulants are managed by balancing the risk of bleeding engendered by maintaining the patient on the agent through the procedure versus the risk of a thromboembolic event if the agent is discontinued in the periprocedure period [7]. In general, aspirin and NSAIDs can be continued safely in all patients having EGD. Recommendations for the management of anticoagulants and antiplatelet agents around the time of endoscopy provide guidance for those performing EGD [8]. Similarly, guidelines for the use of antibiotic prophylaxis in endoscopy provide direction for this situation; the vast majority of patients having EGD have no indication for antibiotic prophylaxis [9].

One final and sometimes underemphasized component of procedure preparation is assessment of the patient's sedation needs and risks prior to the examination [10–12]. This includes taking a complete history of factors that might make sedation more difficult, such as prior difficulties with sedation, narcotic or benzodiazepine use, diminished mental capacity, and agitation or severe anxiety. It also includes considering whether the patient has any characteristics that pose an increased risk for aspiration (e.g., ascites, non-empty stomach, active bleeding), difficult airway management (e.g., obesity, non-visibility of the uvula), or increased cardiopulmonary complications of endoscopy (e.g., co-morbidity, obesity, older age).

Procedure for Esophagogastroduodenoscopy

A complete EGD may be broken down into its component parts, including:

- Intubation
- Oropharyngeal examination
- Esophageal examination
- Examination of the gastroesophageal junction
- Stomach examination, including retroflexion
- Traversing the pylorus
- Passage to the distal duodenum
- Duodenal examination
- Tissue sampling.

Intubation

Patients are typically placed on their left side for EGD, and their neck is flexed forward. A simulation of the maneuver that will be necessary to traverse the mouth towards the upper esophageal sphincter is recommended to assure proper orientation of all equipment. The upper endoscope is introduced into the mouth under direct visualization, allowing for images of the tongue, other structures in the mouth and ultimately the hypopharynx. The endoscopist gets a view of the epiglottis, the vocal cords, both piriform sinuses, and the arytenoid cartilages

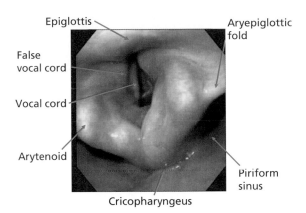

Figure 6.1 Structures of the oropharynx seen during esophagogastroduodenoscopy.

(Figure 6.1). The cricopharyngeus muscle and orifice to the esophagus are located posteriorly, seemingly between the piriform sinuses. The endoscope is therefore passed posteriorly towards the upper esophageal sphincter (UES, or cricopharyngeus muscle), which is at the level of the thyroid cartilage, 15–18 cm from the incisors. The UES is passed under direct visualization, often with the assistance of air insufflation and a gentle amount of pressure. Care must be taken to avoid intubation of a Zenker diverticulum, which exists in some patients, and is an outpouching of the posterior oropharynx just proximal to the UES, caused by decreased compliance of the UES. Care must also be taken in case the patient has a proximal esophageal stricture, which could make esophageal intubation difficult or with increased risk.

Esophagus and Gastroesophageal Junction

The examination continues with the tubular esophagus, a structure about 25 cm in length. Examination of the esophagus should be carried out slowly and with adequate air insufflation to assure complete visualization. Elements to note include color of the mucosa, evidence of erythema, erosions, ulcers, strictures or diverticula.

The gastroesophageal junction is typically about 40 cm from the incisors. Landmarks to differentiate the esophagus from the stomach are sometimes difficult due to movement of these organs during the examination, but the endoscopist should try to identify the top of the gastric folds as representing the place of the gastroesophageal junction. This region is also characterized by the

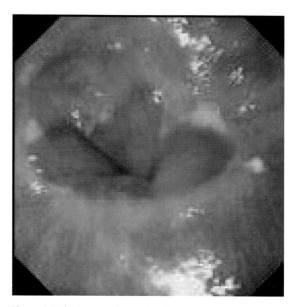

Figure 6.2 The squamocolumnar junction.

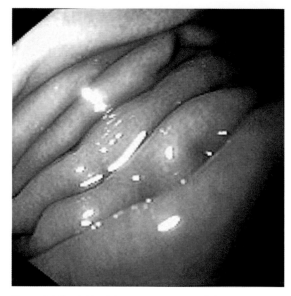

Figure 6.3 The folds of the greater curvature of the stomach seen on esophagogastroduodenoscopy.

squamocolumnar junction, an area where the squamous epithelial lining of the esophagus meets the columnar lining of the stomach. Because this mucosal type transition zone is seldom even along the circumference of the lumen, it is also referred to as the Z-line. The endoscopist can see this demarcation as a color change, with the columnar mucosa of the stomach being darker and having a more "salmon" color (Figure 6.2). This is also the region of the lower esophageal sphincter, a muscular structure that is found at the level of the gastroesophageal junction, but which of course cannot be seen endoscopically.

The endoscopist may recognize a hiatus hernia, where some portion of the stomach has herniated through the esophageal hiatus in the crural diaphragm. In this situation, the columnar-lined mucosa and top of the gastric folds will be seen proximal to the extrinsic narrowing of the lumen caused by the diaphragmatic pinch. Hiatus hernias may also be seen on retroflexed examination of the stomach (see below).

Stomach

Once past the region of the gastroesophageal junction, the endoscope enters the stomach. The initial visualization is usually the relatively large folds of the greater curvature of the stomach (Figure 6.3). A diagram of the

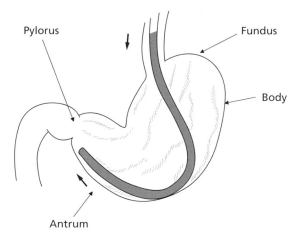

Figure 6.4 Depiction of the insertion of the endoscope into the stomach.

different "portions" of the stomach demonstrates that the exam usually proceeds along the lesser curve of the stomach towards the pylorus (Figure 6.4).

Tips for successful examination of this part of the body include avoiding full insufflation of the stomach upon entering, which may induce retching or belching. A pool of fluid typically is seen in the fundus upon entering the stomach; suctioning this fluid improves visualization of the area, but may induce suction artifacts. In fact, it is incumbent on the endoscopist to examine the mucosa throughout the upper gastrointestinal tract prior to contact between the endoscope and the mucosa, as endoscope trauma may lead to visual abnormalities. Particular attention should be paid to the area of the angularis along the lesser curvature, as it is often the site of pathology.

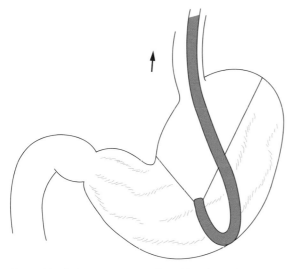

Figure 6.5 Blind spot at gastroesophageal junction and retroflexion.

Retroflexion of the flexible endoscope allows for adequate visualization of the proximal stomach and gastroesophageal junction, an area that may be "blind" to the initial direct examination (Figure 6.5). The technique involves:
• Gastric distension
• Advancing the endoscope to the mid-stomach, to the region of the angularis along the lesser curvature in the antrum
• Turning the endoscope dials all the way "up" so as to achieve an approximately 140–160° bend at the tip of the endoscope
• Many recommend "locking the wheels" of the endoscope to increase stiffness of the tip of the endoscope
• Withdrawing the endoscope in order to advance—this has the effect of drawing the gastroesophageal junction closer to the field of view (Figure 6.6)
• Rotate to obtain a 360° view.

Hiatus hernias are particularly easy to see when the endoscope is in the retroflexed position (Figure 6.7).

It is important to note that items placed through the endoscope's accessory channel, such as a biopsy forceps, may be difficult to use when the endoscope is in the retroflexed position. Care also must be paid to ensure that the retroflexed endoscope does not get stuck in a hiatus hernia or in the esophagus.

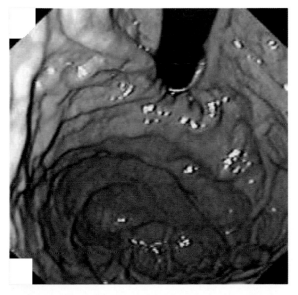
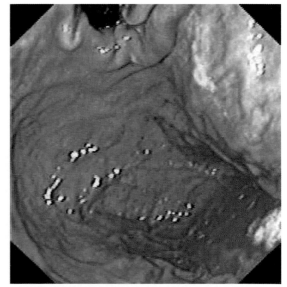

Figure 6.6 Retroflexed views of gastroesophageal junction and proximal stomach.

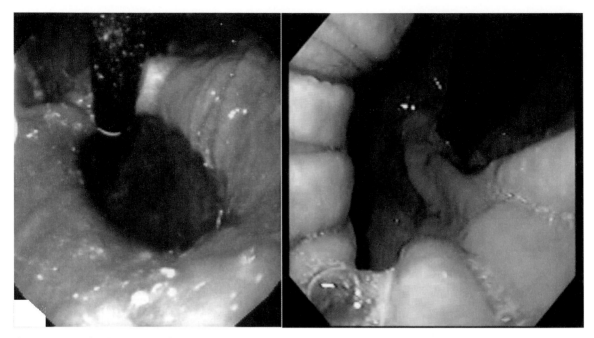

Figure 6.7 Hiatus hernia seen in retroflexion.

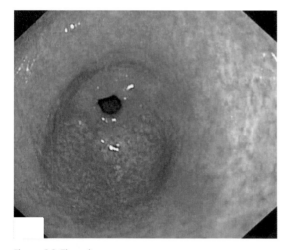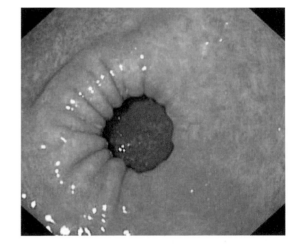

Figure 6.8 The pylorus.

Pyloric Intubation

The pylorus is passed by direct visualization of the lumen separating the stomach from the duodenum (Figure 6.8). Air insufflation is sometime required to "open" the pylorus for passage of the endoscope, and patience is sometimes necessary in situations of a particularly active or motile pyloric region. Some patients have unusual "J-shaped" stomachs, and this may increase the difficulty of success in intubating the pylorus. Attempts to traverse the pylorus in such a patient may result in significant bowing and looping of the instrument and increased pressure on the stomach wall.

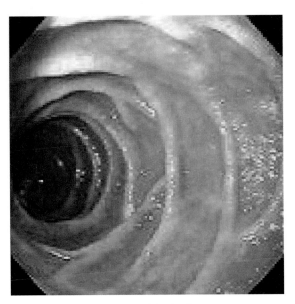

Figure 6.9 The second portion of the duodenum seen on esophagogastroduodenoscopy.

Duodenum

Initial entry into the duodenum through the pylorus leads to the duodenal bulb. Once in the bulb, examination continues by turning to the right, which moves the endoscope posteriorly, following the path of the duodenum. Further right turns lead inferiorly and caudally and into the descending duodenum. Withdrawal of the endoscope here paradoxically leads to antegrade progress distally in the duodenum. The duodenal bulb is often devoid of characteristic features, while the descending duodenum has distinctive circular rings (valvulae conniventes) (Figure 6.9). However, raised bumps and polypoid areas may be encountered, representing either prominent Brunner glands or hetertopic foci of gastric mucosa. The ampulla of Vater, the region in the second portion of the duodenum where the common bile duct and pancreatic duct empty into the duodenum, may be seen on "standard" EGD; a more complete examination of this area of the duodenum is possible using a side-viewing endoscope.

Tissue Sampling

Tissue sampling is an integral part of many EGD procedures [13,14]. In fact, training guidelines emphasize the requirement that anyone performing diagnostic EGD masters standard techniques of tissue sampling. Biopsies,

brushings of the mucosal surface or polypectomy specimens obtained during procedures are sent to the pathologist for analysis.

It is useful for the endoscopist to give the pathologist "the picture", including details such as the clinical history, specimen-specific location and appearance, and a specific question to be answered. Including the endoscopy report and photographs of the area in question are very helpful to the pathologist.

The technique of tissue sampling is usually fairly straightforward; a biopsy forceps is placed though the accessory channel of the endoscope, advanced to the target area and the forceps opened and closed to obtain a pinch biopsy. Many forceps have a "spike", which allows for the acquisition of more than one sample at a time.

One specialized technique bears mentioning. The tubular esophagus may be difficult to obtain biopsy samples in because the forceps comes out of the accessory channel parallel to the wall of the esophagus. This problem can be solved by the "turn-in" technique, where the tip of the endoscope is turned to be more perpendicular to the wall of the esophagus (or anywhere in the upper gastrointestinal tract where this is an issue), allowing for a more direct angle in which to obtain a biopsy. This technique may be augmented by suctioning of the mucosa into the biopsy forceps before tissue acquisition, allowing for a larger sample to be obtained with each bite of the biopsy forceps.

Photodocumentation and Reporting

A key element of every endoscopic procedure is the generation of a complete report to delineate the extent of the tissue examined and all normal and abnormal findings encountered. When possible, clear photodocumentation can greatly enhance this component of the procedure.

Troubleshooting Common Problems in Esophagogastroduodenoscopy

Several problems present frequent issues in EGD. These include:

1 Some examinations prove to be difficult because the stomach is excessively motile. While patience and some additional time may be all that is necessary to allow the bowel to "quiet" and allow the entire exam to be

Table 6.2 Pearls for successful esophagogastroduodenoscopy.

Begin to retroflex in the antrum to better view angularis

Use body movements to facilitate passage to descending duodenum

Remove endoscope slowly to view upper esophagus and cords

Master "turn-in" techniques for esophageal biopsy

Refine precision and technique on routine cases

Increase efforts in preprocedure preparation to ensure that safety measures are maximized and that the EGD is done only for appropriate indications

While making the visual assessment and deciding what sampling to perform, endoscopists should always keep in mind the clinical questions that prompted the procedure in the first place

completed, the use of medications to "calm" the bowel, including glucagon, has been advocated by some.

2 Excessive mucus and bubbles may obscure the view of portions of the upper GI tract during endoscopy; adequate washing using an irrigating syringe or irrigating device is often sufficient. Mucolytic agents, such as *N*-acetylcysteine, or agents that lower surface tension of bubbles, such as simethicone, may be useful.

3 Residual material in the stomach needs to be cleared for adequate visualization; again copious irrigation often is sufficient. Prokinetic agents such as intravenous erythromycin (250 mg) or intravenous metoclopramide (10 mg) 30–90 min prior to endoscopy may facilitate passage of retained debris or blood. Residual gastric contents not only impede complete visualization but also increased the risk of the complication of aspiration.

4 Abnormal anatomy, such as J-shaped stomach or the presence of the stomach in the chest may make completion of EGD more difficult. Specific maneuvers, such as changing the patient's position or the application of external abdominal pressure to "splint" the stomach may facilitate instrument passage in some situations.

Take-home points (see also Table 6.2)

- EGD should be performed only for accepted indications; guidelines of appropriate indications for EGD are available.
- All EGD must be of high quality; there are many critical components to completing a high-quality examination of the upper gastrointestinal tract.

- Adequate preparation of patients for EGD is crucial to the success of the procedure; specific recommendations are available for many issues likely to arise including informed consent, sedation needs and risk assessment, the management of patients on antiplatelet agents and anticoagulants, and the use of prophylactic antibiotics.
- EGD requires visualization of key landmarks as well as recognition and characterization of common abnormalities.
- Key portions of the examination include intubation of the esophagus, evaluation of the tubular esophagus, visualization of the stomach in both the antegrade and retroflexed views, intubation of the pylorus, and examination of the duodenum.
- Inspect the oropharynx and perform a retroflexed view in the stomach of the gastroesophageal junction in all examinations.
- Examine the esophagus slowly enough to allow for detection of subtle irregularities in color and mucosal surface pattern.
- Photodocument key landmarks and any abnormalities.
- Tissue sampling techniques, including biopsy, brushings, and polypectomy, must be mastered to maximize the yield of EGD.
- Fully assess landmarks and complete a thorough mucosal inspection before performing tissue sampling, which might obscure the visual field.
- Acquire sufficient numbers of biopsy samples for the diagnostic question and provide clear communication to the pathologist of the particular clinical information and question to be addressed.

References

1 American Society for Gastrointestinal Endoscopy. Appropriate use of gastrointestinal endoscopy. *Gastrointest Endosc* 2000; **52**: 831–7.

2 Cotton PB, Hawes RH, Barkun A, *et al.* Excellence in endoscopy: Towards practical metrics. *Gastrointest Endosc* 2006; **63**: 286–91.

3 Bjorkman DG. Measuring the quality of endoscopy. *Gastrointest Endosc* 2006; **58**: S1–S38.

4 Zuckerman MJ, Shen B, Harrison ME 3rd, *et al.* Informed consent for GI endoscopy. *Gastrointest Endosc* 2007; **66**: 213–8.

5 Plumeri PA. Informed consent for gastrointestinal endoscopy in the 90's and beyond. *Gastrointest Endosc* 1994; **40**: 379.

6 Faigel DO, Eisen GM, Baron TH, *et al*. Preparation of patients for GI endoscopy. *Gastrointest Endosc* 2003; **57**: 446–50.

7 Eisen GM, Baron TH, Dominitz JA, *et al*. Guidelines on the management of anticoagulation and antiplatelet therapy for endoscopic procedures. *Gastrointest Endosc* 2002; **55**: 775–9.

8 Zuckerman M, Hirota W, Adler D, *et al*. ASGE guideline: the management of low-molecular-weight heparin and nonaspirin antiplatelet agents for endoscopic procedures. *Gastrointest Endosc* 2005; **61**: 189–94.

9 Banerjee S, Shen B, Baron TH, *et al*. Antibiotic prophylaxis for GI endoscopy. *Gastrointest Endosc* 2008; **67**: 791–8.

10 Lichtenstein DR, Jagannath S, Baron TH, *et al*. Sedation and anesthesia in GI endoscopy. *Gastrointest Endosc* 2008; **68**: 815–26.

11 Sharma VK, Nguyen CC, Crowell MD, *et al*. A national study of cardiopulmonary unplanned events after GI endoscopy. *Gastrointest Endosc* 2007; **66**: 27–34.

12 Cohen LB, Delegge MH, Aisenberg J, *et al*. AGA Institute review of endoscopic sedation. *Gastroenterology* 2007; **133**: 675–701.

13 Faigel DO, Eisen GM, Baron TH, *et al*. Tissue sampling and analysis. *Gastrointest Endosc* 2003; **57**: 811–16.

14 Cohen J. The impact of tissue sampling on endoscopy efficiency. *Gastrointestinal Endosc Clin N Am* 2004; **14**: 725–34.

CHAPTER 7

Complications of Esophagogastroduodenoscopy

Herbert C. Wolfsen

Division of Gastroenterology and Hepatology, Mayo Clinic, Jacksonville, FL, USA

Summary

Currently open-access endoscopy and increasing attention to upper gut disease have dramatically increased the number of patients referred for endoscopy. Although there are a paucity of controlled data available, there are some reports of complications associated with EGD, including those associated with sedation and topical anesthetics, cardiovascular complications, infections related to contaminated equipment or transmission of microorganisms from the gut to the bloodstream or other organs and prostheses, perforation, bleeding, and complications associated with percutaneous endoscopic gastrostomy, including endoscope entrapment and aspiration. Generally, most complications of EGD are related to sedation in diagnostic endoscopy and perforation or bleeding, associated with therapeutic EGD. This chapter will focus on the adverse events associated with standard EGD, with an emphasis on the immediate recognition of complications and adverse events.

Case

In February 2008, the Southern Nevada Health District and Nevada State Bureau of Licensure and Certification, along with the Centers for Disease Control and Prevention, determined that unsafe injection practices, related to the administration of anesthesia medication, might have exposed 40 000 patients to the blood of other patients at the Endoscopy Center of Southern Nevada. The process of redrawing medications in multiple patients contaminated the medication vials with blood from previous patients. Some cases of acute hepatitis C have been identified in relation to this incident. This unfortunate situation underlines the importance of paying careful attention to details associated with the preprocedural evaluation, the use and administration of sedation medications, and anticipation and management of complications associated with EGD.

Introduction

In the past, most patients undergoing esophagogastroduodenoscopy (EGD) had severe symptoms such as bleeding, obstruction, and concern about malignancy as an indication for undergoing EGD. However, the widespread availability of open-access endoscopy and increasing awareness of upper GI disorders, such as gastroesophageal reflux disease, Barrett esophagus, and *Helicobacter pylori* infection, have dramatically increased the number of patients undergoing EGD [2]. Improvements in gastrointestinal endoscopic training, as well as endoscopic design improvements, with the development of smaller caliber and more flexible instruments, are expected to improved endoscopy outcomes, and reduces the rate of complications [3,4]. This chapter describes the complications associated with EGD that are not described in other chapters in this volume.

Reports of Complications

Endoscopic complications were addressed extensively during the 1970s and 1980s in several large, retrospective studies [5–7]. Reported complication rates varied widely, including rates of perforation ranging from 0.008 to 0.11%. Two studies were important because of their methodology, procedure description, and stratification

Practical Gastroenterology and Hepatology: Esophagus and Stomach, 1st edition. Edited by Nicholas J. Talley, Kenneth R. DeVault and David E. Fleischer. © 2010 Blackwell Publishing Ltd.

[6,8,9]. These studies reported overall complication rates of 0.13% and 0.24%, perforation rates of 0.03% to 0.1%, and mortality rates of 0.005% to 0.03%. Fleischer evaluated prospectively endoscopic complications over a 1-year period, including diagnostic and therapeutic EGD, colonoscopy, and endoscopic retrograde cholangiopancreatography [10]. He found an overall complication rate of 1.9% in 3287 procedures, primarily in therapeutic procedures. Generally, investigators agree that the risks of endoscopy have decreased over time, although sampling error and selection bias are of concern with many of these previous studies [11–13].

Increasingly, greater numbers of patients are undergoing endoscopic procedures in open-access endoscopy centers, without previous gastroenterology consultation. Some anticipate an increase in complication rates with an increase of patients seeking these procedures in the open-access centers [14–17]. Love reviewed the trend toward open-access endoscopy and found that by reducing the cost associated with subspecialty examination and barium radiography, this practice would enhance cost-effective management of dyspepsia [15]. This Canadian study was a prospective audit of more than 14 000 procedures. There was a reported perforation rate of 0.05% in patients undergoing diagnostic EGD. In the study, 30% of the patients were older than 70 years, and many were considered high-risk patients, and almost 30% of the gastrointestinal endoscopists in this study performed fewer than 200 procedures annually. In a prospective study of endoscopic complications in 214 patients who were 85 years or older, Clark *et al.* only found one complication in the 64 patients who underwent EGD. It was tachyarrhythmia in one patient (1.6%) who underwent emergent endoscopy for gastrointestinal bleeding [18]. In a Germany study, Sieg *et al.* followed 94 gastroenterologists and internists as they performed a total of 110 469 upper endoscopies, with an overall complication rate of 0.009%. The perforation rate was 0.0009%, and the rate of significant hemorrhage was 0.002%. The overall mortality rate for EGD was 0.0009%, with a rate of cardiorespiratory complications of 0.005%. The overall complication rate for diagnostic and therapeutic procedures was lower for gastroenterologists compared with internists. Most of the adverse events associated with diagnostic endoscopy were attributed to use of sedative medications [19].

In a recent prospective Mayo Clinic study, investigators looked for complications among 13 000 upper gastrointestinal tract endoscopic procedures performed between 1999 and 2002 [13]. They noted a total of seven complications, with an overall complication rate of 0.055%. These procedures were performed in ambulatory patients at an open-access endoscopy unit. It was recommended that patients discontinue their use of aspirin and non-steroidal anti-inflammatory drugs for 10–14 days before their procedure, although this approach is more stringent than current guidelines. There was no procedure-related mortality, cardiopulmonary complications were noted in two patients, and perforation occurred in five patients. The risk associated with routine diagnostic endoscopy of the upper gastrointestinal tract, with or without biopsy, was 0.018% (two complications in 11 114 procedures). The risk of perforation associated with dilation of the esophagus was 0.15% (two cases in 1300 procedures). These complication rates compared favorably with those previously reported.

Physicians Insurers Association of America data sharing project reviewed 610 gastrointestinal endoscopy malpractice cases to learn more about endoscopy-associated malpractice claims. "Improper performance" was alleged in 54% of claims and "diagnosis error" in 24% of claims. Of 121 claim files alleging a diagnostic error, 74 (61%) pertained to missed malignancies, of which 69% were colorectal. Of 147 claims alleging iatrogenic injury, 140 (95%) involved perforation or similar direct injury to the gastrointestinal tract. Problems with consent were alleged in 44% of 158 endoscopy-related claim files, alleging additional associated issues [20].

Specific Aspects and Complications of EGD

Preparation for EGD begins with the informed consent, defined as the voluntary agreement by a person, with a functional capability for decision making, to make an informed choice about allowing an action proposed by another person to be performed on him or herself [21]. Over the past years, informed consent has undergone a transformation from an ethical concept to a legal doctrine. The essential elements of disclosure using either standard should include the patient's pertinent medical diagnosis and test results, the nature of the proposed procedure, and the reason the procedure is being suggested, the benefits of the procedure, as well as the risks and complications of the procedure, including the relative incidents and severity that would be material to the patient's decision. Other aspects of the preprocedure evaluation include consideration of medical co-morbidities, current medication usage, and history of substance abuse, medication allergies and intolerances, including latex allergy [1,22,23].

It is recommended that patients ingest no solids for at least 6 h, and no liquids other than a sip of water to take necessary medications for at least 4 h before the EGD procedure. If a gastroduodenal motility problem is suspected, then longer periods of fasting may be needed, as well as limiting the amount of solid food in the previous meal period. In some procedures, topical pharyngeal anesthetic is applied, usually in the form of a benzocaine spray or other topical agent. Although, there have been case reports of life-threatening reactions, such as methemoglobinemia, they are very unusual. For diabetic patients, particularly those using oral hypoglycemic medications and insulin, it is recommended that the long-acting forms of these medications should be held the day of the procedure. However, the use of basal insulin is usually necessary to prevent blood sugar levels from rising excessively. It is recommended to hold short-acting insulin the day of the procedure.

Cardiovascular Events

Lee and colleagues at Duke University studied cardiovascular complications associated with EGD in a retrospective evaluation of a computerized data base of all endoscopies performed between 1988 and 1992, numbering 21 946 procedures [24]. During this time period, nine women and 22 men denoted acute cardiovascular complications, including vasovagal reaction in 24 patients, supraventricular tachycardia in four patients, myocardioinfarction in two patients, and congestive heart failure in one patient. Overall, the rate of acute cardiovascular complications after endoscopy was 0.14% and serious complications occurred exclusively in the setting of known underlying heart disease [25]. American Society for Gastrointestinal Endoscopy (ASGE) guidelines are available describing the appropriate monitoring of patients during endoscopy [22]. These guidelines recommend that a history and physical examination be performed prior to any procedure in order to identify factors that portend a higher risk associated with endoscopy. A detailed review of the medication history, including pre-

vious substance abuse, should be obtained to identify drugs that may interact adversely with sedatives used during the anticipated procedure. Further, the endoscopist and his/her assistants must be trained to identify potential complications and monitor patients carefully during the procedure, and throughout the recovery period.

Infections

Infectious complications associated with EGD may be related to transmission of microbes from patient to patient by means of contaminated endoscopes, equipment, or devices [26]. Alternatively, transmission of microbes from the gut during endoscopy may occur by means of the bloodstream to other organs or prostheses [27,28]. In order to prevent infectious complications of transmission of microbes, it is critically important to follow strict guidelines for the reprocessing of endoscopes and reusable instruments, as well as strict adherence to guidelines prohibiting the use of one-time-use-only drugs and devices, and storing the endoscopes in a vertical hanging position to facilitate drainage of any excess fluid. Several ASGE guidelines describe endoscope reprocessing and infection control during EGD [29,30].

The second type of infectious complication associated with endoscopy is the translocation of microbes to sites distant from the gut, such as infection of vascular grafts or prostheses or endocarditis [27,28,31]. Bacteremia is estimated to occur in zero to 8% of EGD procedures, and more frequently in patients undergoing esophageal dilation (12 to 20%) or variceal band ligation (mean 25%) or sclerotherapy (0–52%, mean 14.6%). This bacteremia is usually short lived and not associated with infectious complications. These statistics compare with bacteremia associated with routine daily activities, such as brushing and flossing of teeth, which are associated with transient rates of bacteremia above 20%. In this context, therefore, the infectious risk for patients undergoing EGD is considered trivial and provides a strong rationale for not routinely administering antibiotic prophylaxis prior to endoscopic procedures (Table 7.1) [32,33].

Perforation

Perforation during diagnostic EGD is unusual, with the reported frequency between 0.02 and 0.2%. Perforation can occur in the proximal esophagus, as well as anatomic lead points, such as the piriform sinus or an esophageal

Table 7.1 Guidelines for antibiotic prophylaxis for esophagogastroduodenoscopy. (Adapted from [1].)

Clinical diagnosis	Endoscopic procedure	Goal of prophylaxis	Periprocedural antibiotic prophylaxis
All cardiac conditions	Any endoscopic procedure	Prevention of infectious endocarditis	Not indicated
Synthetic vascular graft and other non-valvular cardiovascular devices	Any endoscopic procedure	Prevention of graft or device infection	Not recommended
Prosthetic joints	Any endoscopic procedure	Prevention of septic arthritis	Not recommended
Cirrhosis with acute gastrointestinal bleeding	Required for all patients, regardless of endoscopy	Prevent infectious complications	Recommended
All patients	Percutaneous endoscopic gastrostomy placement	Prevention of tube related infections	Recommended

or cricopharyngeal diverticulum. Altered anatomy, previous surgery or treatment, as well as the presence of tissue abnormality, such as dysplasia, acute injury, or neoplasia, may increase the risk of a perforation. In such settings, the mortality of an iatrogenic esophageal perforation may be high. The risk of perforation is higher in patients undergoing therapeutic EGD procedures, including dilation of stenoses, stent placement, and achalasia treatment. Perforation of the upper gut is often associated with severe pain, shortness of breath, tachycardia, fever, and leukocytosis. Chest crepitus is often not initially detectable. The chest X-ray is also frequently normal and does not exclude the presence of a perforation. In a patient with severe pain after a procedure, especially involving a malignant stricture, a water-soluble contrast barium X-ray and contrast-enhanced chest CT scan are recommended. The use of barium radiography is to be avoided since it is associated with severe mediastinitis. Management may include attempts at endoscopic closure of the perforation, conservative management, or surgery [32,34]. In the digital video files that accompany this chapter (Videos 2 and 3) is a case presentation of complex stricture dilation procedures associated with childhood lye ingestion. The second video case presentation describes the use of capsule endoscopy and double-balloon enteroscopy to detect a jejunal adenocarcinoma in a patient with anemia and occult enteric bleeding.

Bleeding

Bleeding after EGD is also rare. The rate of hemorrhage associated with EGD is reportedly 0.15%, and the use of aspirin or non-steroidal anti-inflammatory medications does not appear to increase this risk. ASGE guidelines suggest that routine endoscopy with or without biopsy may be performed in patients using these medications without modification. Previous surveys have reported safe EGD procedures having been performed in patients with severe thrombocytopenia and a platelet count as low as 20 000. Procedures associated with mucosal biopsy or more invasive endoscopy may necessitate platelet transfusions in patients with platelet counts lower than 20 000.

Aspiration

Other rare complications include the risk of aspiration of gastric refluxate. This risk may be reduced by avoiding the use of topical benzocaine, minimizing air insufflation, meticulously aspirating gastric contents, as well as maintaining elevation of the bed and preventing excessive sedation.

Performing EGD procedures in a patient with active bleeding can be a dangerous situation. Previous studies have found aspiration occurring in 1–4% of EGD procedures in patients with massive upper gut bleeding.

Incarceration

Incarceration or entrapment of an endoscope during EGD is also a rare event. Intubation with a second endoscope is recommended to apply pressure to the curved portion of the endoscope to allow it to straighten into the stomach. Both endoscopes may then be removed uneventfully [32,35,36].

Take-home points

- The key to avoiding complications of EGD is to anticipate them and to recognize the source of risk.

- Risk can be reduced by carefully reviewing the patient's history. It also requires assessment of: his/her risks and/or benefits for endoscopy; alternatives to endoscopy; careful consideration of medical co-morbidity; medication use and history of substance abuse; and allergies.

- Attention should be paid to: fasting prior to EGD; adjustment of medications (e.g., oral hypoglycemic drugs, insulin); and modifying techniques for endoscopy in pediatric, pregnant and elderly patients.

- Informed consent is a procedure that emphasizes that the physician is responsible for explaining the procedure with its benefits and risks in terms that the patient can understand.

- Infectious complications occur by utilizing contaminated equipment and transmission of microorganisms from the gut to the bloodstream or the target organ.

- In addition to patient risk, procedural risk can be divided into those that have standard or higher risk. Examples of some that have higher risk are percutaneous endoscopic gastrostomy, dilation of malignant stenoses, foreign body retrieval, endoscopic removal of foreign body, hepatobiliary procedures, and endoscopic hemostasis.

References

1 Banerjee S, Shen B, Baron TH, *et al*. Antibiotic prophylaxis for GI endoscopy. *Gastrointest Endosc* 2008; **67**: 791–8.

2 DeVault KR, Castell DO. Updated guidelines for the diagnosis and treatment of gastroesophageal reflux disease. The Practice Parameters Committee of the American College of Gastroenterology. *Am J Gastroenterol* 1999; **94**: 1434–42.

3 Faigel DO, Pike IM, Baron TH, *et al*. ASGE/ACG Taskforce on Quality in Endoscopy. Quality indicators for gastrointestinal endoscopic procedures: an introduction. *Gastrointest Endosc* 2006; **63**: S3–9.

4 Pollack MJ, Chak A. Quality in endoscopy: it starts during fellowship. *Gastrointest Endosc* 2008; **67**: 120–2.

5 Schiller KF, Cotton PB, Salmon PR. The hazards of digestive fibre-endoscopy: a survey of British experience. *Gut* 1972; **13**: 1027.

6 Silvis SE, Nebel O, Rogers G, *et al*. Endoscopic complications. Results of the 1974 American Society for Gastrointestinal Endoscopy Survey. *JAMA* 1976; **235**: 928–30.

7 Colin-Jones DG, Cockel R, Schiller KF. Current endoscopic practice in the United Kingdom. *Clin Gastroenterol* 1978; **7**: 775–86.

8 Dawson J, Cockel R. Oesophageal perforation at fibreoptic gastroscopy. *BMJ (Clin Res Ed)* 1981; **283**: 583.

9 Davis RE, Graham DY. Endoscopic complications: the Texas experience. *Gastrointest Endosc* 1979; **25**: 146–9.

10 Fleischer D. Monitoring the patient receiving conscious sedation for gastrointestinal endoscopy: issues and guidelines. *Gastrointest Endosc* 1989; **35**: 262–6.

11 Hart R, Classen M. Complications of diagnostic gastrointestinal endoscopy. *Endoscopy* 1990; **22**: 229–33.

12 Newcomer MK, Brazer SR. Complications of upper gastrointestinal endoscopy and their management. *Gastrointest Endosc Clin N Am* 1994; **4**: 551–70.

13 Wolfsen HC, Hemminger LL, Achem SR, *et al*. Complications of endoscopy of the upper gastrointestinal tract: a single-center experience. *Mayo Clin Proc* 2004; **79**: 1264–7.

14 Clarke GA, Jacobson BC, Hammett RJ, *et al*. The indications, utilization and safety of gastrointestinal endoscopy in an extremely elderly patient cohort. *Endoscopy* 2001; **33**: 580–4.

15 Love J. Value of gastroscopy without a prior consultation. *Can J Gastroenterol* 1997; **11** (Suppl. B): 82B–6B.

16 Maroy B, Moullot P. Safety of upper gastrointestinal endoscopy with intravenous sedation by the endoscopist at office: 17,963 examinations performed in a community center by two endoscopists over 17 years. *J Clin Gastroenterol* 1998; **27**: 368–9.

17 Lukens FJ, Wolfsen HC. The impact of screening colonoscopy in an open-access endoscopy unit. *Endonurse* 2002; **2**: 22–3.

18 Clark CS, Kraus BB, Sinclair J, *et al*. Gastroesophageal reflux induced by exercise in healthy volunteers. *JAMA* 1989; **261**: 3599–601.

19 Sieg A, Hachmoeller-Eisenbach U, Eisenbach T. Prospective evaluation of complications in outpatient GI endoscopy: a survey among German gastroenterologists. *Gastrointest Endosc* 2001; **53**: 620–7.

20 Gerstenberger PD, Plumeri PA. Malpractice claims in gastrointestinal endoscopy: analysis of an insurance industry data base. *Gastrointest Endosc* 1993; **39**: 132–8.

21 Zuckerman MJ, Shen B, Harrison ME, 3rd, *et al*. Informed consent for GI endoscopy. *Gastrointest Endosc* 2007; **66**: 213–18.

22 Waring JP, Baron TH, Hirota WK, *et al*. Guidelines for conscious sedation and monitoring during gastrointestinal endoscopy. *Gastrointest Endosc* 2003; **58**: 317–22.

23 Qureshi WA, Rajan E, Adler DG, *et al*. ASGE Guideline: Guidelines for endoscopy in pregnant and lactating women. *Gastrointest Endosc* 2005; **61**: 357–62.

24 Lee JG, Leung JW, Cotton PB. Acute cardiovascular complications of endoscopy: prevalence and clinical characteristics. *Dig Dis* 1995; **13**: 130–5.

25 Gangi S, Saidi F, Patel K, *et al.* Cardiovascular complications after GI endoscopy: occurrence and risks in a large hospital system. *Gastrointest Endosc* 2004; **60**: 679–85.

26 Schembre DB. Infectious complications associated with gastrointestinal endoscopy. *Gastrointest Endosc Clin N Am* 2000; **10**: 215–32.

27 Nelson DB. Infectious disease complications of GI endoscopy: Part I, endogenous infections. *Gastrointest Endosc* 2003; **57**: 546–56.

28 Nelson DB. Infectious disease complications of GI endoscopy: part II, exogenous infections. *Gastrointest Endosc* 2003; **57**: 695–711.

29 Banerjee S, Shen B, Nelson DB, *et al.* Infection control during GI endoscopy. *Gastrointest Endosc* 2008; **67**: 781–90.

30 Banerjee S, Nelson DB, Dominitz JA, *et al.* Reprocessing failure. *Gastrointest Endosc* 2007; **66**: 869–71.

31 Nelson DB. Recent advances in epidemiology and prevention of gastrointestinal endoscopy related infections. *Curr Opin Infect Dis* 2005; **18**: 326–30.

32 Ginzburg L, Greenwald D, Cohen J. Complications of endoscopy. *Gastrointest Endosc Clin N Am* 2007; **17**: 405–32.

33 Mergener K, Baillie J. Complications of endoscopy. *Endoscopy* 1998; **30**: 230–43.

34 Quine MA, Bell GD, McCloy RF, *et al.* Prospective audit of upper gastrointestinal endoscopy in two regions of England: safety, staffing, and sedation methods. *Gut* 1995; **36**: 462–7.

35 Koch DG, Arguedas MR, Fallon MB. Risk of aspiration pneumonia in suspected variceal hemorrhage: the value of prophylactic endotracheal intubation prior to endoscopy. *Dig Dis Sci* 2007; **52**: 2225–8.

36 Rudolph SJ, Landsverk BK, Freeman ML. Endotracheal intubation for airway protection during endoscopy for severe upper GI hemorrhage. *Gastrointest Endosc* 2003; **57**: 58–61.

CHAPTER 8

Advanced Esophagogastroduodenoscopy Techniques

Heiko Pohl, Stuart Gordon, and Richard I. Rothstein

Section of Gastroenterology and Hepatology, Dartmouth Hitchcock Medical Center, Lebanon, NH, USA

Summary

Esophagogastroduodenoscopy (EGD) has evolved from a purely diagnostic technique based on imaging to an advanced technology that facilitates complex therapeutic interventions. This chapter covers technologies that enhance visualization to improve diagnostic accuracy and focuses on several therapeutic techniques not fully covered in companion chapters. In particular, advanced interventions that this chapter will review include the device and technique evolution for endoscopic treatment of gastroesophageal reflux disease (GERD) and obesity, as well as enteroscopy and polypectomy of the stomach and duodenum. Training and mastering advanced EGD techniques requires sufficient background experience with standard diagnostic endoscopy and routine procedures (such as biopsy and esophageal dilation), and a detailed knowledge of the normal appearance and pathological changes of the upper GI tract. Learning advanced endoscopic procedures can be part of routine fellowship training and advanced fellowship training, or may be acquired through mentoring and on-going continuing professional education.

Case

A 42-year-old female who works at a New England medical center has had reflux with substernal burning, regurgitation, and bloating for 15 years. Belching most predictably relieves her symptoms. She has been treated with antacids, H_2-blockers, proton pump inhibitors, and prokinetic agents with only moderate success. Esophageal motility testing reveals a very low lower esophageal sphincter (LES) pressure and some ineffective motility in the distal esophagus. Impedance testing shows both increased acid and non-acid reflux despite a twice daily proton pump inhibitor (PPI) dose. She had a gastric emptying study which shows delayed emptying at 2 and 4h. She was referred to a surgeon experienced in laparoscopic fundoplications who recommended surgery but the patient was reluctant to undergo an operation that may leave her without the ability to "belch." Her husband is a biomedical engineer who is aware of some of the "newer" endoscopic treatments for GERD. She and her husband come to see the gastroenterologist at her medical center who is known to have a good knowledge of advances in endoscopy. The husband pulls out a list from behind the plastic pocket protector in his right shirt pocket and asks the gastroenterologist whether she is a candidate for a Stretta procedure; an Enteryx procedure; a Gatekeeper procedure; an Endocinch procedure; a plicaton; an Esophyx procedure; a Medigus system procedure; or the TOGA system treatment?

Definition

Advanced EGD techniques include all techniques beyond the usual white-light visual inspection and biopsy sampling of the mucosa. During standard gastroenterology fellowships and in most surgical residency training programs, trainees become familiar with routine endoscopic

Practical Gastroenterology and Hepatology: Esophagus and Stomach, 1st edition. Edited by Nicholas J. Talley, Kenneth R. DeVault and David E. Fleischer. © 2010 Blackwell Publishing Ltd.

diagnostic procedures and learn the techniques of tissue biopsy, and guidelines have been established for minimum number of procedures to be performed by the trainee in order to enable competency and maximize safety. The American Society for Gastrointestinal Endoscopy (ASGE) makes a distinction between basic and advanced procedures because the latter procedures are more complex, more technically demanding to perform, and carry a higher risk of complications [1]. Procedures such as foreign body extraction, luminal dilation, and treatment of gastrointestinal bleeding are learned to varying degrees, depending upon the exposure to these cases and adequate numbers of cases for a quality learning experience. During routine fellowships or residencies, exposure to advanced diagnostic imaging is quite variable and does not carry particular training recommendations by the national societies. Endoscopic therapies such as endoscopic mucosal resection (EMR), stenting, mucosal ablation, polypectomy of the stomach or duodenum, treatment of achalasia, use of argon plasma coagulation for treatment of vascular ectasias, and use of cryosprays are among the many techniques to which a trainee may be exposed or possibly perform, although typically these would be more likely learned in additional advanced endoscopic training beyond the standard preliminary programs. Likewise, training in endoscopic ultrasonography and endoscopic retrograde cholangiopancreatography (ERCP) may be part of some routine GI fellowships, but mostly these advanced techniques will be learned in additional months to years of special fellowship training. The emerging field of natural orifice translumenal endoscopic surgery (NOTES), currently in evolution, will have its own set of hybrid endoscopic and surgical knowledge base requirements and training recommendations. Advanced endoscopic procedures can be divided into diagnostic and therapeutic techniques. ASGE guidelines provide detailed information on the role of EGD for conditions that may require the use of advanced endoscopic techniques, including surveillance of premalignant conditions [2], upper GI bleeding [3,4], and GERD [5]. Therapeutic techniques are often restricted to the available tools that can be passed through a 2.8 mm working channel of a diagnostic upper endoscope or a 3.7 mm working channel of therapeutic endoscopes. Special endoscopes with two working channels with the above diameters or one large 4.5 mm working channel are also available. Instruments and

Table 8.1 Advanced esophagogastroduodenoscopy techniques.

Diagnostic adjuncts
　Chromoendoscopy
　Narrow-band/multiband imaging
　Spectroscopy
　In vivo microscopy
Therapeutic adjuncts
　Injection therapy
　Thermal therapy
　Mechanical therapy
　Combined therapy
　Enteroscopy
　Antireflux procedures
　Anti-obesity procedures

accessories can be used for mucosal spraying, magnified and microscopic visualization, *in vivo* microscopy, mucosal or intravascular injection, clipping, rubber banding, and thermal applications, and for numerous other advanced procedures. Some advanced therapeutic interventions employ cutting, stapling, suturing, dilating, injecting, or deployment of implantable devices.

In this review, we will focus on enhanced diagnostic techniques and several therapeutic procedures, as listed in Table 8.1.

Diagnostic Techniques

Endoscopic diagnostic techniques have evolved to improve detection of intralumenal lesions. In concert with high resolution endoscopy (HRE), these are anticipated to increase the detection rates of gastrointestinal lesions. Most of these advances over standard white-light endoscopy are not only important for performance of advanced therapeutic endoscopy, but will find a utility in general endoscopic practice. Techniques that can enhance contrast imaging include spraying dye onto the mucosa (chromoendoscopy), using optical filters (NBI) or computerized image analysis (FICE), or magnifying the image by using mechanical or electronic lenses (zoom endoscopy, *in vivo* microscopy).

Chromoendoscopy

Chromoendoscopy uses agents that are either sprayed onto the mucosa, or in some techniques injected submucosally, to enhance contrast of a dysplastic lesion. For topical application, a special spraying catheter or a standard ERCP cannula can be employed to provide uniform mucosal coating. Chromoendoscopic agents include absorbable substances such as methylene blue and contrasting substances such as indigo carmine, Lugol solution, and acetic acid. In the upper GI tract, these agents have been primarily applied to improve detection of dysplasia in Barrett esophagus or in the stomach.

Methylene blue is a commonly used dye that is sprayed on to the mucosa for enhanced detection of superficial lesions or added to a saline solution for submucosal injection (where it stains the submucosal and deeper layers to assist in endoscopic mucosal resection and submucosal dissection). It is absorbed by the uppermost cell layer and taken up by the nucleus. It is less absorbed by dysplastic cells and thus may result in improved visualization of superficial dysplastic lesions. For detection of Barrett dysplasia (Figure 8.1a,b; Video 4), however, studies have not consistently shown a clear diagnostic benefit with sensitivities around 50% and specificities between 50 and 85%, nearly similar to flipping a coin [6].

Indigo carmine is a sulfonic acid sodium salt that is not absorbed, but can accumulate in the intercellular space in the upper cellular layer, and hence enhance

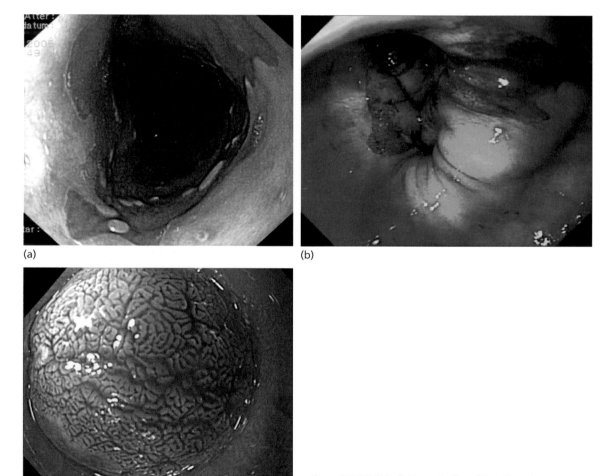

(a)

(b)

(c)

Figure 8.1 (a) White-light examination of Barrett esophagus, no dysplasia. (b) Chromoendoscopy of Barrett esophagus using methylene blue, no dysplasia. (c) Barrett esophagus with high magnification endoscopy and acetic acid.

abnormal architecture. There is no evidence that indigo carmine alone will improve diagnostic accuracy for the detection of dysplasia in the upper GI tract.

Congo red is a diazo-dye and stains acid-secreting gastric mucosa. It has therefore been employed for the detection of early gastric cancer and to evaluate the recovery of gastric mucosa after *Helicobacter pylori* eradication [7]. It is more commonly utilized in Asian countries where there is a higher incidence of gastric cancer.

Lugol solution is an iodine disinfectant. It is employed in the detection of esophageal squamous cell carcinoma. Normal esophageal epithelium stains brown because of its glycogen content, while dysplastic tissue does not stain and therefore appears pale. Screening with this solution has yielded an increased detection rate when compared to standard endoscopy and an improved definition of neoplastic margins [8].

 Acetic acid has also been used to enhance contrast in patients with Barrett esophagus (Video 5, Figure 8.1c). Acetic acid leads to a reversible edema of the mucosa lasting several minutes, and can highlight the irregular surface architecture, which is a feature of neoplastic change. Studies that have examined the accuracy of acetic acid application to diagnose Barrett metaplasia and dysplasia have reported variable results [9].

Narrow-band Imaging/Flexible Spectral Imaging Color Enhancement

To improve macroscopic recognition of dysplastic or inflammatory changes, standard endoscopic imaging can be modified using special software that filters and/or enhances certain spectra of light, essentially chromoendoscopy without the use of dyes. This can permit an "on-the-fly push-button" availability of mucosal contrast imaging that avoids the need for cumbersome and time-consuming spray techniques.

 Narrow-band imaging (NBI) filters the longer red light waves from the white light spectrum and selects shorter wave lengths for display. NBI uses narrow spectra of blue light (440-460nm) and green light (540–560 nm). Hemoglobin preferentially absorbs red light and reflects blue light. NBI therefore better contrasts the superficial details of the mucosa including small capillaries (Figure 8.2a,b; Video 6). In theory, neoplastic lesions with irregular vasculature may therefore be more readily detected (Figure 8.2c,d). However, NBI alone does not necessarily improve neoplasia detection rate, but the combination with zoom

endoscopy (at a 115-fold increase in magnification) has shown some promising results in the detection of Barrett dysplasia (Figure 8.3; Video 7) [10].

Flexible spectral imaging color enhancement (FICE) uses the white-light endoscopic image and creates a computer generated color image based on different wave lengths. Similar to NBI, this computed virtual chromoendoscopy may enhance mucosal and vascular patterns. Limited evaluation in the upper GI tract suggests some benefit in imaging gastric cancer.

Spectroscopy

Autoimmunfluorescence imaging is a technique that relies on the detection of light emission that varies based on the nature of the imaged tissues. Fluorescence happens when molecules and atoms absorb shorter, high-energy wavelength light and emit relatively lower-energy, longer wavelength light. It contrasts inflammatory and neoplastic areas from other normal mucosa. This technique has shown a high sensitivity for neoplasia but a poor specificity [11]. Combining techniques with a highly sensitive identification of a suspicious area ("red flag") followed by a highly specific test (i.e., NBI zoom) may be an optimal stepwise approach to improve detection of precancerous lesions [11].

Optical coherence tomography is considered the optical equivalent to ultrasound. It uses the information obtained from the reflection of light waves by different tissues. Studies in the upper GI tract have primarily determined feasibility.

In vivo Microscopy

In vivo microscopy systems have been developed over the recent years. These include confocal laser microscopy (CLM) and light microscopy technologies and provide a resolution that can produce *in vivo* images at a cellular level (nuclei). Confocal laser microscopy creates images from the reflection of a laser beam that varies dependent on different tissue characteristics. Several studies have examined the yield for the detection of high grade dysplasia in Barrett esophagus using either the integrated or the probe based CLM system (Figures 8.4a,b and 8.5a,b) and reported sensitivities and specificities between 75–93% and 88–98%, respectively [12,13]. Light endocytoscopy, similar to a conventional microscope, incorporates a magnification system that allows 450 to 1100-fold magnification. The technique requires prior tissue staining

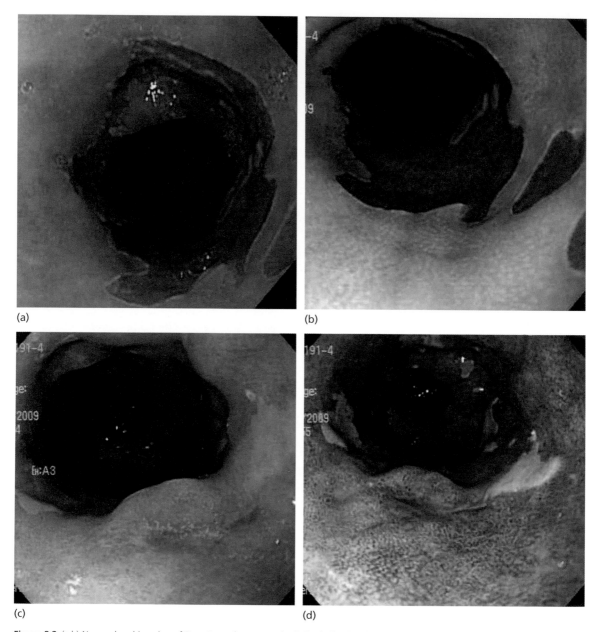

(a)

(b)

(c)

(d)

Figure 8.2 (a,b) Narrow-band imaging of Barrett esophagus, no dysplasia. (c,d) White-light and narrow-band imaging of Barrett esophagus with a nodule representing an intramucosal cancer.

(i.e., with methylene blue). This technique had not been shown to improve detection of Barrett dysplasia (Figure 8.4c) [14], but may be beneficial in detection of squamous cell neoplasia [15] and celiac disease (Figure 8.6) [16].

Additional Thoughts on Imaging

The performance of detailed advanced imaging techniques, especially when applying magnification or microscopic technology, requires a stable field of view. A transparent distal cap (2 or 4 mm depth) (Video 8),

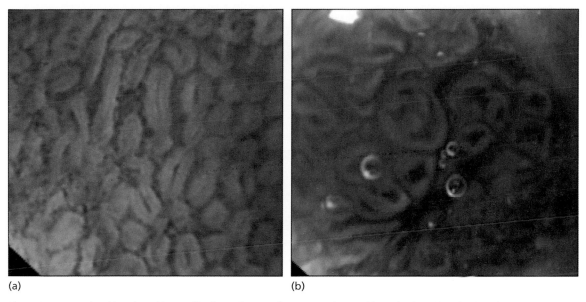

(a)   (b)

Figure 8.3 Narrow-band imaging with magnification endoscopy of Barrett esophagus without dysplasia (a) and with high-grade dysplasia (b).

attached to the tip of the endoscope minimizes mucosal movement and stabilizes the field of view. These widely available caps have proven useful for other diagnostic and therapeutic procedures as explained elsewhere.

For many of the above mentioned diagnostic techniques, a significant benefit has not been firmly established. Although advanced imaging may enhance recognition of neoplastic or dysplastic tissue, the taking of biopsies will continue to be the gold standard for diagnosis. While the development and use of new technologies adds excitement and interest for endoscopists (and the companies that create the technologies), the widespread acceptance of these modalities into routine and advanced endoscopic practice, and payment for same, will require additional studies that clearly show the additional diagnostic and clinical benefit of their use compared to conventionally available techniques.

Therapeutic Techniques

Injection Therapy

Injection therapy involves the delivery of a substance under endoscopic guidance into a specific area. Control of bleeding has been one of the main indications of endoscopic injection therapies. The most common cause of non-variceal upper gastrointestinal bleeding is peptic ulcer disease at about a 50–70% frequency [17]. Injection of epinephrine 1:10 000 into an ulcer effectively controls active bleeding in approximately 95% of patients and reduces the risk of recurrent bleeding in high-risk ulcers (active bleeding, visible vessel, adherent clot) [4]. Bleeding cessation is thought to be caused by vascular constriction as well as a tamponade from the injected volume. A larger injection volume is more effective then lower volumes, and at least 15 mL should be used [18]. The technique involves injecting around the bleeding site in the ulcer. Having only the tamponade effect, it is not surprising that NaCl has been shown to be effective in controlling peptic ulcer bleeding, but with a higher rebleeding rate than epinephrine. Other substances as ethanol (98%) or fibrin have also been used with some benefit, however, these substances have not been shown to be superior to epinephrine injection [19–21].

Sclerosing agents, such as 3% sodium tetradecyl sulfate, sodium morrhuate, or ethanolamine oleate have been used for the treatment of esophageal varices. These agents are placed into and around esophageal varices by

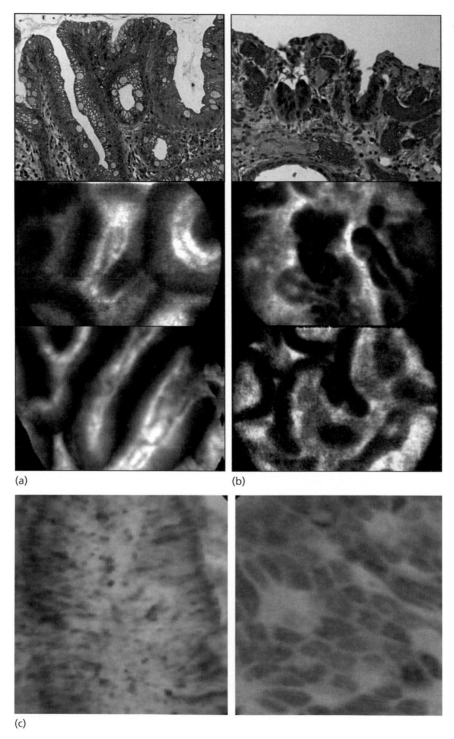

(a)   (b)

(c)

Figure 8.4 Barrett mucosa in HE staining and *in vivo* probe confocal laser microscopy images without dysplasia (a) and with high grade dysplasia (b). (c) Examination of Barrett mucosa without dysplasia with endocytoscopy and prior methylene blue staining in 450 × and 1100 × magnification.

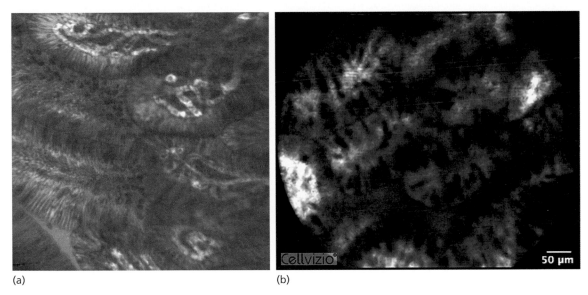

(a)   (b)

Figure 8.5 (a) Examination of normal duodenal mucosa with the confocal laser microscopy system integrated into the endoscope (Pentax). (b) Examination of normal duodenal mucosa with the probe-based confocal laser microscopy system (Cellvizio).

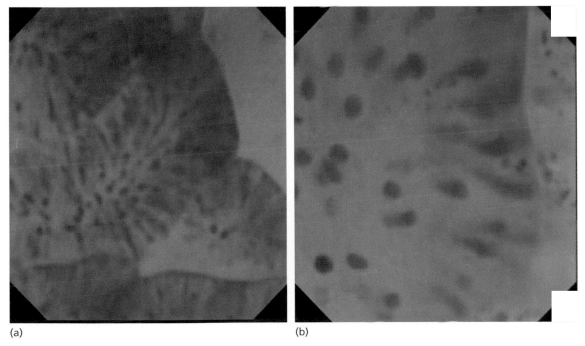

(a)   (b)

Figure 8.6 Examination of normal duodenal mucosa with probe-based endocytoscopy after methylene blue staining in 450 × (a) and 1100 × magnification (b).

injection using the standard 5-mm endoscopic needle, typically at a tangential angle to the esophageal wall. Although effective in treating bleeding varices in 70–80%, post-treatment esophageal stricturing depending on the agent used may reach 33%. Sclerosing agents are therefore not recommended as the first-line therapy [3]. They may be used in patients with active bleeding and impaired visualization; however, no study has rigorously examined this approach.

The sclerosing agent cyanoacrylate (*N*-butyl-2-cyanoacrylate), when injected, seems to be an effective treatment for bleeding gastric fundic and cardiac varices and can reduce the rebleeding rate [22]. Cyanoacrylate is a compound agent requiring the injection of two substances, which will form an expanding polymer within the bleeding varix. There is a reported risk of 1% for pulmonary emboli [22]. Cyanoacrylate has also been used for the treatment of bleeding esophageal varices when endoscopic visualization is poor and in the setting of severely impaired coagulation, however, there have been no studies evaluating the use of this agent as a rescue approach in such patients. Because *N*-butyl-2-cyanoacrylate is not available in the United States, its analog 2-octyl-cyanoacrylate has been studied, but available data are limited.

The use of endoscopic injection for delivery of medication has been mainly for two indications in clinical practice. Botulinum toxin injection has been used for the treatment of achalasia, mainly for patients who are not candidates for surgery or pneumatic balloon treatment. Botulinum toxin type A affects neuromuscular function by binding to receptor sites on motor nerve terminals and inhibiting the release of acetylcholine with subsequent reduction in resting tone and contractile strength of the involved muscle. The procedure involves using a 5-mm sclerotherapy needle, injection of 1 mL (20 units) into the muscular layer in four quadrants at the gastroesophageal junction, plus one additional injection so that 100 units are administered. It is important to identify the endoscopic appearance of gastroesophageal junction, so that the injection can be just above the squamocolumnar junction (1 to 2 cm) at that level, and the needle angled at about 45°. It is not clear that there is an optimal specific target area for injection at the distal esophagus, where in achalasia patients, the lower esophageal sphincter has a somewhat longer length. Injection of botulinum toxin has provided clinical symptom benefit in 64–100% of patients [23]. Symptom response lasts typically for 6 to 11 months, and repeated treatment is generally required to provide on-going benefit. This therapy is therefore infrequently used when a patient may be a candidate for more invasive treatment because it does not provide definite long-term benefit compared to balloon dilatation or surgical myotomy. Botulinum toxin has also been used in selected patients with other esophageal and gastric motility disorders such as a hypercontractile esophagus or for symptom improvement in gastroparesis.

Steroid injection into recurrent benign esophageal strictures has been used in an attempt to decrease the need for recurrent dilatation. The method involves use of a 5-mm sclerotherapy needle and steroid suspension (i.e., triamcinalone 50 mg/5 mL) placed into the strictured region in 0.5 to 1 mL divided injections. A small, randomized trial has found a decreased need for repeat dilatation in the steroid treated group (13%) compared to those not given steroid injection (60%) [24].

Local endoscopic injection of chemotherapeutic agents had been examined in gastric cancer patients in the 1980s. More recently, studies have examined the use of injected chemotherapeutic agents or radioisotope seeds [25] as a palliative treatment for patients with advanced pancreatic cancer. It is possible that endoscopic application of radiochemotherapy or biologic agents may become part of a multimodal cancer treatment in the future.

Submucosal Lifting

Submucosal injection is routine part of endoscopic mucosal resection or submucosal dissection for removal of mucosal neoplastic lesions in the esophagus, stomach, small intestine, and colon. It is most commonly used to assist in the resection of larger colonic polyps, but can be similarly used for lesions in the upper gastrointestinal tract such as gastric or duodenal polyps (Figure 8.7a,b). The injection may provide important information about whether a lesion may be completely resectable ("lifting sign") with clean deep margins. Submucosal injection creates a resection safety cushion by separating the mucosal lesion from the deeper muscular layer. The target lesion is often initially outlined by using superficial cautery and creating a "dotted line" around it with adequate margins. NaCl with a small amount of methylene blue is commonly used as the injectate, and enough is placed beneath the lesion to create a fully lifted target

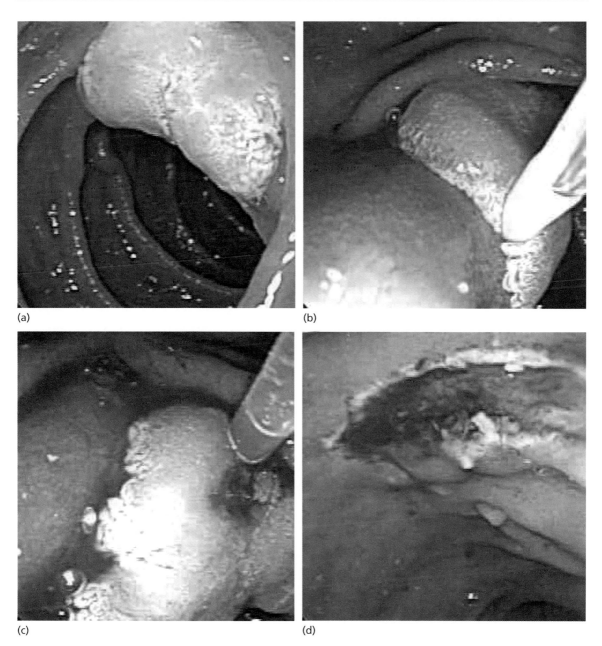

(a)   (b)

(c)   (d)

Figure 8.7 Submucosal injection and snare resection of a duodenal adenoma. (a) Duodenal polyp, (b) saline lift injection, (c) polyp engaged in snare, (d) after snare resection.

area. Other agents such as dextrose, hyaluronic acid, and methyl cellulose may provide a more sustained lifting effect [26]. Dilute epinephrine (1 : 100 000) can be added in an attempt to prevent mucosal bleeding after resection, although this has not been formally studied.

Thermal Therapy (Heat, Electrocautery, Argon, Heater Probe, Laser)

Electrocauterization is most commonly applied for control of bleeding, often from a peptic ulcer. Two different technologies are available—the monopolar probe

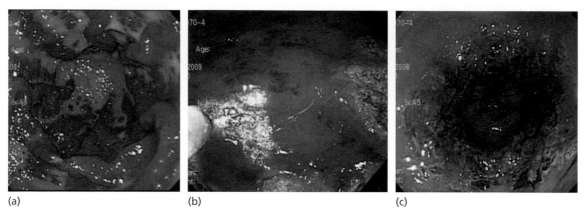

(a)   (b)   (c)

Figure 8.8 Argon plasma coagulation for treatment of gastric antral vascular ectasia (GAVE). (a) gastric antrum with typical mucosal changes of vascular extasia, (b) argon plasma coagulation, (c) after coagulation treatment.

and the bipolar probe. The monopolar device requires a grounding pad to be placed on the patient and current flows from probe to pad. The safer bipolar device has alternating positive and negative polarity built into the distal working end such that the patient does not need to be grounded and the current has a limited and defined course through tissues. These therapeutic tools can be passed through the working channel of a regular endoscope (7 F OD catheter probe) or through the larger working channel of therapeutic endoscopes (10 F OD catheter probe). The probe is placed with pressure on the suspected bleeding vessel (coaptive coagulation) and current is applied. There is successful control of bleeding in 80–100% and a decrease in the rebleeding rate compared to that from ulcers not treated with electrocautery [4]. Electrocoagulation can be used in combination with injection therapy, and this dual therapy for control of bleeding has been reported to be more efficient than monotherapy in reducing rebleeding rates [4].

Argon plasma coagulation (APC), in which a specialized probe allows conduction of high-frequency thermal energy through fluid electrons in an argon plasma arc, is performed by placing the instrument tip just above the target lesion. Indications for APC include coagulation for hemostasis and tissue destruction; the latter can be useful around the perimeter of resected polyps. The advantage of APC is that it is a non-contact coagulation which allows for rapid treatment of large or diffuse lesions, with a lower risk of deep luminal wall injury. It is most com-

monly used as the treatment of choice for bleeding from arteriovenous malformation and the treatment of gastric antral vascular ectasia (GAVE, watermelon stomach) (Figure 8.8a–c) [4]. APC is also used for ablation of adenomatous polyps or for palliative ablation of obstructing tumors. Such therapy is reserved for highly selected patients and requires repeated sessions for success.

Radiofrequency ablation (RFA), cryotherapy, and photodynamic therapy have been used successfully for the ablation of Barrett intestinal metaplasia and for esophageal neoplasia and are discussed elsewhere in this volume. These techniques require specific devices and adequate training for the best outcomes of efficacy and safety. RFA has also been used for the treatment of GAVE with good medium-term success [27].

Nd:YAG laser for treatment of bleeding peptic ulcers or destruction of obstructing tumor masses has become less popular with the development of the newer technologies discussed above. Laser therapies require a major capital investment and technically the coagulation depth is difficult to control. Laser is still preferred in some centers for palliative ablation of obstructing tumor masses. It can also be helpful in very selected patients to facilitate the removal of metal stents.

Mechanical Therapy
Banding
Banding, or rubber band ligation, is primarily used for treatment of esophageal varices. A cap is mounted at the tip of the endoscope. After passing the scope to the level

of the esophageal varices, a varicose vein is suctioned into the cap, and a small rubber band is then deployed around the varix by turning a control wheel that pulls the band off the cap and onto the varix. The ligated portion of the varix will necrose and fall off within a short time. This technique will successfully treat more than 90% of patients who present with an active esophageal variceal bleed [3]. Multiple and successive sessions will eradicate esophageal varices, which will decrease the risk of recurrent variceal bleeding (secondary prophylaxis) [3]. More recently, it has been shown that variceal ligation is probably at least equivalent to non-selective β-blocker for primary prophylaxis of variceal bleeding [28].

Banding has also been used for treatment of bleeding from Dieulafoy lesions and GAVE. Banding can also be used to enable endoscopic mucosal resection, and this technique, in which tissue is captured, banded, and hot snare resected, is discussed elsewhere in this volume.

Clipping
Several mucosal clips are commercially available and they differ in the number of arms (two or three), in their length and opening angle, and in the mechanics of deployment (ability to re-open after closure). Clips are most commonly used for treatment of bleeding ulcers. They have been shown to be equivalent to coaptive coagulation as a single treatment. However, combination treatment with two modalities (i.e., clip and injection) is superior to monotreatment [4].

With an acceptance in performing mucosal resections of larger lesions, the risk of perforation is increasing, and closure of mucosal defects has employed the use of endoscopic clips. Clips have been used in an attempt to prevent a perforation or to close iatrogenic perforations and fistulae with variable success [29]. Clips have also been used to assist with endoscopic mucosal dissection by transiently attaching the edge of a partially resected area to the opposite luminal wall for enhanced submucosal exposure and visualization.

Clips can also be used to attach the tip of a jejunal feeding tube to the small bowel wall to prevent dislodging of the tube or to anchor self-expanding stents to try to prevent migration.

Stents
A variety of luminal stents are available for clinical use. These are uncovered, partially covered, or completely covered. Stents in the upper GI tract are primarily used for palliative treatment of a malignant esophageal or duodenal obstruction [30]. Placement of duodenal stents for obstruction from pancreatic cancer may decrease the need for a palliative gastrojejunostomy, however, stent occlusion rate is high and there has been no study yet comparing palliative stent versus surgery in assessing overall survival and quality of life for these patients. Stents have also been used to cover fistulae and they are the treatment of choice for the management of malignant esophageal fistulae [30].

Combined Therapy
Snare Polypectomy
With similarity to colon polyps, adenomatous polyps in the upper GI tract have the potential for malignant transformation and should be resected. Using a snare with coagulation can safely remove smaller lesions. Duodenal polyps should be removed using injection and submucosal lifting because of the thin duodenal wall and a higher risk of perforation (Figure 8.7a–d). For larger lesions, endoscopic mucosal resection and endoscopic submucosal dissection techniques should be used, which are described in detail elsewhere.

Enteroscopy

Recently, several new techniques became available to assist in the endoscopic evaluation of the small intestine. Historically, a pediatric colonoscope or a specialized enteroscope was used with or without an overtube and a push technique was performed. Typically, the small intestine could only be visualized to about 80 cm beyond the pylorus [31]. Double or single balloon enteroscopies use an overtube with integrated balloon(s) that when inflated may allow fixation and pulling of the small intestine onto the endoscope and can facilitate deeper exploration [31,32]. Double balloon enteroscopy can be performed from above and below, allowing complete or near-complete visualization of the small intestine. A novel technique employs a newly designed overtube with integrated, raised spiral elements at the distal end. When turned, the overtube feeds small intestine onto the endoscope. This technique requires a trained assistant to turn the overtube. Fast and deep visualization has been reported; however, occasional mucosal trauma may occur [33]. All enteroscopes allow therapeutic interventions through a working channel.

Endoscopic Antireflux Therapies

A number of endoscopic antireflux procedures have been developed for the treatment of GERD. These techniques involve the application of radiofrequency (RF) thermal energy, injection or implantation of biopolymers or other bulking agents, and endoluminal suturing/plication. While the development of a variety of endoscopic devices and procedures for GERD therapy is a testament to creativity and entrepreneurship, the reality is that most have not been successful commercial endeavors due to issues with efficacy, durability, safety, and lack of clinical acceptance by endoscopists. The latter problem was exacerbated by the unwillingness of industry and other funding sources to adequately support the needed research to determine the optimization of devices and techniques and to generate comparative data. This inhibited regulatory approval, and ultimately reimbursement, without which these technologies could not be successfully developed and available for clinical use. Nonetheless, it is important to highlight the evolution of this technology, which played a significant role in the further development of advanced intralumenal therapies and translumenal therapies (NOTES).

Thermal Therapy

The Stretta™ (Curon Medical, Sunnyvale, CA) system, no longer available, delivered low-power, temperature-controlled RF energy to the gastroesophageal (GE) junction. The system employed a 20-French balloon-basket single-use catheter with four radially distributed, curved, 25 gauge, 5.5-mm long, nickel-titanium thermocoupled needles, and this was passed over a guidewire that was placed after initial endoscopic inspection of the esophagus and stomach. Ports in the catheter could provide cold water irrigation during the procedure to reduce mucosal heating and prevent surface tissue injury. The RF generator was a computerized control module unit that delivered specific defined energy to the needle electrodes. The Stretta™ procedure involved applying thermal RF treatment in four antegrade rings that straddled the GE junction from 1 cm above to just beneath the squamocolumnar junction in 0.5-cm increments. The procedure, done

typically under conscious sedation in the outpatient setting, required about 45 min to complete. One important effect of this treatment was to reduce the frequency of transient lower esophageal sphincter relaxations, an important mechanism in the pathophysiology of GERD.

A sham-controlled study of 64 GERD patients showed that RF treatment to be superior to sham for control of heartburn symptoms and improvement in quality of life at 6 months after the intervention [34]. Interestingly, although there were more Stretta-treated versus sham subjects who responded to the intervention (defined as >50% improvement in GERD quality of life score) at 6 months (61 vs. 30%), and more treated versus sham who were without daily heartburn symptoms at this follow-up interval (61 vs. 33%), no differences in reduction of daily medication use were evident between the groups. There were also no differences in esophageal acid exposure times between the two groups at 6 months.

Injection and Implantation Techniques

Enteryx™ (Boston Scientific, Natick, MA) which is no longer available for clinical use, was a biocompatible polymer consisting of 8% ethylene vinyl alcohol mixed with tantalum powder that provided for radiographic opacification, in a solution of dimethyl sulfoxide. It changed from a liquid to a spongy mass once injected into tissue, and the targeted area for injection was just above the z-line at the GE junction. The procedure, which was done in an outpatient setting under conscious sedation, required a special 4-mm, 23-gauge injector needle and the use of fluoroscopy to observe the areas of implantation. The standard procedure involved the placement of 1 mL or more of volume circumferentially around the GE junction until about 6 to 8 mL of Enteryx™ was implanted intramuscularly. The procedure was repeatable if symptom control was inadequate, but not reversible.

An international multicenter study of 85 patients treated with Enteryx™ demonstrated cessation of PPI use in 74% of treated subjects at 6 months and, at 12-month follow-up, 70% of these subjects had significant improvements in objective measure of acid reflux; however, pH normalization was encountered in only 38.8% of patients at 12 months, although the LES was approximately 1 cm longer after therapy [35]. In the treated cohort, there was no effect on the incidence or severity of esophagitis after treatment. The GERD-HRQL scores after Enteryx™ were comparable with those obtained on antisecretory medications. Complications included chest pain (92%) that resolved within 14 days in 83% of affected individuals and dysphagia (20%) that resolved within 2 to 12 weeks. Concerns about safety, including a death related to Enteryx™ injection into the aortic wall, led to withdrawal of the procedure from the market.

The Gatekeeper™ (Medtronic, Minneapolis, MN) Reflux Repair System attempted to restrict the diameter of the distal esophagus by submucosal implantation of polyacrylonitrile-based hydrogel implants. The device consisted of a 16-mm overtube-type instrument through which a videogastroscope was passed for visualization of the procedure. Suction was used to draw mucosal tissue at the GE junction into multiple, shallow holes in the distal part of the Gatekeeper instrument to stabilize the target field. A 1-mm diameter flexible endoscopic injector needle and a 1-mm trocar needle catheter were employed through another channel in the overtube to prepare the submucosal region for implantation of the prosthesis. Usually, four to six implants were placed in a radial fashion during one treatment session. This implantation technique was repeatable and reasonably reversible, although bleeding could occur with removal, which required the careful use of a needle knife to incise over the implant before suctioning it into a cap mounted on the tip of the gastroscope.

Pooled data from two prospective non-randomized trials report data for 68 patients treated with this method. At 6 months, time with pH less than 4.0 improved from 9.1 to 6.1% (n = 45, p < 0.05), LES pressure was slightly higher, and GERD-HRQL scores went from 24 to 5 (p < 0.01). Two adverse events occurred: one patient suffered a pharyngeal perforation, and severe postprandial nausea was reported in another that resolved after endoscopic removal of the prostheses [36]. An international multicenter sham-controlled trial was started for this device, but was subsequently cancelled before completion and the device is no longer available.

Durasphere™ (Carbon Medical Technologies, St. Paul, MN) is an FDA approved injectable agent that has been useful in the treatment of urinary incontinence. It consists of carbon-coated beads ranging from 90 to 212 μm suspended in a water-based gel. This agent was recently used to treat 10 GERD patients who had it injected submucosally at the z-line in four quadrants using a standard endoscopic sclerotherapy needle [37]. The patients were followed for 12 months and five of them required retreatment within 90 days for poor symptom control. At the end of the study, the patients were found to have a significant reduction in DeMeester scores (from 44.5 to 26.5) and four of nine patients had normal pH testing. The material and bulk effect was observed to be still in place at endoscopy 1 year later and adverse events such as substernal pain and difficulty belching were minor and transient. Obviously, further data are needed, including a randomized controlled trial.

Suturing, Plicating, or Stapling Devices

The EndoCinch™ (BARD-Davol, Billerica, MA) suturing device is inserted via an overtube, and consists of a sewing capsule attached to the distal tip of a standard videogastroscope which contains a cavity into which a tissue fold can be suctioned. A handle is attached to the biopsy port of the endoscope and controls the advance of a hollow-core suturing needle. A Treasury tag (T-tag) is back-loaded into the hollow-core needle, and is captured into the tip of the capsule after being driven forward by a stiff wire pushed through the hollow needle. The needle is reloaded and a second area of tissue can be captured. The two captured areas are drawn together to create a tissue plication by using a catheter that cuts the suture as it delivers a cinching element to bring together the suture ends at the luminal surface. Typically two or three plications are created at a treatment session, and can be fashioned in a linear, circumferential, or helical pattern, although no strong benefit has been demonstrated for the selected placement pattern. The sutures are mainly placed into the submucosal layer and infrequently go transmurally.

A sham-controlled, randomized study, available published as an abstract, demonstrated improved heartburn frequency at 3 months post treatment for the EndoCinch group (69 vs. 31%, p = 0.03) [38]. There was no significant difference in heartburn severity (81 vs. 50%), regurgitation (53 vs. 56%), or bothersome scores (75 vs. 50%). More subjects in the gastric plication group discontinued their daily acid suppressing medications compared to sham treatment (75 vs. 25.0%, p = 0.01). However, no difference was found comparing use of acid suppressive medications (56 vs. 25%). Acid exposure significantly improved in the EndoCinch versus sham groups (pH difference: −4.0 vs. + 1.0, p = 0.03), but normalized only in two (12.5%) treated patients. The study did not detect a difference between treated and sham patients on LES pressure or quality of life measures. A second sham controlled study demonstrated reduced acid-inhibitory drug use, improved GERD symptoms and improved the quality of life at 3 months compared with a sham procedure. No difference in reduction of esophageal acid exposure was seen after endoscopic treatment compared to sham procedure. Due to suture loss the effects only persisted up to 12 months. Concerns about durability of clinical effect have limited the usefulness of this technique, but it remains the most safe of the GERD endotherapies. It is one of the few remaining approved endoscopic therapies available for clinical use.

The Endoscopic Suturing Device (ESD™) (Cook Medical, Bloomington, IN), which consisted of an external accessory channel, a flexible Sew-Right device, and a flexible Ti-Knot device, was only briefly available. An external accessory channel was attached to a flexible endoscope and provided the access for the Sew- Right and Ti-Knot devices. The flexible Sew-Right device was a dual-needle system that uses a single suture loop to create the tissue plication. The target tissue was aspirated into a suction chamber and a needle with suture was then passed through the tissue collected within the chamber. A continuous single suture loop was used to stitch two adjacent areas in the proximal stomach to form the plication. As for the EndoCinch technique, typically two or three plications were placed during a single treatment, which took about 45 min to perform. Studies revealed early loss of the sutures. At 6 months only 5% of the sutures were found *in situ* and no significant changes in reflux esophagitis or 24-h pH monitoring were observed (median pH <4/24 h, 9.9 vs. 12.3%; p = 0.60) [39]. LES sphincter pressure was unchanged (median lower esophageal sphincter pressure 7.2 mmHg vs. 9.9 mmHg; p = 0.22). PPI use was not improved either. The same poor outcomes mainly related to early loss of the sutures was confirmed by other investigators.

The NDO Plicator™ (NDO Surgical, Mansfield, MA) was a sophisticated instrument that was advanced into the stomach over a Savary guidewire and retroflexed for placement of full-thickness sutures for serosa-to-serosa apposition at the GE-junction using pre-tied, suture-based implants (Figure 8.9; Video 9). Visualization was accomplished using a 5.9-mm flexible endoscope inserted

through a dedicated channel in the instrument. The system included the plicator instrument, a helical tip tissue retracting catheter, and pretied pledgeted suture implants. The total procedure time was about 10 to 20 min to form a single plication and the procedure was done in an outpatient setting with conscious sedation or with monitored propofol when required. Although one full-thickness plication was successful to control symptoms, as discussed below, newer data suggest that placement of two or three implants may be preferable to optimally restructure the GE junction.

A sham-controlled trial randomly assigned 159 patients to either plication (n = 78) or a sham procedure (n = 81) [40]. The percentage reduction in esophageal pH time less than 4 was significantly improved in the plication group (7 vs. 10% compared with baseline) but not in the sham group (10 vs. 9%). There were no perforations or deaths. Four patients required hospitalization for postprocedure pain and one required exploratory laparoscopy 3 months after the procedure for persistent abdominal pain. In a long-term cohort followed for 5 years after receiving full-thickness plications, there appeared to be stability of effect after an initial reduction in clinical improvement during the first year.

The NDO device is no longer available for commercial use, although it was clearly quite promising and showed significant effect with reasonable safety.

The briefly studied Syntheon Anti Reflux Device (ARD™) (Syntheon, Miami, FL) placed a titanium implant into the cardia to create full-thickness serosal-to-serosal apposition, similarly to the Plicator. The ARD™ instrument differed from the Plicator in that the device could be passed alongside any endoscope, and controlled independently, rather than requiring an endoscope to be passed and confined within the plicating instrument. A catheter-based tissue retractor was passed through the endoscope biopsy channel to pull the gastric wall into the opened jaws of the ARD™. The titanium implant was deployed as the jaws closed, creating a full-thickness pleat. Results of a multicenter clinical trial have been published in abstract form [41]. Seventy GERD patients were treated, and 57 had been followed for a minimum of 6 months at the time of publication. GERD-HRQL, improved by 50% or more in 79% of the subjects. At 6 months, 33 of 52 individuals (63%) stopped all antisecretory therapy and the implants were all found to be in place on follow-up endoscopy. One gastric perfora-

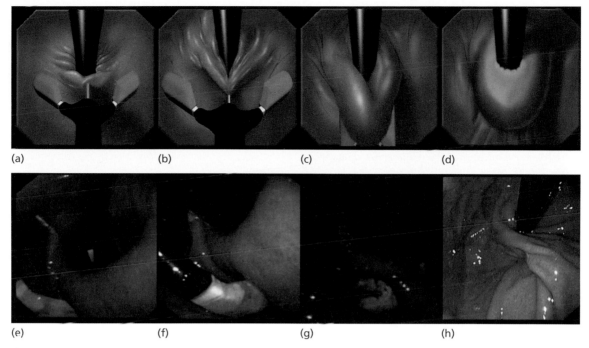

Figure 8.9 NDO plicator. Plication process in schematic (a–d) and endoscopic view (e–h). A 5.9-mm flexible endoscope is inserted through a dedicated channel in the plicator instrument. Components include a helical tip for tissue retraction and pretied pledgeted suture implants (c). Cardia opening before (e) and following the plication (h). (Images courtesy of Dr Daniel von Renteln and Dr Karel Caca.)

tion occurred requiring surgical repair. Despite superb engineering and design, the ARD™ was not brought forward to commercialization.

EsophyX™ (Endogastric Solutions, Redmond, WA) is a large overtube-type device with an insertion channel for a videogastroscope. and the system is designed to create a 270° circumferential endoscopic plication at the angle of His. The technique uses a helical retractor to engage and manipulate tissue at the fundus. After tissue grasping and fixation, double-sided T-tags can be passed through a double layer full-thickness plication. The method involves the placement of about six to 14 sutures to create a near circumferential gastroplication of 180–260°. The device can be used to reduce small hiatal hernias. EsophyX is CE marked and available in Europe, and recently received FDA clearance in the United States. No randomized controlled data has been reported to date. Early clinical experience found that at the study endpoint, median GERD-HRQL scores, improved by 67% and 9/17 patients (82%) were still off their PPI medications, whereas normalization of the pH was seen

in 63%. Recent 2-year data were published by the same group, which included 14 of the initial 19 patients, suggesting durability of the altered anatomy and continued safety [42].

The seemingly reasonable clinical outcomes above were reported from one single center, and the results from a US pilot study in eight patients do not appear as promising [43]. Half of the treated patients did not get clinical benefit from the procedure, and in one patient there was disruption of the sutures. Two patients could be off PPIs and another two were on reduced doses of the medication. Obviously, much further study is needed, including a prospective randomized, controlled trial.

The Medigus™ system (Medigus SRS, Omer, Israel), only now entering into human clinical study, consists of a specialized video echoendoscope with an integrated surgical stapler. The stapling cartridge is located on the shaft of the scope and the anvil is at the tip. B-shaped 4.8-mm staples are fired under ultrasound guidance to create an anterior, full-thickness 180° fundoplication.

One survival porcine study has been published to date using this device in which 12 animals successfully underwent the procedure and were survived for 6 weeks. The mean procedure time was 12 min, and all of the fundoplications appeared to be in place at the end of the study [44]. This complex and fascinating technology shows the ingenuity of device developers to solve the technological challenges for an endoscopic GERD treatment approach.

Another new treatment device, which uses endoscopic stapling technology, is the TOGa™ system (Satiety, Palo Alto, CA, which was initially developed to create a transoral gastroplasty for bariatric treatment. It has recently been evaluated in an animal model for the treatment of GERD [45]. Further study is pending for its utility in endoscopic GERD treatment.

Endoscopic treatment has typically targeted PPI-dependent GERD patients who have small (<3 cm) or no hiatal hernias, and who do not have severe esophagitis or Barrett esophagus. Most of the available data on endoluminal GERD therapies suggest that endoscopic interventions produce significant, but often short-term, improvements in GERD-related quality of life and reduction of antireflux medication intake. Despite symptomatic improvement in the majority of studies, acid exposure was not significantly reduced and LES pressure was not improved. One problem in interpreting these data is that many of the early reported studies, and even the randomized, controlled trials, reflected results obtained on the investigators' learning curves. The devices were initially studied for safety and not efficacy, and therefore treatments were not optimized. Since there is a substantial gap between the need for life-long antisecretory drug use and surgical therapy for GERD, a safe and effective minimally invasive endoscopic antireflux therapy would have an important niche in the clinical armamentarium for GERD treatment.

Endoscopic Treatment for Obesity

Primary Treatment

Devices are available for the primary treatment of obesity, as an alternative to pharmaceutical and diet approaches, or surgical intervention. The endoscopic treatments generally involve placement of a bezoar like a balloon, compartmentalization of the stomach by intralumenal suturing or stapling, or placement of a barrier sheath so that ingested food will bypass the duodenum. In addition to weight loss, the barrier technology may be valuable in the management of diabetes.

Despite the lack of treatment effect demonstrated in a randomized, controlled prospective trial of the early air-filled Garren–Edwards intragastric balloon (American Edwards Labs, Irvine, CA), later-developed, intragastric, liquid-filled balloons have been shown to promote weight loss in the short term. Recent data are available for longer-term outcomes after treatment with the second-generation intragastric balloon for 6 months followed by no structured weight maintenance program offered after balloon removal. With individuals followed for at least 2.5 years, the weight loss and maintenance appeared successful for about one-quarter of subjects, but some were retreated with balloons and some with medications during the follow-up interval [46]. The implanting of removable intragastric bezoars is appealing, with proposed mechanisms of decreased hunger and increased postcibal satiety, but further studies are required to determine the true effect of this intervention, and the balloons are not approved for use in the United States.

Compartmentalization of the stomach can be done endoscopically using devices that can staple or stitch. An example is the TOGA™ device (Satiety, Palo Alto, CA) that is under current clinical study, in which a type of endoscopic lesser-curve serosa-to-serosa gastric sleeve can be created by bringing together the opposite side walls of the proximal stomach and a restrictive pouch formed. A dedicated novel instrument is used, along with a viewing videogastroscope. There is a learning curve, as for all the complex new endoscopic interventions, but it is easily reached and the results of international pilot studies for outcomes and safety have been encouraging. Twenty-one patients were studied in the first human multicenter study and at 6 months after the procedure, the endoscopy showed persistent full or partial stapled sleeves, however gaps were seen in 13 patients. At 1, 3, and 6 months the excess weight loss (EWL) averaged 16.2, 22.6, and 24.4% respectively [47]. It is important that the tissue apposition involve full thickness fastening in order to create a durable compartmentalization, which is a problem with the more superficial suturing devices such as EndoCinch™ (BARD-Davol, Billerica, MA) when used for this bariatric purpose. Future refinement of the compartmentalization techniques need to address the issue of gaps in the staple line to maximize effectiveness.

The EndoBarrier™ (GI Dynamics, Watertown, MA) and the ValenTx sheath (ValenTx, Carpinteria, CA) are two new devices that can effectively isolate swallowed food from the duodenal lining and deliver the ingesta to the jejunum. As for surgical gastrojejunal bypass, numerous metabolic sequelae manifest as weight loss and altered insulin metabolism. In the former, the sheath is anchored in the duodenal bulb with a barbed self expanding metal stent, and the procedure is typically performed in an anesthesia-monitored outpatient setting with fluoroscopic guidance. In the pivotal trials, the sheath was placed for 3 months, and then removed easily by hooking a suture at the proximal end of the stent, creating a conical shape which can fit into a special hood attached to the distal end of the videogastroscope. Initial porcine studies suggested safety of the implant and demonstrated the ease of removal and initial human use showed the ability of the device to effect weight loss. A recently published, randomized controlled trial showed weight loss in the treated group versus sham, and improvement in hemoglobin A1C levels and diabetic subjects reduced or stopped using their oral hypoglycemic medications during the trial, an effect that began within 1 week of placing the barriers [48]. At 12 weeks, the average % EWL was 22.1 ± 8% for the device group and 5.3 ± 6.6% for the control group (p = 0.02).

For the other device, the sheath is anchored at the gastroesophageal junction using eight transmural implants which can be manipulated to release the sheath after a fixed interval of deployment. This technique more closely mimics the gastric bypass since there is no stomach reservoir for ingested food. It bypasses the duodenum and has been shown to be reasonably safe and effective in the first human feasibility study. Data were presented in abstract form on 12 subjects at the 2009 Digestive Disease Week [49]. Obviously, more investigation is required to understand the true effectiveness and safety of these creative devices.

After gastrojejunal bypass surgery, a number of endoscopic opportunities may present for performing advanced procedures. In addition to endoscopic treatment of bleeding from postoperative ulceration, closure of fistulae and staple line dehiscence may be undertaken. Endoscopically sutured closure of dilated stomas in patients who have regained weight post-bypass, controversial due to lack of demonstrated durability, has been reported to offer some patients a chance at follow-up weight loss, and a randomized trial of EndoCinch™ (BARD-Davol, Billerica, MA) stomal closure was recently completed, although the results are not yet available. Other suturing devices have also been used for this purpose in feasibility pilot trials, suggesting a potential alternative to a surgical re-do operation. Gastric pouch reduction, as with StomaphyX™ (Endogastric Solutions, Redmond, WA), has also been suggested for postoperative weight loss in subjects with a large proximal gastric pouch and, although there is no randomized sham-controlled trial, there have been some anecdotal successes. This area of bariatric management calls for rigorous study before any recommendations can be made for incorporation in routine clinical practice.

Final Thoughts

As for all of the possible advanced endoscopic procedures, only some examples of which have been presented in this chapter, adequate training is key. For fellows in training, they can seek out mentors during the initial or advanced training years. For clinicians in academic or private practice, exposure to advanced techniques and devices can occur at locations such as the hands-on training courses at the American Society for Gastrointestinal Endoscopy Institute for Training and Technology Center or at national and regional societal meetings, at live courses, and at academic and sophisticated clinical centers. Simulation is an area we did not discuss in this segment but has been helpful in getting novice endoscopists to rapidly advance along the learning curve for routine endoscopic procedures and may have a role in learning advanced procedures [50]. There is certainly a role for gaining familiarity with new devices and techniques in an animal lab before beginning human clinical work, and a clear need for mentoring and feedback for the individual at any learning level (fellow to seasoned endoscopist) who wishes to add new advanced endoscopic procedures to their clinical armamentarium. In the end, best-practice training in advanced procedures is about learning new skills to provide added patient benefit while maximizing safety as the techniques are added to standard clinical practice.

Take-home points

- The diagnostic accuracy of EGD can be enhanced by new technologies such as chromoendoscopy and narrow-band imaging.

- Current endoscopic techniques lack sufficient accuracy to reliably identify areas of dysplasia; however new technologies, such as *in vivo* microscopy may assist in detection of dysplastic lesions.

- Several new methods which improve the technique of enteroscopy offer promise of better visualization and treatment of small bowel lesions.

- Although polypectomy during colonoscopy is a standard procedure in routine endoscopic practice, a review of the basic principles and techniques for polypectomy in the stomach and duodenum may enhance outcomes.

- Endoscopic therapies for gastroesophageal reflux disease appear promising, but have not been optimized for adequate durability.

- Endoscopic interventions for treating obesity are under current investigation and may be clinically useful adjuncts or alternatives for weight management and for treating diabetes.

References

1 American Society for Gastrointestinal Endoscopy. Principles of training in gastrointestinal endoscopy. From the ASGE. *Gastrointest Endosc* 1999; **49**: 845–53.

2 Leighton JA, Shen B, Baron TH, *et al.* ASGE guideline: endoscopy in the diagnosis and treatment of inflammatory bowel disease. *Gastrointest Endosc* 2006; **63**: 558–65.

3 Qureshi W, Adler DG, Davila R, *et al.* ASGE Guideline: the role of endoscopy in the management of variceal hemorrhage, updated July 2005. *Gastrointest Endosc* 2005; **62**: 651–5.

4 Adler DG, Leighton JA, Davila RE, *et al.* ASGE guideline: The role of endoscopy in acute non-variceal upper-GI hemorrhage. *Gastrointest Endosc* 2004; **60**: 497–504.

5 Lichtenstein DR, Cash BD, Davila R, *et al.* Role of endoscopy in the management of GERD. *Gastrointest Endosc* 2007; **66**: 219–24.

6 Ragunath K, Krasner N, Raman VS, *et al.* A randomized, prospective cross-over trial comparing methylene blue-directed biopsy and conventional random biopsy for detecting intestinal metaplasia and dysplasia in Barrett's esophagus. *Endoscopy* 2003; **35**: 998–1003.

7 Shaw D, Blair V, Framp A, *et al.* Chromoendoscopic surveillance in hereditary diffuse gastric cancer: an alternative to prophylactic gastrectomy? *Gut* 2005; **54**: 461–8.

8 Dubuc J, Legoux JL, Winnock M, *et al.* Endoscopic screening for esophageal squamous-cell carcinoma in high-risk patients: a prospective study conducted in 62 French endoscopy centers. *Endoscopy* 2006; **38**: 690–5.

9 Meining A, Rosch T, Kiesslich R, *et al.* Inter- and intra-observer variability of magnification chromoendoscopy for detecting specialized intestinal metaplasia at the gastro-esophageal junction. *Endoscopy* 2004; **36**: 160–4.

10 Kara MA, Ennahachi M, Fockens P, *et al.* Detection and classification of the mucosal and vascular patterns (mucosal morphology) in Barrett's esophagus by using narrow band imaging. *Gastrointest Endosc* 2006; **64**: 155–66.

11 Kara MA, Bergman JJ. Autofluorescence imaging and narrow-band imaging for the detection of early neoplasia in patients with Barrett's esophagus. *Endoscopy* 2006; **38**: 627–31.

12 Pohl H, Rosch T, Vieth M, *et al.* Miniprobe confocal laser microscopy for the detection of invisible neoplasia in patients with Barrett's oesophagus. *Gut* 2008; **57**: 1648–53.

13 Kiesslich R, Gossner L, Goetz M, *et al.* In vivo histology of Barrett's esophagus and associated neoplasia by confocal laser endomicroscopy. *Clin Gastroenterol Hepatol* 2006; **4**: 979–87.

14 Pohl H, Koch M, Khalifa A, *et al.* Evaluation of endocytoscopy in the surveillance of patients with Barrett's esophagus. *Endoscopy* 2007; **39**: 492–6.

15 Tomizawa Y, Abdulla HM, Prasad GA, *et al.* Endocytoscopy in esophageal cancer. *Gastrointest Endosc Clin N Am* 2009; **19**: 273–81.

16 Pohl H, Rosch T, Tanczos BT, *et al.* Endocytoscopy for the detection of microstructural features in adult patients with celiac sprue: a prospective, blinded endocytoscopy-conventional histology correlation study. *Gastrointest Endosc* 2009; **70**: 933–41.

17 Jutabha R, Jensen DM. Management of upper gastrointestinal bleeding in the patient with chronic liver disease. *Med Clin North Am* 1996; **80**: 1035–68.

18 Park CH, Lee SJ, Park JH, *et al.* Optimal injection volume of epinephrine for endoscopic prevention of recurrent peptic ulcer bleeding. *Gastrointest Endosc* 2004; **60**: 875–80.

19 Rutgeerts P, Rauws E, Wara P, *et al.* Randomised trial of single and repeated fibrin glue compared with injection of polidocanol in treatment of bleeding peptic ulcer. *Lancet* 1997; **350**: 692–6.

20 Chung SC, Leong HT, Chan AC, *et al.* Epinephrine or epinephrine plus alcohol for injection of bleeding ulcers: a prospective randomized trial. *Gastrointest Endosc* 1996; **43**: 591–5.

21 Aabakken L. Current endoscopic and pharmacological therapy of peptic ulcer bleeding. *Best Pract Res Clin Gastroenterol* 2008; **22**: 243–59.

22 Park WG, Yeh RW, Triadafilopoulos G. Injection therapies for variceal bleeding disorders of the GI tract. *Gastrointest Endosc* 2008; **67**: 313–23.

23 Pasricha PJ, Ravich WJ, Hendrix TR, *et al*. Intrasphincteric botulinum toxin for the treatment of achalasia. *N Engl J Med* 1995; **332**: 774–8.

24 Ramage JI, Jr, Rumalla A, Baron TH, *et al*. A prospective, randomized, double-blind, placebo-controlled trial of endoscopic steroid injection therapy for recalcitrant esophageal peptic strictures. *Am J Gastroenterol* 2005; **100**: 2419–25.

25 Jin Z, Du Y, Li Z, *et al*. Endoscopic ultrasonography-guided interstitial implantation of iodine 125-seeds combined with chemotherapy in the treatment of unresectable pancreatic carcinoma: a prospective pilot study. *Endoscopy* 2008; **40**: 314–20.

26 Yamamoto H, Yahagi N, Oyama T, *et al*. Usefulness and safety of 0.4% sodium hyaluronate solution as a submucosal fluid "cushion" in endoscopic resection for gastric neoplasms: a prospective multicenter trial. *Gastrointest Endosc* 2008; **67**: 830–9.

27 Gross SA, Al-Haddad M, Gill KR, *et al*. Endoscopic mucosal ablation for the treatment of gastric antral vascular ectasia with the HALO90 system: a pilot study. *Gastrointest Endosc* 2008; **67**: 324–7.

28 Khuroo MS, Khuroo NS, Farahat KL, *et al*. Meta-analysis: endoscopic variceal ligation for primary prophylaxis of ocsophageal variceal bleeding. *Aliment Pharmacol Ther* 2005; **21**: 347–61.

29 Qadeer MA, Dumot JA, Vargo JJ, *et al*. Endoscopic clips for closing esophageal perforations: case report and pooled analysis. *Gastrointest Endosc* 2007; **66**: 605–11.

30 Ross WA, Alkassab F, Lynch PM, *et al*. Evolving role of self-expanding metal stents in the treatment of malignant dysphagia and fistulas. *Gastrointest Endosc* 2007; **65**: 70–6.

31 May A, Nachbar L, Schneider M, Ell C. Prospective comparison of push enteroscopy and push-and-pull enteroscopy in patients with suspected small-bowel bleeding. *Am J Gastroenterol* 2006; **101**: 2016–24.

32 Tsujikawa T, Saitoh Y, Andoh A, *et al*. Novel single-balloon enteroscopy for diagnosis and treatment of the small intestine: preliminary experiences. *Endoscopy* 2008; **40**: 11–5.

33 Buscaglia JM, Dunbar KB, Okolo PI, 3rd, *et al*. The spiral enteroscopy training initiative: results of a prospective study evaluating the Discovery SB overtube device during small bowel enteroscopy (with video). *Endoscopy* 2009; **41**: 194–9.

34 Corley DA, Katz P, Wo JM, *et al*. Improvement of gastroesophageal reflux symptoms after radiofrequency energy: a randomized, sham-controlled trial. *Gastroenterology* 2003; **125**: 668–76.

35 Johnson DA, Ganz R, Aisenberg J, *et al*. Endoscopic implantation of enteryx for treatment of GERD: 12-month results of a prospective, multicenter trial. *Am J Gastroenterol* 2003; **98**: 1921–30.

36 Fockens P, Bruno MJ, Gabbrielli A, *et al*. Endoscopic augmentation of the lower esophageal sphincter for the treatment of gastroesophageal reflux disease: multicenter study of the Gatekeeper Reflux Repair System. *Endoscopy* 2004; **36**: 682–9.

37 Ganz RA, Fallon E, Wittchow T, Klein D. A new injectable agent for the treatment of GERD: results of the Durasphere pilot trial. *Gastrointest Endosc* 2009; **69**: 318–23.

38 Rothstein RI, Hynes ML, Grove MR, Pohl H. Endoscopic gastric plication (EndoCinch) for GERD: a randomized, sham-controlled, blinded, single-center study. *Gastrointest Endosc* 2004; **59**: P111.

39 Schiefke I, Neumann S, Zabel-Langhennig A, *et al*. Use of an endoscopic suturing device (the "ESD") to treat patients with gastroesophageal reflux disease, after unsuccessful EndoCinch endoluminal gastroplication: another failure. *Endoscopy* 2005; **37**: 700–5.

40 Rothstein R, Filipi C, Caca K, *et al*. Endoscopic full-thickness plication for the treatment of gastroesophageal reflux disease: a randomized sham-controlled trial. *Gastroenterology* 2006; **131**: 704–12.

41 Ramage JI, Rothstein RI, Edmundowicz S, *et al*. Endoscopically placed titanium plicator for GERD: pivotal phase—preliminary 6-month results. *Gastrointest Endosc* 2006; **63**: AB126.

42 Cadiere GB, Van Sante N, Graves JE, *et al*. Two-year results of a feasibility study on antireflux transoral incisionless fundoplication using EsophyX. *Surg Endosc* 2009; **23**: 957–64.

43 Bergman S, Mikami DJ, Hazey JW, *et al*. Endolumenal fundoplication with EsophyX: the initial North American experience. *Surg Innov* 2008; **15**: 166–70.

44 Kauer WK, Roy-Shapira A, Watson D, *et al*. Preclinical trial of a modified gastroscope that performs a true anterior fundoplication for the endoluminal treatment of gastroesophageal reflux disease. *Surg Endosc* 2009; **23**: 2728–31.

45 Jobe BA, O'Rourke RW, McMahon BP, *et al*. Transoral endoscopic fundoplication in the treatment of gastroesophageal reflux disease: the anatomic and physiologic basis for reconstruction of the esophagogastric junction using a novel device. *Ann Surg* 2008; **248**: 69–76.

46 Dastis NS, Francois E, Deviere J, *et al*. Intragastric balloon for weight loss: results in 100 individuals followed for at least 2.5 years. *Endoscopy* 2009; **41**: 575–80.

47 Deviere J, Ojeda Valdes G, Cuevas Herrera L, *et al*. Safety, feasibility and weight loss after transoral gastroplasty:

First human multicenter study. *Surg Endosc* 2008; **22**: 589–98.

48 Tarnoff M, Rodriguez L, Escalona A, *et al*. Open label, prospective, randomized controlled trial of an endoscopic duodenal-jejunal bypass sleeve versus low calorie diet for pre-operative weight loss in bariatric surgery. *Surg Endosc* 2009; **23**: 650–6.

49 Swain P, Rumbaut RA, Gonzalez LT, *et al*. First clinical experience with a novel endoscopic device that mimics the roux-en-y gastric bypass procedure. *Gastrointest Endosc* 2009; **69**: AB187.

50 Mahmood T, Darzi A. The learning curve for a colonoscopy simulator in the absence of any feedback: no feedback, no learning. *Surg Endosc* 2004; **18**: 1224–30.

CHAPTER 9
Esophageal Dilation Technique

David A. Johnson

Division of Gastroenterology, Eastern VA Medical School, Norfolk, VA, USA

Summary

Esophageal strictures, which can develop from a variety of benign or malignant etiologies, frequently require dilation for symptomatic management of dysphagia. There are a number of options available for successful dilation of most strictures and adjunctive techniques reserved for more "refractory" cases. It is key, before any dilation is performed, to fully understand the underlying cause and anatomy of the stricture. Careful selection of the technique for dilation and establishing the goals for the diameter of the luminal restoration are important because, in each case, these factors may need to be altered to suit the etiology and pathology of the stricture.

Case

A 58-year-old woman presents with a 3-month history of intermittent, but not progressive, solid food dysphagia. Food seems to "catch" in the mid-sternal area. She has not noted this with liquids or soft foods but has symptoms in particular with meat, fresh vegetables, bread, and pasta. She has no significant history of heartburn. Her medications are alendronate and a multivitamin. She rarely uses aspirin or other non-steroidal anti-inflammatory drugs.

Her physical exam is normal. The physician alertly notes that the patient is taking a bisphosphonate and is concerned about a pill-induced stricture. Barium X-ray is considered but, as this seems to be a non-complex stricture, she is referred for endoscopy. Goals of therapy are discussed and the target is to re-establish normal dietary habits.

Endoscopy shows a luminal narrowing which is estimated (using the open biopsy forceps) to be 14 mm. The stricture is in the mid-esophagus and there is no evidence of esophagitis. A hydrostatic balloon is chosen and dilation performed using the graduated 15–18 mm dilator. Care is taken to deflate the stomach before the dilation, as well as to deflate the balloon between size increments to assess for mucosal disruption. With the 18-mm balloon, there is a slight mucosal tear in the area of luminal narrowing.

The patient is counseled to avoid her bisphosphonates for a month and to discuss alternative therapy with her primary physician. She is given a proton pump inhibitor for 8 weeks and advised to follow a soft diet, cutting food into small pieces for several weeks and then to slowly advance to a more normal diet as tolerated.

Introduction

Esophageal strictures are a problem frequently encountered by endoscopists and can be divided in numerous ways. They can be categorized according either to the histology or their number, or to the degree of resistance in treating them. Therefore, some use categories such as benign versus malignant, single versus multiple, or simple versus complex. Management of the stricture usually involves definition of the cause of dysphagia and treatment. For centuries, the mainstay of therapy has been esophageal dilation. This dates back to the 17th century when carved whalebones were used to treat achalasia. Bougienage was first reported in the early 1800s and, since then, the equipment to treat esophageal strictures has evolved considerably to include flexible bougies, wire-guided dilators, and through-the-scope balloons.

The etiologies of benign strictures include gastroesophageal reflux esophagitis, Schatzki ring, radiation injury, caustic ingestion, nasogastric intubation with acid reflux, primary or secondary pill-induced injury,

Practical Gastroenterology and Hepatology: Esophagus and Stomach, 1st edition. Edited by Nicholas J. Talley, Kenneth R. DeVault and David E. Fleischer. © 2010 Blackwell Publishing Ltd.

anastomotic stricture with related ischemia or history of an anastomotic leak, "ringed" strictures associated with eosinophilic esophagitis, and several rare disorders. Malignant strictures may develop as a result of local tumor growth or metastatic disease or from an extraesophageal mass that creates extrinsic compression.

In patients with stricture-related complaints, dysphagia for solids is the typical complaint. In general, these patients do not experience liquid dysphagia, which is more evident with motility-related disorders such as achalasia. The goal for dilation should be determined by using the patient's dietary habits and nutritional needs as factors in the treatment plan. The plan for difficult esophageal strictures should not be simply scheduling the dilation.

The mainstay of treatment for benign esophageal strictures is dilation. In the selection of the dilation plan for each patient, it is important to differentiate the structural characteristics between esophageal strictures that are simple and those that are more complex [1–3] (Table 9.1). Further discussion on this topic is found in Chapter 37.

Categories of Esophageal Dilators

There are three basic categories of esophageal dilators that are currently in use: bougies filled with mercury or tungsten (e.g., Maloney dilators), wire-guided polyvinyl dilators (e.g., Savary–Gilliard), and through-the-scope (TTS) balloon dilators. The expansive force generated by these dilators differs, based on the delivery of the device as well as the mechanisms of action. To attain effective dilation of a stricture, radial dilation is key. For both the bougies and the wire-guided dilators, this radial dilation is exerted as the dilator is passed, although there is also, by the very nature of the passage, longitudinal shear force exerted. These longitudinal shear forces are not exerted with the balloon dilators—provided that they are held, during the dilation, in a static position within the stricture. Theoretically, there may be less risk for perforation with the TTS balloons but, to date, no clear advantage in safety or efficacy has been demonstrated [4]. There are certain circumstances, however, in which a longitudinal shearing force should be avoided, such as strictures caused by epidermolysis bullosa, or in cases in which a tracheoesophageal puncture voice prosthesis is present.

Table 9.1 Categories and characteristics of strictures.

	Simple	Complex
Allow passage of endoscope	Yes	No (typically)
Length	Short (≤2 cm)	Long (>2 cm)
Focal	Yes	No
Angulation/irregularity	No	Yes (typically)
Etiology (examples)	Peptic Schatzki ring Anastomotic Pill-induced	Radiation Caustic ingestion Malignancy Photodynamic therapy
Preferred dilation method	Balloon or rigid dilator	Rigid dilator
Fluoroscopy	Rarely needed	Recommended

In these cases, balloon dilation should be the preferred method [2,5].

Technique of Dilation

Endoscopy/Fluoroscopy

After review of any imaging studies that may have been done, esophagoscopy is carried out to further carefully define the anatomy of the stricture. This should include an estimate of the lumen diameter to assist with selecting the appropriate initial dilator size. This measurement is estimated by using an open biopsy forceps in the narrowest lumen of the stricture (standard open biopsy jaws = 7–8 mm). Selection of the first dilator to pass is typically 1–2 mm larger than the estimated lumen diameter. Correlation of estimated luminal size with the dilator size is equated by 1 mm = 3 French. Savary dilators are passed over a guidewire positioned with its spring tip in the distal stomach. Bougienage may be done with fluoroscopy, although there is evidence that this can be done in selected cases safely without radiologic guidance [6].

Fluoroscopy is helpful and recommended for most complex stricture dilations and a requisite for positioning of the balloon for achalasia dilation. The balloon dilators can be filled with contrast, although water is commonly used alternatively, and the "waist" imposed by the stricture on the balloon is evident and should be resolved with a successful dilation. If a guidewire is used for assisting passage/positioning of the dilator, care should be taken to insure that there is a gentle bowing of the guidewire following the greater curvature toward the antrum. Care should be taken during placement and passage of the dilators to avoid a straight-on impact of the wire into the greater curvature or a "knuckling" of the spring portion of the distal portion of the guidewire, whereby direct force can be passed and potentially increase a wire-related perforation risk.

Dilation Procedure

Savary–Gilliard-type Dilators

The mouthpiece can be removed for dilation and lubrication applied to the lips to minimize resistance of passage. When a mouthpiece is in place, the dilator may be forced to enter perpendicular to the posterior pharyngeal wall and must therefore follow a 90° turn against the posterior pharyngeal wall to enter the hypopharynx. This sharp angle of the dilator as it traverses between oropharynx and hypopharynx may cause considerable pressure on the tissues anterior to the cervical spine which, accordingly, increases the risk of pain, contusion, or possible crush injury with perforation. This may be a particular problem when large-diameter dilators are used because these have a greater resistance to bending. By removing the mouthpiece and moving the dilator shaft into one corner of the mouth, the potential for pressure-related injury can be minimized, by keeping the extraoral segment of the dilator shaft elevated (in the direction of the upper posterior molars) and more parallel to the axis of the hypopharyngeal lumen. Antegrade dilation force should be directed more closely into the direct lumen axis between the hypopharynx and stricture beyond. This "in-axis" orientation allows the operator to more accurately appreciate the true stricture resistance rather than sensing an angulated bending resistance of the dilator impinging against the posterior pharyngeal wall [7].

The patient head position should be chin neutral or down, and never extended with the head back. This flexed position reduces the natural cervical spine lordosis and helps to open the hypopharynx. Although most endoscopists prefer not to insert their fingers into the patient's mouth, with passage of either Savary or Maloney dilators, the oropharyngeal curve can also be reduced by

using the index and middle fingers, as positioned in the oropharynx, guiding the dilator with anterior displacement. The shaft of the dilator should be gripped firmly for pushing with the thumb and first three fingertips of the right hand, and not by a full, closed, tight hand grasp. This technique provides a better tactile sensation with which to judge stricture or other structural resistance during dilator passage. Complete passage of the full dilator diameter through the stricture should be assessed using fluoroscopy, or distance measurement numbers on the dilator shaft. During passage of over-the-wire dilators, either the operator or an assistant should provide slight wire retraction, avoiding antegrade or retrograde wire displacement. This is most easily assured by fluoroscopic observation or distance marks etched on the Savary-type guidewire. Dilators should be removed slowly and carefully following each passage, with particular care in the area of the oropharyngeal curve.

Balloon Dilators

Balloon dilation should be done only in strictures in which the balloon dilator can be positioned to traverse the entire stricture and the exact anatomy of the stricture has been defined by endoscopy or X-ray. Dilation with the balloon still contained within the stricture potentially may introduce a "shoulder effect" with an asymmetric delivery of the radial dilation and theoretically increase the risk for perforation. Complex strictures do not respond well to hydrostatic, TTS dilators. These dilators work well for over 90% of simple, benign, usually reflux-related distal esophageal strictures, and rings [7].

With a long track record, pneumatic balloon dilation remains one of the most effective first-line therapies for achalasia. Currently, the Rigiflex pneumatic dilator is the most widely used system for achalasia, but similar devices are available from other manufacturers. The polyethylene balloon comes in three sizes that inflate to fixed diameters of 30, 35, and 40 mm. This system offers a safety advantage over earlier compliant latex balloons that delivered variable diameters depending on inflation pressure.

Typically, a stepwise approach using the Rigiflex system starts with a 30-mm balloon for the first session. If no improvement is noted in follow-up (by standing column on barium study), the patient can be brought back for repeat dilation sessions next with a 35-mm and then at a later date if needed with a 40-mm balloon for patients with no response. This graduated approach has yielded an overall 93% response rate to dilation over a mean follow-up period of 4 years and has become an accepted methodology of treatment [8]. The option for surgical myotomy should be discussed and offered to patients before dilation. Injection of botulinum toxin is more commonly used in elderly patients, those who have significant medical problems, or those who are not candidates for surgical or endoscopic more definitive treatments [9].

Before the balloon is positioned, the endoscopist should be careful to fully decompress the stomach. When the balloon is inflated, if there is over-distension of the stomach and retching against the tightly occluded esophagogastric junction, there may be significant risk for related esophageal barotraumas. The balloon is then positioned in the stricture—ideally with the central portion of the balloon corresponding to the central point of the stenosis. This is confirmed by use of endoscopy or fluoroscopy, or both. Before insufflation, the proximal margin of the balloon is positioned at the tip of the endoscope and the shaft of the balloon dilator grasped firmly (at the biopsy port of the endoscope) by the endoscopist's fingers. With achalasia dilation, typically this is done without reinsertion of the endoscope so the operator needs to firmly grasp and hold the shaft of the balloon at the entrance through the bite block. As the balloon is inflated, there is a tendency for the balloon to move—usually pulling down antegrade. There is no standard yet established for defining the optimal duration of balloon dilation. Typically, a duration of 30–60 s is adequate with 60 s being more standard for achalasia dilation. For achalasia dilation, the initial pressure at the "waist" on the balloon should be noted and, if effective dilation has been achieved, this "waist" should no longer be evident with the second insufflations performed at the same session.

For the TTS balloons, deflation of the balloon between sequential dilations is advised so as to assess the level of mucosal trauma and better direct the progression rate for sequential dilation. Care should be taken to limit further dilation during that session once a minor mucosal disruption is evident.

Rate of Dilation

The standard teaching of the "rule of three" has proven effective and safe as a guide to the number of dilators passed per session [7,10,11]. This means that, in a single

Table 9.2 Tolerable diet consistency relates directly to lumen diameter.

Esophageal lumen (mm)	Type of diet*
7	Liquid/pureed
10	Pureed/soft†
13	Soft†
15	Modified with exclusions‡
18	Regular with care

*In all cases emphasis on appropriately cutting food, paced chewing and swallowing, foods to avoid, and the importance of liquid flushes.
†Soft diet with emphasis to cut food into small pieces.
‡Exclusion of tough meat, hard raw vegetables (e.g., carrot), hard fresh fruits (e.g., apple), large bites of doughy bread, or pasta, fruit or vegetable skin (e.g., potato).
A grading system for dysphagia is shown in Chapter 37, Table 37.2.

session, no more than three dilators of progressive/sequential size are passed once moderate or greater resistance is evident. The initial dilators passed with no or mild resistance do not count in the total of three. Care should be taken, however, in complex strictures—in particular due to radiation, caustic ingestion, anastomosis/ischemia, and malignancy—because these strictures typically are transmural and tend to crack or fracture with dilation, hence with a greater risk of perforation. There is also a higher risk of perforation in patients with eosinophilic esophagitis. This is in contrast to the mucosal disruption seen with dilation of simple strictures, e.g., peptic strictures or the Schatzki ring. Accordingly, the rate of dilation should be carefully planned to meet the needs and defined goals for each patient. The optimal lumen diameter goal is determined primarily by etiology, pathologic features, duration, stricture lumen diameter, and the patient's dietary needs and preferences. In general, diet tolerance may be predicted based on the luminal diameter as shown in Table 9.2 [7].

Adjuncts to Dilation

Although there are no controlled trials addressing removal of foreign material involved in anastomosis-related strictures (e.g., staples, suture), it is reasonable to remove these if relatively feasible. Conceivably, these materials may contribute to ongoing inflammation and scaring from a foreign body effect on the tissue.

Intramural steroid injections have been used in refractory strictures with variable success reported [12,13]. This topic is addressed in Chapter 37.

Retrograde Dilation

In some cases, standard endoscopic management of esophageal strictures is impossible particularly when a guidewire cannot be positioned via an antegrade approach through the stricture. This may be particularly evident in the proximal esophagus of patients who have received radiation for head and neck cancers. In these cases, an "endoscopic rendezvous" approach can be employed—typically in concert with the otolaryngologist [14,15]. This is accomplished by introducing a small-diameter endoscope through a mature PEG (percutaneous endoscopic gastrostomy) tract and advancing it in a retrograde fashion into the esophagus until the stricture is identified. A flexible guidewire can be passed through the stricture and, using direct visualization (endoscopy or rigid laryngoscope), grabbed on the proximal side of the stricture by the assisting physician. In some cases, a thin membrane is present that precludes its passage. In these patients, a stiffer guidewire, with/without assist using a needle knife, can be used to puncture the membrane. Clearly these maneuvers require extreme skill and knowledge of the anatomy because creation of a false channel must be avoided. Once wire passage is achieved, the stricture is dilated over the guidewire in either an antegrade or a retrograde fashion using a balloon or Savary-type dilator.

One practical way is to use an open biopsy forceps in the narrowest lumen of the stricture to determine the size.

- No clear difference in effectiveness has been reported for the Savary–Gilliard-type dilators and through-the-scope balloon dilators for the treatment of benign esophageal strictures.

- The tactile sensation of stricture resistance during antegrade dilation is important for the selection of successive dilator sizes and determination of the pace of dilation.

- Complex strictures do not respond well to hydrostatic, TTS dilators. These dilators work well for over 90% of simple, benign, usually reflux-related distal esophageal strictures, and rings.

- Rarely are complex strictures safely responsive to a single dilation session, so the patient must understand that gradual dilation during a regularly scheduled series of appointments is indicated.

- Intervals between the initial series of dilation sessions are best kept between 2 and 4 weeks. After the goal for presumed optimum diameter has been reached, the intervals are increased based on the patient's opinion of dysphagia relief.

- The etiology and complexity of the stricture should be established as a guide to therapy. Technique, equipment, and target for luminal restoration may need to be altered to suit the pathology of the stricture and goals for the patient.

References

1 Siersema PD. Treatment options for esophageal strictures. *Nat Clin Pract Gastroenterol Hepatol* 2008; **5**: 142–52.

2 Lew RJ, Kochman ML. A review of endoscopic methods of esophageal dilation. *J Clin Gastroenterol* 2002; **35**: 117–26.

3 Pereira-Lima JC, Ramirez RP, Zamin Jr I, *et al.* Endoscopic dilation of benign esophageal strictures: report on 1043 procedures. *Am J Gastroenterol* 1999; **94**: 1497–501.

4 Hernandez LV, Jacobsen JW, Harris MS. Comparison among the perforation rates of Maloney, balloon, and Savary dilation of esophageal strictures. *Gastrointest Endosc* 2000; **51**: 460–2.

5 Anderson SH, Meenan J, Williams KN, *et al.* Efficacy and safety of endoscopic dilation of esophageal dilation of esophageal strictures in epidermolysis bullosa. *Gastrointest Endosc* 2004; **59**: 28–32.

6 Raymondi R, Pereira-Lima JC, Valves A, *et al.* Endoscopic dilation of benign esophageal strictures without fluoroscopy: experience of 2750 procedures. *Hepatogastroenterology* 2008; **55**: 1342–8.

Take-home points

- The initial step in management of patients with an esophageal stricture, after a thorough history and physical examination, can be either an esophagogram or endoscopy. An esophagogram has the advantage of defining the anatomy and eliminating surprises that might be found if endoscopy alone is the first step. Endoscopy, however, has the advantage that both diagnosis (including biopsy) and therapy can be performed with one test.

- Esophagoscopy should include an estimate of the lumen diameter in selecting the appropriate initial dilator size.

7 Boyce HW. Dilation of difficult benign esophageal strictures. *Am J Gastroenterol* 2005; **100**: 744–5.

8 Waltzer N, Hirano I. Achalasia. *Gastroenterol Clin North Am* 2008; **37**: 807–25.

9 Kadakia SC, Wong RK. Graded pneumatic dilation using Rigiflex achalasia dilators in patients with primary esophageal achalasia. *Am J Gastroenterol* 1993; **88**: 34–8.

10 Kochman ML. Minimization of risks of esophageal dilation. *Gastrointest Endosc Clin North Am* 2007; **17**: 47–58.

11 Standards of Practice Committee (ASGE) Egan JV, Baron TH, Adler DG, *et al.* Esophageal dilation. *Gastrointest Endosc* 2006; **63**: 755–60.

12 Altintas E, Kacar S, Tunc B, *et al.* Intralesional steroid injection in benign esophageal strictures resistant to bougie dilation. *J Gastroenterol Hepatol* 2004; **19**: 1388–91.

13 Ramage JI Jr, Rumalla A, Baron TH, *et al.* A prospective, randomized, double-blind, placebo-controlled trial of endoscopic steroid injection therapy for recalcitrant esophageal peptic strictures. *Am J Gastroenterol* 2005; **100**: 2419–25.

14 Bueno R, Swanson SJ, Jaklitsch MT, *et al.* Combined antegrade and retrograde dilation: a new endoscopic technique in the management of complex esophageal obstruction. *Gastrointest Endosc* 2001; **54**: 368–72.

15 Lew RJ, Shah JN, Chalian A, *et al.* Technique of endoscopic retrograde puncture and dilatation of total esophageal stenosis in patients with radiation-induced strictures. *Head Neck* 2004; **26**: 179–83.

CHAPTER 10
Endoscopic Mucosal Resection

Hendrik Manner and Oliver Pech

Department of Gastroenterology and Hepatology, Horst Schmidt Klinik (HSK), Wiesbaden, Germany

Summary

The term endoscopic mucosal resection (EMR), also known as endoscopic resection, refers to an endoscopic procedure during which tissue acquisition occurs by electrosurgical incision of both mucosa and submucosa. The two most common EMR techniques are: (i) cap technique ("suck" and cut); and (ii) band ligation (ligate and snare). EMR has been shown to be effective and safe in patients with high-grade intraepithelial neoplasia (HGIN) and mucosal carcinoma of the esophagus (squamous cell carcinoma and Barrett carcinoma). For these lesions, the risk of lymph node metastasis is very low and the procedure may obviate the need for esophagectomy, which has a higher morbidity and mortality. Endoscopic submucosal dissection (ESD) is an attractive, new treatment approach with the ability to provide *en bloc* resection of larger neoplastic lesions. Both EMR and ESD should be performed by experienced endoscopists.

Case

A 54-year-old male with the histological diagnosis of low-grade intraepithelial neoplasia (Tables 10.1 and 10.2) was referred to the endoscopy unit for further diagnostics. Esophagogastroduodenoscopy (EGD) revealed a type IIa+c lesion (Table 10.3) within a short-segment Barrett esophagus (Figure 10.1a). The diagnosis of early Barrett cancer was made. Metastatic disease was ruled out by the initial staging protocol. Diagnostic EMR with a ligation device was performed (Figure 10.1b,c). The pathological assessment revealed a well-differentiated mucosal Barrett cancer without signs of lymphangio- or venous invasion (PT1M2, G1, L0, V0, R0 at the basal and lateral margins of the lesion). The patient had a normal check-up examination at regular intervals after the procedure and, to date, there is no residual disease or new neoplasm.

Preinterventional Staging

When EMR is being considered, the neoplastic lesion should be carefully evaluated, including the determination of the gross tumor type. The Paris Classification

Practical Gastroenterology and Hepatology: Esophagus and Stomach, 1st edition. Edited by Nicholas J. Talley, Kenneth R. DeVault and David E. Fleischer. © 2010 Blackwell Publishing Ltd.

(Table 10.3) is commonly used for endoscopic tumor classification. It is often useful to employ high-resolution endoscopes with additional types of imaging to best evaluate the primary lesion and search for multifocal neoplasia.

In esophageal squamous cell carcinomas (SCC), chromoendoscopy (CE) with iodine solution (1–2%) enables detection of synchronous lesions. In Barrett esophagus, the current gold standard is still four-quadrant biopsy of the Barrett segment but new methods, such as contrast enhancement with acetic acid together with magnification endoscopy, and virtual CE (narrow-band imaging, multiband imaging or computed virtual chromoendoscopy), are widely used in experienced hands and may shorten examination time. In early gastric cancer, indigo carmine 0.5% with or without acetic acid is used for CE.

Conventional endoscopic ultrasound (EUS) and miniprobe-EUS are carried out for evaluation of T and N stage. In general, diagnostic EMR can be carried out when infiltration of the lamina muscularis propria has been ruled out by EUS. If the specimen shows submucosal tumor infiltration, the patient can be referred for esophagectomy. EUS is superior to computed tomography for lymph node staging [1]. Abdominal imaging (CT, endoscopic ultrasound) is performed to rule out

Table 10.1 Alternative terms for premalignant and superficial carcinoma of the esophagus.

WHO preferred terminology	Non-WHO terminology
Low grade intraepithelial neoplasia (LGIN)	Low grade dysplasia (LGD)
If lower third only involved = mild dysplasia	
Lower two-thirds involved = moderate dysplasia	
High-grade intraepithelial neoplasia (HGIN)	High-grade dysplasia
All thirds involved = severe dysplasia	
Intramucosal carcinoma	Carcinoma *in situ*

Table 10.2 Intramucosal carcinoma based on depth of invasion.

$T_1 m_1$	Intraepithelial neoplasia
$T_1 m_2$	Involves lamina propria
$T_1 m_3$	Involves muscularis mucosae
$T_1 sm_1$	Involves upper third of submucosa
$T_1 sm_2$	Involves middle third of submucosa
$T_1 sm_3$	Involves lower third of submucosa

Table 10.3 Japanese morphological system (Paris Classification) for gross endoscopic appearance of tumors.

Type I: Polypoid type

Type II: Flat type
   (a) flat, elevated type
   (b) flat, level type
   (c) flat, depressed type

Type III: Excavated type

metastatic disease before EMR. For early gastric cancer, abdominal CT, and chest radiography are part of the staging protocol.

Overview of Methods and Technology

EMR of early neoplastic lesions is used both as a diagnostic tool and as a definitive treatment method

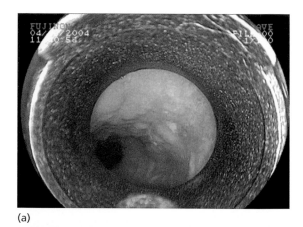

(a)

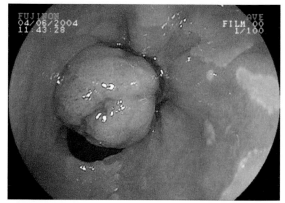

(b)

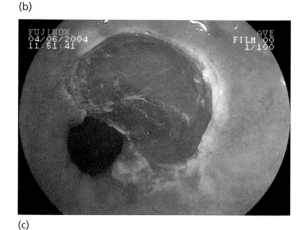

(c)

Figure 10.1 (a) Type IIa+c lesion (view through ligation device). (b) Pseudopolyp containing neoplastic lesion. (c) Endoscopic view of resection area after *en bloc* resection.

when the cancer meets certain criteria in which the risk of lymph node metastasis is negligible. The aim of EMR must always be complete resection of the neoplastic tissue.

Endoscopic Mucosal Resection (EMR)

EMR with the "suck-and-cut" technique (SCT) is routinely used in the West. Using either a cap or a ligation device, both mucosa and submucosa are sucked into a cap or tube, and the pseudopolyp created is resected using a snare.

In EMR with the cap technique, a transparent plastic cap (e.g., Olympus MAJ-295) is attached to the end of the endoscope. After submucosal injection under the target lesion, the lesion is sucked into the cap and resected with a diathermy snare. Prior marking of the borders of the lesion with electrocautery is recommended in order to be able to identify the borders even after injection.

When using one of the various ligation systems available [2–4], the target lesion is sucked into the cylinder of the ligation device without prior submucosal injection, and a rubber band is then released to create a pseudopolyp. After this, the endoscope can be withdrawn and reintroduced in order to remove the ligation cylinder and introduce the snare, or the snare can be introduced through the ligation device. There is no significant difference in the maximum diameter of the resected specimen achieved by ligation or cap resection. The major drawback of EMR with SCT is that, in the majority of cases, only small lesions with a diameter of less than 20 mm can be resected *en bloc* with tumor-free lateral margins. Larger lesions can usually be resected completely with the piecemeal technique, but this method is associated with a relevant recurrence rate, and pathological assessment is more difficult.

Endoscopic Submucosal Dissection (ESD)

Using the new technique of ESD, larger-size specimens can be removed in comparison with conventional EMR: The size of resected specimens can extend to more than 10 cm in diameter. A fascinating *en bloc* R0 resection rate for gastric neoplasias of more than 90% has been reported in experienced hands [5]. On the other hand, there is a substantial complication rate (perforation, bleeding), long procedure times, and a slow learning curve, together with low experience of this procedure in the West.

Before the ESD procedure, the lesion's borders are marked with electrocautery. Submucosal injection (e.g., with hyaluronic acid or saline with epinephrine) is carried out, and the mucosa surrounding the lesion is circumferentially cut outside the markings. Finally, the submucosal connective tissue is dissected with a special knife (e.g., IT knife or flush knife).

Indications for Endoscopic Mucosal Resection

Indications and contraindications of EMR in patients with SCC and Barrett cancer are summarized in Table 10.4.

Early Squamous Cell Carcinoma

It must be kept in mind that for cancers invading the lamina muscularis mucosa (M3), the risk of lymph node metastasis (LNM) is 1.9–10%. These cancers should only be treated with EMR if no further risk factors are present (poor grade of differentiation/lymph vessel or vein infiltration/high grade of tumor cell dissociation) [6,7]. In older patients with greater co-morbidity, the surgical

Table 10.4 Indications for endoscopic mucosal resection in esophageal neoplasia.

	Indication	Expanded indication*
Barrett neoplasia	HGIN, mucosal cancer, size <20 mm, no risk factors†, macroscopic type I, IIa, b, c	Carcinoma >20 mm, multifocal cancer, sm1 infiltration without risk factors
Squamous cell neoplasia	HGIN, mucosal cancer, no risk factors†, macroscopic type I, IIa, b, c	Lesion >20 mm, multifocal cancer

*EMR only in highly experienced centers and/or under study conditions.
†Risk factors: lymph vessel invasion (L1), venous infiltration (V1), low tumor differentiation (G3).
HGIN, high-grade intraepithelial neoplasia.

Table 10.5 Publications on endoscopic mucosal resection for early Barrett neoplasia with treatment of at least 30 patients.

First author [Ref.]	Patients (n)	EMR technique	Minor complications (%)	Major complications (%)	Complete response (%)	Follow-up (months)	Recurrence rate (%)
Ell [2]	64	L	Minor bleeding (12.5)		82.5	12	14
Behrens [11]	44	L/PDT	Minor bleeding (9.3)		97.7	38	17.1
Peters [12]	39	Circumferential C		Perforation (2.6) Major bleeding (2.6) Strictures (26)	95	11	0
Ell [13]	100	L	Minor bleeding (10)		98	36.7	11
Pech [14]	349	L/PDT/L+PDT/APC	Minor bleeding, slight stenosis, odynophagia, sunburn (16.6)	Major bleeding (0.6)	86	63.6	21.5

APC, argon plasma coagulation; C, endoscopic mucosal resection with cap device; L, endoscopic mucosal resection with ligation device; PDT, photodynamic therapy.

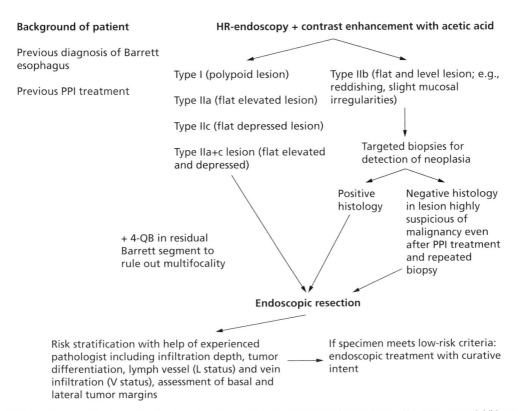

Figure 10.2 Algorithm for detection and endoscopic mucosal resection of early Barrett adenocarcinoma. PPI, proton pump inhibitors; 4-QB, four-quadrant biopsies.

risk has to be balanced against the relatively low risk of LNM.

Early Barrett Carcinoma

Before EMR with a curative intent (Table 10.5), risk stratification should be carried out in accordance with known risk factors (differentiation grade, lymph vessel/venous infiltration, infiltration depth (M1–M3/M4)) and with the help of a highly experienced pathologist.

Limitations for EMR should be submucosal (sm) infiltration or infiltration of the lamina muscularis mucosa in combination with another risk factor. Cancers showing an incipient "low-risk" sm invasion might be eligible for EMR in experienced hands [8].

Recurrent or metachronous neoplasia may occur after initial EMR. Successful repeated endoscopic treatment is possible in the majority of patients. Ablation of the residual Barrett segment with radiofrequency ablation (RFA), argon plasma coagulation (APC) or circumferential EMR (relevant stricture rate) of the whole Barrett segment is used to reduce recurrence rates.

An algorithm for the use of EMR in patients with early Barrett carcinoma is given in Figure 10.2.

Early Gastric Cancer

Gotoda *et al.* [9]. clarified the risks of LNM and proposed criteria of indications for EMR of early gastric cancer (Table 10.6). Western experience with EMR in early gastric cancer is limited [10].

Table 10.6 Japanese criteria for endoscopic mucosal resection in early gastric cancer.

Mucosal cancer
Differentiated adenocarcinoma
No lymphatic–vascular invasion (L0)
If ulcer finding: tumor size <3 cm
Without ulcer findings: irrespective of tumor size

Undifferentiated mucosal cancer
L0
Without ulcer findings
Tumor <2 cm

sm1 invasion, <500 μm
Differentiated adenocarcinoma
L0
Tumor <3 cm

Take-home points

- A precise preinterventional staging protocol is required to select the right patients for EMR.
- Different pathologic staging systems are used to define the histopathology of superficial premalignant and malignant lesions of the gastrointestinal tract. They are explained in Tables 10.2 and 10.3.
- In Western hands, EMR with both the cap technique and the ligation technique are effective for premalignant lesions and in early esophageal cancer. Western experience is still limited in endoscopic treatment of early gastric cancer and the ESD procedure.
- Both preinterventional staging and endoscopic treatment should be performed by experienced endoscopists.
- The histological work-up of the EMR specimen—performed by a highly-experienced pathologist—is used for risk stratification and to determine if endoscopic therapy can be carried out with a curative intent.
- All patients should undergo a strict follow-up program to enable detection and treatment of metachronous and/or recurrent lesions. Almost all secondary lesions can be treated successfully using repeated endoscopic therapy.

References

1 Pech O, May A, Günter E, *et al.* The impact of endoscopic ultrasound and computed tomography on the TNM staging of early cancer in Barrett's esophagus. *Am J Gastroenterol* 2006; **101**: 2223–9.

2 Ell C, May A, Gossner L, *et al.* Endoscopic mucosal resection of early cancer and high-grade dysplasia in Barrett's esophagus. *Gastroenterology* 2000; **118**: 670–7.

3 Ell C, May A, Wurster H. The first reusable multiple-band ligator for endoscopic hemostasis of variceal bleeding and mucosal resection. *Endoscopy* 1999; **31**: 738–40.

4 Soehendra N, Seewald S, Groth S, *et al.* Use of modified multiband ligator facilitates circumferential EMR in Barrett's esophagus (with video). *Gastrointest Endosc* 2006; **63**: 847–52.

5 Onozato Y, Ishihara H, Iizuka H, *et al.* Endoscopic submucosal dissection for early gastric cancers and large flat adenomas. *Endoscopy* 2006; **38**: 980–6.

6 Pech O, May A, Gossner L, *et al.* Curative endoscopic therapy in patients with early esophageal squamous-cell carcinoma or high-grade intraepithelial neoplasia. *Endoscopy* 2007; **39**: 30–5.

7 Pech O, May A, Rabenstein T, *et al*. Endoscopic resection of early oesophageal cancer. *Gut* 2007; **56**: 1625–34.

8 Manner H, May A, Pech O, *et al*. Early Barrett's carcinoma with "low-risk" submucosal invasion: long-term results of endoscopic resection with a curative intent. *Am J Gastroenterol* 2008; **103**: 2589–97.

9 Gotoda T, Yanagisawa A, Sasako M, *et al*. Incidence of lymph node metastasis from early gastric cancer: estimation with a large number of cases at two large centers. *Gastric Cancer* 2000; **3**: 219–25.

10 Manner H, Rabenstein T, May A, *et al*. Long-term results of endoscopic resection in early gastric cancer: the Western experience. *Am J Gastroenterol* 2009; **104**: 566–73.

11 Behrens A, May A, Gossner L, *et al*. Curative treatment for high-grade intraepithelial neoplasia in Barrett's esophagus. *Endoscopy* 2005; **37**: 999–1005.

12 Peters FP, Kara MA, Rosmolen WD, *et al*. Stepwise radical endoscopic resection is effective for complete removal of Barrett's esophagus with early neoplasia: a prospective study. *Am J Gastroenterol* 2006; **101**: 1449–57.

13 Ell C, May A, Pech O, *et al*. Curative endoscopic resection of early esophageal adenocarcinomas (Barrett's cancer). *Gastrointest Endosc* 2007; **65**: 3–10.

14 Pech O, Behrens A, May A, *et al*. Long-term results and risk factor analysis for recurrence after curative endoscopic therapy in 349 patients with high-grade intraepithelial neoplasia and mucosal adenocarcinoma in Barrett's oesophagus. *Gut* 2008; **57**: 1200–6.

CHAPTER 11

Ablation of Upper Gastrointestinal Neoplasia

Virender K. Sharma

Arizona Center for Digestive Health, Phoenix, AZ, USA

Summary

Barrett esophagus, a complication of reflux disease, is a precancerous condition resulting in esophageal adenocarcinoma. Regular endoscopic surveillance has been the standard of care for the management of Barrett esophagus. Minimally-invasive ablative treatments, such as ablation using the Halo[360] ablation system, cryoablation, photodynamic therapy and endoscopic mucosal resection and submucosal dissection, offer newer treatment options for patients with Barrett esophagus with and without dysplasia and for patients with early-stage esophageal cancer. Endoscopic mucosal resection and submucosal dissection offer resective options and photodynamic therapy offers an ablative option for early-stage gastric cancer. The patients treated with these minimally invasive treatments need to continue surveillance as determined by their baseline disease stage. With longer-term follow-up and demonstration of safety and efficacy, it may not be necessary to have continued surveillance after treatment.

Case

A 54-year-old Caucasian male had symptoms of esophageal reflux for 20 years. Initially, the symptoms responded to over-the-counter medications, but when they persisted he saw his primary-care physician who referred him to a gastroenterologist for endoscopy. At the time of endoscopy, he was found to have a 6-cm segment of Barrett with no nodules. Four quadrant biopsies were taken at 2-cm intervals and on several of the biopsies high-grade dysplasia was found. The patient returned to his primary-care physician who referred him to a thoracic surgeon. The thoracic surgeon described the operation and scheduled him for surgery. Prior to having that surgery, the patient's niece, who was a medical student, reported that in Journal Club they had recently discussed a paper in the *New England Journal* that described radiofrequency ablation for high-grade dysplasia with encouraging results. The medical student encouraged the patient to look into this. He saw a second gastroenterologist who described the risks and benefits of radiofrequency ablation and explained to him he would need to have staging with endoscopic ultrasound and a CT scan. The patient underwent those tests and the disease was felt to be localized. The patient then underwent radiofrequency ablation and, after two treatments, was told that there was no residual Barrett or dysplasia. The patient was maintained on a twice-daily dose of proton pump inhibitors and at the follow-up examination at 1 year he remained free of Barrett or dysplasia.

Introduction

Barrett esophagus (BE) is a complication of chronic gastroesophageal reflux disease (GERD) (see Chapter 31). Recurrent mucosal injury from chronic exposure to refluxed acid and bile results in a change from the normal squamous mucosa to a specialized intestinal mucosa with

Practical Gastroenterology and Hepatology: Esophagus and Stomach, 1st edition. Edited by Nicholas J. Talley, Kenneth R. DeVault and David E. Fleischer. © 2010 Blackwell Publishing Ltd.

goblet cells. BE is the precursor lesion in a majority of cases of esophageal adenocarcinoma, one of the fastest growing cancers in the USA and other Western nations. The National Cancer Institute Surveillance, Epidemiology and End Results (SEER) program reported the incidence of esophageal cancer to be greater than for any other cancer in the USA. The greatest rise has been predominantly seen in white men (>350% since the mid-1970s). SEER has also reported a small but significant increase in women and African Americans [1].

On the other hand, distal gastric cancer has been showing a constant decline in incidence in the USA and Western nations, mainly attributable to decline in the prevalence of *H. pylori* infection. However, prevalence of gastric cancer worldwide has remained stable. Although advances in endoscopic resective therapies have been made for the management of early-stage gastric neoplasia, the current chapter will mainly focus on endoscopic ablative treatments for esophageal neoplasia, including dysplasia.

Epidemiology of Barrett Esophagus and Risk of Esophageal Cancer

Approximately 10% of patient undergoing endoscopy for chronic GERD symptoms will have BE. Older, white men with long-standing acid reflux are at highest risk of development of BE. Chronic and nighttime heartburn portend BE and esophageal adenocarcinoma (EAC). The traditional view that BE progresses from metaplasia to low-grade dysplasia (LGD) to high-grade dysplasia (HGD) and then to cancer has been supplanted by recent reports of BE progressing directly to HGD or esophageal adenocarcinoma. The risk of developing esophageal cancer in patients with BE is 0.4% per patient-year [2].

Endoscopic Treatments for Upper Gastrointestinal Neoplasia

Thermal ablation with monopolar and bipolar diathermy probes has been investigated as possible treatment for upper gastrointestinal metaplasia, dysplasia and cancer. Lasers such as CO_2, Nd:YAG and KTP have been reported as effective therapy of upper GI neoplasias. The depth of penetration and amount of thermal ablation of tissue is correlated to wavelength. The Nd:YAG generally has a depth of penetration to 4 mm, whereas KTP and argon reach about 1 mm. Argon plasma coagulation (APC) is a non-contact electrocoagulation device that uses a high-frequency monopolar current which is conducted to tissue via an ionized argon gas and is used for hemostasis and tissue ablation. The depth of tissue penetration depends on the power setting of the generator, the argon gas flow rate, the application's duration, and the distance between the probe tip and tissue. APC is supposed to have a more superficial depth of tissue injury than laser; however, unintentional contact with the mucosa may cause deeper tissue damage [3].

Thermal ablation techniques are simple to use, relatively widely available and inexpensive; however, they are highly operator dependent, require long procedure durations and multiple session to treat larger surface areas of neoplastic tissue. Energy delivery in these techniques is operator controlled, which may result in uneven energy application and non-uniform ablation. Under-ablation results in residual neoplastic tissue and buried Barrett, while excessive depth of ablation results in complications such as perforation, bleeding and stricture formation. Laser devices require a large, upfront capital investment and additional training for safe operation. Due to these limitations, traditional thermal ablation techniques have not gained wide-spread application for treatment of upper gastrointestinal neoplasia.

Radiofrequency ablation (RFA) using the Halo ablation system offers a safe and effective ablative treatment of Barrett mucosa with and without dysplasia. With an FDA-approved endoscopically-guided, bipolar, RFA catheter, Barrett ablation can be performed at the time of upper endoscopy (Figure 11.1a, b). Animal and human studies prove that achieving complete circumferential ablation of esophageal epithelium without subsequent stricture formation is possible with the RFA system. Automated regulation of the energy density delivered to the tissue via the bipolar electrode array helps limit the depth of injury to the epithelium and lamina propria.

Patients with flat (non-nodular) BE with and without dysplasia are eligible for RFA treatment. In patients with non-dysplastic Barrett, at 12 months (n = 69; mean 1.5 sessions), a complete response (CR) for BE with circum-

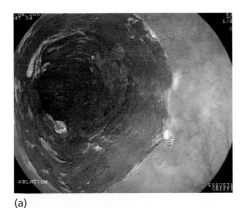

(a)

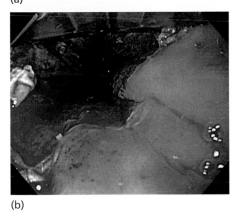

(b)

Figure 11.1 (a) Postablation image of long-segment Barrett esophagus after circumferential ablation with the Halo³⁶⁰ electrode. The ablated mucosa sloughs off and over time is replaced by normal squamous epithelium. (b) Postablation image of short-segment Barrett esophagus after focal ablation with the Halo⁹⁰ electrode. The Halo⁹⁰ electrode is seen at the 12° clock position in the endoscopic image. The ablated mucosa sloughs off and over time is replaced by normal squamous epithelium.

ferential ablation was achieved in 70% of patients. A follow-up study in the same group of patients reported CR of 98% at 2.5 year follow-up with addition of focal ablation [4]. There were no strictures and no buried glandular mucosa. In patients with flat dysplasia, preliminary results show high CR (>90%) for ablation of both LGD and HGD. Patients with nodular disease have been effectively treated with combination of EMR followed by RFA. A randomized, sham-controlled trial of RFA in patient with LGD and HGD resulted in complete ablation (intention to treat) of dysplasia in 91% of patients in LGD and 81% patient in HGD subgroups. There was significantly less cancer (1.2% vs. 9.3%; p < 0.05) and less progression to higher grades (3.6% vs. 16.3%; p < 0.05) in the treatment compared to the sham group [5]. It is performed as an outpatient procedure and is fairly well tolerated. Adverse events, including chest pain and dysphagia, are usually mild and resolve within a week in most patients. Other rare complications include strictures (~2–6% of patients), bleeding and perforation.

Low-pressure spray cryoablation using liquid nitrogen is another newer ablative technique for Barrett esophagus. Cryoablation device components include: (i) liquid nitrogen tank; (ii) electronic console for monitoring and control of liquid nitrogen release; (iii) a dual foot pedal for control of liquid nitrogen release and heating of the catheter; and (iv) a multilayered 7–9 F open-tipped catheter for spraying super-cold nitrogen gas through an upper endoscope. Liquid nitrogen cryoablation induces apoptosis and causes cryonecrosis at low temperatures (−76°C to −158°C), which results in transient ischemic injury followed by immune-mediated destruction of Barrett epithelium. Initial trials using this device show promising results in treatment of both nodular and non-nodular HGD and early-stage esophageal cancer [6].

Photodynamic therapy (PDT) is FDA-approved and is a significantly superior treatment to endoscopic surveillance in the eradication of HGD and the prevention of progression to esophageal adenocarcinoma [7]. PDT is a two-stage process in which a photosensitizer (Porfimer-Na), which accumulates in the metaplastic and dysplastic tissue of BE, is administered intravenously. When exposed to non-thermal red laser light at 630 nm, the Porfimer-Na absorbs the light energy, resulting in a porphyrin-excited state yielding singlet oxygen [O] that induces ischemic necrosis of metaplastic and dysplastic tissue in BE (Figure 11.2a, b). Unfortunately, PDT is not without serious complications. All patients undergoing PDT become extremely photosensitive and are advised to avoid direct sun-exposure for at least 1 month. Despite these warning, severe photosensitive reactions have been reported in 7% patients undergoing PDT. Stricture formation is another major complication of PDT and is reported in 40% of the patients, 8% of which are severe. Other adverse effects reported with PDT include

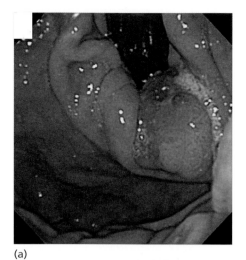

(a)

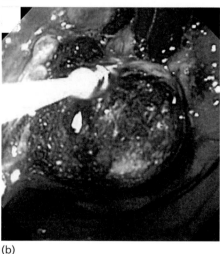

(b)

Figure 11.2 (a) An endoscopic image of the cardia in the retroflex position that reveals a 2-cm T1N0M0 cardia cancer. (b) The same tumor 48 h after photodynamic therapy (PDT) treatment. The tumor has undergone ischemic necrosis after PDT ablation. PDT fiber that is used to deliver the laser light to the tumor is seen in the image.

vomiting, chest pain requiring narcotics, fever, mediastinitis and pleural effusions.

Endoscopic mucosal resection (EMR) is an endoscopic technique to resect nodular lesions in the gastrointestinal tract (Figure 11.3a, b) (see Chapter 10). This has been effectively used to resect nodular high-grade dysplasia and early esophageal cancer. Various techniques, such as lift and cut with or without submucosal

injection and with or without a cap device, or ligate and cut technique, have been used to perform EMR. Alone or in conjunction with other endoscopic ablative therapy, EMR is effective for the treatment of nodular high-grade dysplasia or early esophageal cancer. Larger lesions can be piecemeal resected and completely removed. Residual flat neoplasia can be treated using ablative techniques. EMR is performed as an outpatient procedure and is well tolerated. Chest pain and transient dysphagia are rare. Complications include bleeding (1–2%), stricture formation and perforation. Prior ablative therapy, radiation therapy or resection of more than 50% of the circumference increase the risk of stricture formation. EMR is recommended for treatment of *all* nodular lesions for more accurate diagnosis and staging, and treatment (Figure 11.3c) [8].

Endoscopic submucosal dissection (ESD) is a technique used for *en bloc* resection of upper gastrointestinal lesions. ESD is more commonly used in far-east and south-east Asia and requires special electrosurgical devices to successfully complete the procedure. ESD requires lifting the lesion with saline and then mechanically lifting and dissecting the complete lesion in one piece. A few centers in the US have performed ESD using a needle knife to resect large, superficial upper gastrointestinal tumor. ESD is associated with better margin clearance and decrease local recurrence of the tumor. However, ESD is time-intensive and complications, including bleeding, perforation and stricture formation, occur frequently. However, most ESD complications can be managed conservatively without the need for surgery [8].

Endoscopic Management of Barrett with No or Low-Grade Dysplasia

Once diagnosed, BE requires surveillance, because studies have shown EAC can be diagnosed earlier and at a more treatable stage. Because of these results, patients over 50 years of age with chronic GERD symptoms merit endoscopy to screen for BE. Once diagnosed, patients with BE should undergo endoscopic examination with four quadrant biopsies every 3 years to detect dysplasia and early esophageal cancer. LGD requires yearly surveillance. HGD, confirmed by two pathologists, is an indication for esophagectomy to prevent progression to esophageal cancer [2].

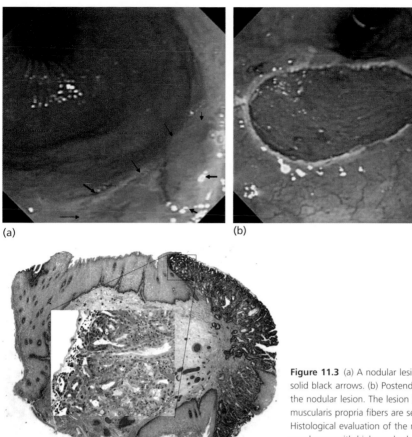

(a)

(b)

(c)

Figure 11.3 (a) A nodular lesion in the distal esophagus marked by solid black arrows. (b) Postendoscopic mucosal resection image of the nodular lesion. The lesion is resected in toto and the superficial muscularis propria fibers are seen in the base of the resection. (c) Histological evaluation of the resected lesion revealed Barrett esophagus with high-grade dysplasia and intramucosal cancer at the edges of the nodule. The inset shows a magnified view of the intramucosal cancer that is completely resected.

Emergence of safe and effective ablative techniques such as RFA has increased the interest in ablation as possible management strategy for early-stage Barrett esophagus. Preliminary results show that complete eradication of Barrett epithelium is possible with decrease in progression to higher grade [4,5]. Ablation has also been shown to be cost effective [9]. However, data on cancer prevention are lacking and require long-term prospective trials.

Endoscopic Management of Barrett with High-Grade Dysplasia

Traditionally, HGD has been managed with esophagectomy; however, the procedure is associated with significant morbidity and a small but finite mortality. Complications include anastomotic strictures (20–40%) and leaks (3–39%), recurrent laryngeal nerve paresis (3–16%) and death (2–10%). Other long-term complications include gastroparesis, loss of esophageal and lower esophageal sphincter functions resulting in severe gastroesophageal reflux disease and regurgitation of gastric contents.

Ablative therapies such as PDT, RFA and cryoablation have been shown to be effective in eradicating HGD and preventing progression to cancer without the associated morbidity and mortality of an esophagectomy [5–7]. PDT and cryoablation are effective in eradicating nodular HGD, while RFA is ineffective against nodular Barrett and requires the addition of EMR to eliminate any nodular disease [8]. Patients undergoing ablative therapy still need to undergo periodic surveillance, although at a reduced interval.

Endoscopic Management of Early-stage Esophageal Cancer

Esophagectomy remains the mainstay of treatment of early-stage esophageal cancer. However, some patients who are unwilling or, due to significant co-morbidity, unable to undergo surgical resection can be effectively managed with endoscopic treatments. EMR or PDT alone, or as combination therapy have yielded promising results in the management of early-stage esophageal cancer. In a prospective, multicenter, cohort study Canto *et al.* reported their experience with 80 patients (70% male; mean age 73 years) who underwent PDT for T1N0M0 esophageal cancers (mean follow up 29 months, range 6–82). Three-quarters of the patients had PDT alone. The complete response rate for PDT with EMR (95.4%) was comparable to PDT alone (89.7%, p = 0.67). Subsquamous dysplasia or cancer was found in five (6%) patients after PDT and strictures developed in nine patients (11.2%). The 5-year survival of evaluable patients was 97% and there were no procedural or cancer-related deaths in this cohort of patients. May *et al.* reported their experience in 115 patients with intraepithelial neoplasia (n = 19) or early-stage esophageal cancer (n = 96) treated with EMR (n = 70), PDT (n = 32), both (n = 10), or APC (n = 3). Complete remission was achieved in 98%; 30% had metachronous recurrence. Thirteen patients died over a median 3-year follow-up; only one was a cancer-related death. Recently, using the SEER database, we have reported comparable outcomes in patient with early-stage esophageal cancer treated with endoscopic therapy or surgery [10]. These data suggest that minimally invasive endoscopic therapies maybe a good alternative to eophagectomy for management of early-stage esophageal cancer.

Endoscopic Management of Early-stage Gastric Cancer

Distal gastric cancer has been decreasing in the West and subtotal gastrectomy remains the mainstay of treatment of early-stage gastric cancer. Multiple, large and long-term studies show that ESD is effective in successful resection of early-stage gastric cancer with results comparable to surgery [11]. PDT and cryoablation can also be used for ablation of early-stage gastric cancer although high-quality, long-term data are lacking.

Take-home points

- Upper GI cancers around the gastroesophageal junction are rising at an epidemic rate.
- Surgery remains the standard of care for the management of resectable esophageal and gastric cancers.
- Endoscopic therapy has an emerging role for the management of dysplasia and early-stage (T1) esophageal and gastric cancer.
- Combination of resective and ablative techniques have yielded outcome comparable to surgery in patients with early-stage (T1) esophageal cancer.
- Accurate staging of cancer using endosonography and PET-CT is imperative for optimal results from endotherapy.
- Advances in safe and effective endoscopic therapies may make endoprevention of esophageal cancer a reality.
- Ablative therapy may have role in palliation of malignant dysphagia; however, self-expanding metal stents remain the palliative treatment of choice.

References

1　Spechler S. Clinical practice. Barrett esophagus. *N Engl J Med* 2002; **346**: 836–42.

2　Wang KK, Sampliner RE. Updated guidelines 2008 for the diagnosis, surveillance and therapy of Barrett's esophagus. *Am J Gastroenterol* 2008; **103**: 788–97.

3　Sampliner RE. Endoscopic ablative therapy for Barrett's esophagus: current status. *Gastrointest Endosc* 2004; **59**: 66.

4　Fleischer DE, Overholt BF, Sharma VK, *et al.* Endoscopic ablation of Barrett's esophagus: a multicenter study with 2.5-year follow-up. *Gastrointest Endosc* 2008; **68**: 867–76.

5　Shaheen NJ, Sharma P, BF Overholt, *et al.* A randomized, multicenter, sham-controlled trial of radiofrequency ablation (RFA) for subjects with Barrett's esophagus (BE) containing dysplasia. *N Engl J Med* 2009; **360**: 2277–88.

6　Johnston MH, Eastone JA, Horwhat JD, *et al.* Cryoablation of Barrett's esophagus: a pilot study. *Gastrointest Endosc* 2005; **62**: 842–8.

7　Overholt BF, Lightdale CJ, Wang KK, *et al.* Photodynamic therapy with porfimer sodium for ablation of high-grade dysplasia in Barrett's esophagus: international, partially blinded, randomized phase III trial. *Gastrointest Endosc* 2005; **62**: 488–98.

8 Kantsevoy SV, Adler DG, Conway JD, *et al.* Prepared by: ASGE Technology Committee. Endoscopic mucosal resection and endoscopic submucosal dissection. *Gastrointest Endosc* 2008; **68**: 11–18.

9 Das A, Wells C, Kim HJ, *et al.* An economic analysis of endoscopic ablative therapy for management of nondysplastic Barrett's esophagus. *Endoscopy* 2009; **41**: 400–8.

10 Das A, Singh V, Fleischer DE, Sharma VK. Comparison of endoscopic treatment and surgery in early esophageal cancer: an analysis of surveillance epidemiology and end results data. *Am J Gastroenterol* 2008; **103**: 1340–5.

11 Ono H, Kondo II, Gotoda T, *et al.* Endoscopic mucosal resection for treatment of early gastric cancer. *Gut* 2001; **48**: 225–9.

CHAPTER 12

Benefits and Delivery of Enteral Nutrition

Stephen A. McClave

Division of Gastroenterology/Hepatology, University of Louisville School of Medicine, Louisville, KY, USA

Summary

For the critically ill patient, initiation of early enteral nutrition (EN) is an important therapeutic strategy which can change their course of hospitalization. If started soon after admission to the Intensive Care Unit (ICU) and if provided with sufficient dosage, early EN can be expected to reduce infectious morbidity, decrease risk for multiorgan failure, and shorten ICU and hospital length of stay (compared to parenteral nutrition or standard therapy with no nutrition support). Obstacles to delivery of EN should be avoided, risk for gut ischemia should be carefully differentiated from clinical ileus, and use of gastric residual volume should not be misinterpreted as an effective deterrent against aspiration pneumonia. The gastroenterologist/endoscopist has a number of innate skills to bring to the table for the provision of EN. If partnered with a nurse or clinical dietitian, such a combination of talent can lead to a highly effective nutrition support team.

Case

A 52-year-old female with diabetes, hypertension, and strong family history of coronary artery disease is admitted with severe abdominal pain to the intensive care unit. She has radiographic and laboratory signs suggesting acute pancreatitis. There is no evidence of gall stones on the studies. She appears ill and in addition to fluid balance, management of her glucose and insulin, and pain control, the issue of nutrition is raised. The issue of enteral versus parenteral nutrition is the major focus of conversation among the various consultants. The arguments for utilizing enteral nutrition focused upon a more natural nutritional supplementation and the safety benefits. The arguments for parenteral nutrition addressed the fact that she is diabetic and may have gastroparesis and therefore enteral feeding would require jejunal tubes placed either orally or as a jejunostomy. A gastroenterologist with expertise in nutrition is called to resolve the matter.

Introduction

Compared to parenteral nutrition (PN) or standard therapy (STD) where no nutrition support is provided,

Practical Gastroenterology and Hepatology: Esophagus and Stomach, 1st edition. Edited by Nicholas J. Talley, Kenneth R. DeVault and David E. Fleischer. © 2010 Blackwell Publishing Ltd.

delivery of early enteral nutrition (EN) in the critical care setting has been shown to improve patient outcome. Gastroenterologists have an inherent knowledge of gut physiology and have the endoscopic skills to place enteral access devices. As a result of these factors, the makeup of a nutrition support team has shifted over the past decade. Early on, the nutrition support team was comprised of a surgeon who could place central intravenous lines and a pharmacist who could compound the PN. Now the team is better comprised of a physician, hopefully with knowledge of gastrointestinal physiology and endoscopic skills to achieve enteral access, along with a dietitian or a nurse that can aid in the delivery of early EN. An algorithm for the initiation of EN is given in Figure 12.1.

Outcome Benefits from Enteral Nutrition

A wide variety of studies in the literature support the existence of a "window of opportunity" for early enteral feeding in the critical care setting [1–3]. This window of opportunity opens shortly after the patient is admitted to the Intensive Care Unit (ICU) and may remain open for

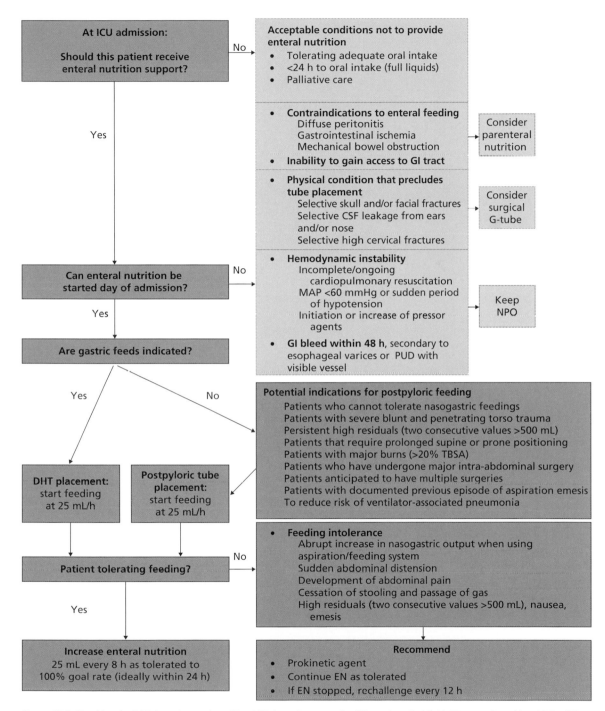

Figure 12.1 Algorithm for initiation of enteral nutrition. ICU, intensive care unit; CSF, cerebrospinal fluid; EN, enteral nutrition; NPO, nil by mouth; MAP, mean arterial pressure; PUD, peptic ulcer disease; TBSA, total body surface area; DHT, Dobhoff tube.

up to 48–72 h. If enteral access is achieved and enteral feeding started during this time period, the EN has the chance to actually improve patient outcome by reducing infection, multiple organ failure, duration of mechanical ventilation, length of hospitalization, and, in some disease processes, even mortality [4–6]. If there are delays in initiating EN, then the window of opportunity closes. The patient still may require nutrition support with EN, but the opportunity to actually change outcome may be lost. This window of opportunity is supported by at least four distinct bodies of literature in the published record.

Early versus Delayed Enteral Nutrition

In one group of studies, early EN was compared to delayed EN, with the average cutoff being 36 h. Two meta-analyses showed that feeds started within 36 h of admission to the ICU, reduced infection by 55% ($P = 0.006$) and shortened hospital length of stay by 2.2 days ($P = 0.0004$), with a trend toward reduced mortality by as much as 35% ($P = 0.06$) compared to feeds started after that time point [2,5].

Early Enteral Nutrition versus Standard Therapy

Another body of literature looks at early EN versus STD therapy, where the patient receives no specialized nutrition therapy and is on their own to advance gradually to an oral diet. A meta-analyses in elective surgery and surgery critical care patients, randomized on the operating table to either aggressive use of the oral route or EN through placement of a feeding tube the next day versus STD therapy, showed that early enteral feeding postoperation reduced infection by 28% ($P = 0.03$) and hospital length of stay was reduced by 0.84 days ($P = 0.0001$) [7]. A second meta-analysis in severe acute pancreatitis, again where patients were randomized on the table at the time of surgery for complications of pancreatitis to either EN or STD therapy the first day post-operatively, delivery of early EN reduced mortality by 74% compared to STD therapy ($P = 0.06$) [8].

Cumulative Caloric Balance

Yet another group of studies in the literature supporting the window of opportunity relates to the concept of cumulative caloric deficit. For each day that a patient resides in the ICU, he or she expends a certain number of calories. Any delay in initiating enteral feeding results in the development of a caloric deficit. In a study from Europe, Villet showed that the greater the caloric deficit, the greater the likelihood for complications [9]. Hospital length of stay, increasing infections, and longer duration of mechanical ventilation all correlate to increasing cumulative energy deficit ($P < 0.04$ for all endpoints) [9]. This type of study has been criticized for the fact that the greater the severity of illness for a particular ICU patient, the more difficult it is to deliver EN.

Impact of Enteral Nutrition Protocols

A fourth body of literature, which involves the impact of feeding protocols on delivery of EN and patient outcome, refutes this criticism. In other words, any strategies that increase delivery of EN in these critically ill patients who are difficult to feed, reduces the cumulative calorie deficit and improves outcome. In this last body of literature, patients or medical centers are randomized to use or not to use a feeding protocol. Typically, the protocol identifies a patient who is nil per os (NPO), orders a tube to be placed, feeds to be initiated, and raises the value for gastric residual volume. Use of an EN protocol typically provides a number of parameters that results in an increase in the number of patients fed over the first week of hospitalization, an increase in the percent of goal calories infused, and a reduction in cessation of EN delivery. In a study from Louisville, patients were randomized to one of two separate trauma teams [10]. In the study, team residents received targeted physician education regarding a number of strategies to improve delivery of EN. Specifically, they were asked to substitute a full liquid diet for any clear liquid diet ordered, to minimize periods that patients were kept NPO, to order volume-based feeds (where nurses could increase the rate of EN if patients lost feeding time during diagnostic tests or bedside procedures), and to be aware of the increasing caloric deficit. The control team was given no such instructions. As a result of the targeted education, the number of days patients were on clear liquid diet was nearly eliminated and the mean caloric deficit was reduced by 23% [10]. As a result of this difference, patients on the team that received targeted physician education had a decreased length of stay in the ICU of 1.7 days ($P = 0.13$), the number of patients infected was reduced by over half (23.6% versus 10.6%, $P = 0.10$), and the mean Denver Multi-Organ Failure Score was reduced significantly from 0.45 ± 0.1 to 0.20 ± 0.8 ($P < 0.05$) compared respectively to those patients on the control service [10]. In a second study from Canada, entire hospitals were randomized to an intervention center or a control center based on the degree to which the Canadian Practice Guidelines were introduced into patient care [11]. At intervention centers, the hospital personnel were tested for their delivery of EN, educated as to the details of the Canadian Practice Guidelines [2], and then retested after the educational period. In control centers, they simply received the Canadian Practice Guidelines with no specific education or testing strategies. As a result of the more comprehensive strategy, study centers succeeded at increasing the number of days that patients were on EN in the first week (6.7 versus 5.4 days, $P = 0.04$), reducing hospital length of stay by 10 full days (25 versus 35 days, $P = 0.003$), and significantly decreasing mortality by 10% (from 37 to 27%, $P = 0.058$) compared to the control centers [11].

Physiologic Mechanism of Enteral Nutrition Benefit

In the past, the benefit of nutrition support by either the enteral or parenteral route was thought to be related to prevention of protein energy malnutrition and support of the stress response in critical illness [12]. The specific value of even small amounts of EN was thought to be related to its ability to maintain villous height and to protect against bacterial translocation. Clinicians believed that increases in permeability during critical illness allowed bacteria to cross the intestinal epithelium and migrate to distant sites, where colonization could lead to systemic infection, pneumonia, and organ failure. Assessment of nutritional risk and therefore adequacy of therapy focused on nitrogen balance and normalization of "visceral proteins", such as prealbumin, transferrin, and albumen. Subsequent studies showed that many of these early beliefs were flawed [4,13,14]. Decreases in visceral protein levels have been shown to be overwhelmingly related to the stress response, increases in vascular permeability, and reprioritization of hepatic protein synthesis. Villous atrophy is much more prevalent in animal studies involving mice and rats and happens to a much more limited extent in humans. While increasing permeability is a huge issue in critical illness, bacteria do not need to translocate beyond the lamina propria and do

not even have to be alive to exert an inflammatory response on systemic immunity. Meeting caloric requirements and achieving a positive nitrogen balance become more of an issue later in hospitalization; there are not the mechanisms for impact on outcome seen in the first week [13,15].

The key issues in the benefit of early EN relate to maintenance of gut integrity, prevention of increased permeability, and down-regulation of systemic inflammatory responses [4,16,17] (Table 12.1). In the fed state, the mass of gut-associated lymphoid tissue (GALT) is maintained, production and release of secretory IgA (which help coat bacteria in the gastrointestinal tract) is sustained, and good intestinal contractility helps keep the overall number of lumenal bacteria in check [6,13,18]. Blood flow to the gut is increased and the production of trophic substances such as bile salts, gastrin, and short-chain fatty acids maintain the health of intestinal epithelium [6]. Failure to feed increases gut permeability, a phenomenon which is time dependent and related to disease severity [6,19] (Table 12.2). With increasing degrees of critical illness, the permeability changes are greater and in some disease processes, such as burns, may move to within 4–6 h of admission to the hospital [1]. Consequences of increased permeability are risk for systemic infection and multiple organ failure [1,3,17]. In a

Table 12.1 Physiologic benefits of early enteral nutrition.

Increased intestinal contractility through stimulation of bombesin and motilin

Stimulation and release of secretory IgA

Stimulation of enteric trophic agents—bile salts, gastrin

Support of comensal bacterial

Maintenance of gut integrity and tight junctions between epithelial cells

Support of the mass of GALT (gut-associated lymphoid tissue)

Support of MALT (mucosal-associated lymphoid tissue) at distant sites—lung, liver, kidneys, lacrimal glands

Increase in splanchnic intestinal blood flow

Stimulation and relapse of anti-inflammatory Th2 subset of CD4 helper lymphocytes into the systemic circulation

Expression of MadCAM adhesion molecules which allows homing of GALT cells back to the intestinal lamina propria

Table 12.2 Consequences of gut disuse in critical illness.

Reduced intestinal blood flow with increased risk for ischemia/reperfusion injury

Decreased intestinal contractility

Bacterial overgrowth, emergence of pathogens such as pseudomonas, and increased adherence of bacteria to the intestinal epithelium

Increased intestinal permeability

Release of inflammatory cytokines into the lymphatic system and subsequent passage to pulmonary capillary beds

Increased activation of macrophages, neutrophils, intestinal epithelial cells, and other components of the innate immune system contributing to SIRS

Stimulation and release into the systemic circulation of proinflammatory Th1 CD4 helper lymphocytes contributing to SIRS

Expression of ICAM and E-selectin which allows activated neutrophils to pass out of the vascular space into the pulmonary alveoli

Reduction in mass of GALT and MALT tissue

SIRS, systemic inflammatory response syndrome; ICAM, intercellular adhesion molecule; GALT, gut-associated lymphoid tissue; MALT, mucosal-associated lymphoid tissue.

prospective burn study, Ziegler showed that patients who became infected had increased permeability (as measured by lactose–mannitol ratios in the urine) [3]. Those patients who remained uninfected throughout their hospitalization showed no increases in permeability, as did controls with no burns [3]. In a prospective cohort study of ICU patients, Doig showed that increases in gut permeability on admission correlated directly with increased risk for multiple organ failure [17]. Increases in gut permeability affect both the innate and acquired immune system, leading to the systemic inflammatory response syndrome (SIRS) [17]. Macrophages of the innate immune system contained within the lamina propria are more likely to become activated in the absence of enteral feeding. Neutrophils flowing through the splanchnic circulation can become primed by these macrophages, and then go out to distant sites such as the liver, lung, and kidneys, and generate an inflammatory response [4]. With the acquired immune system, lack of feeding leads to the generation of a Th1 population of CD4 helper lymphocytes which subsequently lead to an inflamma-

tory response and increased production of tumor necrosis factor, and interlukin-12 [13]. In contrast, delivery of EN alters the subset populations that emerge from the gut, promoting a Th2 line of CD4 helper lymphocytes which go on to produce interlukin-4, interlukin-10, and transforming growth factor-β, all of which down-regulate inflammation [20]. There is an interesting lymphatic conduit of inflammation between the gut and the lung [14]. Increases in permeability and the opportunity for enteric bacteria to engage the immune system, results in the release of inflammatory cytokines into the lymphatic channels. These inflammatory mediators move through the thoracic duct, out to the systemic circulation, and into the first capillary bed following their exit from the gut (which happens to be in the lung) [14]. Thus maintenance of gut integrity helps protect against respiratory failure, adult respiratory distress syndrome, and ventilatory-associated pneumonia [14]. Whether or not the patient receives early EN even affects the pattern of adhesion molecules that are released, which in turn determines outcome consequences [21]. Failure to feed a critically ill patient leads to increased release of intercellular adhesion molecule (ICAM) and E-selectin in the lungs, which allow activated polymorphonucleocytes to pass out of the vascular space into the alveoli and lead to respiratory failure [21]. Feeding the patient suppresses release of these adhesion molecules and helps trap the neutrophils within the vascular space. At the level of the gut, failure to provide EN down-regulates release of MadCAM, which traps GALT cells in the vascular space, preventing their return to the intestinal epithelium [13]. Providing EN increases MadCAM levels, which allows these cells to exit the vascular space and return to the lamina propria, providing greater defense against subsequent bacterial antigen [13].

The net effect of enteral feeding is to maintain the mass of GALT tissue, prevent increases in permeability, and down-regulate inflammatory immune responses, all of which favorably impacts patient outcome.

Gap Between Beliefs and Clinical Practice

An unfortunate gap exists between the strength of the literature supporting a benefit of EN and the beliefs of health-care providers in the value of EN for their patients with actual clinical practice where there is gross under-utilization and poor delivery of EN. In a university-based hospital setting, one study showed that 21.9% of patients admitted to the hospital remained NPO for 3 days or longer, with a mean duration of 5.2 days and a range of up to 16 days [22]. A second study at the same institution indicated that once feedings were initiated, a variety of factors lead to poor delivery [23]. Physicians tended to order a mean of only 65% of goal calories every day of hospitalization, a fact related to slow ramp-ups of the rate, cutting the concentration of the formula, and a reluctance to reach goal calories in a timely fashion. Cessation of EN was shown to occur in the vast majority of patients for an average of 20% of the infusion time, such that patients only received 80% of the prescribed volume of EN. The net effect of these errors was that patients only received approximately 50% of goal volume [23]. What is even more concerning is there has been little improvement over the past decade. The above mentioned study from Louisville showed specifically that in 1999 a mean 51.6% of goal calories was infused daily in the ICU setting [23]. A year later, a survey of all ICUs in Canada revealed a similar number, that patients received 55.6% of goal calories [24]. Over the next 6 years, the Canadian Practice Guidelines were developed and integrated into use all over Canada [2]. A repeat survey in January 2007 indicated that the average volume of EN infused remained unchanged at a mean 51.3% of goal calories, despite these efforts (NE Jones, R Dhaliwar, A Day, M Wang, X Jiang, DK Heyland, unpublished)

The importance of sufficient delivery of EN relates to the fact that its clinical benefits may be dose dependent. In an animal model, 50% of caloric requirements were required to maintain gut integrity and prevent increases in permeability [25]. In bone marrow transplant patients, an identical percent of requirements (50%) was required to maintain integrity and prevent increases in permeability (which in turn led to adverse outcome and systemic infection) (Demeo M, Personal Communication). In a prospective burn study by Ziegler, mentioned earlier, burn patients who developed infection received 40% of caloric requirements, whereas those burn patients who remained uninfected throughout hospitalization received 64% of caloric requirements [3]. While the exact dose required to achieve the benefits of EN may vary from one patient to the next and from one disease process to the next, it is evident that more than 50–60% of caloric

requirements may need to be infused, especially in the first few days of hospitalization, to achieve the clinical benefits from EN.

Strategies to Promote Delivery of Enteral Nutrition

Concern for ileus is a major roadblock to delivering EN. However, ileus is a vague, poorly understood process. In all practicality, ileus may represent little more than a "plumbing problem" involving segmental contractility and requiring alternative strategies for achieving and maintaining enteral access. In the absence of intestinal obstruction, clinicians should be encouraged to "feed an ileus" and be fairly aggressive in evaluating segmental contractility of the gut, determining at what level within the gut that EN needs to be infused, and whether or not the stomach needs to be simultaneously decompressed. Studies have shown that the presence of bowel sounds do not correlate to small bowel functional status. Borborygmi, abdominal pain, distension, flatus, passage of stool, are all surrogate markers of bowel function that do not correlate well to findings on formal manometric testing. Return of bowel function is the same whether an operative procedure is open or laparoscopic. The surgical factors that would be thought to affect the duration of colonic ileus (such as length of time of operation, amount of postoperative analgesia, degree of bowel handling, and duration of bowel exposure) surprisingly have little predictable impact. As studies have shown, aggressive early feeding after surgery, compared to postoperative fasting, can be expected to reduce hospital length of stay, overall infections, and risk of anastomotic leaks, even though vomiting may be increased [7]. Thus clinicians can be fairly aggressive in their efforts to minimize ileus and promote delivery of EN. Close scrutiny and correction of electrolytes help promote contractility, as does reassessment and reduction of sedation and analgesia. Naloxone 8 mg in 10 cc of saline may be infused through the feeding tube at 6-h intervals to reduce the effect of the opioid narcotics at the level of the bowel with minimal interruption of systemic analgesia [26]. In a study of critically ill patients receiving Fentanyl to reduce resistance to mechanical ventilation, patients were randomized to an infusion of naloxone or placebo through the feeding tube every 6 h [26]. For study patients given Naloxone, the amount of EN was increased significantly, gastric residual volumes were decreased significantly, and pneumonia was reduced from 56 to 34% ($P = 0.04$), compared to controls receiving placebo [26]. Minimizing the duration of ileus can be achieved by making patients NPO after 4:00 AM for early morning tests or continuing to deliver EN through radiologic tests that do not require NPO status. In a prospective study of patients with pancreatitis, minimizing the duration of ileus prior to initiating feeds improved tolerance of EN [27]. If the duration of ileus exceeded 6 days, no patients tolerated EN and all had to be placed on PN. Minimizing the ileus to less than 48 h resulted in a 92% tolerance once EN was initiated [27]. Promoting expertise in small bowel placement of feeding tubes can be done through bedside procedures by a dietitian or nurse, or through deep jejunal access by an endoscopist for patients with more severe ileus.

In a setting of sepsis, hypotension, or hypoxemia, delivery of EN must be done with caution because of the risk of ischemic bowel. The complication of bowel infarction is rare, occurring in less than 1% of patients receiving EN [28]. If clinicians are aggressive in the use of EN, sudden changes in blood pressure or oxygen levels in the blood can lead to cascade events that precipitate ischemia. Sudden changes in perfusion pressure or oxygen content first cause injury to the tips of the intestinal villi, which leads to reduced absorption of formula. Reduced contractility and bacterial overgrowth results in fermentation of unabsorbed formula, leading to gas production and distension of the intestinal wall. With increased pressure, there is decreased mucosal perfusion, and, ultimately, reduced transmural perfusion leading to bowel infarction. In a patient who is hypotensive, hypoxic, or at risk for bowel ischemia, EN should be held if the clinician is initiating pressor therapy, increasing the dose of vasopressive agents, or adding a second or third agent to the first. It may be acceptable to feed in hypotension in a patient on pressor therapy if they have been stable for 24 to 48 h and/or the clinician has begun decreasing the dose of these agents. Feedings may be started after the patient has been fully resuscitated, as evidenced by a mean arterial pressure above 65 mmHg, a mixed venous oxygen pressure ($P\bar{v}O_2$) above 60 mmHg, and a central venous pressure between 8 and 12 mmHg. Feeds would need to be held in the patient on pressor therapy if any sign of intolerance develops, such as increases in naso-gastric output, abdominal distension, new abdominal pain, or the cessation of passing flatus or stool.

Establishing an EN protocol promotes nutrient delivery (Table 12.3). A protocol which orders chlorhexidine mouthwash and aggressive oral hygiene twice per day may reduce ventilator-associated pneumonia. Having a low threshold for initiating prokinetic therapy, such as metoclopramide or erythromycin, promotes contractility and tolerance. Increasing the gastric residual volume (at which there is automatic cessation of EN) promotes

Table 12.3 Best practices for optimum nasogastric feeding.

1 Elevate head of bed 30–45° at all times

2 Scrutinize and correct electrolyte abnormalities (especially K⁺, Ca⁺⁺, Mg⁺⁺, and phosphate)

3 Initiate proton pump inhibitor IV every 8 h

4 Place nasal bridle
   Place 12 Fr NG tube into stomach
   Secure tube to bridle
   Confirm position by abdominal KUB radiograph

5 Initiate EN feeds with small peptide formula 1.0 full strength at 25 mL/h
   Advance by 25 mL/h every 12 h as tolerated to goal
   State goal feeds: _____ Kcal/d, infused at final rate ____ mL/h

6 Chlorhexidine mouthwash with good oral hygiene nursing care twice per day

7 Check GRV every 4 h
   Return all contents <500 mL to the patient
   Determine volume formula for each GRV by refractometry
   [GRV × (BV_aspirated/BV_full formula)]

8 If GRV > 400 mL initiate the following:
   Continue EN at the current rate
   Turn patient to right lateral decubitus position if possible for 30 min
   Begin metoclopramide 10 mg IV every 6 h
   Begin naloxone 8 mg in 10 mL saline per tube every 6 h
   Recheck GRV in 4 h

9 Only if 2nd GRV 4 h later is >400 mL, hold EN
   Recheck GRV every 2 h and restart EN when GRV is <400 mL
   If no other signs of intolerance, restart at same rate
   If other evidence of intolerance is present, consider reducing rate by 25 mL/h when GRV < 400 mL (or to baseline 25 mL/h)

10 If tube in small bowel and GRV > 50 mL, recheck position of tube by abdominal KUB radiograph. Consider switching to aspirate/feed NJ tube

NG, nasogastric; NJ, nasojejunal; EN, enteral nutrition; GRV, gastric residual volume; KUB, kidney, ureter, bladder; BV, Brix value.

delivery. Also, a high residual volume is often an isolated event (>80% of occasions) [29]. Ordering that EN be withheld only after a second elevated gastric residual volume 4 h later helps promote delivery [29].

Use of pharmaconutrition, in which immune modulatory agents are added to the standard enteral formula, may lead to even better outcome benefits [30]. Such formulas contain agents such as arginine (a direct immune stimulant), glutamine (which can maintain gut integrity and promote release of heat shock proteins), selected antioxidants (such as selenium, vitamin E, and vitamin C), and a mix of anti-inflammatory lipids (such as omega-3 fish oil and borage oil). Pharmaconutrition formulas have been shown to have the most consistent benefit in patients undergoing major elective surgery, where their use results in a reduction in infections from 45 to 74%, organ failure up to 79%, and length of stay in the ICU and hospital from 1.6 to 3.4 days, compared to standard formulas [30]. The benefit is more variable and less pronounced in the medical ICU patients on mechanical ventilation, where the net effect in a recent meta-analysis was shown to be limited to a reduction in hospital length of stay of 0.33 days ($P = 0.06$) and ICU length of stay of 0.36 days ($P = 0.05$) [2].

Increased utilization of gastric feeding in the ICU setting may help promote earlier initiation of EN. Clinicians have the perception that small bowel feeds are better tolerated and result in a reduction in pneumonia compared to gastric feeding. Formal studies have shown that while displacing the level of infusion lower down in the GI tract from the stomach to the small bowel probably does significantly reduce gastroesophageal reflux, and possibly aspiration of gastric contents into the lungs, the actual incidence of pneumonia is probably not reduced [31]. An early meta-analysis by Heyland of gastric versus small bowel feeds showed a significant 24% reduction in pneumonia with use of small bowel feeds [32]. Two subsequent meta-analyses, however, failed to show a significant difference [33,34]. This discrepancy can be explained by the fact that pneumonia in the ICU setting may be more closely related to aspiration of contaminated oropharyngeal secretions than reflux and aspiration of gastric contents [35]. The perception of better tolerance of small bowel feeds by clinicians is based upon the observed difference in gastric residual volumes, where small bowel feeds will have 50% lower residual volume than gastric feeds [36]. Gastric residual volumes,

however, are a poor marker of gastric emptying and are inaccurate in predicting risk of aspiration. Greater utilization of gastric feeds can be expected to result in earlier initiation of EN, by a mean of 16 h (with a range of up to 20 h) sooner than small bowel feeds [33]. Eventually, postpyloric feeds catch up, such that the time to reach goal is no different between the two routes of feeding, the mean percent of goal calories infused is no different, and the overall mean daily caloric intake is the same [33]. Thus, gastric feeds may lead to initiation of EN 1 day earlier than postpyloric feeds.

As mentioned in the section above on benefits of EN, development and instigation of an EN protocol serve to increase delivery of EN and improve patient outcome. Such a protocol should lead to achievement of enteral access, early initiation of formula infusion, rapid ramp-ups in rate, elevation of residual volume, authorization for nurses to initiate prokinetic agents, and provision of good oral hygiene.

Modification of Techniques for Deep Jejunal Access

Despite all of these strategies to promote early EN, a need for gastroenterologists and endoscopists exists to help manage the most difficult patients. Those patients with such disease processes as severe acute pancreatitis, trauma, or burns are the ones with the greatest disease severity, the most profound SIRS response, and the most persistent ileus. These patients require special techniques for deep jejunal access in order to facilitate delivery of EN. While a discussion of each of the techniques for nasoenteric and percutaneous placement of small bowel feeding tubes is beyond the scope of this chapter, a number of important caveats can be made.

Whether a tube is placed into the small bowel by blind bedside technique or by endoscopy, a nasal bridle should be utilized to secure the tube. A nasal bridle may be fashioned through the use of 5 French neonatal feeding tubes or through a commercial magnet system that allows the positioning of a ribbon in one nares, around the nasal septum, and out the other nares. Subsequent placement of the feeding tube, securing it by tape to the nasal bridle, virtually eliminates displacement (in one study, reducing displacement from 44% down to 4%, $P < 0.05$) [37].

Having a variety of techniques at one's disposal maximizes options for achievement of deep jejunal access in any number of clinical situations. A transnasal 5.5 mm diameter neonatal gastroscope or a pediatric colonoscope are the "work horses" of a busy tube service. The endoscopist should be capable of placing nasojejunal tubes at the bedside in the ICU without fluoroscopic guidance. Transport out of the ICU to the radiology or endoscopy suite results in a fourfold increase in risk of pneumonia and at least a twofold increase in the risk of some kind of mishap (such as new dysrhythmia, hypotension, or cardiopulmonary arrest) [38,39].

Repositioning the site for percutaneous endoscopic gastrostomy (PEG) tubes helps facilitate subsequent conversion to a percutaneous endoscopic gastrojejunostomy (PEGJ) if evidence of gastroparesis develops and intolerance ensues. Displacing the site from the normal left upper quadrant of the abdomen down lower to the patient's right side close to the umbilicus positions the PEG tube in the gastric antrum. In this position, there is a greater surface area and a shorter, more perpendicular approach to the gastric lumen than the more traditional site in the left upper quadrant. This new position does not appear to interfere with the falciform ligament or the antral grinding mechanism of the stomach. The combination of cutting the PEG down short to 10–15 cm with the new positioning of the tube site on the right side near the umbilicus promotes a greater length of jejunal tube within the small bowel. Specific techniques for converting a PEG to a PEGJ are discussed elsewhere (Video 10).

For more permanent deep jejunal access, a direct percutaneous endoscopic jejunostomy (DPEJ) tube should be placed. Successful placement is facilitated in thin patients with a low or normal body mass index (BMI) and in those patients who have had previous surgery (such as surgery for peptic ulcer disease) in which the duodenum has been brought out of the retroperitoneum and a reanastomosis has been made in a Billroth I or II fashion. For DPEJs in particular, a smaller (15–18 French) PEG tube with a smaller profile for the internal bolster should be utilized. In contrast to standard PEG where the choice for using the Ponsky pull technique or the Sachs–Vine push technique is inconsequential, the original Ponsky pull technique should be utilized for DPEJ. The length of the plastic leader on the end of the PEG tube used for the Sachs–Vine push technique may

not be sufficient to reach the site for small bowel access when placing the DPEJ.

The most important aspect for successful achievement of deep jejunal access is the promotion and marketing of the tube service. Expanding the practice by partnering with dieticians and nurses who can do bedside postpyloric placement helps reduce the workload that may be imposed on an endoscopist. These partners may be trained to monitor feeding tubes and identify complications before they cascade into problems that necessitate surgical intervention. Availability and making time in the endoscopic schedule for tube placement are necessary, as critical care specialists are sensitive to the timing for initiation of EN and the need to avoid delays in tube placement.

Conclusion

Gastroenterologists can play a key role in facilitating delivery of EN. By learning the techniques for enteral access placement, monitoring development of complications, and assessing ongoing tolerance of enteral nutrition, these clinicians promote EN therapy and the practice of a nutrition support team.

Take-home points

- A "window of opportunity" exists shortly after admission to the ICU during which achievement of enteral access and initiation of early enteral nutrition (EN) favorably alters patient outcome.

- The benefit of early EN is well documented in the literature by studies involving early versus delayed feeding, early EN versus standard therapy (no nutrition support), cumulative calorie deficit, and impact of EN feeding protocols.

- The physiologic benefits of early EN relate to maintaining gut integrity, sustaining the mass of gut-associated lymphoid tissue, and down-regulating systemic immune responses.

- Failure to provide early EN leads to increased gut permeability, a conduit of inflammatory mediators passing from the GI tract to the lung, and up-regulation of innate and acquired immune responses (SIRS), with clinical risk for organ failure and systemic infection.

- The most consistent outcome benefits from early EN involve decreased infectious morbidity, reduced risk for multiorgan failure, shortened duration of mechanical ventilation, and decreased ICU and hospital length of stay.

- Obstacles to delivery of early EN include concern for ileus, inappropriately low gastric residual volumes (GRVs), cessation of EN for diagnostic tests and bedside procedures, and inadvertent dislodgement of the tube.

- Delivery of EN may be promoted by early initiation and rapid ramp-up to goal rate, effectively securing the tube, "feeding an ileus", raising the cut-off level for GRVs, providing good oral hygiene, elevating the head of the bed, and having a low threshold for use of prokinetic agents.

References

1 Peng YZ, Yuan ZQ, Xiao GX. Effects of early enteral feeding on the prevention of enterogenic infection in severely burned patients. *Burns* 2001; **27**: 145–9.

2 Heyland DK, Dhaliwal R, Drover JW, *et al.* Canadian Critical Care Clinical Practice Guidelines Committee. Canadian clinical practice guidelines for nutrition support in mechanically ventilated, critically ill adult patients. *J Parenter Enteral Nutr* 2003; **27**: 355–73.

3 Ziegler TR, Smith RJ, O'Dwyer ST, *et al.* Increased intestinal permeability associated with infection in burn patients. *Arch Surg* 1988; **123**: 1313–9.

4 Jabbar A, Chang WK, Dryden GW, McClave SA. Gut immunology and the differential response to feeding and starvation. *Nutrit Clin Pract* 2003; **18**: 461–82.

5 Marik PE, Zaloga GP. Early enteral nutrition in acutely ill patients: A systematic review. *Crit Care Med* 2001; **29**: 2264–70.

6 Kudsk KA. Importance of enteral feeding in maintaining gut integrity. *Tech Gastro Endoscopy* 2001; **3**: 2–8.

7 Lewis SJ, Egger M, Sylvester PA, Thomas S. Early enteral feeding versus "nil by mouth" after gastrointestinal surgery: systematic review and meta-analysis of controlled trials. *BMJ* 2001; **323**: 773–6.

8 McClave SA, Chang WK, Dhaliwal R, Heyland DK. Nutrition support in acute pancreatitis: a systematic review of the literature. *J Parenter Enteral Nutr* 2006; **30**: 143–56.

9 Villet S, Chiolero RL, Bollmann MD, *et al.* Negative impact of hypocaloric feeding and energy balance on clinical outcome in ICU patients. *Clin Nutr* 2005; **24**: 502–9.

10 Franklin GA, McClave SA, Rosado S, *et al.* Targeted physician education positively impacts delivery of nutrition support and patient outcome. *J Parenter Enteral Nutr* 2007; **31**: S7–8.

11 Martin CM, Doig GS, Heyland DK, *et al.*; Southwestern Ontario Critical Care Research Network. Multicentre, cluster-randomized clinical trial of algorithms for critical-care enteral and parenteral therapy (ACCEPT). *Can Med Assoc J* 2004; **170**: 197–204.

12 Bistrian BR, Blackburn GL, Vitale J, *et al.* Prevalence of malnutrition in general medical patients. *JAMA* 1976; **235**: 1567–70.

13 Kudsk KA. Current aspects of mucosal immunology and its influence by nutrition. *Am J Surg* 2002; **183**: 390–8.

14 Deitch EA. Role of the gut lymphatic system in multiple organ failure. *Curr Opin Crit Care* 2001; **7**: 92–8.

15 Braunschweig CL, Levy P, Sheean PM, Wang X. Enteral compared with parenteral nutrition: a meta-analysis. *Am J Clin Nutr* 2001; **74**: 534–42.

16 Fink MP. Why the GI tract is pivotal in trauma, sepsis, and MOF. *J Crit Illness* 1991; **6**: 253–69.

17 Doig CJ, Sutherland LR, Sandham JD *et al.* Increased intestinal permeability is associated with the development of multiple organ dysfunction syndrome in critically ill ICU patients. *Am J Respir Crit Care Med* 1998; **158**: 444–51.

18 Dobbins WO. Gut immunophysiology: a gastroenterologist's view with emphasis on pathophysiology. *Am J Physiol* 1982; **242**: G1–8.

19 Ammori BJ, Leeder PC, King RF, *et al.* Early increase in intestinal permeability in patients with severe acute pancreatitis: correlation with endotoxemia, organ failure, and mortality. *J Gastrointest Surg* 1999; **3**: 252–62.

20 Spiekermann GM, Walker WA. Oral tolerance and its role in clinical disease. *J Pediatr Gastroent Nutr* 2001; **32**: 237–55.

21 Fukatsu K, Lundberg AH, Hanna MK, *et al.* Increased expression of intestinal P-selectin and pulmonary E-selectin during intravenous total parenteral nutrition. *Arch Surg* 2000; **135**: 1177–82.

22 Franklin G, McClave SA, Lowen C, *et al.* Physician-delivered malnutrition: Why do patients remain NPO or on clear liquids in a university hospital setting? *J Parenter Enteral Nutr* 2006; **30**: S32–3.

23 McClave SA, Sexton LK, Spain DA, *et al.* Enteral tube feeding in the intensive care unit: Factors impeding adequate delivery. *Crit Care Med* 1999; **27**: 1252–6.

24 Heyland DK, Schroter-Noppe D, Drover JW, *et al.* Nutrition support in the critical care setting: current practice in Canadian ICUs–opportunities for improvement? *J Parenter Enteral Nutr* 2003; **27**: 74–83.

25 Nelson JL, Alexander JW, Gianotti L, *et al.* High protein diets are associated with increased bacterial translocation in septic guinea pigs. *Nutrition* 1996; **12**: 195–9.

26 Meissner W, Dohrn B, Reinhart K. Enteral naloxone reduces gastric tube reflux and frequency of pneumonia in critical care patients during opioid analgesia. *Crit Care Med* 2003; **31**: 776–80.

27 Cravo M, Camilo ME, Marques A, Pinto Correa J. Early tube feeding in acute pancreatitis. A prospective study. *Clin Nutrit* 1989; **8** (Suppl.): 14.

28 Scaife CL, Saffle JR, Morris SE. Intestinal obstruction secondary to enteral feedings in burn trauma patients. *J Trauma* 1999; **47**: 859–63.

29 McClave SA, Snider HL, Lowen CC, *et al.* Use of residual volume as a marker for enteral feeding intolerance: prospective blinded comparison with physical examination and radiographic findings. *J Parenter Enteral Nutr* 1992; **16**: 99–105.

30 Montejo JC, Zarazaga A, Lopez-Martinez J, *et al.*; Spanish Society of Intensive Care Medicine and Coronary Units. Immunonutrition in the intensive care unit. A systematic review and consensus statement. *Clin Nutr* 2003; **22**: 221–33.

31 Heyland DK, Drover JW, MacDonald S, *et al.* Effect of post-pyloric feeding on gastroesophageal regurgitation and pulmonary microaspiration: results of a randomized controlled trial. *Crit Care Med* 2001; **29**: 1495–501.

32 Heyland DK, Drover JW, Dhaliwal R, Greenwood J. Optimizing the benefits and minimizing the risks of enteral nutrition in the critically ill: role of small bowel feeding. *J*

Parenter Enteral Nutr 2002; **26** (6 Suppl.): S51–5; discussion S56–7.

33 Marik PE, Zaloga GP. Gastric versus post-pyloric feeding: a systematic review. *Crit Care* 2003; **7**: R46–51.

34 Ho KM, Dobb GJ, Webb SA. A comparison of early gastric and post-pyloric feeding in critically ill patients: A meta-analysis. *Intens Care Med* 2006; **32**: 639–49.

35 Bonten MJ, Gaillard CA, van Tiel FH, *et al.* The stomach is not a source for colonization of the upper respiratory tract and pneumonia in ICU patients. *Chest* 1994; **105**: 878–84.

36 Davies AR, Froomes PR, French C, *et al.* Nasojejunal feeding leads to less gastric residual volume than nasogastric feeding in critically ill patients (abstract). *Am J Respir Crit Care Med* 2000; **161**: A92.

37 Brand CP, Mittendorf EA. Endoscopic placement of nasojejunal feeding tubes in ICU patients. *Surg Endosc* 1999; **13**: 1211–14.

38 Smith I, Fleming S, Cernaianu A. Mishaps during transport from the intensive care unit. *Crit Care Med* 1990; **18**: 278–81.

39 Kollef MH, Von Harz B, Prentice D, *et al.* Patient transport from intensive care increases the risk of developing ventilator-associated pneumonia. *Chest* 1997; **112**: 765–73.

CHAPTER 13

Foreign Bodies in the Esophagus and Stomach

Gregory G. Ginsberg

Division of Gastroenterology, University of Pennsylvania Health Systems, Philadelphia, PA, USA

Summary

Foreign bodies in the esophagus and stomach are comprised of intentionally and unintentionally ingested foreign objects (IFO) and food bolus impactions (FBI). Esophageal and gastric IFO/FBIs are fairly common conditions prompting gastroenterological consultation. While most IFO/FBIs resolve with no sequelae, they may result in life-threatening consequences. A number of conditions can promote clinical presentation with IFO/FBIs. This chapter reviews the evaluation and management of patients with suspected IFO/FBI with an emphasis on the endoscopic tools and techniques for relief from IFO/FBI in the esophagus and stomach.

Case

An edentulous, 52-year-old, alcoholic male goes with some of his drinking buddies to see the world champion Philadelphia Phillies play. They are eating and drinking and having a good time. While sipping his fifth beer and eating his second Philly Dog , Shane Victorino comes to the plate with the Phillies trailing 5–3 in the sixth and hits a basesloaded triple to put the Phillies ahead. In his excitement he gulps down the hotdog and, before the "Flyin' Hawaiian" can get to third base, he feels the hotdog stick in the area of his lower esophagus. It does not pass despite further attempts to "float it down" with more brew. His buddies attempt the Heimlich maneuver but there is no improvement. An hour later, with the Phillies comfortably ahead 9–5 in the ninth, they take him to the closest hospital.

At the time of the evaluation he develops more chest discomfort and, despite retching and vomiting, the hotdog seems to remain lodged in his esophagus. Radiographs of the chest and abdomen show no abnormalities and his lab work is normal, except for elevated transaminases. The emergency room physician calls the gastroenterologist on call who assesses the patient and decides to perform an endoscopy because the patient is having difficulty with his secretions. In addition, the patient is inebriated so he asks that the procedure be done with anesthesiology support. Prior to the procedure he reviews the plan he will likely pursue with the Endoscopy Team and makes certain that all the needed endoscopic accessories are at hand. At the time of the procedure he sees the partially digested hot dog lodged in the patient's distal esophagus, seemingly impacted at 37 cm. He is not able to guide the endoscope around the food into the lower esophagus.

He is comforted that the patient's airway is protected and he uses a "banding device" to suction the hotdog into the cap and removes it from the esophagus. He then examines the area where the "dog" had been lodged and finds a Schatzki ring. He then dilates the ring and schedules the patient for follow-up in his office. The patient does not keep the appointment but the physician feels that the cause of the food impaction has been defined and sends a letter to the patient and his primary caregiver defining the next steps.

Practical Gastroenterology and Hepatology: Esophagus and Stomach, 1st edition. Edited by Nicholas J. Talley, Kenneth R. DeVault and David E. Fleischer. © 2010 Blackwell Publishing Ltd.

Introduction

Foreign bodies in the esophagus and stomach are comprised of intentionally and unintentionally ingested foreign objects (IFO) and food bolus impactions (FBI). Esophageal and gastric IFO/FBIs are fairly common GI emergencies, occurring with an estimated 16 cases per 100 000 population. Most (80–90%) of IFO/FBIs pass spontaneously, however, 10–20% require endoscopic and 1% operative intervention. Moreover, there is risk for serious consequences, including perforation and death [1].

Epidemiology

Foreign object ingestion occurs most commonly in children, particularly those between ages 6 months and 3 years [2]. Children's natural oral curiosity leads to placing objects in the mouth. Coins are the most common IFO in children but other frequently swallowed objects include small toys, crayons, hair accessories, etc.

Unintentional IFO occurs in adults with compromised oral sensation attributed to dental prosthetics, including the swallowing one's own dentures (Figure 13.1). Unintentional IFO occurs in adults with altered mental status, including dementia and inebriation. Certain occupations, such as roofers, carpenters, and seamstresses, are at risk of accidental IFO when nails or pins are held in the mouth.

Intentional IFO occurs most commonly in incarcerated adults and psychiatric patients seeking some secondary gain [3]. These patients not uncommonly ingest multiple objects, do so on multiple occasions, and often ingest the most complex foreign bodies.

Esophageal FBI tends to occur in patients with underlying predisposing structural or functional esophageal pathology [4]. The most common underlying esophageal pathology contributing to FBI are peptic strictures, Schatzki rings and, increasingly, eosinophilic esophagitis [5]. Other contributor causes of esophageal food impactions are altered surgical anatomy secondary to esophagectomy, fundoplication, or bariatric surgery and motility disorders, such as achalasia and diffuse esophageal spasm. Cultural and regional dietary habits influence esophageal food ingestion complications. Fish bone injuries are more common in countries along the Pacific Rim,

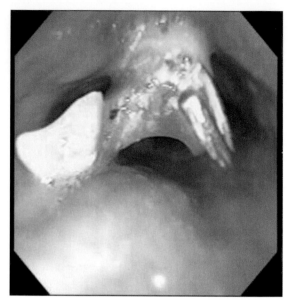

Figure 13.1 Accidentally ingested dental bridge work lodged in the mid-esophagus.

whereas meat impactions, including hot dogs, pork, beef, and chicken, are more common in the United States [6].

Pathophysiology

Perforation and obstruction from IFO/FBI can occur in any part of the digestive tract but are more apt to occur in areas of physiologic narrowing, acute angulation, anatomic sphincters, or prior surgery. In the hypopharynx short, sharp objects such as fish bones and toothpicks may lacerate or become lodged. Once in the esophagus there are four areas of noted narrowing, including the upper esophageal sphincter, level of the aortic arch, level of the main stem bronchus, and the gastroesophageal junction where food boluses and true foreign bodies become lodged. These areas all are true luminal narrowings of 23 mm or less.

History and Physical Examination

The history from children or non-communicative adults is often unreliable. The majority of gastric and up to

20–30% of esophageal foreign bodies in children are asymptomatic. Most of these present having been witnessed or suspected by a parent, caregiver or older sibling. However, in up to 40% of cases there is no history of a witnessed ingestion [7]. Symptoms are thus often subtle in children presenting as drooling, not wanting to eat, and failure to thrive.

For communicative adults, history of the timing and type of ingestion is usually reliable. Patients are able to relate exactly what they ingested, when they ingested it and symptoms of pain or/and obstruction. Patients with esophageal FBI are symptomatic with complete or intermittent obstruction. They are unable to drink liquids or retain their own oral secretions. Sialorrhea is common. Ingestion of an unappreciated, small, sharp object, including obscured fish or animal bones, may cause odynophagia or a persistent foreign body sensation due to mucosal laceration.

The type of symptoms can aid in determining if an esophageal foreign object is still present or not. If the patient presents with dysphagia, odynophagia, or dysphonia there is an 80% likelihood a foreign body is present, causing at least partial obstruction. Symptoms of drooling and inability to handle secretions are indicative of a near total obstruction of the esophagus. If the symptoms are only retrosternal chest pain or pharyngeal discomfort, less than 50% of these patients will still have a persistently present IFO/FBI.

Patient localization of where an ingested foreign object is lodged is poorly accurate, with only a 30–40% correct localization in the esophagus and essentially a 0% accuracy for foreign bodies in the stomach [8]. Once in the stomach, small intestine, and colon the patient will not report symptoms unless a complication occurs, such as obstruction, perforation, or bleeding caused by the foreign body.

Physical examination does little to secure the diagnosis or location of a retained foreign body. However, physical examination is crucial to identify already developed complications related to foreign body ingestion. Assessment of the patient's airway, ventillatory status, and risk for aspiration are crucial prior to initiating therapy to remove an IFO/FBI. A neck and chest exam looking for crepitus, erythrema, and swelling can suggest a proximal perforation. An abdominal exam should be performed to evaluate for signs of perforation or obstruction.

Diagnosis

Radiography

Plain films of the chest and abdomen are recommended in patients presenting with suspected FBI to determine the presence, type, number, and location of foreign objects present. Both anteroposterior films and lateral films are needed as lateral films will aid in determining if a foreign body is in the esophagus versus the trachea and may detail foreign bodies that are obscured by overlying spine in AP films. Bi-planar neck films are recommended if there is a suspected object or complication in the hypopharynx or cervical esophagus (Figure 13.2) Plain films are also useful in identifying complications such as free air, aspirations, or subcutaneous emphysema.

However, radiography is unable to diagnose radiolucent objects such as plastic, glass, or wood and may miss small bones or metal objects. The false-negative rate for plain film investigation of IFOs is as high as 47% with false-positive rates up to 20%. Thus anyone with a continued clinical suspicion or symptoms should undergo further clinical investigation [9].

Contrast radiographic studies are not recommended in the evaluation of IFO/FBIs. Aspiration of hypertonic contrast agents in patients with complete or near complete esophageal obstruction may lead to aspiration pneumonitis [10]. Further, oral radiographic contrast agents may delay or impair the performance of a therapeutic endoscopic intervention by interfering with endoscopic visualization. Finally, even if a barium study is considered normal an endoscopy is still recommended if symptoms persist or the suspicion of a foreign body is high.

Advanced imaging such as computed tomography (CT) or magnetic resonance imaging rarely is needed in the diagnosis of GIFBs. However, CT has been found to detect foreign bodies missed by other modalities [11] and may aid in detecting complications of foreign body ingestion such as perforation or abscess prior to the use of endoscopy [12].

Endoscopy

Flexible endoscopy is the most precise means to diagnose suspected IFO/FBI. This ensures a near 100% diagnosis accuracy for objects within the reach of the endoscope, including non-radio-opaque objects and objects obscured by overlying bony structures not seen by radiography.

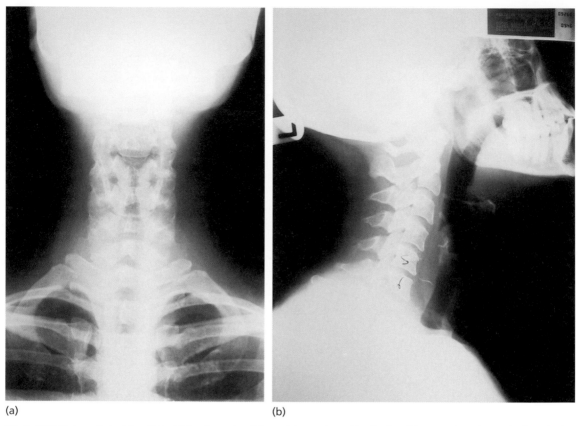

(a)   (b)

Figure 13.2 Posteroanterior (a) and lateral (b) radiographs of the neck in a patient with a foreign object sensation. The retained metal wire is seen only on the lateral film anterior to cervical vertebrae 5–6.

Endoscopy also provides the most accurate diagnosis of underlying pathology that may have contributed to IFO/FBI and mucosal injury that may have resulted. Of course, diagnostic endoscopy is also linked to therapeutic endoscopy to remove or treat IFO/FBI.

Treatment

Flexible endoscopy has become the treatment of choice for management of IFO/FBI because it is safe and highly efficacious. Multiple, large series have reported the success rate for endoscopic treatment to be greater than 95% with complication rates of less than 5% [13–16]. The risk for complications is increased when sharp objects are ingested, when multiple objects are ingested, and when the ingestion is intentional as opposed to accidental.

As most IFO/FBI pass spontaneously without causing symptoms it is important to understand the indications and timing for endoscopic intervention. Generally, all foreign bodies lodged in the esophagus require urgent intervention. The risk for an adverse outcome from an esophageal foreign body or food impaction is directly related to the time the object or food dwells in the esophagus [17]. Ideally, no object should be left in the esophagus for greater than 24 hours.

Once in the stomach most ingested objects will pass spontaneously and the risks of complications is much lower, thus making observation acceptable except in the notable circumstances described as follows. Sharp and pointed objects are associated with perforation rates as high as 15–35% [17]. Longer objects, more than 5 cm in length, and round objects more than 2 cm in diameter also may not be passed and should be removed from the stomach with an endoscope at presentation or if they have not progressed in 3–5 days. If a more complex or sharp object has progressed beyond the stomach and cannot be retrieved, periodic radiographs should be obtained to document progression through the GI tract [18]. The patient should then be followed for any symptom suggestive of obstruction or perforation such as fever, tachycardia, abdominal pain, or distension.

The type of sedation selected to facilitate endoscopy in the management of food impactions and ingested foreign objects should be individualized. While conscious sedation is adequate for the treatment of most food impactions and simple foreign bodies in the adult population, anesthesia assistance may be required for uncooperative patients or patients who have swallowed multiple, complex objects.

Availability of, and familiarity with, multiple endoscopic retrieval devices for the removal of foreign bodies and food impactions is valuable. A grasping forceps, polypectomy snare, Dormia basket and retrieval net should be available. Oroesophageal overtubes allow protection of the airway, multiple exchanges of the endoscope and mucosal protection during retrieval of sharp or pointed objects. A commercially available 50-cm overtube enables retrieval of sharp and complex objects from the stomach, bypassing the lower esophageal sphincter. An alternative adjunct for extraction of sharp objects is a latex protection hood which fits onto the tip of the endoscope.

Food Bolus Impaction

Food impaction is the most common ingested "foreign body" in the United States. Given that food boluses may pass spontaneously, the need for endoscopic intervention is based on the persistence of symptoms. Patients with signs of complete or near complete obstruction with drooling or excessive salivation should undergo urgent endoscopy. Endoscopic intervention should be performed, at the latest, within 24 h of onset of symptoms and more ideally within the first 6–12 h. Increased risk for complications is thought to be proportional to duration of esophageal food impaction [19–21].

 Most FBIs can be safely relieved with a gentle push using air insufflation and the tip of the endoscope [22] (Video 11). Before an FBI is pushed an attempt should be made to steer the tip of the endoscope around the food bolus. Generally, if the endoscope can be passed around the FBI and into the stomach the bolus can be disrupted and can be safely pushed into the stomach without dif-

ficulty. This also allows assessment of any obstructive esophageal pathology beyond the food impaction. Even if the endoscope can not steer around the food impaction, *gentle* pushing pressure can be safely attempted. Larger boluses of impacted meat must be broken apart with the endoscope or an accessory prior to safely pushing the smaller pieces into the stomach.

Food impactions that cannot be gently pushed into the stomach must be dislodged and withdrawn. Retrograde removal can be achieved with various retrieval devices including snares, baskets, and forceps. Initial manual disruption of the food bolus into smaller pieces typically makes removal easier. An oroesophageal overtube is again useful in such cases as it protects the airway and allows multiple exchanges of the endoscope during retrieval. A dedicated food bolus retrieval net can be useful in removing large pieces of food without the use of an overtube because the food can be satisfactorily secured within the net, thus reducing the risk of aspiration of the ingestate.

Transparent plastic hoods or caps like those used to perform variceal band ligation and endoscopic mucosal resection have been used successfully for the removal of large, tightly impacted meat boluses. With the cap secured to the tip of the endoscope, the device can be used to suction the food into the vacuum chamber and then withdraw the bolus per os.

If an esophageal stricture or Schatzki ring is present after the food bolus is cleared it can be safely and effectively dilated concurrently if circumstances allow. More often, dilation is delayed for 2–4 weeks, during which time patients should be prescribed proton pump inhibitor therapy. When multiple esophageal rings are present, biopsies should be obtained to evaluate for eosinophillic esophagitis.

Sharp and Pointed Objects

Ingested sharp/pointed objects include such items as fish and animal bones, toothpicks, dental bridgework, pins and needles, broken glass and razorblades. Sharp/pointed objects are the most likely ingested foreign objects to cause a perforation and/or need for operative management. Sharp/pointed objects retained in the esophagus are considered a medical emergency and should be removed expeditiously. Moreover, any sharp/pointed object within the reach of the endoscope should be removed if it can be safely executed. When removing sharp/pointed objects the foreign body should be grasped and oriented so that the pointed end trails on withdrawal to reduce the risk of perforation and mucosal laceration

For sharp and pointed objects retrieval is best achieved with a grasping forceps, polypectomy snare, or biliary stone retrieval basket. All of these devices can secure the object and orient it as described above. Use of a 25-cm or 50-cm overtube should be considered to protect the esophagus and oropharynx. Long, pointed objects can be grasped and directed into the overtube, and then the entire assembly, including the sharp/pointed object, the endoscope, and the overtube, are removed in unison (Figure 13.3).

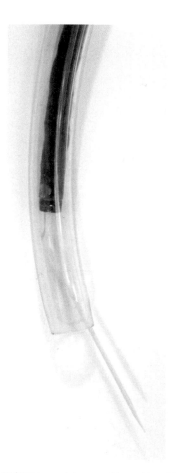

Figure 13.3 Endoscope-overtube assembly used to retrieve long, sharp and pointed objects while avoiding mucosal and mural injury. The object should be withdrawn into the overtube and then the entire assemble removed as one.

An alternative to an overtube for the extraction of sharp and pointed objects is a retractable latex hood that can be affixed to the tip of the endoscope. When the endoscope is pulled back through the lower esophageal sphincter the hood flips over the grasped object and protects the mucosa during withdrawal.

Though associated with an increased risk of perforation, most sharp or pointed objects beyond reach of the endoscope will pass unimpeded and be eliminated through the GI tract without complication. Because of the increased risk of perforation, sharp/pointed objects should be followed by serial daily radiographs to ensure progression. If a sharp/pointed object fails to progress over 3 days, operative intervention should be considered.

Long Objects

Ingested objects longer than 5–10 cm have difficulty passing through the pylorus and duodenal sweep and can get hung up, causing obstruction or perforation at these locations. The most commonly ingested long objects are pens, pencils, toothbrushes, and eating utensils. Grasping forceps and polypectomy snares are the most commonly used devices to secure and long objects. Long objects should be grasped at one end and oriented longitudinally to permit removal. For extraction of long objects use of the 50-cm overtube–endoscope assembly, as described above, should be considered.

Blunt Objects—Coins, Button Batteries, Magnets, and Bread Tabs

Small, blunt objects such as pieces of toys and coins are the most common objects ingested by children. Button battery and magnet ingestions are uncommon but pose unique potential dangers. Blunt objects in the esophagus should be removed promptly. Impacted coins can result in pressure necrosis of the esophageal wall, resulting in perforation and fistula. Any size coin can become lodged in the esophagus of children but ingested coins, in particular dimes and pennies measuring 17 and 18 mm, will usually pass through the adult esophagus.

Polyp retrieval nets allow secure capture and removal of most ingested blunt objects. Grasping forceps and biliary stone retrieval baskets are also effective. Blunt objects in the esophagus may be pushed into the stomach where there is more room to negotiate.

Once a small, blunt object enters the stomach, conservative outpatient management is appropriate in most patients. Exceptions to this include patients with surgically altered digestive tract anatomy and those who have ingested large, blunt objects. In adults, the pylorus will allow passage of most blunt objects up to 25 mm in girth, which includes all coins except half-dollars (30 mm) and silver dollars (38 mm). Otherwise, once in the stomach a regular diet may be resumed with radiographic monitoring every 1 to 2 weeks to confirm progression or elimination. If after 3–4 weeks a blunt object has not passed, endoscopic removal should be performed [23].

Button disc batteries are now contained in many small toys and electronic devices accessible to young children. Because batteries contain alkaline solution, liquification necrosis can occur when lodged in the esophagus. Button battery ingestion occurs most commonly in younger children but as few as 10% will be symptomatic. Therefore any clinical suspicion of a button battery in the esophagus should prompt investigation. Grasping forceps and snares are generally ineffective for button disc battery removal but use of retrieval net permits successful extraction in close to 100%. Once in the stomach or small intestine button batteries rarely cause clinical problems and can be observed radiographically with 85% passing within 72 h [24].

Small, brightly colored, coupling magnets have become popular as children's toys. Ingested magnets within the reach of the endoscope should also be removed on an urgent basis. While a single magnet will rarely be a cause of symptoms, concern exists if multiple magnets are ingested or if magnets were ingested with other metal objects. This can result in magnetic attraction and coupling between interposed loops of bowel with subsequent pressure necrosis, fistula formation, and bowel perforation [25,26]. Removal should be performed urgently when the magnets are more apt to be within reach of a standard endoscope and can be achieved with grasping forceps, retrieval net or basket. Magnetic attraction to metallic retrieval devices may ease the task of removal.

Bread tabs or bread bag clips are another otherwise seemingly innocuous blunt object that when ingested (usually unknowingly) have been associated with a high risk for gastrointestinal tract complications [27]. Bleeding, bowel obstruction, and perforation have all been described. The small bowel is the most common site of impaction where the arms of the clip tenaciously grasp the mucosa. Management is problematic in that ingestion is typically not detected until complications arise. Bread bag clips are radiolucent and as such are not detected by conventional radiography. When recognized at endoscopy an attempt at removal is justified using a gasping forceps, however, operative intervention is commonly required.

Narcotic Packets

Ingested packets of illicit narcotics in the GI tract present in two general groups, "body stuffers" and "body packers". Body stuffers refers to drug users or traffickers who, in an effort to avoid detection, quickly ingest small amounts of drugs, but in poorly wrapped or contained packages that are prone to leakage. Body packers are the "mules" used by drug smugglers to ingest large quantities of carefully prepared packages intended to withstand GI transit [28]. These patients may present with intestinal obstruction because of the packages or symptoms related to the drug ingested. The later may result in serious toxicology and death in 5% [29].

Suspected patients are typically uncooperative and accompanied by law enforcement agents. Diagnosis is initiated with plain film radiology or CT scan with multiple round or tube-shaped packets seen. Endoscopic removal is contraindicated due to the high risk of package perforation resulting toxicological emergency. Observation on a clear liquid diet is recommended. Operative intervention is indicated when bowel obstruction or drug leakage are suspected.

Complications

IFO/FBI in the esophagus have the highest incidence of overall adverse events with the complication rate being directly proportional to the duration the object is lodged in the esophagus. Serious complications of esophageal foreign bodies include perforation, abscess, mediastinitis, pneumothorax, fistula formation, and cardiac tamponade.

While the reported complication rate associated with endoscopic removal of gastrointestinal foreign bodies and food impactions is low ($0^-1.8\%$) it is thought to be much higher in practice [4,16]. While perforation is the most feared complication, aspiration and sedation-related cardiopulmonary complications may also occur.

Features that increase the risk for complications include removal of sharp and pointed objects, an uncooperative patient, multiple ingestions, deliberate ingestions, and extended duration of time from food impaction or foreign body ingestion [30].

Take-home points

- Esophageal and gastric ingested foreign objects (IFO) and food bolus impactions (FBI) are fairly common conditions prompting gastroenterological consultation.

- Foreign object ingestion occurs most commonly in children, particularly those between ages 6 months and 3 years.

- Perforation and obstruction from IFO/FBI can occur in any part of the digestive tract but are more apt to occur in areas of physiologic narrowing, acute angulation, anatomic sphincters, or prior surgery.

- Plain films of the chest and abdomen are recommended in patients presenting with suspected FBI to determine the presence, type, number, and location of foreign objects present.

- Flexible endoscopy is the most precise means to diagnose and treat suspected IFO/FBI.

- The risk for complications is increased when sharp objects are ingested, when multiple objects are ingested, and when the ingestion is intentional as opposed to accidental.

- Generally, all foreign bodies lodged in the esophagus require urgent intervention.

- Once in the stomach, most ingested objects will pass spontaneously.

- Before attempting to remove a foreign body, it is valuable for the endoscopist to practice the anticipated removal with the endoscopic team, utilizing the expected endoscopic accessories and, if possible, an object that is identical to or similar to the foreign body.

References

1 Eisen GM, Baron TH, Dominitz JA, *et al.* Guideline for the management of ingested foreign bodies. *Gastrointest Endosc* 2002; **55**: 802–6.

2 Chen MK, Beierle EA. Gastrointestinal foreign bodies. *Pediatr Ann* 2001; **30**: 736–42

3 O'Sullivan ST, McGreal GT, Reardon CM, *et al.* Selective endoscopy in management of ingested foreign bodies of the upper gastrointestinal tract: is it safe? *Int J Clin Pract* 1997; **51**: 289–92.

4 Vicari JJ, Johanson JF, Frakes JT. Outcomes of acute esophageal food impaction: success of the push technique. *Gastrointest Endosc* 2001; **53**: 178–81.

5 Kerlin P, Jones D, Remedios M, *et al.* Prevalence of eosinophillic esophagitis in adults with food bolus obstruction of the esophagus. *J Clin Gastroenterol* 2007; **41**: 356–61.

6 Lin HH, Lee SC, Chu HC, *et al.* Emergency endoscopic management of dietary foreign bodies in the esophagus. *Am J Emerg Med* 2007; **25**: 662–5.

7 Muniz AE, Joffe MD. Foreign bodies, ingested and inhaled. *JAAPA* 1999; **12**: 23–46.

8 Lee J. Bezoars and foreign bodies of the stomach. *Gastrointest Endosc Clin North Am* 1996; **6**: 605–19.

9 Ciriza C, Garcia L, Suarez P, *et al.* What predictive parameters best indicate the need for emergent gastrointestinal endoscopy after foreign body ingestion? *J Clin Gastroenterol* 2000; **31**: 23–8.

10 Mosca S, Manes G, Martino L, *et al.* Endoscopic management of foreign bodies in the upper gastrointestinal tract: report on a series of 414 adult patients. *Endoscopy* 2001; **33**: 692–6.

11 Takada M, Kashiwagi R, Sakane M, *et al.* 3D-CT Diagnosis for ingested foreign bodies. *Am J Emerg Med* 2000; **18**: 192–3.

12 Silva RG, Ahluwaiia JP. Asymptomatic esophageal perforation after foreign body ingestion. *Gastrointest Endosc* 2005; **61**: 615–9.

13 Wong KKY, Fang CX, Tam PHK. Selective upper endoscopy for foreign body ingestion in children: an evaluation of management protocol after 282 cases. *J Pediat Surg* 2006; **41**: 2016–18.

14 Katsinelos P, Kountouras J, Paroutoglou G, *et al.* Endoscopic techniques and management of foreign body ingestion and food bolus impaction in the upper gastrointestinal tract: A retrospective analysis of 139 cases. *J Clin Gastroenterol* 2006; **40**: 784–9.

15 Conway WC, Sugawa C, Ono H, *et al.* Upper GI foreign body: An adult urban emergency hospital experience. *Surg Endosc* 2007; **21**: 455–60.

16 Mosca S. Management and endoscopic techniques in cases of ingestion of foreign bodies. *Endoscopy* 2000; **32**: 232–3.

17 Henderson CT, Engel J, Schlesinger P. Foreign body ingestion: Review and suggested guidelines for management. *Endoscopy* 1987; **19**: 68–71.

18 Macgregor D, Ferguson J. Foreign body ingestion in children: an audit of transit time. *J Accid Emerg Med* 1998; **15**: 371–3.

19 Ginsberg GG. Management of ingested foreign objects and food bolus impactions. *Gastrointest Endosc* 1995; **41**: 33–8.

20 Chaves DM, Ishioka S, Felix VN, *et al.* Removal of a foreign body from the upper gastrointestinal tract with a flexible

endoscope: a prospective study. *Endoscopy* 2004; **36**: 887–92.

21 Smith MT, Wong RKH. Foreign bodies. *Gastrointest Endosc Clin N Am* 2007; **17**: 361–82.

22 Vicari JJ, Johanson JF, Frakes JT. Outcomes of acute esophageal food impaction: success of the push technique. *Gastrointest Endosc* 2001; **53**: 178–81.

23 Rebhandl W, Milassin A, Brunner L, *et al.* In vitro study of ingested coins: leave them or retrieve them? *J Pediat Surg* 2007; **42**: 1729–34.

24 Litovitz TL, Schmitz BF. Ingestion of cylindrical and button batteries. An analysis of 2382 cases. *Pediatrics* 1992; **89**: 1992.

25 Alzakem AM, Soundappan SSV, Jefferies H, *et al.* Ingested magnets and gastrointestinal complications. *J Paediatr Child H* 2007; **40**: 497–8.

26 Gastrointestinal injuries from magnet ingestion in children—United States, 2003–2006. *MMWR* 2006: 1296–300.

27 Morrissey SK, Thakar SJ, Weaver ML, Farah K. Bread bag clip ingestion: a rare cause of upper gastrointestinal bleeding. *Gastroenterol Hepatol* 2008; **4**: 409–500.

28 Pidoto RR, Agliata AM, Bertolini R, *et al.* A new method of packaging cocaine for international traffic and implication for the management of cocaine body packers. *J Emerg Med* 2002; **23**: 149–53.

29 June R, Aks SE, Keys N, *et al.* Medical outcome of cocaine bodystuffers. *J Emerg Med* 2000; **18**: 221–4.

30 Tokar B, Cevik A, Ihan H. Ingested gastrointestinal foreign bodies: predisposing factors for complications in children having surgical or endoscopic removal. *Pediatr Surg Int* 2007; **23**: 135–9.

CHAPTER 14
Endoluminal Surgery (NOTES)

C. Daniel Smith

Department of Surgery, Mayo Clinic, Jacksonville, FL, USA

Summary

Natural orifice transluminal endoscopic surgery (NOTES) is an extension of endoluminal surgery and is a novel technique using the body's natural orifices to access the peritoneal or thoracic cavity to perform operations. The goal is to perform these intraperitoneal or intrathoracic operations safely through a natural orifice, perhaps even outside the operating room setting, and to avoid the pain and recovery associated with incisions and any potential complications such as wound infection or herniation. NOTES became possible due to the advances in therapeutic endoscopy and a 2003 video from India showing an appendectomy performed through a transoral approach. The American Society of Gastrointestinal Endoscopy (ASGE) and the Society of American Gastrointestinal and Endoscopic Surgery (SAGES) collaborate through the Natural Orifice Surgery Consortium for Assessment and Research (NOSCAR) to help guide the safe and responsible development and implementation of NOTES. Research into NOTES focuses on the barriers to safe NOTES introduction. Recent human experiences with NOTES, particularly transvaginal cholecystectomy, are fueling intense interest in human applications. Many remain skeptical about its viability as a new surgical technique.

Definitions

Although natural orifice translumenal endoscopic surgery (NOTES) is an extension of endoluminal surgery, the terms "NOTES" and "endoluminal surgery" define different approaches and deserve differentiation.

Endoluminal surgery is simply operations performed within the lumen of the gastrointestinal tract through an endoscope. Over the past two decades the term "endoluminal surgery" has been used to describe a variety of approaches to managing gastrointestinal conditions using some form of endoscopy—flexible intraluminal endoscopy, laparoscopy, or a combination of both. Initially, endoluminal surgery simply described what is now considered very basic therapeutic endoscopy and was limited to interventions such as polypectomy and ligation of esophageal varices. As the capabilities of therapeutic endoscopy advanced, it came to include transluminal approaches such as transgastric approaches for pancreatic pathology or full-thickness excision for rectal disease. At this point endoluminal surgery was limited to interventions within the lumen of the gastrointestinal (GI) tract or to immediate peri-intestinal structures.

Concurrent with the development of the interventional capabilities of flexible endoscopy, the modern use of laparoscopy was evolving and GI surgeons began to use endoluminal surgery to describe transperitoneal laparoscopic access to the GI tract for resection and management of intraluminal conditions not readily managed with a transorally passed flexible endoscopic. Most uses were focused on gastric access and management of gastric pathology or transgastric access to pancreatic pathology.

Most recently, endoluminal surgery describes surgical procedures performed with a flexible endoscope without ever entering the peritoneal cavity. Current examples include procedures such as antireflux surgery or bariatric surgery. Put differently, the current use of the term "endoluminal surgery" defines surgical procedures that

Practical Gastroenterology and Hepatology: Esophagus and Stomach, 1st edition. Edited by Nicholas J. Talley, Kenneth R. DeVault and David E. Fleischer. © 2010 Blackwell Publishing Ltd.

can now be performed entirely within the lumen of the GI tract. This is in contrast to NOTES, which by definition is leaving the GI tract to enter the peritoneal or thoracic cavity to perform extraluminal procedures.

NOTES History

The concept of using a flexible endoscope to exit the lumen of the GI tract, thereby gaining access to structures outside the GI tract, is not particularly new. Endoscopic management of pancreatic pseudocysts was developed in the 1980s and likely represents the first use of NOTES [1]. Similarly, transanal approaches for full-thickness resection of rectal tumors was first described in 1986 [2]. In the early 2000s a surgeon performed a laparoscopic cholecystectomy and then made a gastrostomy to remove the gall bladder through the patient's mouth using a flexible endoscope. At that time, the concept of breaching the GI tract to gain access to the peritoneal cavity was largely rejected.

In 2003, a video produced from India showing an appendectomy performed via a transoral, transgastric approach using a flexible endoscope was informally circulated around the world. This provoked many thought leaders to rethink this novel concept and soon after the concept of performing intraperitoneal procedures through natural orifices, i.e., NOTES, was officially introduced [3].

Since that time there has been an increased interest in NOTES evidenced by the proliferation of citations in the medical literature dealing with the topic (Figure 14.1). Of the 162 citations in the English literature through 2008, approximately 40% are position papers, commentaries, editorials, or review articles. The remainder are small series of animal work and case reports in humans. Only a few publications actually deal with the foundational issues of NOTES (see below).

NOTES Principles

The concept of NOTES is a novel technique using the body's natural orifices to access the peritoneal or thoracic cavity to perform surgery. The goal is to perform intraperitoneal or intrathoracic surgery safely through a natural orifice, perhaps even outside the operating room

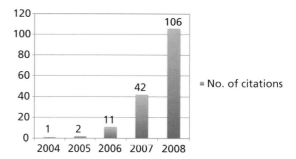

Figure 14.1 NOTES (natural orifice transluminal endoscopic surgery) citations in medicine through 2008.

setting, and to avoid the pain and recovery associated with incisions and any potential complications such as wound infection or herniation.

Since 2003 there has been considerable dialogue and effort toward NOTES. To address this emerging concept, a working group consisting of expert laparoscopic surgeons from the Society of American Gastrointestinal and Endoscopic Surgeons (SAGES) and a group of expert interventional endoscopists representing the American Society for Gastrointestinal Endoscopy (ASGE) came together for a meeting in July 2005. This group identified itself as the Working Group on Natural Orifice Transluminal Endoscopic Surgery, later to be more formalized through an official ASGE and SAGES collaboration, the NOSCAR (Natural Orifice Surgery Consortium for Assessment and Research) Joint Committee [4]. The overriding goal of this collaboration is to provide guidance and oversight of NOTES techniques and the related research required to define and overcome the barriers to the safe introduction of NOTES [5,6].

Before NOTES can be adopted as a favorable alternative to existing surgical interventions, several barriers need to be overcome [5,6]:

• Techniques for safe transluminal access to the peritoneal and thoracic cavity
• Secure closure of the viscus used for peritoneal and thoracic access
• Prevention of infection from contamination of cavity entered
• Manipulation of tissue including dissection, ligation, suturing, and anastomosis
• Development of a new platform of tools and devices for performing tasks
• Management of intraoperative complications

• Understanding of the physiology of NOTES and the impact on the patient
• Standards for training and credentialing in NOTES.

Much of the guidance provided by NOSCAR and efforts in research have been to address these barriers. However, enthusiasm for bringing the proposed benefits of NOTES to patients as soon as possible has led to significant work in showing the feasibility and safety of NOTES as reported in multiple case reports of human NOTES.

NOTES Development

Under the guidance of NOSCAR and with money provided by industry, over 50 research grants have been awarded to study NOTES. Research activities have focused largely on the barriers outlined above and feasibility studies assessing the ability to perform specific procedures using NOTES. With this, there is preliminary experience related to the identified barriers, and nearly every operation currently performed laparoscopically has now been performed in animal models using NOTES techniques [7–15]. Research has also focused on the physiology of NOTES and the fundamental issues of closure of the necessary luminal perforation [16–23].

It is important to note that most of these procedures are being performed using existing instruments for therapeutic endoscopy. These instruments and device platforms are not able to safely and efficiently perform the tissue manipulation needed to safely complete a procedure. Therefore, most of the NOTES procedures that have been performed today use a hybrid technique where laparoscopy is also employed to facilitate completion of the procedure. This has been true for much of the animal work and nearly all of the human NOTES that have been performed. These hybrid procedures serve as a bridge until devices can be developed to allow full procedures exclusively via NOTES.

Human use of NOTES was initially limited to procedures where a gastrostomy was performed for other reasons, thereby allowing the use of an flexible endoscope to be orally passed during the operation into the abdominal cavity, primarily for diagnostic purposes and to show the feasibility of NOTES in humans [24]. It did not take long for innovative surgeons to prospectively perform NOTES procedures in humans and, in 2007, the first

NOTES cholecystectomy was performed in a human [25] using a transvaginal approach.

Several teams have now performed NOTES procedures in humans [26]—most being transvaginal cholecystectomy. To monitor the progress in human NOTES and to consolidate experiences for the purposes of outcome reporting, NOSCAR has started a global registry of human NOTES procedures.

Future of NOTES

Not surprisingly, there has been considerable controversy surrounding the development of NOTES, especially for performing common procedures such as laparoscopic cholecystectomy that are currently done safely and efficiently. Many have expressed concern that NOTES is taking something that is fairly easily accomplished with laparoscopy and making it complicated and unsafe [27–29]. There is also considerable concern that the current healthcare climate will not tolerate the increased costs that would inevitably be associated with developing this new approach for surgical procedures, and that the proposed benefits would be nominal at best.

Although all of this speaks against NOTES having any significant future in surgical care, there are some potential exceptions. First, there remain surgical procedures where the morbidity of access into the body's cavity remains significant, e.g., access to the thoracic cavity carries considerable morbidity even when accomplished using thoracoscopy. Therefore NOTES approaches to the chest may provide a differential benefit that warrants development along these lines.

Second, the prospect that NOTES procedures can be performed outside a hospital operating room could carry significant benefits in regions where operating rooms are not readily available or are too expensive to maintain, e.g., the use of NOTES in developing countries may allow access to surgical care where it would not otherwise be available due to the absence of an operating room resource [29].

Clearly, the future of NOTES remains very unclear. There is little reason to think that at this time NOTES will have the overwhelming impact on surgery that was seen with the introduction and development of modern laparoscopy. That said, there will remain a core group of innovative surgeons and gastroenterologists who will and should continue to develop this concept. With the right circumstances NOTES promises to be a true revolution in surgery that could transform how surgical care is delivered.

Take-home points

- Today, endoluminal surgery defines operations performed within the lumen of the gastrointestinal tract through an endoscope and includes such procedures as antireflux procedures, mucosal excision or ablation of pathology such as Barrett esophagus, and some bariatric procedures.

- Natural orifice transluminal endoscopic surgery (NOTES) defines the use of flexible endoscopy through a natural orifice to gain access to the peritoneal or thoracic cavity to perform intraperitoneal surgical procedures such as cholecystectomy.

- NOSCAR is a joint effort between the ASGE and the SAGES to help guide the responsible development and implementation of NOTES.

- NOTES promises incisionless surgery with associated benefits in accelerated recovery and cosmesis.

- Several concerns related to NOTES serve as barriers to widespread adoption.

- There are limited data to substantiate current claims as to the benefits of NOTES.

- As NOTES procedures may avoid the requirement of a full operating room needed for transperitoneal or transthoracic surgery, NOTES may have great potential in developing countries where the infrastructure of full operating rooms does not exist.

References

1 Dohmoto M, Rupp KD. Endoscopic drainage of pancreatic pseudocysts. *Surg Endosc* 1992; **6**: 118–24.

2 Buess G, Theiss R, Gunther M, Hutterer F, Pichlmaier H. Endoscopic surgery in the rectum. *Endoscopy* 1985; **17**: 31–5.

3 Kalloo AN, Singh VK, Jagannath SB, *et al.* Flexible transgastric peritoneoscopy: a novel approach to diagnostic and therapeutic interventions in the peritoneal cavity. *Gastrointest Endosc* 2004; **60**: 114–17.

4 Natural Orifice Surgery Consortium for Assessment and Research. Available from: www.nosccar.org (accessed February 12, 2010).

5 Rattner D, Kalloo A, Group ASW. ASGE/SAGES Working Group on Natural Orifice Transluminal Endoscopic Surgery White Paper, October 2005. *Gastrointest Endosc* 2006; **63**: 199–203.

6 Rattner D, Kalloo A, Group ASW. ASGE/SAGES Working Group on Natural Orifice Transluminal Endoscopic Surgery, October 2005. *Surg Endosc* 2006; **20**: 329–33.

7 Kantsevoy SV, Jagannath SB, Niiyama H, *et al.* Endoscopic gastrojejunostomy with survival in a porcine model. *Gastrointest Endosc* 2005; **62**: 287–92.

8 Sclabas GM, Swain P, Swanstrom LL. Endoluminal methods for gastrotomy closure in natural orifice transenteric surgery (NOTES). *Surg Innov* 2006; **13**: 23–30.

9 Lima E, Rolanda C, Pego JM, *et al.* Third-generation nephrectomy by natural orifice transluminal endoscopic surgery. *J Urol* 2007; **178**: 2648–54.

10 Ryou M, Fong DG, Pai RD, Tavakkolizadeh A, Rattner DW, Thompson CC. Dual-port distal pancreatectomy using a prototype endoscope and endoscopic stapler: a natural orifice transluminal endoscopic surgery (NOTES) survival study in a porcine model. *Endoscopy* 2007; **39**: 881–7.

11 Whiteford MH, Denk PM, Swanstrom LL. Feasibility of radical sigmoid colectomy performed as natural orifice translumenal endoscopic surgery (NOTES) using transanal endoscopic microsurgery. *Surg Endosc* 2007; **21**: 1870–4.

12 Hagen ME, Wagner OJ, Swain P, *et al.* Hybrid natural orifice transluminal endoscopic surgery (NOTES) for Roux-en-Y gastric bypass: an experimental surgical study in human cadavers. *Endoscopy* 2008; **40**: 918–24.

13 Noguera JF, Dolz C, Cuadrado A, Olea JM, Vilella A. Transvaginal liver resection (NOTES) combined with minilaparoscopy. *Revista Espanola de Enfermedades Digestivas* 2008; **100**: 411–15.

14 Woodward T, McCluskey D 3rd, Wallace MB, Raimondo M, Mannone J, Smith CD. Pilot study of transesophageal endoscopic surgery: NOTES esophagomyotomy, vagotomy, lymphadenectomy. *J Laparoendosc Adv Surg Tech A* 2008; **18**: 743–5.

15 Vitale GC, Davis BR, Vitale M, Tran TC, Clemons R. Natural orifice translumenal endoscopic drainage for pancreatic abscesses. *Surg Endosc* 2009; **23**: 140–6.

16 Bergstrom M, Swain P, Park PO. Measurements of intraperitoneal pressure and the development of a feedback control valve for regulating pressure during flexible transgastric surgery (NOTES). *Gastrointest Endosc* 2007; **66**: 174–8.

17 von Delius S, Huber W, Feussner H, *et al.* Effect of pneumoperitoneum on hemodynamics and inspiratory pressures during natural orifice transluminal endoscopic surgery (NOTES): an experimental, controlled study in an acute porcine model. *Endoscopy* 2007; **39**: 854–61.

18 Arezzo A, Repici A, Kirschniak A, Schurr MO, Ho CN, Morino M. New developments for endoscopic hollow organ closure in prospective of NOTES. *Minimally Invasive Therapy & Allied Technologies: Mitat* 2008; **17**: 355–60.

19 Buck L, Michalek J, Van Sickle K, Schwesinger W, Bingener J. Can gastric irrigation prevent infection during NOTES mesh placement? *J Gastrointest Surg* 2008; **12**: 2010–14.

20 Dray X, Gabrielson KL, Buscaglia JM, *et al.* Air and fluid leak tests after NOTES procedures: a pilot study in a live porcine model (with videos). *Gastrointest Endosc* 2008; **68**: 513–19.

21 Kantsevoy SV. Infection prevention in NOTES. *Gastrointest Endosc Clinics North Am* 2008; **18**: 291–6; ix.

22 Levy LC, Adrales G, Rothstein RI. Training for NOTES. *Gastrointest Endosc Clinics North Am* 2008; **18**: 343–60; x.

23 McGee MF, Schomisch SJ, Marks JM, *et al.* Late phase TNF-alpha depression in natural orifice translumenal endoscopic surgery (NOTES) peritoneoscopy. *Surgery* 2008; **143**: 318–28.

24 Marks JM, Ponsky JL, Pearl JP, McGee MF. PEG "rescue": a practical NOTES technique. *Surg Endosc* 2007; **21**: 816–19.

25 Bessler M, Stevens PD, Milone L, Parikh M, Fowler D. Transvaginal laparoscopically assisted endoscopic cholecystectomy: a hybrid approach to natural orifice surgery. *Gastrointest Endosc* 2007; **66**: 1243–5.

26 Sodergren MH, Clark J, Athanasiou T, Teare J, Yang GZ, Darzi A. Natural orifice translumenal endoscopic surgery: critical appraisal of applications in clinical practice. *Surg Endosc* 2009; **23**: 680–7.

27 Pomp A. Notes on NOTES: The emperor is not wearing any clothes. *Surg Endosc* 2008; **22**: 283–4.

28 Rosch T. Who votes for NOTES? *Gut* 2008; **57**: 1481–6.

29 Smith CD. A critical assessment of NOTES: a pessimistic view from an optimist. *J Laparoendosc Adv Surg Tech A* 2008; **18**: 665–7.

PART 3

Other Diagnostic Modalities

CHAPTER 15
Radiologic Approach to Diagnosis in the Upper Gastrointestinal Tract

Stephen W. Trenkner and James E. Huprich

Division of Radiology, Mayo Clinic, Rochester, MN, USA

Summary

The widespread availability of endoscopy and the advent of cross-sectional imaging have reduced the utilization of barium studies of the upper gastrointestinal tract. Nevertheless, the esophagram has remained an important study for the evaluation of dysphagia, hiatal hernias, and postoperative fundoplications. Contrast studies of the stomach also remain vital for evaluating postoperative anatomy, such as morbid obesity procedures. CT and MR have more limited uses for evaluating the upper gastrointestinal tract.

Case

An 88-year-old female with dysphagia underwent an upper endoscopy. No abnormalities were described. The patient was sent for esophageal motility studies which were also normal. Eventually, the patient underwent an esophagram and a web was seen in the proximal esophagus. The patient was then referred for repeat upper endoscopy with dilation. The patient underwent dilation through the endoscope at the level of the web. 12 mm, 15 mm, and 18 mm balloons were used. The patient was discharged from the Endoscopy Suite, but returned to the Emergency Room 8h later with increasing chest pain. The Emergency Room physician ordered an esophagram with a water-soluble contrast agent. A small leak of contrast was seen at the area where the web had been identified. Because of the patient's age and co-morbidities, she was treated with antibiotics, analgesics, and a nasogastric aspirate. She was followed by thoracic surgery. The patient's pain diminished and her vital signs and laboratory tests were normal. After 10 days, the nasogastric tube was removed and a water-soluble contrast esophagram was performed. No leak was noted and immediately afterwards a barium esophagram was performed to make certain that there was in fact no leakage. None was seen. The patient resumed a soft diet and was discharged.

Esophagus

Techniques

The primary imaging study of the esophagus is the barium esophagram [1]. It is performed with the patient standing (double-contrast) and lying down (single-contrast). It evaluates the structure of the esophagus and cardia and to some extent swallowing, esophageal peristalsis, and gastroesophageal reflux. Occasionally, the patient is given a 13-mm barium tablet to evaluate the diameter of strictures. Swallowing marshmallows is rarely helpful.

When the swallowing mechanism is of primary concern, the esophagram should be performed in conjunction with a modified barium swallow/video esophagram [2]. The modified barium swallow is done with the assistance of a speech pathologist or occupational therapist. The swallow is evaluated with both

Practical Gastroenterology and Hepatology: Esophagus and Stomach, 1st edition. Edited by Nicholas J. Talley, Kenneth R. DeVault and David E. Fleischer. © 2010 Blackwell Publishing Ltd.

liquids and solids. When an abnormality is detected, the therapists are invaluable in retraining the patient to swallow safely.

The esophagram is excellent for evaluating perforations and postoperative anatomy. In these cases, water-soluble contrast is used and is followed by barium if the initial study is negative for perforation.

Computed tomography (CT) plays a limited role in the evaluation of the esophagus. It can be used to stage esophageal cancer and to evaluate abnormalities extrinsic to the esophagus. In the case of an esophageal lipoma, CT is diagnostic.

Dysphagia

Dysphagia is the feeling of difficulty passing liquids or solids from the mouth to the stomach [1]. The abnormality may be structural or functional and involve any part of the anatomy between the mouth and gastric cardia. When ordering studies it is important to remember that patients are not always able to localize the level of obstruction [3]. An obstructing lesion in the distal esophagus or cardia may be perceived in the neck. Conversely, a proximal obstructing lesion is rarely referred distally. Therefore, patients with symptoms in the neck need an evaluation of swallowing followed by an esophagram if necessary. If the symptoms are perceived in the chest, only an esophageal evaluation is usually needed.

While endoscopy is superior for evaluating reflux esophagitis, and provides the opportunity for biopsies, the barium studies provide an excellent overview of swallowing and the esophagus. The esophagram is also excellent for defining the size and type of hiatal hernia (sliding, paraesophageal or mixed). The esophagram is also superior to endoscopy for detecting Schatzki rings (mucosal rings), which are a common cause of dysphagia [4].

Imaging after Antireflux Surgery

In the past decade, there has been an 8 to 10-fold increase in the number of laparoscopic antireflux procedures performed. Approximately, 50% of patients have persistent or new symptoms within 3 months following surgery and 2–17% will eventually have objective evidence of failed antireflux surgery. Managing these patients has occupied a significant portion of the gastroenterologist's practice. Barium studies play an important role in the evaluation of these challenging patients. Familiarity with these techniques is important for a successful patient outcome.

The purpose of antireflux surgery is to restore the function of the lower esophageal sphincter (LES) and return the gastroesophageal junction (GEJ) to an intra-abdominal location. Fundoplication types can be divided into: (i) complete (Nissen) and (ii) partial fundoplications (e.g., Belsey, Toupet, Dor). Partial fundoplications can further be divided into anterior or posterior types depending upon the location of the plication. The choice of fundoplication type depends upon many factors. In general, complete wraps (e.g., Nissen) provide better protection against reflux but have a higher incidence of dysphagia, especially in patients with poor esophageal function.

The successful radiographic evaluation of patients with fundoplications depends upon proper technique and a thorough knowledge of the surgical anatomy. The radiologist must be familiar with double-contrast upper gastrointestinal series (UGI) techniques for the proper evaluation of these patients. It is important for the gastroenterologist to consult with the radiologist prior to the exam to insure a successful outcome.

Complete and partial fundoplications each have characteristic radiographic appearances. In both types, a soft tissue density representing the wrap is seen in the gastric fundus (Figure 15.1). The fundic soft tissue density appears larger in the case of a complete versus partial wrap. In both cases, the esophageal lumen appears narrowed as it passes through the wrap. Since the wrap completely surrounds the esophagus in a complete fundoplication, the esophageal lumen appears centered within the wrap. In partial fundoplications, the lumen is eccentrically located within the wrap, either anteriorly, in posterior fundoplications, or posteriorly, in anterior fundoplications. In all cases, the wrap should be located below the diaphragm, indicating an intra-abdominal location. One other very important radiographic sign of an intact fundoplication is the absence of any portion of the stomach or hiatal hernia above the wrap. The radiographic features of an intact fundoplication are stated in Table 15.1.

Radiographic changes during the first 3 months following antireflux surgery may cause concern if one is not aware of their temporary nature. In the early postoperative period, there is delayed emptying of barium from the esophagus as a result of swelling. The soft tissue density in the gastric fundus may appear quite large initially—approximately the size of an apricot. The soft tissue

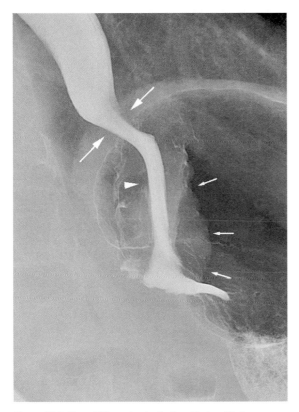

Figure 15.1 Normal Nissen fundoplication. Barium-filled esophageal lumen (arrowhead) is slightly narrowed as it passes through the wrap, represented by the soft tissue density in the gastric fundus (small arrows). Note that the wrap is located entirely below the diaphragmatic hiatus (large arrows) and no hiatal hernia or any portion of the gastric fundus is seen above the wrap.

Table 15.1 Signs of intact fundoplication on barium swallows.

Soft tissue density (wrap) within the gastric fundus

Wrap located below the diaphragm

Slightly narrowed esophageal lumen passes centrally (in complete fundoplications) or eccentrically (partial fundoplication) within the soft tissue density

No stomach (or hiatal hernia) above the wrap

density shrinks over the following months to less than half the original size. During the first few days after surgery the stomach may be somewhat dilated, reflecting temporary delayed gastric emptying. Recognition of

these normal transient changes can be reassuring to the patient.

The diagnosis of failed antireflux surgery is based upon persistent or new symptoms associated with an anatomical or physiological abnormality. Various classifications of types of anatomical failure, based upon barium studies, have been published [5–7]. However, if one adheres to the simple criteria listed in Table 15.1, most cases of anatomical failure can be recognized.

Dysphagia persisting more than 3 to 6 months after a fundoplication may be caused by a wrap that is too tight. Diagnosis is usually difficult. However, findings of delayed emptying of the esophagus in the upright position and an excessively long luminal narrowing may provide clues to the diagnosis.

The most common finding of fundoplication failure is the appearance or reappearance of a hiatal hernia. In most cases, portions of the wrap remain intact, causing an asymmetrical, sometimes bizarre appearance (Figure 15.2). With complete disruption of the wrap and failure of the hiatal closure, a larger hiatal hernia may result. Herniation of an intact wrap above the diaphragm is less common but may be more difficult to diagnose, especially if there is no associated hiatal hernia. In these cases CT or MR may be of value in demonstrating the supradiaphragmatic location of the wrap (Figure 15.3).

Stomach

Techniques
The major imaging study of the stomach is the UGI. It is an evaluation of the mouth to the duodenal/jejunal junction. It therefore incorporates the esophageal evaluation discussed previously but also includes an evaluation of the stomach and duodenum. Like the esophagram, it is a biphasic technique including double and single contrast [8]. When perforation is suspected, water-soluble contrast is used.

CT plays a secondary role in gastric imaging. It can be used to stage gastric malignancies and is helpful in defining intramural tumors, such as gastrointestinal stromal tumors (GIST) and extrinsic abnormalities.

Major Indications
Barium evaluation of the stomach is less clinically relevant than the esophagram. The UGI is often ordered

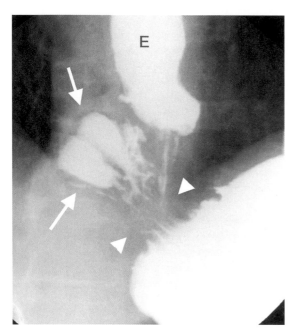

Figure 15.2 Disrupted Nissen fundoplication. Barium filling a bizarrely-shaped paraesophageal hernia (arrows) located above the diaphragmatic hiatus (arrowheads) adjacent to the esophagus (E). Note the absence of the normal soft tissue density in the gastric fundus indicating herniation of the disrupted wrap through the hiatus into the chest.

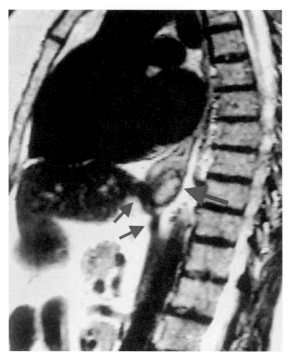

Figure 15.3 Intrathoracic herniation of fundoplication. This patient experienced severe dysphagia several months after laparoscopic Nissen fundoplication. Endoscopy and barium studies showed an intact wrap. This sagittal MR image through the diaphragmatic hiatus demonstrates the fundoplication (large arrow) to be located above the diaphragm (small arrows). (Reproduced from *Journal of Gastroenterology & Hepatology* 2000; **15**: 1221.)

when an esophagram is all that is needed. Endoscopy has largely replaced the UGI for evaluating the gastric mucosa.

Probably, the current leading indication for an UGI is to evaluate the postoperative stomach. With the decline in partial gastrectomies for ulcers, evaluation is now mainly for morbid obesity procedures. The two main procedures are the Roux-en-Y gastric bypass (RYGBP) and laparoscopic adjustable gastric banding (LAGB) [9].

The RYGBP consists of a small gastric pouch that is attached to the Roux limb. Further down, the Roux limb is anastomosed to the jejunum. The UGI is excellent for evaluating the major complications, including obstructions and fistulas between the gastric pouch and bypassed stomach (Figure 15.4).

The LAGB is an inflatable silicone band that is surgically placed around the proximal stomach. The band is connected to a subcutaneous port, allowing inflation and deflation of the band. Inflating the band narrows the proximal stomach, restricting food intake. Adverse

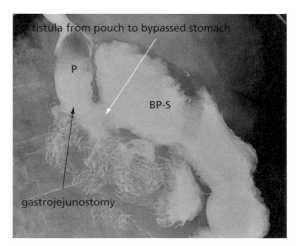

Figure 15.4 Roux-en-Y gastric bypass with large area of breakdown in the staple line between the gastric pouch (P) and bypassed portion of the stomach (BP-S).

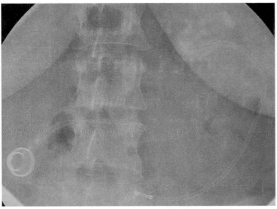

(a)

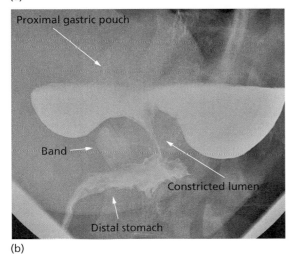

Proximal gastric pouch

Band

Constricted lumen

Distal stomach

(b)

Figure 15.5 (a) Laparoscopic adjustable gastric banding on plain film. (b) Slipped laparoscopic adjustable gastric banding. Almost no stomach is seen above the band in normal cases.

symptoms occur when the band is too tight or there is slippage of the stomach above the band (Figure 15.5). Both are easily assessed with an UGI.

Take-home points

- When difficulty with swallowing is the indication for a contrast study of the esophagus, the patient should undergo a modified barium swallow/video esophagram with the assistance of a speech pathologist.

- Obstructing lesion in the distal esophagus or proximal stomach may be perceived by the patient to be causing difficulties in the neck. A proximal obstructing lesion is rarely referred distally.
- Imaging of the esophagus and proximal stomach is helpful to assess patient complaints after antireflux surgery.
- The signs of an intact fundoplication include wrap within the gastric fundus; wrap located below diaphragm; centrally narrowed esophageal lumen; and no stomach above the wrap.
- The most common finding of a fundoplication failure is the appearance or reappearance of a hiatal hernia.
- The leading indication for an upper gastrointestinal series is to evaluate the postoperative stomach.
- The two main procedures performed for morbid obesity are Roux-en-Y gastric bypass and laparoscopic adjustable gastric banding.

References

1 Levine MS, Rubesin SE. Radiologic investigation of dysphagia. *Am J Roentgenol* 1990; **154**: 1157–63.
2 Logemann JA. Role of the modified barium swallow in management of patients with dysphagia. *Otolaryngol Head Neck Surg* 1997; **116**: 335–8.
3 Wilcox CM, Alexander LN, Clark WS. Localization of an obstructing esophageal lesion: is the patient accurate? *Dig Dis Sci* 1995; **40**: 2192–6.
4 Ott DJ, Chen YM, Wu WC, *et al.* Radiographic and endoscopic sensitivity in detecting lower esophageal mucosal ring. *Am J Roentgenol* 1986; **147**: 261–5.
5 Horgan S, Bogetti D, *et al.* Failed antireflux surgery: What have we learned from reoperations? *Arch Surg* 1999; **134**: 809–17.
6 Saik R, Peskin G. The study of fundoplication disruption and deformity. *Am J Surg* 1977; **134**: 19–22.
7 Thoeni R, Moss A. The radiographic appearance of complications following Nissen fundoplication. *Radiology* 1979; **131**: 17–21.
8 Levine MS, Rubesin SE, Herlinger H, Laufer I. Double-contrast upper gastrointestinal examination: technique and interpretation. *Radiology* 1988; **168**: 593–602.
9 Trenkner SW. Imaging of morbid obesity procedures and their complications. *Abdom Imaging* 2009; **34**: 335–44.

CHAPTER 16

Esophageal Motility Testing

Jason R. Roberts and Donald O. Castell

Division of Gastroenterology and Hepatology, Medical University of South Carolina, Charleston, SC, USA

Summary

Since its inception more than a half century ago, esophageal motility testing has undergone continuous evolution. Although pressure has been the standard by which esophageal function is measured, today multichannel intraluminal impedance (MII) allows for a truer assessment of function through bolus movement. Despite many technologic innovations, the underlying principles of proper esophageal function are unchanged. A minimum pressure has to be generated in the esophageal body in a peristaltic sequence with appropriate lower esophageal sphincter (LES) relaxation for a normal swallow to occur. The use of combined MII–manometry (MII–EM) and high-resolution manometry (HRM) aid the physician in determining if any deviation from this normal pattern explains the patient's symptoms.

Introduction

Esophageal motility testing has traditionally been performed by obtaining pressure measurements of the muscular contractions usually initiated by a swallow inducing primary peristalsis. Over the years, the common placement for pressure sensors were at 5-cm intervals, usually beginning with a distal sensor at the lower esophageal sphincter (LES) and proximal sensors at 5, 10, 15, and 20 cm above [1]. The functional "effectiveness" of the contraction wave was implied based on these pressure measurements, with this information often supplemented by functional data obtained during a barium esophagram [2]. Recently, evolving technology has provided the opportunity to measure intraluminal pressures at each centimeter from the upper stomach to the lower pharynx providing "high-resolution" manometric (HRM) studies. Over the past 5 years, the addition of electrical impedance measurements (discussed below) provided a functional assessment, potentially replacing the need for barium studies (Figure 16.1). Thus, esopha-geal testing in the 21st century now has the potential to provide more complete motility assessment in the hope of identifying a possible esophageal etiology for the patient's presenting symptoms. The primary indication for esophageal motility testing over the past 50 years has been in the evaluation of the patient with dysphagia and, less commonly, chest pain, although recently more tests are being done to evaluate esophageal function prior to endoscopic or surgical therapy for gastroesophageal reflux. A summary of indications for motility testing are listed in (Table 16.1).

Equipment

Early esophageal motility testing was performed using either a small water- or air-filled balloon or, more commonly, with a series of orifices filled or constantly perfused with water. Over the past 25 years, technological advances have provided miniaturized solid-state transducers that have been shown to record similar pressures as the water-filled systems and obviate the need for this component. Accurate esophageal pressure recordings can be obtained with either technique. A major advantage introduced with solid-state transducers was the circumferential transducer which provided an average of

Practical Gastroenterology and Hepatology: Esophagus and Stomach, 1st edition. Edited by Nicholas J. Talley, Kenneth R. DeVault and David E. Fleischer. © 2010 Blackwell Publishing Ltd.

Table 16.1 Suggested clinical indications for motility testing.

Evaluation of patients with non-obstructive dysphagia
   Pharyngeal and upper esophageal sphincter abnormalities
   Primary esophageal motility disorders (e.g., achalasia)
   Secondary esophageal motility disorders (e.g., scleroderma)

Evaluation of patients with possible gastroesophageal reflux
disease
   Assist in placement of pH probe
   Evaluate lower esophageal sphincter pressure (e.g., poor
     treatment response)
   Evaluate defective peristalsis (particularly before fundoplication)

Evaluation of patients with non-cardiac chest pain
   Primary esophageal motility disorders
   Pain response to provocative testing

Evaluation of generalized gastrointestinal tract disease
   Scleroderma

Exclude esophageal etiology for suspected anorexia or bulimia
nervosa

pressure generated around the esophagus [3]. This was a particular advantage in recording a single pressure within both the upper and lower esophageal sphincters with their well-known radial asymmetry. A limitation of a single recording sensor within the sphincter is produced by axial movement of both the upper esophageal sphincter (UES) and lower esophageal sphincter (LES) during swallowing. To circumvent this problem, a 6-cm sleeve design developed by Dent and colleagues allows continuous placement within a sphincter moving during swallowing [4]. However, the sleeve is limited by a recording in only one direction, thus failing to provide an average overall squeeze pressure. The newer, high-resolution catheters have multiple recording sites in the area of the LES (and UES), perhaps making appropriate placement easier and more accurate. The major advantage of a water perfused catheter is a less expensive, disposable form. Fortunately, the more expensive solid-state catheters have proven to be quite durable over many years. A more

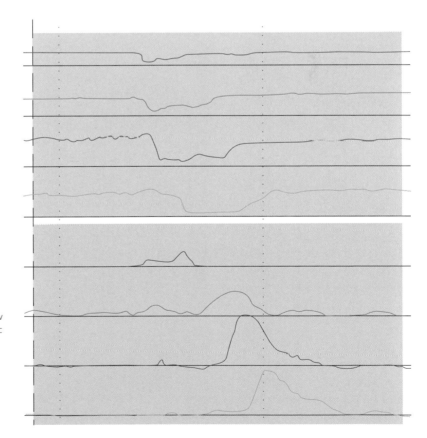

Figure 16.1 Normal swallow during combined MII–EM testing. This swallow illustrates a typical, "normal" peristaltic sequence. The top four channels are impedance, showing a drop in impedance with the swallow with a return to baseline after the bolus passes. The lower four channels are pressure channels and show the corresponding peristaltic wave.

recent innovation is a disposable manometry catheter which uses small balloons at appropriate testing sites that are air filled and calibrated for accurate pressure measurement. Essentially, all systems today use computerized recording and analysis [5].

Acquisition

Patients are generally studied after a 5–6 h fasting period. The catheter and its transducers (whether internal or external) are calibrated to a known pressure and gently inserted transanally so that at least the distal pressure sites are located within the stomach. A quiet gastric baseline pressure is first obtained and a recording site is slowly withdrawn across the LES. This "pull through" or LES "profile" is preferably obtained by gently withdrawing the catheter in 0.5-cm intervals while allowing three to four quiet respirations at each station [6]. As the catheter continues to move across the sphincter, the pressure inversion point (PIP) should be identified just before pressure drops to an esophageal level. The PIP is the point at which the respiratory phasic pressure changes from intra-abdominal in type (up with inspiration) to intrathoracic in type (down with inspiration). Anatomically, this indicates the level of the diaphragm.

Next, the distal recording sensor is placed in the LES high-pressure zone and an esophageal baseline pressure obtained in the more proximal recording sites. Traditionally, 5-mL water swallows are given 10 times, via a handheld syringe, with 20–30 seconds separating each swallow [7]. In our laboratory at the completion of the testing swallows, the distal pressure sensor is slowly withdrawn across the PIP to provide the opportunity for a second measurement of the LES high-pressure zone [8].

The protocol for HRM is somewhat different in that the catheter has sufficient number and spacing of monitoring sites to allow a simultaneous measurement of pressures in the UES, esophageal body, and LES. The usual protocol does not have a specific sphincter pull through, but simply places the catheter in the appropriate position, with swallows to follow (Figure 16.2). This simplified approach seems to allow quicker data acquisition, but one must remember that there are fewer robust normal data on this technique compared to older, more established methodology.

Measurements and Normal Values

Normal values for esophageal manometry were obtained from a series of 95 volunteer subjects [9]. Resting pressure of both the LES and UES are obtained by slow pull through using the gastric and esophageal pressures as baseline standard. The assessment of relaxation of the sphincters requires that the recording transducer be carefully positioned to account for proximal movement of these sphincters during swallowing. A relaxation residual pressure should be obtained and also referenced to gastric and esophageal baseline. Esophageal peristaltic pressures have focused mainly on amplitude and duration of the contraction wave in the smooth muscle segment of the distal half of the esophagus [8]. Traditionally, the average value for the pressures obtained at 5 and 10 cm above the LES is termed the distal esophageal amplitude (DEA) and represents a measure of this smooth muscle region. A pressure trough is commonly found, normally in the muscle transition area above this distal segment, often seen on the recording site located 15 cm proximal to the LES [10,11]. The velocity of the peristaltic sequence in the smooth muscle region is usually obtained by measuring the timing between the *onset* of the major upstroke at the two distal sites. It is important to remember that reported velocities of around 8 cm/s become ineffective in bolus movement and most like should be considered "simultaneous". Most normal values were defined using water-perfused manometry equipment, some were reconfirmed with solid-state catheters and there is ongoing (incomplete) work toward obtaining adequate normal date with the newer high-resolution and impedance-based systems. The most commonly accepted definitions for esophageal motility disorders (discussed in more detail in Chapter 34) are presented in Table 16.2.

Bolus Transit Assessment

Over the past 5 years, new technology has provided the opportunity to assess transit function simultaneously with pressure measurements. Intraluminal electrical impedance measurements, obtained as change in alternating current measured between adjacent metal rings spaced at 2 cm distance, provides the basis for this measurement [12]. When liquid with ionic content travels

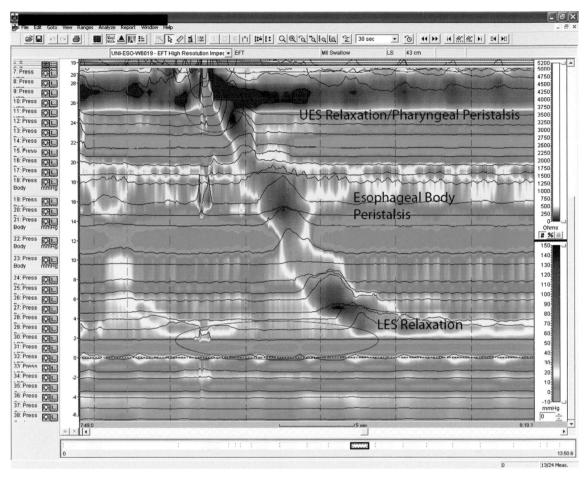

Figure 16.2 Swallow sequence with high resolution testing. This peristaltic sequence measured with a high-resolution catheter shows an adequate evaluation of the upper esophageal sphincter/pharyngeal area, esophageal body, and lower esophageal sphincter with a single swallow of liquid.

Table 16.2 Manometric features of accepted esophageal motility disorders (see Chapter 34 for details)

	Resting LES pressure	LES relaxation	Peristalsis	Peristaltic amplitude
Achalasia	High or normal	Incomplete	Absent (may appear simultaneous)	Low or normal
Distal esophageal spasm	Low, normal or high	Complete	>10% simultaneous with some normal	Normal or high
Nutcracker esophagus	Normal or high	Complete	Normal	High
Scleroderma-like aperistalsis (also seen in severe GERD)	Low	Complete	Absent	Low
Ineffective esophageal motility	Low or normal	Complete	Normal or absent	Low or absent in >50% of swallows
Hypertensive LES	High	Complete	Normal	Normal
Incomplete LES relaxation	Low, normal, or high	Incomplete	Normal	Normal

GERD, gastroesophageal reflux disease; LES, lower esophageal sphincter.

	Liquid	Viscous
Impedance		
Total bolus transit time (s)	12.5	12.5
Smooth muscle transit time 10–5 cm (s)	10.5	8.5
Percent complete bolus transit	≥80%	≥70%
Manometry		
Resting lower esophageal pressure (mmHg)	10–45	10–45
Esophageal body amplitude (mmHg)	≥30	≥30
Distal esophageal amplitude (mmHg)	≤220	≤204
Distal onset velocity (cm/s)	≤8	≤7
Number of ineffective swallows	≤50%	≤60%
Number of simultaneous swallows	≤10%	≤10%
Residual lower esophageal sphincter pressure (mmHg)	≤8	≤11.7

Table 16.3 Normal values for combined MII–EM testing.

across the measuring site, the enhanced current flow results in a decrease in the impedance (resistance) value. This ability to detect the transient presence of liquid has developed into catheters with multiple recording sites that accurately record liquid movement either antero-grade or retrograde within the esophagus. Thus, multi-channel intraluminal impedance (MII), with recording sites straddling pressure transducers at 5, 10, 15, and 20 cm above the LES, has provided the opportunity to add an assessment of esophageal function into the motil-ity laboratory. The major advantages of this technology for motility testing are that it provides a functional measure on the same swallow from which pressure is obtained while eliminating the need for radiation expo-sure. As a complement to standard pressure-related motility testing, a series of 10 liquid swallows (usually normal saline) is tested followed by 10 swallows using a more viscous test solution. Normal values for combined impedance manometry MII–EM are shown in Table 16.3.

Provocative Testing

Since esophageal motility testing has evolved as a tech-nique to help ascertain potential motility abnormalities underlying patients' symptoms, the concept of manipu-lating the esophagus to produce or "provoke" symptoms has been suggested. Originally, detecting acid reflux-related symptoms was performed using the acid infusion "Bernstein" tests [13]. This has been essentially replaced by the excellent techniques now available to record ambulatory acid reflux events and compare with sponta-neously occurring symptoms. A major clinical question that persists, however, is the potential relationship of spontaneously recurring symptoms, usually chest pain or dysphagia, suspected as being produced by esophageal dysmotility. The use of intravenous edrophonium, injected as a mechanism to produce increased magnitude of the esophageal peristaltic contraction, has been uti-lized for many years [14,15]. In many centers, after com-pleting the baseline esophageal studies, the patient is sequentially given an intravenous injection of saline fol-lowed by a series of approximately six swallows in a single-blinded fashion [8]. The edrophonium is injected in a dose of 80 μg/kg, followed by a series of wet swallows. The test is considered positive if the patient notes pain or a sensation of dysphagia during the swallow testing. Although no direct outcome studies have been pub-lished, a positive response to edrophonium is believed to provide evidence that the esophagus is a *likely* source of the patient's symptom. Unfortunately, at least in the United States, edrophonium is no longer available and this testing has been halted in most centers.

Take-home points

- Esophageal manometry is beneficial in non-obstructive dysphagia, in selected patients with chest pain, and in patients being considered for endoscopic or surgical reflux therapy.

- Solid-state catheters are more expensive than water-infused but are more durable.

- Circumferential measurement of sphincter pressures are preferred.

- Combined manometry and impendence testing (MII–EM) adds an additional measurement of esophageal function with bolus transit.
- Normal manometric ranges are based on the 5th and 95th percentiles in 95 healthy volunteers.
- Provocative testing using edrophonium must be combined with a control substance and involve patient blinding.
- Proper acquisition is key to obtaining interpretable manometry data.
- Axial movement of the LES makes relaxation measurements during test swallows difficult with single transducer sites.
- As a rule, MII–EM and high-resolution studies should be read with the goal of under-calling borderline abnormalities.

References

1 Dodds WJ. Instrumentation and methods for intraluminal esophageal manometry. *Arch Intern Med* 1976; **136**: 515–23.

2 Hewson EG, Oh DJ, Dalton CB, *et al.* Manometry and radiology. Complementary studies in the assessment of esophageal motility disorders. *Gastroenterology* 1990; **89**: 626–32.

3 Pursnani K, *et al.* Comparison of lower oesophageal sphincter pressure measurements using circumferential vs unidirectional transducers. *Neurogastroenterol Motil* 1997; **9**: 177–77.

4 Dent J, Chir B. A new technique for continuous sphincter pressure measurement. *Gastroenterology* 1976; **71**: 263–7.

5 Wilson JA, Pryde A, Macintyre CC, *et al.* Computerized manometric recording: an evaluation. *Gullet* 1991; **1**: 87–91.

6 Welch RW, Drake ST. Normal lower esophageal sphincter: a comparison of rapid vs slow pull-through techniques. *Gastroenterology* 1980; **78**: 1446–51.

7 DeVault K, Castell JA, Castell DO. How many swallows are required to establish reliable esophageal peristaltic parameters in normal subjects? An on-line computer analysis. *Am J Gastroenterol* 1987; **82**: 754–7.

8 Roberts J, Freeman J, Castell D. Everyone Deserves a Second Chance: Validation of a Double LESP Profile Technique [Abstract]. In: American College of Gastroenterology Annual Scientific Meeting; 2009 Oct 23–28. San Diego, CA. Charleston (SC), 2009: 439.

9 Richter JE, Wu WC, Johns DN, *et al.* Esophageal manometry in 95 healthy adult volunteers. *Dig Dis Sci* 1987; **32**: 583–92.

10 Clouse RE, Staiano A. Topography of normal and high-amplitude esophageal peristalsis. *Am J Physiol* 1993; **268**: G1098.

11 Clouse RE, Staiano A. Topography of the esophageal peristaltic pressure wave. *Am J Physiol* 1991; **261**: G677.

12 Tutuian R, Vela MF, Shay SS, Castell DO. Multichannel intraluminal impedance in esophageal function testing and gastroesophageal reflux monitoring. *J Clin Gastroenterol* 2003; **37**: 206–15.

13 Bernstein LM, Baker LA. A clinical test for esophagitis. *Gastroenterology* 1958; **34**: 760–81.

14 London RL, Ouyang A, Shape WJ, *et al.* Provocation of esophageal pain by ergonovine or edrophonium. *Gastroenterology* 1981; **81**: 10–14.

15 Richter JE, Hackshaw BT, Wu WC. Edrophonium. A useful provocative test for esophageal chest pain. *Ann Intern Med* 1985; **103**: 14–21.

CHAPTER 17
Ambulatory Reflux Monitoring

Philip O. Katz[1] and Ellen Stein[2]

[1] Jefferson Medical College, Philadelphia, PA, USA
[2] Division of Gastroenterology, Albert Einstein Medical Center, Philadelphia, PA, USA

Summary

Prolonged ambulatory reflux monitoring is an important tool in evaluating patients with gastroesophageal reflux disease (GERD) symptoms. Although current clinical practice guidelines favor empiric trials of proton pump inhibitors before pH testing or endoscopy to diagnose GERD, esophageal pH testing is recommended in patients with persistent symptoms despite acid-suppressing therapy and in patients who are considering antireflux surgery. In many circumstances the decision to test the patient on or off therapy is problematic and one of debate among experts. Off-therapy testing allows for a diagnosis of abnormal esophageal acid exposure and assessment of the relationship of symptoms and acid reflux. On-therapy testing can assess the effect of therapy, the relationship of reflux, and the remaining symptoms, and, if impedance is added to pH, the presence of non-acid reflux. This chapter reviews the options available for ambulatory reflux monitoring, as well as the potential benefits in the clinical arena.

Case

A 46-year-old woman reported with what she described as "bad GERD." Her symptoms consisted of a burning sensation in her mouth and posterior pharynx that tended to occur after meals. This had been present for the past year. There was no associated dysphagia, nor did she have burning or discomfort in her retrosternal region or her abdomen, and did not describe symptoms consistent with regurgitation. Her primary care physician had started her on omeprazole 20 mg daily with no change in her symptoms. An otolaryngologist had noted redness of her posterior vocal folds and changed her medications to esomeprazole 40 mg taken twice daily before her breakfast and evening meals. She noted no improvement with this change and was referred to a gastroenterologist.

Technical Aspects of Reflux Monitoring

Prolonged reflux monitoring is performed over a 24-h monitoring period with either a transnasal catheter, used to record pH, or the newly designed catheter that records

Practical Gastroenterology and Hepatology: Esophagus and Stomach, 1st edition. Edited by Nicholas J. Talley, Kenneth R. DeVault and David E. Fleischer. © 2010 Blackwell Publishing Ltd.

multichannel intraluminal impedance and pH (MII-pH) simultaneously [2]. Alternatively, prolonged pH monitoring can be performed with a telemetry capsule [3] affixed to the esophageal wall using a suction device and pin placed endoscopically. This allows for a longer monitoring period of 48 h. Catheter-based pH monitoring utilizes an antimony or glass electrode placed transnasally, with the esophageal electrode placed 5 cm above the manometrically located lower esophageal sphincter. This 5-cm level is a consensus measurement designed to allow for monitoring of 24-h pH without movement of the electrode into the stomach. In appropriate clinical circumstances, multielectrode monitoring can be performed with a distal esophageal electrode (5-cm location) and a proximal esophageal electrode placed 15 cm above the lower sphincter. Simultaneous intraesophageal and intragastric pH monitoring can also be performed [4]. In this case, the intragastric electrode is placed 7–10 cm below the manometrically localized lower esophageal sphincter with the esophageal electrodes placed as above. In some clinical situations, hypopharyngeal monitoring may be added, in which case an electrode is placed 1–2 cm above the upper esophageal sphincter. More recently, a new device has been developed (Restec) [5] that may be a more sensitive hypopharyngeal monitor.

Placement of a pH catheter requires technical expertise both to localize the lower esophageal sphincter and upper esophageal sphincter, and to provide appropriate patient comfort that improves tolerability and acceptance [6]. Before catheter placement, activation and calibration are required in appropriate, standardized buffers. Transnasal catheters are usually affixed to the nose or around the ear and connected to a recording device that acquires data at a standardized sampling interval. Data are ultimately downloaded to appropriate computer software for analysis.

Combined MII-pH is performed with a transnasal catheter. The pH electrode is positioned 5 cm above the lower esophageal sphincter, straddled by impedance measuring segments located at intervals of 3, 5, 7, 9, 15, and 17 cm above the lower esophageal sphincter [3]. Catheters are available that allow simultaneous recording of intragastric and intraesophageal pH as well as MII. These catheters require similar technical expertise as placement of a traditional ambulatory pH catheter, are placed in a similar fashion, and connected to a similar appearing recording device. MII-pH requires additional training for interpretation. All software provides a computer printout of results but should be read over manually to remove artifacts and to be certain that all symptoms have been recorded.

The newly developed wireless telemetry capsule measures $6 \times 5.5 \times 25$ mm. It contains an antimony pH electrode and a reference electrode on the distal tip of the capsule, as well as an internal battery and a transmitter contained within the capsule. Data are sent to the external receiver using a radiofrequency signal sampling pH data points at a 6-s interval. The capsule is activated by magnetic switch and calibrated in standardized pH solutions. This device is placed 6 cm above the endoscopically located squamocolumnar line, a position felt to be clinically similar to the reference point of a transnasal electrode [4]. The delivery system is introduced orally to the appropriate position. Suction is applied for 30 s, allowing mucosa to be trapped in a well, subsequent to which a pin is fired detaching the capsule from the delivery device. A key to accomplishing this successfully is to avoid lubricating the capsule, particularly the well. It is the authors' preference to document photographically that the capsule has been deployed successfully and is attached. The key advantage of the wireless telemetry capsule system is the ability to perform prolonged record-

ing. The current software allows for a 48-h study but adaptation of the technology allows for longer recording if the patient returns to the laboratory and the receiver is reprogrammed for an additional 48 h. In addition, it is clear that tolerability and patient acceptance are higher with a telemetry capsule [7,8].

Current software allows for automated analyses of reflux monitoring recordings. The majority of programs record total time esophageal and/or intragastric pH < 4, as well as allowing for a separate recording of upright and recumbent time. This requires "telling the computer" when the individual is recumbent and is accomplished by the person being studied pushing the appropriate button on the recorder. If multiple electrodes are used, the number of reflux episodes can be documented at each position. If MII is added to pH, the software will record total number of reflux episodes, number of acid reflux episodes, and number of non-acid reflux episodes. Almost all software will also calculate the so-called Johnson/DeMeester score, a composite scoring system that includes number of reflux episodes, number of reflux episodes greater than 5 min, and the longest reflux episode. Although many experts believe that overall acid exposure is the most important reportable parameter, others utilize the composite score as their analysis standard. The pattern of reflux, whether upright, recumbent, or both, has minimal importance in the interpretation of most studies [9]; however, it may be pertinent in select clinical situations. Proximal reflux may be important in the genesis of symptoms and some believe that recording proximal events is important in evaluating the patient with supra- or extraesophageal symptoms. The clinical value of routinely analyzing proximal and/or hypopharyngeal reflux is debated [1,10] and, at present, is recommended only on a case-by-case basis.

MII-pH allows for assessment of proximal reflux because of the placement of the impedance electrodes. This technology, as noted above, allows for the differentiation of reflux episodes with pH both below and above 4, offers the clinician the ability to diagnose "abnormal" esophageal acid and non-acid reflux.

Currently, the clinical importance of measuring and assessing the presence of non-acid reflux is debated. Although it makes clinical sense that some patients have symptoms related to non-acid reflux and that this may be responsible for residual symptoms in some patients on optimal antisecretory therapy, the true number of patients in this category is still a subject of study. As such, the optimal use of MII-pH in clinical practice continues to evolve [11–14].

Ambulatory reflux monitoring allows for the assessment of the relationship between symptoms and esophageal reflux. To many, this is the key to the study's interpretation. The strength of this relationship can be evaluated in a global sense, simply determining an overall impression of this relationship, or by using one of the three numeric systems currently published in the literature and discussed subsequently [9].

The first is the symptom index (number of reflux-related symptoms divided by total number of symptom episodes × 100%). A symptom index (SI) of ≥50% is considered positive and suggests that a response to therapy will occur.

The SI does not take into account the number of overall reflux episodes so some would use the symptom sensitivity index (SSI; number of symptom-associated reflux episodes divided by total number of reflux episodes times 100). An SSI of ≥10% is considered positive [9].

The most complicated, and perhaps most accurate, system is the symptom association probability (SAP). The study is divided into 2-min segments and evaluates whether a symptom and acid are present during this segment. Contingency table analysis of four possible outcomes for each segment (acid positive, symptom positive, etc.) is calculated with a value of 95% considered positive [9].

Each of these calculations has been compared with a so-called proton pump inhibitor (PPI) test for sensitivity and specificity, and are respectively: SI 35%, 80%, SSI 74%, 73%, and SAP 65%, 73%.

Finally, one can calculate integrated acidity (integrating the pH and converting it to hydrogen ion concentration for every second of the study). Some believe this to be the most accurate way of analyzing a pH study; however, it has met with limited acceptance and is not widely used in clinical practice [9].

Ultimately, a reflux monitoring study must be interpreted in the light of the clinical scenario. No single measurement can ultimately determine whether or not the patient's symptoms are due to reflux disease. Therefore, much like an ambulatory Holter monitor or even a treadmill test, the combination of the available analyses should be used together with the patient's clinical presentation to interpret the study. An illustration of a reflux episode detected by impedance is shown in Figure 17.1.

Clinical Use of Reflux Monitoring

Using a reflux monitor of any kind is not essential to the primary evaluation and/or treatment of a patient with suspected gastroesophageal reflux disease (GERD) who is responsive to therapy, nor is it needed for patients who have endoscopy-documented erosive reflux disease that responds to typical therapy. The history and observed clinical evidence provide adequate support for the diagnosis of GERD in these patients.

However, there are patients who may need further evaluation including: patients with endoscopy-negative disease (so-called NERD), patients with symptoms resistant, recurrent, or refractory to standard or double-dose therapy, patients with distinct, atypical symptoms such as cough, laryngitis, chest pain, globus, or regurgitation in whom heartburn is infrequent or absent, patients who are seeking surgical or endoscopic corrective procedures to treat their symptoms, and patients who have undergone surgical procedures and are experiencing a recurrence of symptoms. For these patients, a diagnostic and confirmatory test is a vital part of their evaluation (Table 17.1).

The two key questions are:
1 Which of the available technologies should be used?
2 Should the monitoring study be performed on or off antisecretory therapy?

The most comprehensive test is a MII-pH because it can demonstrate both acid and "non-acid" reflux events. However, the telemetry capsule monitor is the simplest and best tolerated test for most patients [3,7,8]. Our approach is to base testing in part on the question being asked. If the clinician seeks to confirm that acid reflux is well controlled on therapy, despite persistent symptoms reported by the patient, then ambulatory pH testing on therapy is indicated. Otherwise, for most of these conditions, testing patients off-therapy has a greater yield of symptoms and reflux events [11], e.g., in patients with low probability of GERD, a negative test off therapy makes GERD an even more unlikely diagnosis [15].

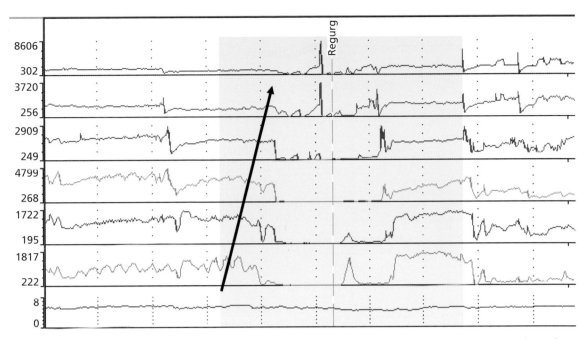

Figure 17.1 This figure focuses on a brief time period during a multichannel intraluminal impedance and pH (MII-pH) study. The y axis of the graph records impedance at separate intervals along the catheter (top lines being proximal and bottom lines being distal), whereas the x axis reveals time in seconds. Along the arrow, the waves of impedance clearly begin to drop in the bottom most lines on the y axis first and then proceed to drop successively up the graph. The arrow points to the distal to proximal direction of the non-acid reflux episode. Temporally, this episode is immediately followed by the patient's experience of a symptom of regurgitation, recorded when the patient pressed the symptoms button. In evaluating MII-pH studies, these temporally associated symptoms and monitor recorded events are tallied to calculate the symptom index (SI), symptom sensitivity index (SSI), and symptom association probability (SAP) scores. The recording along the bottom of the graph measures pH. This pH is static at a value of approximately 6 throughout the time period represented here, so this is a non-acid event.

Specific Clinical Scenarios: How to Evaluate?

The pH monitor

The Patient being Considered for Endoscopic or Surgical Antireflux Procedure, with Negative Endoscopy at Initial Evaluation. Before any surgical or endoscopic options are considered, most guidelines suggest a thorough evaluation to confirm the diagnosis of reflux disease. Esophageal manometry rules out severe motility disorders (scleroderma-like esophagus, achalasia) that may be negatively affected by surgery [16]. Most guidelines suggest that pH monitoring, regardless of method, should be performed to document reflux disease. It is the authors' practice to use telemetry capsule testing with the patient entirely off PPI medication for at least 1 week "before testing." They can take an antacid or H_2-receptor blocker until the evening before testing. A definitive preoperative diagnosis is not only important before surgery but may provide vital information for postoperative evaluation of any complication, such as recurrence of symptoms. Of note, the most important predictors of a successful outcome after laparoscopic Nissen fundoplication are an abnormal pH score before the procedure [16], typical primary symptoms of reflux (heartburn or regurgitation), and symptomatic improvement during a prior trial of acid suppression. Patients who experience recurrent symptoms suspected to be due to GERD after surgery should have a pH study before reinstituting medical therapy [17].

Endoscopy-negative Patients with Symptoms of Reflux who are Reportedly Refractory to PPI Therapy. This is a very common scenario best evaluated with the approach outlined in Figure 17.2. The first step in evaluation of the

Table 17.1 Recommendations for ambulatory esophageal pH, impedance monitoring, and bile acid reflux testing.

pH monitoring is useful:

1 Document abnormal esophageal acid exposure in an endoscopy-negative patient being considered for endoscopic or surgical antireflux procedure

2 Evaluation of endoscopy-negative patients with typical reflux symptoms that are refractory to PPI therapy:
  a pH study done on therapy but consider extended testing with wireless pH system incorporating periods of both off- and on-therapy testing
  b Use of a symptom correlation measure (SI, SSI, or SAP) is recommended to statistically interpret the causality of a particular symptom with episodes of acid reflux
  c Routine proximal or intragastric pH monitoring not recommended

pH monitoring may be useful:

1 Document adequacy of (PPI) therapy in esophageal acid control in patients with complications of reflux disease that include Barrett esophagus

2 Evaluation of endoscopy-negative patients with atypical reflux symptoms that are refractory to twice daily PPI therapy
  a pH study done on bid PPI therapy in patients with high pretest probability of GERD or off therapy in patients with low pretest probability of GERD
  b Use of symptom correlation recommended for selected symptoms that include chest pain
  c Routine proximal or intragastric pH monitoring not recommended

Combined pH monitoring with esophageal impedance monitoring may be useful

1 Evaluation of endoscopy-negative patients with complaints of heartburn or regurgitation despite PPI therapy in whom documentation of nonacid reflux will alter clinical management

2 Utility of impedance monitoring in refractory reflux patients with primary complaints of chest pain or extraesophageal symptoms is unproven

3 Current interpretation of impedance monitoring relies on use of symptom correlation measures (SI, SSI, or SAP)

Bile acid reflux testing may be useful

1 Evaluation of patients with persistent typical reflux symptoms in spite of demonstrated normalization of distal esophageal acid exposure by pH study

2 Bile acid reflux testing equipment currently has very limited commercial availability

Adapted from Hirano and Richter [1].
GERD, gastroesophageal reflux disease; PPI, proton pump inhibitor; SAP, symptom association probability; SI, symptom index; SSI, symptom sensitivity index.

endoscopy-negative patient with persistent refractory reflux symptoms is to confirm that he or she is properly timing the dosing of the PPI. The most commonly used, initially effective dose of once-daily PPI is before breakfast, with a meal 15–30 min after taking the dose. The meal helps activate proton pumps and allows the drug to more effectively inhibit acid. If this initial regimen is unsuccessful, a twice-daily regimen may be tried once before breakfast, once before dinner [4].

If an optimal trial of antisecretory therapy has been tried and symptoms persist, the patient is best served by prolonged reflux monitoring. If the pre-test probability is high (clear history, typical symptoms), a monitoring study should be performed while on PPI therapy, to document success of therapy in control of esophageal acid exposure and to determine if continued symptoms are related to continued reflux events. The likelihood of having abnormal esophageal acid exposure while on PPI is variable, depending on the clinical scenarios and PPI dose. In the authors' experience as a referral practice, about 5% of patients with typical GERD symptoms on twice-daily PPI will have either abnormal esophageal acid exposure or a positive SI with physiologic acid reflux. Other centers have found higher percentages with continued acid reflux. Up to 50% of Barrett esophagus patients will have some reflux at night despite twice-daily PPI. Even if the overall percentage of patients with persistent acid reflux is small, reflux monitoring is helpful in completely taking acid out of the equation or identifying truly refractory patients who may benefit from additional therapy.

Document Adequate Treatment of PPI Therapy in Patients with Barrett Esophagus. The patient with documented Barrett esophagus is at risk of the development of dysplasia and cancer. Although there is little evidence to support the use of routine ambulatory pH monitoring to document adequate acid control in asymptomatic patients, there is evidence that a substantial number will have abnormal esophageal acid exposure despite being asymptomatic [4]. There are no prospective data showing that adequately treating reflux disease will reduce progression, although retrospective case reviews suggesting a decrease in dysplasia in patients on PPI compared with H_2-receptor antagonists or no therapy [18]. In addition, if ablative therapy is undertaken for management of dysplasia, esophageal acid control is likely crucial. Thus,

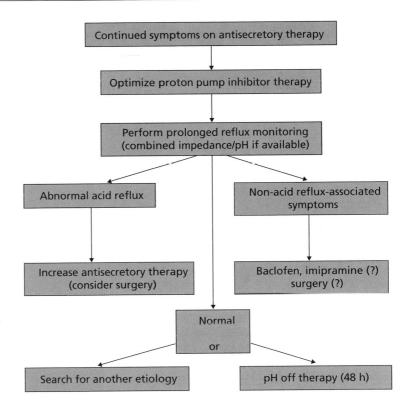

Figure 17.2 Suggested approach to a patient with symptoms suspected to be the result of gastroesophageal reflux who is symptomatic despite antisecretory therapy. This approach is designed to establish whether continued symptoms are due to continued reflux.

it is not unreasonable to do a pH study on therapy to document the effectiveness of treatment. MII-pH studies of patients with Barrett esophagus have shown that these patients have significantly more non-acid reflux events and a higher percentage of non-acid bolus reflux time while supine, as well as an increased amount of acid reflux in the upright and supine positions, although the clinical significance of this finding remains unclear [13].

Evaluate Endoscopy-negative Patients with Extraesophageal or Atypical Symptoms of Reflux that are Refractory to Twice-daily PPI Therapy. The correlation between acid reflux and atypical symptoms has been documented for some patients. Often symptoms of extraesophageal reflux or atypical symptoms of reflux are difficult for patients and physicians to quantify. Cough, chest pain, regurgitation without heartburn, globus, and asthma can be hard to correlate with actual reflux events by history alone. For some of these patients, before embarking on years of therapy for a set of symptoms not traditionally characteristic of acid reflux, documentation of acid or non-acid

reflux events and abnormal acid exposure can be an important step in guiding therapy. A negative MII-pH study on or off PPI can redirect therapeutic options and reassure patients that they do not have acid-related or non-acid-related symptoms. With a positive study, PPI therapy can be continued with confidence that these atypical symptoms are in fact associated with reflux [14]. Of note, testing for extraesophageal symptoms in general has a lower diagnostic yield than testing for more typical reflux symptoms.

Combined pH and Impedance Monitoring

Evaluate endoscopy-negative patients with persistent heartburn or regurgitation despite PPI therapy if the presence of non-acid reflux would help to adjust the therapeutic regimen.

Combined multichannel intraluminal impedance (MII-pH) monitoring augments the evaluation of patients with symptoms suspected to be due to refractory GERD. MII-pH studies in patients on PPI with symptoms suggestive of reflux on PPI therapy have documented the presence of non-acid reflux; however, patient symptoms correlate with recorded non-acid events with variable frequency. If the patient has symptoms caused by non-acid reflux, decisions about therapy are complex because controlled studies on these patients are unavailable. The authors' opinion is that most have some non-acid reflux but few have non-acid reflux events that correlate with symptoms. If warranted, "reflux reduction" can be accomplished with a Nissen fundoplication, endoscopy therapy, lifestyle modifications, or so-called medical therapy. Conceptually medical options include therapies that decrease transient lower esophageal sphincter relaxations, increase lower esophageal sphincter pressure, improve gastric emptying, and decrease visceral sensation and/or reflux. One observational series has shown that laparoscopic Nissen fundoplication can offer a positive outcome in patients with non-acid reflux [19]. It is the authors' clinical impression that surgery is most valuable for patients with regurgitation and possibly for cough [20]. Of note, fundoplication in general is not recommended in patients with symptoms refractory to PPI unless a strong association between their symptoms and non-acid reflux events can be documented. This is particularly true in patients with laryngeal symptoms, because these patients do not appear to respond to surgery if they have failed PPI therapy [21,22].

Ultimately, a thorough evaluation of the GERD patient may require both impedance/pH monitoring on therapy and 48-h Bravo off-therapy to satisfy the patient and referring physician as to the diagnosis (see Figure 17.1). If symptoms are documented to be acid related while on twice-daily PPI therapy, a change or increase in antisecretory therapy is recommended. When pursuing on-therapy testing, MII-pH offers more diagnostic information because the reflux events in both acid and non-acid can be determined [11]. The role of non-acid reflux in producing symptoms is currently an active area of investigation. More recent studies have focused on obtaining information about patients both on and off their therapy through 4-day protocols involving wireless endoscopy, 48 h on and 48 h off therapy. The investigators showed that a longer study time period did improve the detection of reflux events, and they also showed that a resolution of reflux occurred in 95% of patients placed on PPI

therapy. Those authors recommended MII-pH studies for those patients with ongoing symptoms on PPI therapy and either abnormal or normal acid exposure [15]. If the on-therapy test is negative or equivocal.

In the authors' practice, impedance/pH testing would be routinely used in so-called NERD patients for the following reasons (Figure 17.2). If continued acid reflux is demonstrated, antisecretory therapy can be changed, reassessed or increased. Surgery can be considered, although the authors rarely do this until after a new/different medical therapy trial. If non-acid reflux is found to be associated with symptoms, the patient can be offered an explanation for continued symptoms and possible therapy. If no association of symptoms and reflux is seen, acid control is optimal and non-acid reflux frequency is normal (findings in about 70% tested), then it can be confidently said that reflux is not the cause of the symptoms recorded on the test tracing. Thus both patient and referring physician can be reassured.

Case: Conclusion

Given the patient's history, the gastroenterologist felt that a combined impedance/pH test (on medication) was indicated. When the patient presented for this test she was unable to tolerate nasal intubation and refused the test. After additional consultation, it was elected to stop her medications and perform an endoscopy and a "tubeless" pH test. Her symptoms did not change with stopping the PPI, the endoscopy was normal, and the ambulatory pH test showed minimal (1.0% acid) exposure. Her mouth symptoms were present for all of the conscious time during the study and did not appear to be reflux related. Given the negative medication trial and negative pH test, the patient was not felt to have GERD. A very poor sleep habit was discovered and she was started on trazodone 25–50 mg at bedtime with a good improvement in sleep and a partial improvement in her mouth symptoms.

Take-home points

- There are three diagnostic techniques for performing ambulatory reflux monitoring:
  - transnasal catheter pH monitoring
  - telemetry capsule pH monitoring (48-h monitoring)
  - transnasal or multi-channel intraluminal impedance pH monitoring (MII-pH).
- Ambulatory (pH) reflux monitoring is useful clinically to (see Table 17.1):

- ○ document abnormal esophageal acid exposure in a patient being considered for surgical or endoscopic antireflux therapy, especially with negative endoscopy at initial evaluation
  - ○ evaluate endoscopy-negative patients with symptoms suspected to be due to reflux who are "refractory" to PPI therapy
  - ○ evaluate patients with so-called extraesophageal or atypical symptoms of reflux such as cough, asthma, or laryngitis (especially if refractory to PPI therapy). In these patients, if the presence of non-acid reflux is suspected or will alter therapy, consider a combined MII-pH.
- Prolonged (pH) reflux monitoring studies can be evaluated for:
  - ○ time pH < 4 (total, upright, recumbent)
  - ○ Johnson/DeMeester composite score
  - ○ pattern of reflux (upright, recumbent, proximal, hypopharyngeal)
  - ○ symptom association (SI, SSI, or SAP).

References

1 Hirano I, Richter JE, Practice Parameters Committee of the American College of Gastroenterology. ACG practice guidelines. *Am J Gastroenterol* 2007; **102**: 668–685.

2 Tutuian R, Castell DO. Multichannel intraluminal impedance: General principles and technical issues. *Gastrointest Endosc Clin North Am* 2005; **15**: 257–64.

3 Pandolfino JE, Richter JE, Ours T, *et al*. Ambulatory esophageal pH monitoring using a wireless system. *Am J Gastroenterol* 2003; **98**: 740–9.

4 Katz PO. Use of intragastric pH monitoring in gastroesophageal reflux disease. *Gastrointest Endosc Clin North Am* 2005; **15**: 277–87.

5 Gaughan CB, Tang A, Lipham JC, *et al*. Measurement of gastroesophageal reflux in the pharynx: A new technology. *Gastroenterology* 2007; **132**: A-285 (abstract S1946).

6 Gideon RM. Manometry: Technical issues. *Gastrointest Endosc Clin North Am* 2005; **15**: 243–55.

7 Lacy BE, O'Shana T, Hynes M, *et al*. Safety and tolerability of transoral Bravo capsule placement after transnasal manometry using a validated conversion factor. *Am J Gastroenterol* 2007; **102**: 24–32.

8 Maerten P. Ortner M, Michetti P, Dorta G. Wireless capsule pH monitoring: Does it fulfill all expectations? *Digestion* 2007; **76**: 235–40.

9 DeVault KR. Catheter-based pH monitoring: Use in evaluation of gastroesophageal reflux disease symptoms (on and off therapy). *Gastrointest Endosc Clin North Am* 2005; **15**: 289–306.

10 Kahrilas PJ, Quigley EM. Clinical esophageal pH recording: A technical review of practice guideline development. *Gastroenterology* 1996; **110**: 1982–96.

11 Hemmink GJ, Bredenoord AJ, Weusten BL, *et al*. Esophageal pH-impedance monitoring in patients with therapy-resistant reflux symptoms: "On" or "off" proton pump inhibitor? *Am J Gastroenterol* 2008; **103**: 2446–53.

12 Bredenoord AJ, Weusten BL, Timmer R, *et al*. Addition of esophageal impedance monitoring to pH monitoring increases the yield of symptom association analysis in patients off PPI therapy. *Am J Gastroenterol* 2006; **101**: 453–9.

13 Gutschow CA, Bludau M, Vallbohmer D, *et al*. NERD, GERD, and Barrett's esophagus: Role of acid and non-acid reflux revisited with combined pH-impedance monitoring. *Dig Dis Sci* 2008; **53**: 3076–81.

14 Malhotra A, Freston JW, Aziz K. Use of pH-impedance testing to evaluate patients with suspected extraesophageal manifestations of gastroesophageal reflux disease. *J Clin Gastroenterol* 2008; **42**: 271–8.

15 Garrean CP, Zhang Q, Gonsalves N, Hirano I. Acid reflux detection and symptom-reflux association using 4-day wireless pH recording combining 48-hour periods off and on PPI therapy. *Am J Gastroenterol* 2008; **103**: 1631–7.

16 Watson TJ, Peters JH. Evaluation of esophageal function for antireflux surgery. *Gastrointest Endosc Clin North Am* 2005; **15**: 347–60.

17 Campos GM, Peters JH, DeMeester TR, *et al*. Multivariate analysis of factors predicting outcome after laparoscopic Nissen fundoplication. *J Gastrointest Surg* 1999; **3**: 292–300.

18 Vela MF, Tutuian R, Katz PO, Castell DO. Baclofen decreases acid and non-acid post-prandial gastro-oesophageal reflux measured by combined multichannel intraluminal impedance and pH. *Aliment Pharmacol Ther* 2003; **17**: 243–51.

19 Mainie I, Tutuian R, Agrawal A, *et al*. Combined multichannel intraluminal impedance-pH monitoring to select patients with persistent gastro-oesophageal reflux for laparoscopic Nissen fundoplication. *Br J Surg* 2006; **92**: 1483–7.

20 Tutuian R, Mainie I, Agrawal A, *et al*. Nonacid reflux in patients with chronic cough on acid-suppressive therapy. *Chest* 2006; **130**: 386–91.

21 Oelschlager BK, Quiroga E, Parra JD, *et al*. Long-term outcomes after laparoscopic antireflux surgery. *Am J Gastroenterol* 2008; **103**: 280–7.

22 Swoger J, Ponsky J, Hicks DM, *et al*. Surgical fundoplication in laryngopharyngeal reflux unresponsive to aggressive acid suppression: A controlled study. *Clin Gastroenterol Hepatol* 2006; **4**: 433–41.

18

CHAPTER 18
Gastric Motility Testing

Jan Tack

Gastroenterology Section, University of Leuven, Leuven, Belgium

Summary

Tests of gastric motor function include gastric emptying tests, antroduodenal manometry, electrogastrograpy, and tests to study gastric accommodation. Tests of gastric motor function have limited diagnostic specificity, and their impact on management is hampered by the lack of therapeutic alternatives for patients with gastric motor disorders. Gastric emptying tests are most frequently applied clinically, and they may be useful when invasive or experimental therapies for gastroparesis are considered. Antroduodenal manometry is mostly useful in cases of severe, potentially generalized motor disorders. Electrogastrography and tests of gastric accommodation have mainly research applications.

Introduction

In patients presenting with gastrointestinal symptoms, conventional diagnostic approaches such as endoscopy with biopsies, radiological, or biochemical examinations, may identify an underlying abnormality that explains the patient's symptoms. When no such underlying disease can be found, it is often assumed that disorders of gastrointestinal motor or sensory function underlie symptom generation [1].

Symptoms related to feeding may include epigastric pain and burning, early satiation, postprandial fullness, anorexia, belching, nausea, and vomiting. These symptoms, in the absence of organic causes, may suggest a disturbance of gastric function and a number of tests have been developed to study the motor (and sensory) function of the stomach.

Gastric motor disorders can either be primary, that is no apparent underlying cause is present, or secondary, that is they are related to another medical condition of the patient. The primary and secondary gastric motor disorders are listed in Table 18.1. Tests are especially

useful if they have diagnostic specificity (i.e., the outcome of the test may yield a clear diagnosis), and if they are able to explain the patient's symptoms. Diagnostic tests may also determine the choice of therapy, help to predict response to therapy, and predict the long-term prognosis of the underlying condition.

Gastric Motility Testing

Assessment of gastric motor function is generally pursued after the exclusion of structural disease, using esophagogastroduodenoscopy (EGD), radiology, and laboratory testing. The most frequently applied tests of gastric motor function are measurement of gastric emptying rate, gastrointestinal manometry, electrogastrography, and gastric barostat testing.

Gastric Emptying Testing
Measurement of Gastric Emptying Rate
Several techniques are available to quantify gastric emptying of solid or liquid meals, but solid emptying rate is considered clinically most relevant. When evaluating suspected dumping syndrome, assessment of liquid emptying may also be considered. Radionuclide gastric emptying measurement is considered the standard

Practical Gastroenterology and Hepatology: Esophagus and Stomach, 1st edition. Edited by Nicholas J. Talley, Kenneth R. DeVault and David E. Fleischer. © 2010 Blackwell Publishing Ltd.

Table 18.1 Primary and secondary disorders of gastric motor and sensory function.

Primary disorders
    Functional dyspepsia—postprandial distress syndrome
    Functional dyspepsia—epigastric pain syndrome
    Idiopathic gastroparesis
    Chronic idiopathic nausea
    Functional vomiting
    Cyclic vomiting syndrome
    Aerophagia
    Rumination syndrome

Secondary disorders
    Metabolic disorders (diabetes, thyroid dysfunction)
    Postsurgical
    Drug-induced gastric motor disorders
    Central nervous system disorders
    Extrinsic neuropathy
    Intestinal neuropathy
    Intestinal myopathy

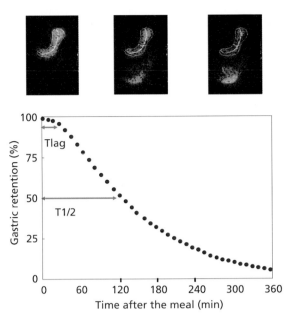

Figure 18.1 Scintigraphic assessment of gastric emptying rate. The presence of the radiolabeled meal is quantified in a region of interest, representing the stomach (upper panels). Presence of the label in the stomach region of interest over time is plotted and allows quantification of gastric half emptying time and lag phase.

method to assess gastric emptying rate. Depending on the label used, solid or liquid emptying can be assessed separately or simultaneously. The solid and/or liquid meal are labeled with a (different) radioisotope. A gamma-camera measures the number of counts in an investigator-determined region of interest (total, proximal or distal stomach, small intestine) for a certain time frame after ingestion of a meal. Mathematical processing involves corrections for distance to the camera and isotope decay, and curve fitting which allows calculation of the half emptying time, the lag phase (period of delay after meal ingestion before emptying starts), and the percentage of labeled meal retention at different time points (Figure 18.1). Although not routinely applied, the technique also has the ability to provide information on distribution within the stomach. Disadvantages include the use of radioactive substances, considerable costs, and the poor level of standardization of meal composition and measuring times over different laboratories. In a recent consensus document, supported by the American Neurogastroenterology and Motility Society and the American Society of Nuclear Medicine, a single standardized protocol for gastric emptying scintigraphy was proposed [2]. One potential drawback of the consensus proposal is the use of an egg replacement meal, which lacks lipids. As it is not uncommon for patients to report symptom aggravation after lipid-rich meals, it is unclear whether

lack of lipids compromises the ability of the meal to detect abnormalities in certain patient groups.

Breath tests can also be used to measure gastric emptying rates. The solid or liquid phase of a meal is labeled with a ^{13}C containing substrate (octanoic acid, acetic acid, glycin, or spirulina) [3]. As soon as the substrate enters the small bowel, it is metabolized with generation of $^{13}CO_2$, which appears in the breath. Breath sampling at regular intervals and mathematical processing of its $^{13}CO_2$ content over time allows calculation of a gastric emptying curve. The advantages of this test are the use of non-radioactive materials and the ability to perform the test outside a hospital setting. Disadvantages are the absence of standardization of meal and substrate. The test is well accepted in Europe, but has not gained clinical application in the USA.

Real-time ultrasonography has also been applied to measure gastric emptying [4]. The method is based on serial measurements of the cross-sectional area of the gastric antrum. In spite of attractive features, such as the non-invasive character, the absence of radiation burden, and the wide-spread availability of the equipment, ultrasonographic determination of gastric emptying rate has the disadvantages of being time-consuming and not suitable for solid meals. Moreover, antral volume is not only determined by gastric emptying rate, but also by redistribution of the meal inside the stomach, for instance in case of impaired accommodation.

The Smartpill® (SmartPill Corporation, Buffalo, New York) is a recently developed, non-digestible capsule which records luminal pH, temperature, and pressure during transit through the gastrointestinal tract with data transmitted to an ambulatory data recorder [5]. The device therefore provides a measure of gastric emptying time, small bowel transit time, and whole gut transit time. Simultaneous manometry studies demonstrated that the return of gastric phase 3 activity is the principal mechanism underlying emptying of the capsule from the stomach after a meal [6]. However, in a US multicenter study, gastric emptying times determined by the Smartpill® capsule correlated well with scintigraphy results, and were able to distinguish between health and gastroparesis with good diagnostic accuracy [7]. Although more large-scale studies are needed, Smartpill® has the potential to offer a non-radioactive, standardized, ambulatory alternative to scintigraphy in case of suspected gastroparesis, while also providing information on the amplitude of contractions and intestinal and colonic transit times as the capsule traverses the rest of the gastrointestinal tract.

Impact of Gastric Emptying Testing
Gastric emptying tests do not have a high diagnostic specificity. Delayed gastric emptying, for instance, can be found in the majority of patients with anorexia nervosa, and several drugs that are commonly used or co-existing neurological or endocrine disorders may affect gastric emptying rate. Hence, a finding of a delayed gastric emptying has limited diagnostic specificity. Similarly, one can find rapid gastric emptying, especially of liquids, in patients with dumping syndrome. However, a diagnosis of dumping syndrome cannot be made on the basis of rapid emptying alone, but requires specific additional tests or observations.

The relationship between gastric emptying rate and symptom pattern is also a matter of controversy. Studies in functional dyspepsia patients found associations between delayed gastric emptying and the presence and severity of symptoms of postprandial fullness, nausea and, vomiting. However, the correlation of delayed emp-

tying with the presence or severity of specific symptoms was weak, limiting its use when aiming at an explanation of symptoms. The impact of establishing abnormalities in gastric emptying on the therapeutic approach is also limited. The limited treatment options for patients with gastric motility disorders eliminates the need for a test to guide choices. Moreover, most studies found no correlation between the severity of delayed emptying and the response to prokinetic therapy.

Routine gastric emptying testing in patients with symptoms suggestive of impaired gastric motility therefore cannot be recommended, but can be applied in patients who fail to respond to initial empiric treatment approaches, especially when more invasive or experimental treatment modalities such as jejunal tube feeding or gastric electrical stimulation are considered.

Electrogastrography
Measurement of Gastric Electrical Rhythm
Cutaneous electrodes placed over the stomach region allow the measurement of gastric electrical activity. This electrogastrogram (EGG) provides information on frequency and regularity of gastric pacemaker activity, as well as on changes in power of the signal after meal ingestion [8].

Impact of Gastric Emptying Testing
The EGG has been advocated to distinguish between patients with normal and delayed emptying, and to explain intractable nausea. However, EGG abnormalities can also be induced through central mechanisms (e.g., vertigo-induced nausea). Furthermore, as EGG findings are unlikely to alter clinical management, EGG remains mainly a research tool.

Gastrointestinal Manometry
Antroduodenal Manometry
Antroduodenal manometry quantifies contractility in regions that determine interdigestive motility and gastric emptying [9]. The technique is only available at a small number of specialized centers, and is mainly used in the evaluation of patients with potentially generalized motility disorders, such as chronic idiopathic intestinal pseudo-obstruction syndromes. The key features that are evaluated on antroduodenal manometry are the number and amplitude of contractions, and their pattern in the interdigestive and in the postprandial state (Figure 18.2).

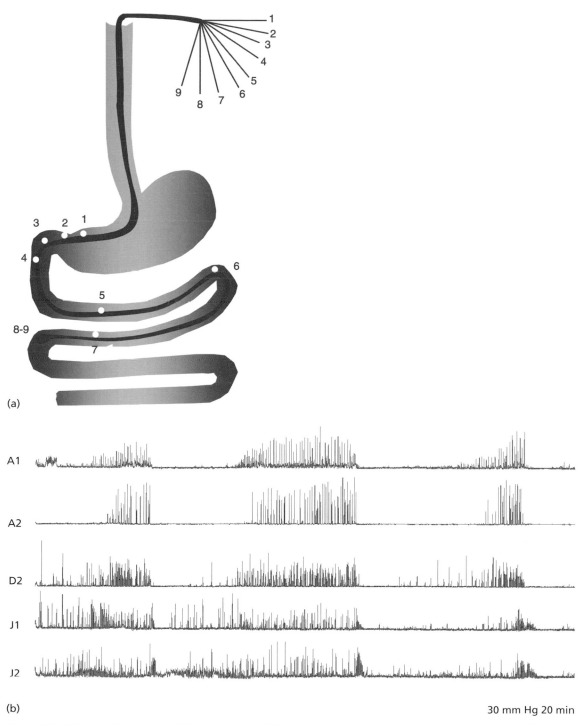

(a)

(b)

30 mm Hg 20 min

Figure 18.2 (a) Principle of antroduodenojejunal manometry, which uses a catheter with manometry ports in the stomach and different parts of the small intestine. (b) Example of interdigestive motility as recorded in the antrum (A channels), duodenum (D channel), and jejunum (J channels) with a catheter as depicted in (a).

So-called clustered contractions may be indicative of mechanical obstruction.

Impact of Antroduodenal Manometry

The finding of antral hypomotility is a non-specific finding, often associated with delayed gastric emptying. In patients with pseudo-obstruction syndrome or in radiation enteropathy, aberrant configuration and migration of intestinal phase 3 are indicators of a major motor disorder. Adequate assessment of interdigestive motility requires a prolonged measurement in the fasting state, and some centers are using 24-h antroduodenojejal manometry which provides a long nocturnal period for optimal evaluation of interdigestive motility. After a standard meal, up to 10 h may be required before return to normal interdigestive motility occurs.

With its ability to diagnose patterns suggestive of intestinal neuropathy (normal contractile strength, but abnormal patterns), intestinal myopathy (decreased contractile strength), retrogradely propagated phase 3 activity, and patterns suggestive of mechanical subobstruction, intestinal manometry has the potential to provide diagnostic specificity and to impact on management choices. This is a highly technical and often challenging procedure, which justifies referral to a specialized center when a provider contemplates the need for this type of testing.

Gastric Accommodation Testing

Methods to Measure Accommodation

The gastric barostat measures changes in tone and sensitivity to distension of the proximal stomach [10]. The procedure is invasive as it requires positioning of a double lumen polyvinyl tube with an adherent plastic bag through the mouth into the stomach. The barostat is the gold standard for measurement of gastric accommodation (meal-induced relaxation of the proximal stomach), which may be impaired in functional dyspepsia, but also in diabetic gastropathy, rumination syndrome, and after antireflux surgery. The gastric barostat can also be used to quantify sensitivity to gastric distension.

A number of other methods to assess gastric accommodation have been proposed. These include tolerance of an oral water or nutrient load, and gastric volume imaging by means of scintigraphy, ultrasound, single positron emission computed tomography (SPECT), or magnetic resonance imaging. Most of these require further validation and additional studies before they can be applied clinically.

Impact of Accommodation Testing

Although impaired accommodation has been associated to early satiation and weight loss, accommodation measurements are also influenced by emotions such as anxiety. In the absence of established therapy for impaired accommodation, measuring accommodation does not influence choice and outcome of therapy, and remains a research tool. The same is true for gastric hypersensitivity, which can also be measured with the barostat.

Take-home points

- The most frequently applied tests of gastric motor function are measurement of gastric emptying rate (scintigraphy or breath test), gastrointestinal manometry, and electrogastrography.

- Gastric emptying testing can be applied to help explain symptoms, but the impact on management is limited.

- In rare or refractory cases, small bowel manometry may lead to specific diagnoses.

- The main limitation to a greater clinical usefulness of gastric motility testing is the lack of therapeutic alternatives.

References

1 Tack J, Talley NJ, Camilleri M, *et al.* Functional gastroduodenal disorders. *Gastroenterology* 2006; **130**: 1466–79.

2 McCallum RW, Nowak T, Nusynowitz ML, *et al*; American Neurogastroenterology and Motility Society and the Society of Nuclear Medicine. Consensus recommendations for gastric emptying scintigraphy: a joint report of the American Neurogastroenterology and Motility Society and the Society of Nuclear Medicine. *Am J Gastroenterol* 2008; **103**: 753–63.

3 Sanaka M, Yamamoto T, Kuyama Y. Retention, fixation and loss of the [13C] label: a review for the understanding of gastric emptying breath tests. *Dig Dis Sci* 2008; **53**: 1747–56.

4 Gentilcore D, Hausken T, Horowitz M, Jones KL. Measurements of gastric emptying of low- and high-nutrient liquids using 3D ultrasonography and scintigraphy in healthy subjects. *Neurogastroenterol Motil* 2006; **18**: 1062–8.

5 Kuo B, McCallum RW, Koch KL, *et al.* Comparison of gastric emptying of a nondigestible capsule to a radio-labelled meal in healthy and gastroparetic subjects. *Aliment Pharmacol Ther* 2008; **27**: 186–96.

6 Cassilly D, Kantor S, Knight LC, *et al.* Gastric emptying of a non-digestible solid: assessment with simultaneous Smart-Pill pH and pressure capsule, antroduodenal manometry, gastric emptying scintigraphy. *Neurogastroenterol Motil* 2008; **20**: 311–9.

7 Rao SS, Kuo B, McCallum RW, *et al.* Investigation of colonic and whole-gut transit with wireless motility capsule and radiopaque markers in constipation. *Clin Gastroenterol Hepatol* 2009; **7**: 537–44.

8 Hutzinga JD. Physiology and pathophysiology of the interstitial cell of Cajal: from bench to bedside II. Gastric motility:

lessons from mutant mice on slow waves and innervation. *Am J Physiol* 2001; **281**: G1119–34.

9 Camilleri M, Bharucha AE, di Lorenzo C, *et al.* American Neurogastroenterology and Motility Society consensus statement on intraluminal measurement of gastrointestinal and colonic motility in clinical practice. *Neurogastroenterol Motil* 2008; **20**: 1269–82.

10 Sarnelli G, Vos R, Cuomo R, *et al.* Reproducibility of gastric barostat studies in healthy controls and in dyspeptic patients. *Am J Gastroenterol* 2001; **96**: 1047–53.

CHAPTER 19
Capsule Endoscopy for Esophageal Disease

Roberto de Franchis

Department of Medical Sciences, University of Milan, Milan, Italy

Summary

Endoscopic screening is recommended for patients with chronic gastroesophageal reflux symptoms to detect the presence of Barrett esophagus, and for cirrhotic patients to detect the presence of esophageal varices. Screening with conventional esophagogastroduodenoscopy (EGD) may be hampered by poor acceptance of the procedure by patients. Esophageal capsule endoscopy is painless, does not require sedation and might constitute a valid alternative to EGD. Studies comparing esophageal capsule endoscopy with EGD in patients with chronic gastroesophageal reflux symptoms and with cirrhosis have given variable results but, overall, esophageal capsule endoscopy has been found to be somewhat inferior to EGD for detecting both Barrett esophagus and esophageal varices. Whether the second-generation esophageal capsule endoscopy and the new ingestion procedure will fill the gap between EGD and esophageal capsule endoscopy remains to be ascertained with new studies.

Case

A 42-year-old man complaining of recent swelling of the abdomen is referred to the liver clinic for further evaluation. Upon questioning, he admits drinking up to 1 liter of hard liquor per day for the past 15 years. Physical examination reveals a swollen abdomen with shifting dullness. His liver chemistries show a slight increase of serum alanine amino transferase (ALT), aspartate amino transferase (AST) and bilirubin, and a modest decrease of serum albumin. Abdominal ultrasound shows a liver slightly reduced in size and the presence of fluid in the peritoneal cavity. After evacuation of the ascites, the patient undergoes liver stiffness measurement, which yields a value of 14 kPa, denoting advanced liver fibrosis. An EGD is proposed to evaluate the presence of varices, but the patient refuses. Esophageal capsule endoscopy is performed, showing large esophageal varices. The patient is discharged on diuretics and β-blockers, and with advice to stop drinking. At a follow-up visit at 6 months the patient is well; he declares that he has stopped drinking and can tolerate β-blockers well; no intra-abdominal fluid is detected on abdominal ultrasound scan and his serum ALT, AST, and bilirubin have returned to normal.

Equipment and Review of Technology

Capsule endoscopy technology has become suitable for the study of the esophagus with the ntroduction of the PillCam ESO (Given Imaging, Yoqneam, Israel) [1,2], a new capsule specifically designed for this organ (Video 12). Like the diagnostic system used for the small bowel capsule, the PillCam ESO diagnostic system consists of three main components: a disposable, ingestible capsule, a data recorder and sensor array, and a workstation with proprietary software for processing and interpreting the endoscopic images. Although the PillCam ESO capsule is

Practical Gastroenterology and Hepatology: Esophagus and Stomach, 1st edition. Edited by Nicholas J. Talley, Kenneth R. DeVault and David E. Fleischer. © 2010 Blackwell Publishing Ltd.

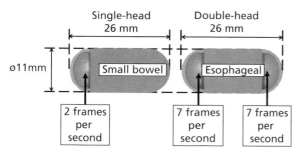

Figure 19.1 Comparison of the characteristics of the small bowel and the esophageal capsule.

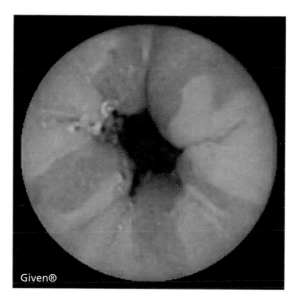

Figure 19.2 Capsule image of Barrett esophagus.

the same size and shape as the small bowel capsule, it differs in that it carries two imagers, one at each end, and each imager captures seven frames per second, instead of two frames per second of the single imager of the small bowel capsule (Figure 19.1). Other important differences concern the duration of capsule battery life (20 min for the esophageal, 8 h for the small bowel capsule) and the sensor array: three sensors applied to the chest wall are used in conjunction with the PillCam ESO as compared to eight sensors applied to the abdominal wall for use with the small bowel capsule. Finally, since fluoroscopic studies have shown that the capsule speed in the esophagus can reach up to 20 cm/s, a special ingestion procedure has been devised to slow down esophageal transit: the patient is instructed to swallow 100 mL of water to clear saliva from the esophagus. The patient then ingests the capsule in a supine position and is allowed to drink up to 10 mL of water to facilitate swallowing. After ingestion, the patient is kept in the supine position for 2 min, then the chest is raised to an angle of 30° for 2 min, and then to 60° for 1 min. The patient is instructed to avoid speaking or moving during this time, after which he/she is allowed to resume normal activity. After 20 min the recording ends, the sensor array, and recorder are removed and the patient is discharged. Preliminary studies have shown that the esophageal capsule can provide good-quality images of the esophagus [1,2] (Figures 19.2 and 19.3).

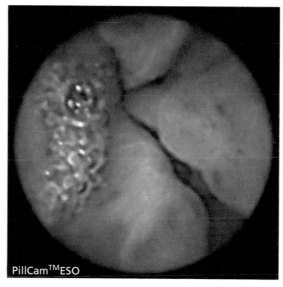

Figure 19.3 Capsule image of large esophageal varices.

Clinical Applications of Esophageal Capsule Endoscopy

The esophageal diseases that most frequently require endoscopy are gastroesophageal reflux disease and its complications (esophagitis, stricture, and Barrett esophagus) and esophageal varices. Indeed, most guidelines recommend endoscopic screening of patients with chronic reflux symptoms [3,4] to detect Barrett esophagus, and of patients with cirrhosis and portal

Table 19.1 Performance characteristics of capsule endoscopy compared with EGD for the diagnosis of suspected Barrett esophagus in patients with chronic gastroesophageal reflux symptoms.

Author, year	Ref.	Number of patients	Failed capsule study* n (%)	Prevalence of Barrett esophagus (%)	Sensitivity (%)	Specificity (%)	PPV (%)	NPV (%)	LR+	LR–	Miss rate† n (%)
Eliakim R et al., 2004	[1]	17	0 (0.0)	n. a.	100	80	92	100	5.0	0	0 (0.0)
Eliakim R et al., 2005	[12]	109	3 (2.7)	31	97	99	97	99	69.2	0.014	1 (3.0)
Lin OS et al., 2007	[13]	95	5 (5.3)	23	67	84	56	89	4.2	0.39	7 (33.3)
Sharma P et al., 2008	[14]	100	6 (6.0)	22‡	67‡	87‡	60‡	90‡	5.1‡	0.38‡	3 (33.3)‡
Galmiche JP et al., 2008	[15]	89	12 (13.5)	13	60	100	100	95	60.0	0.60	4 (40.0)

*Inability to swallow the capsule, rapid esophageal transit or unusable capsule images.
PPV, positive predictive value; NPV, negative predictive value; LR+, positive likelihood ratio; LR–, negative likelihood ratio.
LR+ ≥ 10 and LR– ≤ 0.1 denote "robust" performance.
†Number (%) of patients with suspected Barrett esophagus who would have been missed if the alternative test had been performed instead of EGD.
‡Data refer to 41 patients with GERD symptoms enrolled for screening; this study also included 53 patients enrolled for surveillance of known Barrett esophagus.

hypertension [5–10] to detect the presence of varices. Currently, such screening is done by EGD, which is generally well tolerated but can be perceived as unpleasant, requires conscious sedation in most cases, may lead to decreased work productivity, and has a small but not insignificant risk of complications [11]. All these factors may hamper the adherence to screening programs. An accurate, safe, painless, and convenient alternative imaging procedure would enhance the acceptability of endoscopic screening and might improve compliance.

Capsule endoscopy is painless and does not require sedation, and thus is a potential substitute for EGD; as a consequence, most studies with this device have compared capsule endoscopy and EGD for the diagnosis of Barrett esophagus and esophageal varices.

Performance of Capsule Endoscopy in Patients with Chronic Gastroesophageal Reflux

The role of capsule endoscopy in this setting would be to identify patients with suspected Barrett esophagus, who should then undergo EGD for histological confirmation. Between 2004 and 2008, five papers [1,12–15] have specifically analyzed the diagnostic yield of capsule endos-

copy for the diagnosis of Barrett esophagus and esophagitis in patients with chronic gastroesophageal reflux. These studies proved that esophageal capsule endoscopy is feasible and safe; however, the results, listed in Table 19.1, have been variable; sensitivity and specificity of capsule endoscopy for the diagnosis of Barrett esophagus were excellent in the first two [1,12], but were disappointing in the other three [13–15]. In particular, in the latter three studies, up to 40% of patients with suspected Barrett esophagus would have been missed if capsule endoscopy had been used instead of EGD. Another study [16] examined a mixed population of patients, including cases of reflux esophagitis, hiatus hernia, esophageal varices, Barrett esophagus etc. In this study, the overall diagnostic yield of capsule endoscopy for the detection of esophageal pathology was 62.5% with positive and negative predictive values of 80.0% and 61.1% respectively; the overall agreement between capsule endoscopy and EGD was only moderate (κ = 0.42). In a further study [17], capsule endoscopy was performed in 23 patients with chronic gastroesophageal reflux and in five with cirrhosis refusing conventional EGD. This study confirmed the feasibility and safety of esophageal capsule endoscopy; however, the performance characteristics of the capsule could not be estimated as there was no comparator.

Performance of Esophageal Capsule Endoscopy in Patients with Cirrhosis

In patients with a new diagnosis of cirrhosis, capsule endoscopy could be used as a screening tool to detect the presence of varices: patients with no or small varices at screening endoscopy should enter endoscopic surveillance, while patients with medium-sized or large varices should be treated prophylactically to prevent bleeding. In patients with a previous diagnosis of esophageal varices, capsule endoscopy could be used as a surveillance tool, to detect those patients in whom the varices have increased in size and require prophylaxis.

Four pilot studies [18–21] and a large, multicenter study [22] have examined the potential of the esophageal capsule in comparison with EGD for the diagnosis of esophageal varices. The performance characteristics of capsule endoscopy in these studies are reported in Table 19.2. The pilot studies have shown that the degree of correlation between the capsule and standard EGD in the detection of varices ranges from fair to excellent. The multicenter trial included 288 patients with portal hypertension. The study was designed as a non-inferiority trial using conventional EGD as the gold standard, with the assumption that a difference of 10% or less between EGD and capsule endoscopy for the diagnosis of varices would denote equivalence. There was substantial agreement between capsule endoscopy and EGD for the diagnosis of varices ($\kappa = 0.73$). Capsule endoscopy had a sensitivity of 84% and a specificity of 88% for the detection of varices. The probability of having varices rose from a pretest value of 62.5% to a post-test value of 93%. For the discrimination between medium–large varices and small or no varices, the agreement between capsule endoscopy was also substantial ($\kappa = 0.77$): sensitivity and specificity were 78% and 96% respectively, with a change of the probability of having large varices from a pretest value of 27.4% to a post-test value of 85%. However, since the difference in diagnosing varices was 15.6% in favor of EGD, the study was considered negative.

Patient Satisfaction Assessment

Preprocedure patient anxiety and/or postprocedure satisfaction for capsule endoscopy and EGD were assessed in seven studies [1,12,18–22]: in all, capsule endoscopy was mostly preferred over EGD.

Cost–benefit Analysis of Capsule Endoscopy versus EGD

Two studies [23,24] have analyzed the cost–benefit and the cost–utility ratio of capsule endoscopy for the detection of Barrett esophagus; in both, EGD appeared to be the preferred strategy. One study [25] examined the budget impact of endoscopic screening for esophageal varices in cirrhosis, and concluded that capsule endoscopy screening followed by β-blocker treatment for patients with large varices would be an acceptable strategy. However, all the cost–effectiveness studies carried out so far suffer from the paucity of hard data on which to base the model assumptions.

Conclusions

In most studies comparing the esophageal capsule with standard EGD for the diagnosis of Barrett esophagus, capsule endoscopy appeared to be inferior to EGD. The performance of capsule endoscopy was found to be better for the investigation of esophageal varices than for Barrett esophagus; however, the capsule was still not equivalent to EGD. It should be noted that the capsule study failed in up to 13.5% of patients, owing to: the inability of patients to swallow the capsule; rapid esophageal transit; the presence of bubbles or debris in the esophagus; failure to visualize the entire Z–line; or to technical problems such as failure to record capsule images. In addition, even in technically correct recordings, the agreement between EGD and capsule findings was inconsistent, ranging from near perfect to unsatisfactory. Some of the above problems may be solved in the future: in fact, a new improved esophageal capsule has been recently introduced [26], which features a higher rate of images capture (18 vs. 14 per second), a wider angle of vision (169° vs. 140°) advanced optics and automated light control, which results in capsule images quite similar to those of EGD. In addition, a new ingestion procedure has been devised [27], which decreases the amount of bubbles at the gastroesophageal junction and allows a better visualization of the Z-line. Whether these improvements will fill the gap between the performance of capsule endoscopy and that of EGD remains to be ascertained in future

Table 19.2 Performance characteristics of capsule endoscopy for the diagnosis of esophageal varices in patients with portal hypertension

Author, year	Ref.	Number of patients	Failed capsule study* n (%)	Prevalence of EV (%)	Cut-off (%)	Sensitivity (%)	Specificity (%)	PPV (%)	NPV (%)	LR+	LR-	Miss rate‡ n (%)
Eisen G et al., 2006	[18]	32	0 (0.0)	72	n.a.	100	89	96	100	9.1	<0.1	0 (0)
Lapalus MG et al., 2006	[19]	21	1 (4.8)	75	n.a.	81	100	100	57	>8.75	0.19	3 (19)
Groce JR et al., 2007	[20]	21	1 (4.5)	43	n.a.	78	83	78	83	4.6	0.26	2 (22)
Pena LR et al., 2008	[21]	20	2 (10.0)	95	n.a.	68	100	100	14	> 6.8	0.32	6 (32)
de Franchis R et al., 2008 all varices	[22]	290	2 (0.7)	63	n.a.	84	88	92	77	7.0	0.18	29 (16)
medium–large varices				27	25†	78	96	87	92	19.5	0.23	17 (22)

*Inability to swallow the capsule, rapid esophageal transit or unusable capsule images.

PPV, positive predicting value; NPV, negative predicting value; LR+, positive likelihood ratio; LR−, negative likelihood ratio.

LR+ ≥ 10 and LR− ≤ 0.1 denote "robust" performance.

†25% of the capsule picture frame.

‡Number (%) of patients with varices (or large varices) who would have been missed if the alternative test had been performed instead of EGD.

studies. For the time being, capsule endoscopy can only be recommended for patients unwilling or unable to undergo conventional EGD.

Take-home points

- Endoscopic screening is utilized for patients with chronic gastroesophageal reflux symptoms to detect the presence of Barrett esophagus, and for cirrhotic patients to detect the presence of esophageal varices.

- Esophageal capsule endoscopy is painless, does not require sedation and might constitute a valid alternative to EGD

- A special ingestion procedure, involving patient positioning and sips of water, is utilized to obtain more images of the esophagus.

- Studies comparing esophageal capsule endoscopy with EGD in patients with chronic gastroesophageal reflux symptoms and with cirrhosis have given variable results but, overall, esophageal capsule endoscopy has been found to be somewhat inferior to EGD for detecting both Barrett esophagus and esophageal varices.

References

1 Eliakim R, Yassin K, Shlomi I, et al. A novel diagnostic tool for detecting esophageal pathology: the PillCam oesophageal videocapsule. *Aliment Pharmacol Ther* 2004; **20**: 1083–9.

2 Koslowsky B, Jacob H, Eliakim R, et al. PillCam ESO in esophageal studies: improved diagnostic yield of 14 frames per second (fps) compared with 4 fps. *Endoscopy* 2006; **38**: 27–30.

3 Armstrong D, Marshall JK, Chiba N, et al. Canadian Consensus Conference on the management of gastroesophageal reflux disease in adults: update 2004. *Can J Gastroenterol* 2005; **19**: 15–35.

4 Sampliner RE. Updated guidelines for the diagnosis, surveillance and therapy of Barrett's esophagus. *Am J Gastroenterol* 2002; **97**: 1888–95.

5 de Franchis R. Developing consensus in portal hypertension. *J Hepatol* 1996; **25**: 390–4.

6 Grace ND, Groszmann RJ, Garcia-Tsao G, et al. Portal hypertension and variceal bleeding: an AASLD single topic symposium. *Hepatology* 1998; **28**: 868–80.

7 Jalan R, Hayes PC. UK guidelines on the management of variceal haemorrhage in cirrhotic patients. *Gut* 2000; **46** (Suppl. III): 1–15.

8 de Franchis R. Updating consensus in portal hypertension. *J Hepatol* 2000; **33**: 846–52.

9 de Franchis R. Evolving consensus in portal hypertension. Report of the Baveno IV Consensus Workshop on methodology of diagnosis and therapy in portal hypertension. *J Hepatol* 2005; **43**: 167–76.

10 Garcia-Tsao G, Sanyal AJ, Grace ND, et al. Prevention and management of gastroesophageal varices and variceal hemorrhage in cirrhosis. *Hepatology* 2007; **46**: 922–38.

11 Eisen G, Baron TH, Dominitz J. American Society for Gastrointestinal Endoscopy. Complications of upper GI endoscopy. *Gastrointest Endosc* 2002; **55**: 784–93.

12 Eliakim R, Sharma VK, Yassin K, et al. A prospective study of the diagnostic accuracy of PillCam ESO esophageal capsule endoscopy versus conventional upper endoscopy in patients with chronic gastroesophageal reflux disease. *J Clin Gastroenterol* 2005; **39**: 572–8.

13 Lin OS, Schembre DB, Mergener K, et al. Blinded comparison of esophageal capsule endoscopy versus conventional endoscopy for a diagnosis of Barrett's esophagus in patients with chronic gastroesophageal reflux. *Gastrointest Endosc* 2007; **65**: 577–83.

14 Sharma P, Wani S, Rastogi A, et al. The diagnostic accuracy of esophageal capsule endoscopy in patients with gastroesophageal reflux disease and Barrett's esophagus: a blinded, prospective study. *Am J Gastroenterol* 2008; **103**: 525–32.

15 Galmiche JP, Sacher-Huvelin S, Coron E, et al. Screening for esophagitis and Barrett's esophagus with wireless capsule endoscopy: a multicenter prospective trial in patients with reflux symptoms. *Am J Gastroenterol* 2008; **103**: 538–45.

16 Delvaux M, Papanikolau IS, Fassler I, et al. Esophageal capsule endoscopy in petients with suspected esophageal disease: double blinded comparison with esophagogastroduodenoscopy and assessment of interobserver variability. *Endoscopy* 2008; **40**: 16–22.

17 Sànchez-Yagüe A, Caunedo-'Alvarez A, Garcia-Montes JM, et al. Esophageal capsule endoscopy in patients refusing conventional endoscopy for the study of suspected esophageal pathology. *Eur J Gastroenterol Hepatol* 2006; **18**: 977–83.

18 Eisen G, Eliakim R, Zaman A, et al. The accuracy of PillCam ESO capsule endoscopy versus conventional upper endoscopy for the diagnosis of esophageal varices: a prospective three-center pilot study. *Endoscopy* 2006; **38**: 31–5.

19 Lapalus MG, Dumortier J, Fumex F, et al. Esophageal capsule endoscopy versus esophagogastroduodenoscopy for evaluating portal hypertension: a prospective comparative study of performance and tolerance. *Endoscopy* 2006; **38**: 36–41.

20 Groce JR, Raju GS, Sood GK, et al. A prospective blinded comparative trial of capsule esophagoscopy vs. traditional EGD for variceal screening. *Gastroenterology* 2007; **102** (Suppl. 2): A 802 (abstract).

21 Pena LR, Cox T, Koch AG, *et al.* Study comparing oesopha-geal capsule endoscopy versus EGD in the detection of varices. *Dig Liver Dis* 2008; **40**: 216–23.

22 de Franchis R, Eisen GM, Laine L, *et al.* Esophageal capsule endoscopy for screening and surveillance of esophageal varices in patients with portal hypertension. *Hepatology* 2008; **47**: 1595–603.

23 Gerson L, Lin OS. Cost-benefit analysis of capsule endos-copy compared with standard upper endoscopy for the detection of Barrett's esophagus. *Clin Gastroenterol Hepatol* 2007; **5**: 319–25.

24 Rubenstein JH, Inadomi JM, Brill JV, *et al.* Cost utility of screening for Barrett's esophagus with esophageal capsule endoscopy versus conventional upper endoscopy. *Clin Gastroenterol Hepatol* 2007; **5**: 312–18.

25 Spiegel BMR, Esrailian E, Eisen G. The budget impact of endoscopic screening for esophageal varices in cirrhosis. *Gastrointest Endosc* 2007; **66**: 679–92.

26 Gralnek IM, Adler SN, Koslowsky B, *et al.* Detecting esopha-geal disease with second-generation capsule endoscopy: initial evaluation of the PillCam ESO 2. *Endoscopy* 2008; **40**: 275–9.

27 Gralnek IM, Rabinowitz R, Afik D, *et al.* A simplified inges-tion procedure for esophageal capsule endoscopy: initial evaluation of healthy volunteers. *Endoscopy* 2006; **38**: 913–18.

CHAPTER 20

Unsedated Endoscopy

Deepak Agrawal[1] and Amitabh Chak[2]

[1] University Texas Southwestern Medical Center, Dallas, TX, USA
[2] Division of Gastroenterology, Case Western Reserve University School of Medicine, Cleveland, OH, USA

Summary

The availability of newer, small-caliber videoendoscopes makes unsedated endoscopy an attractive option for the screening of Barrett esophagus, esophageal varices, and gastric cancers. Unsedated endoscopy, via a transnasal or peroral route, is well tolerated, has a diagnostic accuracy similar to standard esophagogastroduodenoscopy (EGD) and leads to substantial cost savings. Preconceived notions on the part of physicians, as well as patients, continue to be an obstacle to the widespread acceptance of this procedure.

Case

A physician who had participated in trials using small-caliber endoscopes during his fellowship opens a practice in a city where there had been no gastroenterologist before and he becomes very busy during the first year. He performs many of the EGDs in his office to increase his efficiency but he has a limited area for recovering patients after a sedated procedure. He offers patients the option of non-sedated or sedated EGDs and about one-third of the patients give the unsedated procedure a try. About half of those like the convenience of not being sedated and tolerate the procedure well. Three years later he moves to a much larger office where recovery space is not a problem, but he finds that many of those who are in surveillance programs for Barrett or who have had family members undergo unsedated endoscopy prefer that approach. At his 10-year anniversary he finds that he is performing about 25% of his office endoscopies with no sedation.

Introduction

Esophagogastroduodenoscopy (EGD) without conscious sedation has been used since the introduction of flexible EGD in 1957, and is commonly performed in many parts

Practical Gastroenterology and Hepatology: Esophagus and Stomach, 1st edition. Edited by Nicholas J. Talley, Kenneth R. DeVault and David E. Fleischer. © 2010 Blackwell Publishing Ltd.

of the world. The development of smaller caliber endoscopes make unsedated endoscopy an increasingly popular option to sedated examinations [1,2]. However, unsedated endoscopy is still not widely accepted in the United States [3].

Equipment

Small-caliber (sc) endoscopes, generally less than 6 mm in diameter, are recommended for unsedated endoscopy. Standard diagnostic upper endoscopes have diameters of 9 to 11 mm with an accessory channel of 2.8 mm (Figures 20.1 and 20.2). The sc-endoscopes suitable for unsedated examinations commercially available through various manufacturers are listed in Table 20.1 (see Video 13).

Recent advances in sc-endoscopes include thinner diameter, four-way angulation, wider viewing angle, and improved CCD chips that provide image quality similar to conventional endoscopes. From the endoscopes listed in Table 20.1, it is apparent that the variables in choosing the endoscope include the length, outer diameter, two-way versus four-way angulation, and the viewing angle. The goal of unsedated endoscopy is maximum patient comfort while achieving maximum diagnostic efficacy. Based mainly on anecdotal data, the most important determinant of patient comfort appears to be

Table 20.1 Small-caliber endoscopes suitable for unsedated examinations.

Company	Model	Outer diameter (mm)	Channel (mm)	Length (mm)	Up/down	R/L	View (degrees)
Olympus	GIF-XP160	5.9	2	1345	180/90	100/100	120
Olympus	GIF-N180	4.9	2	1100	210/90	N/A	120
Olympus	PEF-V	5.3	2	650	–	N/A	–
Pentax	FG-16V	5.3	2	925	180/180	160/160	125
Pentax	EE-1540	5.1	2	600	210/120	N/A	140
Pentax	EG-1540	5.1	2	1050	210/120	N/A	140
Pentax	EG-1840	6	2	1050	210/120	120/120	120
Pentax	EE-1580K	5.1	2	600	210/120	N/A	140
Pentax	EG-1580K	5.1	2	1050	210/120	N/A	140
Pentax	EE-1870K	6	2	1050	210/120	120/120	140
Fujinon	EG-530N	5.9	2	1100	210/90	100/100	120
Fujinon	EG-470N5	5.9	2	1100	210/90	100/100	120
Fujinon	EG-270N5	5.9	2	1100	210/90	100/100	120

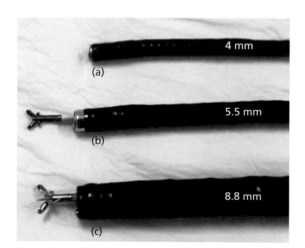

Figure 20.1 A prototype esophagoscope (a) without a biopsy channel; an ultrathin upper endoscope with biopsy channel (b); and. insertion tubes of the standard diagnostic upper endoscope (c). Reproduced courtesy of Olympus America, Inc.

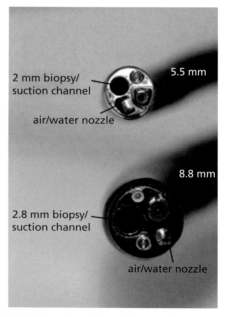

Figure 20.2 *En face* view of tips of the two endoscopes with biopsy channels from Figure 20.1.

the endoscope diameter. Esophagoscopes that are 60 cm in length with diameters of 5 mm or less have been proposed for population screening of esophageal varices and Barrett esophagus. Slightly larger diameter sc-endoscopes with an accessory channel and a full working length of 100 cm or more are useful for a complete examination and obtaining biopsies. Some sc-endoscopes only have two-way angulation. Although these endoscopes can perform a complete EGD, directed biopsies with these instruments can be challenging. Four-way angulation appears to be advantageous in positioning the scope during targeted biopsies [2]. Wider viewing angles are inherently appealing to improve the completeness of the examination but it is unclear if there is a minimal angle of view that is necessary for a complete examination.

Technique

Unsedated EGD can be performed either transnasally or perorally. The procedure must be explained clearly and reassurances offered to the patient to decrease the patient's anxiety and improve tolerance. Topical lidocaine is then used to anesthetize the mucosa. For the transnasal approach, the most patent nostril is identified by visual inspection and then lidocaine or a derivative applied by a cotton-tip applicator or under endoscopic visualization by using a catheter through the accessory channel of the endoscope. Use of topical vasoconstrictors is optional. These are reported to constrict the spongy nasal turbinates and facilitate passage of the endoscope. Oropharygeal spray may be helpful because nasal anesthesia does not significantly alter the laryngeal sensation. For the peroral approach, an oropharyngeal anesthetic spray is recommended.

The procedure can be performed with the patient in either the standard left lateral decubitus position or in the upright position. The procedure should be performed with minimal air insufflation and the endoscope should be moved slowly and gently to decrease patient discomfort. Care must be taken to avoid contact of the endo- scope with the nasal turbinates (see Video 13). Talking to the patient and demonstrating findings on the video monitor may help reassure patients while the procedure is being performed. There is no clear consensus on which route (transnasal vs. peroral) is preferable, although

studies have suggested that the transnasal route is much better tolerated [2,4]. It is likely that the preferred route for unsedated endoscopy is patient specific and some endoscopists recommend letting the patient choose. A biopsy specimen can be obtained with a pediatric biopsy forceps (diameter 1.8 mm) through the smaller accessory channel as required.

Clinical Considerations

Clinical Uses

Unsedated sc-EGD can be performed for all the diagnostic indications of sc-EGD. Major indications include the screening of Barrett esophagus in the United States [5] and gastric cancer screening in countries where gastric cancer prevalence is high. Patients at high risk of complications from sedation are also good candidates for diagnostic unsedated sc-EGD. Therapeutic procedures such as placement of enteral feeding tubes and PEG tubes have also been performed with sc-endoscopes in intensive care unit patients and patients with esophageal strictures.

Feasibility

The feasibility of unsedated EGD, defined as the ability to complete the procedure, ranges from 88% to 98.8% in different studies. The success rates for passage through the pylorus are 100% and intubation of the second portion of the duodenum are reportedly over 92%. These rates are comparable across patient populations in different countries, in males and females. Reasons for inability to perform the procedure include patient intolerance due to excessive gagging when using the peroral route, nasal pain, and narrow nasal passage. Peroral endoscopy can be successful when the transnasal route fails.

Tolerance and Acceptability

The tolerance of unsedated EGD is the most important factor that determines patient acceptance, physician acceptance, and, ultimately, the adequacy and feasibility of the procedure. "Tolerance" is a complex and subjective variable, which can be difficult to measure. It is affected by numerous patient-related factors such as patient age, gender, race, education, preprocedure anxiety and operator-related factors such as prior experience, endoscopy skill, and technical parameters of the endoscope.

The rate of acceptance of a repeat endoscopy can be a surrogate marker of tolerance. In published studies, the rate varies substantially and appears to depend on the nature of the health-care system, geography, and culture, with rates of over 95% reported from Japan and around 70 to 93% from studies in the United States [1,2,4]. In other studies, amongst patients who had both sedated c-EGD and unsedated sc-EGD, 46–87% of patients preferred unsedated EGD. The results of tolerance and acceptance of transnasal versus peroral route have also been contradictory, although in recent studies the transnasal route has been preferred [2,4].

Barriers to Acceptance

The initial acceptance rate of unsedated sc-EGD in research studies is around 52% [6] and its use is still confined to few large academic centers. Sc-endoscopes use the same endoscopy platform as standard endoscopes. Unsedated sc-EGD is easy to learn and perform [7]. Technical considerations should not be a factor for poor acceptance. In one study, the referral for unsedated sc-EGD was poor even with ready availability of trained endoscopists [3]. This suggests that the perception of discomfort by both the patients and the physicians may be a major barrier to the spread of this procedure.

Efficacy

The diagnostic yield of biopsies in unsedated sc-EGD has been found to be similar to that of c-EGD in evaluation for *Helicobacter pylori* diagnosis and eradication, detection and grading of esophageal varices, and detection of Barrett metaplasia and dysplasia. The channel of the small caliber endoscope is 2 mm, necessitating the use of pediatric biopsy forceps. However, studies have reported no difference in precision or efficacy of biopsies using these smaller biopsy forceps.

Complications

Unsedated EGD is a safe procedure. Small case series have suggested a minor complication rate of 0–6.5%. These complications include nasal pain, epistaxis, and vasovagal attacks. Epistaxis is usually mild and easily treated with cotton swab tamponade.

Take-home points

- Unsedated small-caliber EGD is a feasible, effective cheaper alternative to conventional EGD.
- It is well tolerated by most patients, although the overall comfort level may be less than sedated EGD.
- The overall acceptance of this procedure remains poor.
- Physicians should consider unsedated endoscopy as an alternative for patients, especially those at high risk for complications from sedation.

References

1 Sorbi D, Gostout CJ, Henry J, *et al.* Unsedated small-caliber EGD versus conventional EGD: a comparative study. *Gastroenterology* 1999; **117**: 1301–7.

2 Trevisani L, Cifalà V, Sartori S, *et al.* Unsedated ultrathin upper endoscopy is better than conventional endoscopy in routine outpatient gastroenterology practice: A randomized trial. *World J Gastroenterol* 2007; **13**: 906–11.

3 Atkinson M, Das A, Faulx A, *et al.* Ultrathin esophagoscopy in screening for Barrett's esophagus at a Veterans Administration Hospital: easy access does not lead to referrals. *Am J Gastroenterol* 2008; **103**: 92–7.

4 Tatsumi Y, Harada A, Matsumoto T, *et al.* Feasibility and tolerance of 2-way and 4-way angulation videoscopes for unsedated patients undergoing transnasal EGD in GI cancer screening. *Gastrointest Endosc* 2008; **67**: 1021–7.

5 Saeian K, Staff DM, Vasilopoulos S, *et al.* Unsedated transnasal endoscopy accurately detects Barrett's metaplasia and dysplasia. *Gastrointest Endosc* 2002; **56**: 472–8.

6 Faulx AL, Catanzaro A, Zyzanski S, *et al.* Patient tolerance and acceptance of unsedated ultrathin esophagoscopy. *Gastrointest Endosc* 2002; **55**: 620–3.

7 Maffei M, Dumortier J, Dumonceau J. Self-training in unsedated transnasal EGD by endoscopists competent in standard peroral EGD: prospective assessment of the learning curve. *Gastrointest Endosc* 2008; **67**: 410–8.

PART 4

Problem-based Approach to Diagnosis and Differential Diagnosis

CHAPTER 21

General Approach to History Taking and Physical Exam of the Upper Gastrointestinal Tract

Evan S. Dellon[1] and Eugene M. Bozymski[2]

[1] Division of Gastroenterology and Hepatology, Department of Medicine, University of North Carolina School of Medicine, Chapel Hill, NC, USA
[2] Department of Medicine, Division of Gastroenterology and Hepatology, University of North Carolina Medical Center, Chapel Hill, NC, USA

Summary

The history and physical exam remains the cornerstone of the doctor–patient relationship, providing the basis for formulating a differential diagnosis and directing medical decision making. After a thorough history and physical, the physician should be well along in determining the genesis of the patient's problem. This chapter discusses an approach to the history and physical which emphasizes developing a physician–patient rapport and a complete differential by focusing on upper gastrointestinal symptoms that are commonly encountered in the practice of Gastroenterology, including heartburn, dysphagia, nausea and vomiting, abdominal pain, and diarrhea. General approaches to beginning and ending the visit, asking pertinent questions which maximize information yield, and performing a targeted but thorough physical exam are also reviewed.

The history and physical exam (H&P) remains the cornerstone of the doctor–patient relationship, forming the basis of medical decision making. In the current age of rapidly evolving technologies it may seem expedient to proceed directly to testing after a cursory history, but this is a trap that should be avoided. A thorough yet targeted H&P is the best way to construct an appropriate differential diagnosis (DDx) which facilitates judicious use of the numerous testing modalities available. This chapter will discuss an approach to the H&P which emphasizes developing a physician–patient rapport and a complete DDx.

Practical Gastroenterology and Hepatology: Esophagus and Stomach, 1st edition. Edited by Nicholas J. Talley, Kenneth R. DeVault and David E. Fleischer. © 2010 Blackwell Publishing Ltd.

Setting the Stage

A good visit starts with introducing yourself to the patient by making eye contact and shaking their hand. It is not only good practice to wash your hands in the patient's view prior to shaking hands, but also an important part of the National Patient Safety Goals. Then, take a seat at the same level as the patient, preferably without any barriers (such as a desk) between you. The first question is the most important and should be sufficiently open-ended to allow the patient to fully describe their concerns. Possible options include: "What can I help you with?", "What brings you into the office today?", or "I see Dr So-and-so referred you. I've reviewed your records, but I wanted to hear what's been going on from your perspective." It is less advisable to start with a directed or yes/no question because it immediately limits what the patient might tell you.

It is also important to allow the patient to speak without interruption. Data indicate that, on average, physicians interrupt patients after only 18 seconds [1]. This temptation to ask questions immediately should be suppressed. If the patient talks for enough time and you listen carefully, in most cases they will tell you what is wrong with them. After a certain amount of time, directed questions or redirection is appropriate. Experienced clinicians have learned how to do this without appearing to interrupt the patient: "These symptoms seem to have affected your life greatly. Let's go back to the beginning. Can you tell me where exactly the pain was located the very first time it occurred?"

A final, general point is that if there are records to review from prior evaluation, it is best to do this before seeing the patient rather than shuffling though pages when they are talking. Any prior information should certainly play into the overall diagnostic picture, but keeping an open mind is key during the early phase of the H&P. Symptoms should then be explored in depth, with special focus on onset, exacerbating and relieving factors, progression, and other associated factors. A thorough medication history, including over-the-counter drugs and supplements, is imperative given the number of agents available with myriad potential side effects. The remainder of this chapter will review the approach to the H&P for common symptoms of upper GI tract diseases.

Heartburn

Heartburn, a substernal burning sensation that radiates orad, is the cardinal symptom of gastroesophageal reflux disease (GERD). When approaching a patient with this complaint, the symptom must be elicited accurately. Because heartburn is frequently (but perhaps imprecisely) experienced, patients may really mean dysphagia, chest pain, shortness-of-breath, or even abdominal pain when they say that have heartburn [2]. When discussing this complaint, focused questioning should be used to clarify exactly what is meant. Questioning should also attempt to exclude other conditions which might present with central chest pain mimicking heartburn from reflux. For example, when does the symptom occur? If it is postprandial, nocturnal, or exacerbated by lying supine or bending over, then it is more typical of GERD. If it is exertional, then heart disease should be considered. Since symptom overlap may make differentiation difficult,

cardiac evaluation will often be necessary. It is not uncommon for gastroenterologists to pick up unstable angina masquerading as "GERD" [3]. Physical exam is generally normal in the patients with heartburn from GERD, but clues of severe acid exposure (e.g., tooth enamel loss) may be detected.

Dysphagia

When a patient presents with a chief complaint of difficulty swallowing, the H&P should be used to distinguish between oropharyngeal (or transfer) dysphagia and esophageal dysphagia and whether the symptoms most likely represent a structural or motor disease. Dysphagia can be sought by asking the patient whether food "sticks", is "hung-up", or "slows down" after swallowing. Symptoms of difficulty passing the bolus to the back of the mouth or initiating swallowing, regurgitation of food or liquid through the nose, coughing during swallows, or frank aspiration are all suggestive of oropharyngeal dysphagia [4]. If these are elicited, physical exam should search for focal or global neurologic deficits that might suggest an underlying etiology.

Classically, dysphagia to solid foods alone or dysphagia for solids that progresses to solid and liquid dysphagia has been associated with structural disease. In contrast, dysphagia for liquids alone, or for a combination of liquids and solids, is indicative of a motor disorder. The history should construct a careful timeline of the symptoms with attention to specific foods (e.g., meat vs. rice vs. bread), consistencies (e.g., dry vs. soft vs. liquid), and temperature triggers. Dysphagia can appear to be not "progressing" when a patient has adapted by eating smaller bites, softer foods, avoiding certain items altogether, or chewing thoroughly. Risk factors for malignancy (smoking, alcohol, GERD, family history), and systemic signs and symptoms associated with connective tissue diseases should be examined. With the increasing recognition of eosinophilic esophagitis, it is important to inquire specifically about atopic diseases, longstanding dysphagia, or remote episodes of food impaction [5]. While patients often point to a substernal area where they feel food "hanging-up", there can be poor correlation between this localization and a potentially causative structural lesion, particularly for proximal locations [6]. Physical examination is typically unrevealing in patients with esophageal dysphagia except for the finding of tylosis palmaris (hyperkeratosis of the palmar surface of the hands rarely seen with esophageal cancer) but, if a motor disorder is suggested on history, a thorough exam for signs of scleroderma (e.g., sclerodactyly, periungual telangiectasias, shiny skin), arthritis, CREST syndrome, or other signs of connective tissue diseases is mandated. Signs of weight loss and/or the finding of palpable lymphadenopathy are also suggestive of a malignant lesion.

Nausea/Vomiting

The patient complaining of nausea and/or vomiting presents a challenge to the gastroenterologist because these symptoms are non-specific, the potential causes are legion, and evaluation may range from minimal to extensive. Similar to heartburn, the history for nausea and vomiting should initially focus on having the patient explicitly describe what they are experiencing [7]. Nausea is defined as sensation of impending emesis, while the act of emesis is the expulsion of gastric contents. These should be distinguished from reflux, regurgitation, rumination, indigestion, abdominal pain, early satiety, and sitophobia.

Next, the H&P should focus on determining whether these symptoms represent a primary or secondary process, whether they are structural or functional, and whether they might be a side-effect of a medication or supplement. For example, the patient who complains of constant and longstanding nausea alone, with no emesis or associated symptoms, almost certainly has a functional GI disorder. In contrast, worsening postprandial nausea and vomiting associated with abdominal distension that develops in a patient with known Crohn disease may represent obstructive symptoms from a critical intestinal stenosis. The presence of a succussion splash remote from eating on physical exam raises the issue of gastric outlet obstruction or gastroparesis. Extra-GI etiologies, while rare, should be kept in the differential.

Abdominal Pain

Abdominal pain is the most frequent presenting symptom the gastroenterologist encounters [8], and it should

always be evaluated systematically. A complete history includes eliciting information about the acuity of onset, triggering events, location, radiation, quality, progression, and exacerbating and relieving factors. Location can help narrow the DDx to structures in that specific area. The quality of the pain is most useful for characterizing colic, a paroxysmal cramping sensation typical of an intermittently obstructed hollow viscus. Biliary colic is typically localized to the right-upper quadrant or the epigastrium. Pancreatic pain is frequently severe and bores into the mid-back from the epigastric region and may be eased by sitting and leaning forward.

On physical exam, the severity of the patient's symptoms can be correlated with the presence or absence of signs that might require urgent surgical intervention (e.g., guarding or rebound). Another useful finding is that of Carnett sign, a worsening of discomfort with tightening of abdominal musculature [9], which can indicate a musculoskeletal etiology. When functional abdominal pain is a possibility, examination with distraction, the application of abdominal pressure with the stethoscope while "listening" or conducting a conversation with the patient, is invaluable. Finally, it is important to consider non-GI causes of abdominal pain, particularly those which can be life threatening such as an aortic dissection or aneurysm, and mesenteric vascular insufficiency leading to bowel ischemia.

Diarrhea

While many patients who present with diarrhea have a lower GI source, it is important to keep upper GI causes of diarrhea on the DDx in the appropriate clinical context. Malabsorptive diarrhea, either from pancreatic insufficiency, bacterial overgrowth, or celiac disease, can be characterized by steatorrhea. Because many patients do not see frank fat, oil, or grease mixed with their stools, this sign is often difficult to elicit on history [10]. Instead, asking about "peanut-butter" consistency and color of the stool may provide a more "real-world" prompt for the patient. In addition, small bowel sources of diarrhea, such as infectious (*Giardia*, Whipple disease), autoimmune (celiac disease), or malignant (lymphoma) causes, should be kept on the differential and esophagogastroduodenoscopy (EGD) with biopsies pursued when indicated.

Finishing the Visit

After the H&P, it is important to describe your thought processes to the patient, outlining the DDx and options for further diagnosis and treatment, before making recommendations. This allows patient preferences and concerns to be discussed and addressed. It is equally important to summarize the plan going forward, and to ask the patient to repeat their understanding of the next steps required. It may also be useful to ask "is there anything else you'd like to mention today" in order to avoid a "doorknob" moment [11]. A good visit ends with follow-up appointments made when possible, as well as with the understanding that the initial H&P is just the first step in the therapeutic doctor–patient relationship.

Take-home points

- Listening to and talking with the patient are the most important initial diagnostic tests available.

- Ask an open-ended question to allow the patient to describe their symptoms and chief complaints without interruption.

- Ask directed questions to clarify exactly what is meant by each symptom. For example, ensure a patient's "heartburn" means heartburn from reflux and not angina.

- Qualify each symptom by learning about the acuity of onset, triggering events, quality, progression, and exacerbating and relieving factors.

- When discussing difficult topics or relating bad news, it is acceptable to show empathy or emotion. Providing tissues to a tearful patient or touching them on the shoulder can be reassuring in the right setting.

- After the H&P, the tempo of the planned evaluation should match the relative acuity and severity of the patient's symptoms. For example, progressive dysphagia and weight loss over a month requires expedited evaluation, while longstanding chronic abdominal pain may be worked-up more slowly.

- At the end of the visit, summarize the differential diagnosis and evaluation or treatment plan. It is useful to

have the patient repeat their understanding of the plan, since no matter how skilled the physician is at eliciting information on the H&P, the patient must act to carry this plan forward.

- *Lavabo manus meus* (I wash my hands) is a precept that we should always follow and one that we should practice before and between patient encounters.

References

1 Beckman HB, Frankel RM. The effect of physician behavior on the collection of data. *Ann Intern Med* 1984; **101**: 692–6.

2 DeVault KR, Castell DO. Updated guidelines for the diagnosis and treatment of gastroesophageal reflux disease. *Am J Gastroenterol* 2005; **100**: 190–200.

3 Ruigomez A, Garcia Rodriguez LA, Wallander MA, et al. Natural history of gastro-oesophageal reflux disease diagnosed in general practice. *Aliment Pharmacol Ther* 2004; **20**: 751–60.

4 Cook IJ. Diagnostic evaluation of dysphagia. *Nat Clin Pract Gastroenterol Hepatol* 2008; **5**: 393–403.

5 Furuta GT, Liacouras CA, Collins MH, et al. Eosinophilic esophagitis in children and adults: a systematic review and consensus recommendations for diagnosis and treatment. *Gastroenterology* 2007; **133**: 1342–63.

6 Roeder BE, Murray JA, Dierkhising RA. Patient localization of esophageal dysphagia. *Dig Dis Sci* 2004; **49**: 697–701.

7 Quigley EM, Hasler WL, Parkman HP. AGA technical review on nausea and vomiting. *Gastroenterology* 2001; **120**: 263–86.

8 Shaheen NJ, Hansen RA, Morgan DR, et al. The burden of gastrointestinal and liver diseases, 2006. *Am J Gastroenterol* 2006; **101**: 2128–38.

9 Editorial. Abdominal wall tenderness test: could Carnett cut costs? *Lancet* 1991; **337**: 1134.

10 Fine KD, Schiller LR. AGA technical review on the evaluation and management of chronic diarrhea. *Gastroenterology* 1999; **116**: 1464–86.

11 Jackson G. "Oh … by the way …": doorknob syndrome. *Int J Clin Pract* 2005; **59**: 869.

CHAPTER 22
Heartburn and Regurgitation

Joel E. Richter

Department of Medicine, Temple University School of Medicine, Philadelphia, PA, USA

Summary

Heartburn and regurgitation are the cardinal symptoms of gastroesophageal reflux disease (GERD). These complaints usually occur postprandially after "refluxogenic" foods and can be aggravated by exercise or the supine position. Recent studies find the sensitivity of reflux symptoms relatively disappointing for GERD (30–76%) and an unreliable indicator of the severity of erosive esophagitis. This may not be surprising as acid reflux is not the sole mechanism of heartburn symptoms. Other factors include the reflux of bile and weak acid, mechanical stimulation of the esophagus, esophageal hyperalgesia, and psychological co-morbidity.

Heartburn and regurgitation are the cardinal symptoms of gastroesophageal reflux disease (GERD). Heartburn itself is probably the most common gastrointestinal complaint in the Western world. One systematic review [1] identified 31 articles that assessed the period prevalence of heartburn symptoms in the community, reporting on a total of nearly 78 000 patients. In these Western populations, 25% of people reported heartburn at least once a month, 12% at least once per week, and 5% described daily symptoms. However, most languages do not have a direct translation for the word "heartburn" [2]. Most people do not consider heartburn a medical problem and seldom report this complaint to their physicians. For example, a large population survey from Olmsted County, Minnesota [3] found that only 5.4% had seen a physician for their heartburn in the last year, despite describing their symptoms as moderately severe in intensity with a duration of 5 years or more. These subjects seek relief, with over-the-counter antacids accounting for most of the $1 billion dollars-per-year sales in the USA of these non-prescription drugs [4].

Symptom Complex

Heartburn is a commonly used but frequently misunderstood word. It has may synonyms including "indigestion," "acid regurgitation," "sour stomach," and "bitter belching." Heartburn usually is described as burning discomfort experienced behind the breastbone. The term "burning," "hot," or "acidic" sensation typically is used by the patient unless the symptom becomes so intense that pain is experienced. In those situations, the patient commonly complains of both heartburn and pain. Heartburn typically radiates toward the neck, throat, and occasionally the back [5]. Heartburn is particularly aggravated by foods, frequently noted within 1 h of eating and usually after the largest meal of the day. Foods high in fats, sugars, chocolate, onions, and carminatives may aggravate heartburn, usually by reducing lower esophageal sphincter (LES) pressure [6]. Other foods commonly associated with heartburn, including citrus products, tomato-based foods, and spicy foods, do not affect LES pressure but are direct irritants to the esophageal mucosa [7]. This mechanism is independent of pH and probably related to high osmolarity [8]. Many beverages can aggravate heartburn, including citrus drinks, coffee, and alcohol, by means of mixed mechanisms [6]. Wine drinkers may report intermittent heartburn after drinking hearty red wines, but not after drinking delicate white wines.

Practical Gastroenterology and Hepatology: Esophagus and Stomach, 1st edition. Edited by Nicholas J. Talley, Kenneth R. DeVault and David E. Fleischer. © 2010 Blackwell Publishing Ltd.

The supine position frequently aggravates heartburn, especially if subjects eat late in the evening or have bedtime snacks. This sensation occurs within 1 to 2 h of reclining [9] and, in contrast to peptic ulcer disease, does not awaken the person in the early morning. Some patients say their heartburn is more pronounced while lying on the right side [6]. Nighttime heartburn may affect the quality of life in some patients, causing sleep difficulties and impaired next-day function [10]. Maneuvers that increase intra-abdominal pressure may aggravate heartburn, including bending over, lifting heavy objects, and isometric exercises [6]. Recent studies suggest that sleep deprivation as well as psychological or auditory stress may exacerbate heartburn by lowering the threshold for symptom perception rather than by actually increasing the amount of acid reflux [11–13].

Heartburn is frequently accompanied by regurgitation, defined as the perception of flow of refluxed gastric content into the mouth or hypopharynx [5]. The fluid has a bitter, acidic taste, is common after meals, and worsened by stooping or the supine position. Among patients with daily regurgitation, LES pressure is usually low, some have associated gastroparesis, and esophagitis is common, making this symptom more difficulty to treat medically than heartburn. It is important to distinguish regurgitation from "vomiting" and "waterbrash." The absence of nausea, retching, and abdominal contractions should suggest that regurgitation and not vomiting is present. Waterbrash is an uncommon symptom used to describe the sudden filling of the mouth with clear, slightly salty fluid. This fluid is not regurgitated material but rather secretions from the salivary glands as part of the protective vagally mediated reflex from the distal esophagus [14].

Heartburn Symptoms as Predictors of GERD

The accuracy of heartburn and regurgitation in the diagnosis of GERD is difficult to define. Studies are particularly limited by the lack of a gold standard for GERD. A recent systematic review [15] identified seven studies that assessed the accuracy of reflux symptoms in the diagnosis of esophagitis. A total of 5134 patients were included, with 894 (17%) having esophagitis. All studies recruited consecutive patients; three studies evaluated primary-care physicians, three evaluated the accuracy of specialists, and one study evaluated the accuracy of both groups in diagnosing esophagitis. The sensitivity of reflux symptoms was generally disappointing with a range of 30 to 76% (pooled sensitivity 55%: 95% CI 45–68%) and a specificity between 62 and 96%. These results are similar to the much-cited study by Klauser *et al.* [16] where the presence of heartburn had a sensitivity of 78% and a specificity of 60% in a highly selected population referred for esophageal pH monitoring. Finally, *post hoc* analysis of five esophagitis studies involving nearly 12 000 patients found the severity of heartburn was an unreliable indicator of the severity of erosive disease. This was particularly true in the elderly patients over 70 years of age [17].

Mechanisms of Heartburn

The underlying mechanisms of heartburn symptoms are only partially understood. The etiology appears multifactorial, potentially arising from chemostimulation, mechanostimulation or hyperalgesia [18] (Figure 22.1).

Role of Acid Reflux

Acid reflux is critical but not the sole cause of heartburn. This was elegantly demonstrated by esophageal acid perfusion studies by Smith *et al.* [19]. In this double-blind study, 25 patients with heartburn were randomly perfused with eight solutions of different pH (1.0–6.0). An overall positive correlation (R = 0.77) was demonstrated between the time of onset of pain and the pH of the infused solution. Solutions of pH 1 and 1.5 induced heartburn in all patients, but even the pH 6.0 solution produced heartburn in more than 40% of the patients. Ambulatory pH monitoring consistently finds that only a small proportion of acid reflux episodes evoke heartburn. Studies suggest symptom generation is related to the spatiotemporal characteristics of esophageal exposure to the gastric refluxate and the proximal extent of the refluxate [20,21].

The receptor that mediates the sensation of heartburn has not been identified; however, the capsaicin or vanilloid receptor 1 (TRPV1) is a leading candidate. TRPV1 is a cation channel that is expressed by sensory neurons and its activation by heat, acid pH or ethanol may trigger burning pain [22]. Increased expression of TRPV1 has been identified on sensory nerve fibers from patients

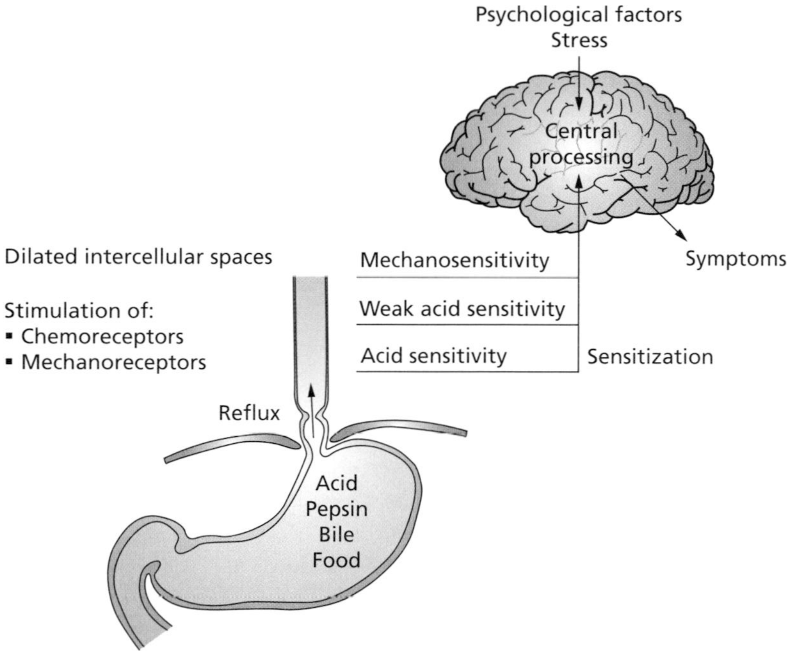

Figure 22.1 Schematic representation of the mechanisms involved in the generation of heartburn. These mechanisms and pathways include activation of chemoreceptors by acid, weak acid, and bile refluxates and mechanoreceptors. Dilated intercellular spaces may facilitate the activation of these receptors. Afferent signaling and perception can be enhanced by sensitization of affluent sensory neurons, central brain processing, psychological factors, and stress Reproduced from [18], with permission from Nature Publishing Group.

with symptomatic esophagitis but not healthy controls [23].

Nerve endings and acid-sensitive ion channels are found in the deepest layer of the esophageal mucosa, which are normally shielded from luminal influences by anatomical barriers. The presence of dilated intercellular spaces (DIS) within the stratified squamous epithelium is now recognized as the earliest lesion in the damaged esophagus. DIS are present in animal models of GERD and in GERD patients, even those with visually normal mucosa [24]. This defect decreases mucosal resistance, allowing the diffusion of acid and luminal contents into the intercellular spaces. Activation of chemosensitive nociceptors occurs with signals transmitted to the brain which generate the perception of heartburn [25]. Some researchers propose that resolution of DIS after proton pump inhibitor (PPI) therapy is the key to heartburn relief [26].

Role of Weakly Acid Reflux

With combined impedance/pH monitoring, esophageal refluxate can be further characterized as acidic (nadir pH <4), weakly acidic (nadir pH 4–7) and non-acidic (nadir pH >7) [27]. Off PPIs, heartburn is most commonly associated with acid reflux, but up to 15% of episodes occur with weakly acidic reflux [28]. High proximal extent of the esophageal refluxate, a low nadir pH and a large pH drop, as well as large reflux volume and prolonged acid clearance times, are more likely associated with heartburn symptoms. On twice-daily PPI therapy, the relationship is modified with studies finding that 17 to 37% of patients have symptom production with non-acid, usually weakly acidic reflux [29,30]. Cough and regurgitation are the most common non-acid associated symptoms [29].

Role of Bile Reflux

Esophageal infusion of bile acids can generate heartburn symptoms, but not with the rapidity and intensity of acid infusion [31]. The likely mechanism is the release of intracellular mediators via damage to lipid membranes [32]. Combined 24-h pH and bilirubin absorbance monitoring (indirect measure of bile) finds that acid and bile reflux occur simultaneously during most reflux episodes, occurring in 100% of patients with complicated Barrett esophagus, 89% of patients with simple Barrett esophagus, 79% of patients with esophagitis, and 50% of patients without esophagitis [33]. Off PPI therapy, Koek *et al.* observed that less than 10% of symptoms were related to bile reflux alone, but the majority of symptoms on BID PPIs were related to bile reflux as compared to acid reflux [34].

Role of Esophageal Mechanical Stimulation

The concept that mechanical stimulation of the esophagus may have a role in heartburn symptoms has attracted increasing support. Esophageal balloon distension, especially in the proximal esophagus, can produce the symptom of heartburn [35]. Researchers postulate that the proximal esophagus has a larger number of mechanoreceptors than the distal esophagus, contributing to the generation of symptoms during reflux events [36]. Acid exposure might also reduce the threshold for mechanoreceptor stimulation [37]. In addition, sustained esophageal contractions are another proposed mechanism to explain the pathogenesis of heartburn. Sustained esophageal contractions represent prolonged contractions of the longitudinal esophageal smooth muscle identified by high-frequency intraluminal ultrasound. Balaban, *et al.* [38]. demonstrated a strong correlations between spontaneous chest pain or chest pain induced by edrophanium chloride and sustained contractions. These contractions did not occlude the esophageal lumen and were not associated with changes in intraluminal esophageal pressure, indicating that the circular muscles are not involved.

Role of Esophageal Hypersensitivity

Esophageal hypersensitivity contributes to heartburn complaints, especially in the subgroup of GERD patients with normal acid exposure, and a close relationship between reflux events and heartburn perception [39,40]. These patients are also hypersensitive to mechanical distension, as shown by balloon studies [39,40]. The proposed mechanisms are complex, but studies suggest altered brain processing (central sensitization) rather than abnormal esophageal wall receptors is key to the development of visceral hypersensitivity [41]. Anxiety and stress contribute to this increased perception of heartburn via both central mechanisms and possibly peripherally by dilated intercellular spaces in the esophageal mucosa [42].

> **Take-home points**
>
> - Heartburn and regurgitation are the cardinal symptoms of GERD.
> - However, the sensitivity of reflux symptoms for GERD is disappointing (30–76%) and unreliable for the severity of esophagitis.
> - Other than acid reflux, the perception of heartburn can be triggered by bile and weak acid reflux, mechanical stimulation of the esophagus, esophageal hyperalgesia, and psychological stress.

References

1 Moayyedi P, Axon ATR. Gastro-oesophageal reflux disease: the extent of the problem. *Aliment Pharmacol Ther* 2005; **22** (Suppl. 1): 11–19.

2 Wong WM, Wong BCY. Definition and diagnosis of gastroesophageal reflux disease. *J Gastroenterol Hepatol* 2004; **19** (Suppl. 3): S26–32.

3 Locke GM, Talley NJ, Fett SL, *et al.* Prevalence and clinical spectrum of gastroesophageal reflux: A population-based study in Olmsted County, Minnesota. *Gastroenterology* 1997; **112**: 1448–53.

4 Shaheen NJ, Hansen RA, Morgan DR, *et al.* The burden of gastrointestinal and liver disease, 2006. *Am J Gastroenterol* 2006; **101**: 2128–38.

5 Vakil N, van Zanten SV, Kahrilas P, *et al.* The Montreal definition and classification of gastroesophageal reflux disease: A global evidence based consensus. *Am J Gastroenterol* 2006; **101**: 1900–20.

6 Kaltenback T, Crockett S, Gersen LB. Are lifestyle measures effective in patients with gastroesophageal reflux disease? *Am J Gastroenterol* 2006; **101**: 2128–38.

7 Price SF, Smithson KW, Castell DO. Food sensitivity in reflux esophagitis. *Gastroenterology* 1978; **75**: 240–6.

8 Feldman M, Barnett C. Relationship between the acidity and osmolality of popular beverages and reported postprandial heartburn. *Gastroenterology* 1995; **108**: 125–31.

9 Fujiwara Y, Machida A, Watanabe Y, *et al.* Association between dinner-to-bedtime and gastroesophageal reflux disease. *Am J Gastroenterol* 2005; **100**: 2633–6.

10 Shaker R, Castell DO, Schoenfeld PS, Spechler SJ. Nighttime heartburn is an underappreciated clinical problem that impacts sleep and daytime function: The results of a Gallup survey conducted on behalf of the American Gastroenterological Association. *Am J Gastroenterol* 2003; **98**: 1487–92.

11 Schey R, Dickman R, Parthasarthy S, *et al*. Sleep deprivation is hyperalgesic in patients with gastroesophageal reflux disease. *Gastroenterology* 2007; **133**: 1787–95.

12 Wright CE, Ebrecht M, Mitchell R, *et al*. The effect of psychological stress on symptom severity and perception in patients with gastroesophageal reflux disease. *J Psychosom Res* 2005; **59**: 415–24.

13 Fass R, Naliboff BD, Fass SS, *et al*. The effect of auditory stress on perception of intraesophageal acid in patients with gastroesophageal reflux disease. *Gastroenterology* 2008; **134**: 696–705.

14 Helms JF, Dodds WJ, Hogan WJ. Salivary response to esophageal acid in normal and patients with reflux esophagitis. *Gastroenterology* 1987; **93**: 1393–9.

15 Moayyedi P, Talley NJ, Fennerty MB, Vakil N. Can the clinical history distinguish between organic and functional dyspepsia? *JAMA* 2006; **295**: 1566–76.

16 Klauser AG, Schindlbeck NE, Muller-Lissner SA. Symptoms in gastro-oesophageal reflux disease. *Lancet* 1990; **335**: 205–8.

17 Johnson DA, Fennerty MB. Heartburn severity underestimates erosive esophagitis in elderly patients with gastroesophageal reflux disease. *Gastroenterology* 2004; **126**: 660–8.

18 Ang D, Sifrim D, Tack J. Mechanisms of heartburn. *Nat Clin Prac Gastroenterol Hepatol* 2008; **5**: 383–92.

19 Smith JL, Opekun AR, Larkai E, *et al*. Sensitivity of the esophageal mucosa to pH in gastroesophageal reflux disease. *Gastroenterology* 1989; **96**: 683–9.

20 Weusten BL, Akkermans LMA, vanBerge-Henegouwen GP, *et al*. Symptom perception in gastroesophageal reflux disease is dependent on spatiotemporal reflux characteristics. *Gastroenterology* 1995; **108**: 1739–44.

21 Cicala M, Emerenziani S, Caviglia R, *et al*. Intra-oesophageal distribution and perception of acid reflux in patients with non-erosive gastro-oesophageal reflux disease. *Aliment Pharmacol Ther* 2003; **18**: 605–13.

22 Holzer P. TRPV1: a new target for treatment of visceral pain in IBS? *Gut* 2008; **57**: 882–4.

23 Matthews PJ, Aziz, Q, Facer P, *et al*. Increased capsaicin receptor TRPV1 nerve fibres in the inflamed human oesophagus. *Eur J Gastroenterol Hepatol* 2004; **16**: 897–902.

24 Malenstein HV, Farre R, Sifrim D. Esophageal dilated intercellular spaces (DIS) and nonerosive reflux disease. *Am J Gastroenterol* 2008; **103**: 1021–8.

25 Barlow WJ, Orlando RC. The pathogenesis of heartburn in nonerosive reflux disaease: a unifying hypothesis. *Gastroenterology* 2005; **128**: 771–8.

26 Calabrese C, Bortolotti M, Fabbri A, *et al*. Reversibility of GERD ultrastructural alteration and relief of symptoms after omeprazole treatment. *Am J Gastroenterol* 2005; **100**: 537–42.

27 Sifrim D, Castell DO, Dent J, *et al*. Gastro-oesophageal reflux monitoring: Review and consensus report on detection and definitions of acid, non-acid, and gas reflux. *Gut* 2004; **53**: 1024–31.

28 Bredenoord AJ, Weusten BLAM, Curvers WL, *et al*. Determinants of perception of heartburn and regurgitation. *Gut* 2006; **55**: 313–18.

29 Zerbib F, Roman S, Ropert A, *et al*. Esophageal pH-impedance monitoring and symptom analysis in GERD: A study in patients off and on therapy. *Am J Gastroenterol* 2006; **101**: 1956–63.

30 Maine I, Tutuian R, Shay S, *et al*. Acid and non-acid reflux in patients with persistent symptoms despite acid suppressive therapy: a multicentre study using combined ambulatory impedance-pH monitoring. *Gut* 2006; **55**: 1398–402.

31 Siddiqui A, Rodriguez-Stanley S, Zubaidi S, *et al*. Esophageal visceral sensitivity to bile salts in patients with functional heartburn and in healthy control subjects. *Dig Dis Sci* 2005; **50**: 81–5.

32 Tack J. Review article: the role of bile and pepsin in the pathophysiology and treatment of gastroesophageal reflux disease. *Aliment Pharmacol Ther* 2006; 24 (Suppl): 10–16.

33 Vaezi MF, Richter JE. Role of acid and duodenogastroesophageal reflux in GERD. *Gastroenterology* 1006; **111**: 1992–9.

34 Koek GH. The role of acid and duodenal gastroesophageal reflux in symptomatic GERD. *Am J Gastroenterol* 2001; **96**: 2033–40.

35 Fass R, Naliboff B, Higaet L, *et al*. Differential effect of long-term esophageal acid exposure on mechanosensitivity and chemoensitivity in humans. *Gastroenterology* 1998; **115**: 1363–73.

36 Patel S, Rao S. Biomechanical and sensory parameters of the human esophagus at four levels. *Am J Physiol Gastrointest Liver Physiol* 1998; **275**: G187–91.

37 Peghini P, Johnston BT, Leite LP, *et al*. Mucosal acid exposure sensitizes a subset of normal subjects to intra-oesophageal balloon distension. *Eur J Gastroenterol Hepatol* 1996; **8**: 978–83.

38 Balaban DH, Yamamoto Y, Liu J, *et al*. Sustained esophageal contraction: A marker of esophageal chest pain identified by intraluminal ultrasonography. *Gastroenterology* 1999; **116**: 29–37.

39 Trimble KC, Pryde A, Heading RC. Lowered esophageal sensory thresholds in patients with symptomatic but not excess gastro-oesphageal reflux: evidence for a spectrum of visceral sensitivity in GORD. *Gut* 1995; **37**: 7–12.

40 Rao SC, Gregersen H, Hayek B, *et al.* Unexplained chest pain: the hypersensitive, hyperactive and poorly compliant esophagus. *Ann Intern Med* 1996; **124**: 950–8.

41 Sarkar S, Hobson AR, Furlong PL, *et al.* Central neural mechanisms mediating human visceral hypersensitivity.

Am J Physiol Gastroentest Liver Physiol 2001; **881**: G1196–202.

42 Naliboff BD, Mayer M, Fass R, *et al.* The effect of life stress on symptoms of heartburn. *Psych Med* 2004; **66**: 426–34.

CHAPTER 23

Chest Pain

Ronnie Fass[1] and Guy D. Eslick[2]

[1] Section of Gastroenterology, Southern Arizona VA Health Care System, Tucson, AZ, USA
[2] Discipline of Surgery, The University of Sydney, Nepean Hospital, Penrith, NSW, Australia

Summary

Noncardiac chest pain (NCCP) is very common, resulting in poor quality of life, reduced work productivity, and significant health-related cost. The presentation of NCCP is indistinguishable from that of ischemic heart disease, so all patients with chest pain should first be evaluated by a cardiologist. Gastroesophageal reflux disease (GERD) is by far the most common cause of esophageal-related NCCP. Consequently, the initial approach should include either the proton pump inhibitor (PPI) test or PPI empirical therapy. In the absence of evidence for GERD, patients should undergo evaluation with esophageal manometry to primarily exclude achalasia. In patients with negative esophageal manometry or evidence of spastic esophageal motor disorder, esophageal hypersensitivity appears to be the main underlying mechanism. In this subgroup of NCCP patients, pain modulators have been demonstrated to be the most efficacious therapeutic strategy. The role of provocative testing has diminished in the last decade due to poor sensitivity and the introduction of PPIs. There is growing evidence about the value of psychological intervention in patients with NCCP in the form of cognitive–behavioral therapy or hypnotherapy.

Case

A 48-year-old woman presents to the emergency room with substernal chest pain. The pain has been present for an hour and is a severe burning sensation. She admits to occasional similar episodes over the past 2–3 months. An initial ECG and chest radiograph were normal. The pain resolved after a single sublingual nitroglycerin dose and a dose of "GI cocktail." She was admitted to the hospital and myocardial infarction was ruled out. An image stress test was normal on the second hospital day, and a gastroenterology consultation was requested.

Introduction

Chest pain is a very common symptom, representing 2–5% of all emergency room presentations [1,2]. The current estimated population prevalence of noncardiac chest pain (NCCP) ranges from 14% (Hong Kong) [3] to 33% (Australia) [4]. There are also very few data on

the natural history of NCCP, but studies suggest that chest pain continues in over 65% of patients 4 years after initial presentation [5]. There are conflicting reports about the long-term prognosis of patients with NCCP. Approximately 14% of all chest pain patients will see a gastroenterologist about their chest pain. The heterogeneous nature of NCCP does not allow easy classification of this complex condition.

Cardiac or Noncardiac Chest Pain?

The differential diagnosis of chest pain can be very challenging. Chest pain is a relatively nonspecific symptom and is linked with a large number of conditions (Figure 23.1). Even though the patient may have seen a cardiologist, it may be important to repeat some of the diagnostic tests that will assist in differentiating between cardiac and noncardiac chest pain. The patient history is the most important part of any chest pain assessment.

Traditionally, assessment of patients is based on the description of the pain, the overall clinical picture, the ECG, and cardiac enzymes including troponin levels.

Practical Gastroenterology and Hepatology: Esophagus and Stomach, 1st edition. Edited by Nicholas J. Talley, Kenneth R. DeVault and David E. Fleischer. © 2010 Blackwell Publishing Ltd.

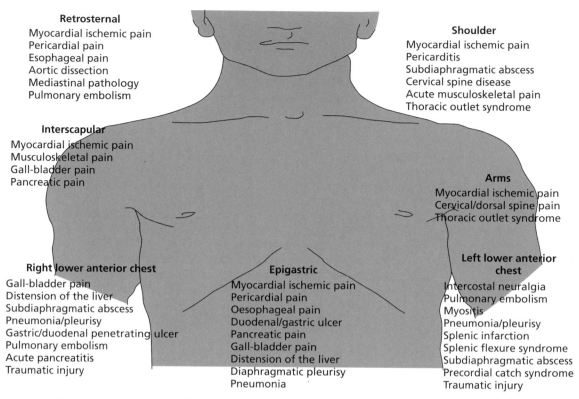

Retrosternal
Myocardial ischemic pain
Pericardial pain
Esophageal pain
Aortic dissection
Mediastinal pathology
Pulmonary embolism

Shoulder
Myocardial ischemic pain
Pericarditis
Subdiaphragmatic abscess
Cervical spine disease
Acute musculoskeletal pain
Thoracic outlet syndrome

Interscapular
Myocardial ischemic pain
Musculoskeletal pain
Gall-bladder pain
Pancreatic pain

Arms
Myocardial ischemic pain
Cervical/dorsal spine pain
Thoracic outlet syndrome

Right lower anterior chest
Gall-bladder pain
Distension of the liver
Subdiaphragmatic abscess
Pneumonia/pleurisy
Gastric/duodenal penetrating ulcer
Pulmonary embolism
Acute pancreatitis
Traumatic injury

Epigastric
Myocardial ischemic pain
Pericardial pain
Oesophageal pain
Duodenal/gastric ulcer
Pancreatic pain
Gall-bladder pain
Distension of the liver
Diaphragmatic pleurisy
Pneumonia

Left lower anterior chest
Intercostal neuralgia
Pulmonary embolism
Myositis
Pneumonia/pleurisy
Splenic infarction
Splenic flexure syndrome
Subdiaphragmatic abscess
Precordial catch syndrome
Traumatic injury

Figure 23.1 Various conditions associated with chest pain.

An important aspect in differentiating cardiac from noncardiac chest pain is the taking of a careful history with an emphasis on discriminatory features. However, due to extensive overlap between cardiac and noncardiac causes of chest pain, reliance on history alone does not provide optimal exclusion of cardiac or noncardiac causes (Table 23.1). Research has suggested that, due to the heterogeneity of chest pain, locations and characteristics that previously used indicators (such as pain traveling down the left arm, generally thought to be indicative of an acute myocardial infarction) should no longer be used [6]. It must be remembered that there is a subset of acute coronary syndrome patients who present without chest pain [7,8].

Differentiating Esophageal from Nonesophageal Causes of NCCP

There can be an overlap of esophageal and nonesophageal causes of chest pain. Patients with documented coro-

nary artery disease are likely to have concomitant chest pain of esophageal origin [9]. Although there are a number of esophageal disorders reported in patients with coronary artery disease, the most common is gastroesophageal reflux [10,11]. Previous research suggests that cardiac manipulation (e.g., coronary angioplasty) can induce esophageal motility abnormalities, but not gastroesophageal reflux [12]. In one study, antianginal treatment became partially ineffective in patients with coronary artery disease who also demonstrated esophageal abnormalities [10]. A case series registered that patients reported a reduction in symptoms related to atrial fibrillation after treatment of gastroesophageal reflux disease (GERD) symptoms with proton pump inhibitor (PPI) therapy, which was verified by combined 24-h pH and ambulatory Holter monitoring [13]. In addition, Lux and colleagues have shown a statistically significant association between ST-segment abnormalities and gastroesophageal reflux or esophageal dysmotility [14]. Thus, the interaction between the heart and

Table 23.1 A comparison of gastrointestinal causes of chest pain.

	Acid reflux	Oesophageal spasm	Peptic ulcer	Gall-bladder disease
Site	Retrosternal	Deep retrosternal	Epigastric	Right hypochondrium
Radiation	Retrosternal Throat	Back	To back (DU)	Below right scapula Tip of right shoulder
Quality	Burning	Constricting	Gnawing	Deep ache
Precipitation	Heavy meals Wine/coffee Lying Bending	Eating hot/cold food and drinks	Eating GU: 30 min DU: 2–3 h	Fatty food
Relief	Standing Antacids	Antispasmodics Nitroglycerine	Antacids	
Associated symptoms	Water brash	Dysphagia	Dyspepsia	Flatulence Dyspepsia

DU, duodenal ulcer; GU, gastric ulcer.
Reproduced with permission from Murtagh J. *General Practice*, 4th edn. New York, McGraw-Hill, 2007.

esophagus in causing chest pain is a complex one, so patients with chest pain should first undergo a thorough diagnostic assessment by a cardiologist and only if negative should they be referred to a gastroenterologist for further evaluation.

Evidence-based Facts about Chest Pain

Increased risk of an acute coronary syndrome is associated with:
- Increasing age
- Chest pain that began 48 hours ago
- Constant pain
- Pressure
- Nausea and vomiting
- Sweating
- Hypotension.

Decreased risk of acute coronary syndrome is associated with:
- Stabbing or sharp pain
- Positional chest pain
- Chest pain reproduced on palpation.

Diagnostic "Pearls"
- Females may present with more subtle and less specific symptoms than males.

- Up to 20% of patients with suspected acute myocardial infarction may also have indigestion.
- Studies have shown that low-risk chest pain patients who undergo an ECG and have cardiac enzymes feel better and have improved activity at 3 weeks.
- Remember that GERD and motility disorders are common in patients both with and without coronary heart disease.
- Some patients may not be able to describe their symptoms adequately or feel that they are not serious.
- Emotional patients with chest pain are less likely to have noninvasive testing (never make decisions on additional investigations based on the patient's manner of presentation).

Esophageal Mechanisms for NCCP

GERD is by far the most common esophageal cause for NCCP, followed by esophageal hypersensitivity and esophageal dysmotility. Figure 23.2 provides an algorithm for NCCP evaluation.

GERD-related Chest Pain
As stated above, GERD is by far the most common cause of NCCP [4]. There are currently several useful diagnostic tests available to assess GERD in patients with NCCP, which include esophagogastroduodenoscopy (EGD),

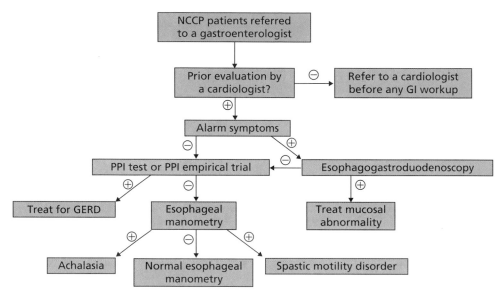

Figure 23.2 Proposed diagnostic evaluation of patients with noncardiac chest pain. NCCP, noncardiac chest pain; PPI proton pump inhibitor; GERD, gastroesophageal reflux disease.

esophageal pH monitoring, esophageal impedance and pH, and the PPI test.

Esophagogastroduodenoscopy

Alarm symptoms such as recent weight loss, dysphagia or odynophagia, decreased appetite, hematemesis, and anemia are important indications for EGD in individuals with NCCP. EGD is ideal for detecting erosive esophagitis, esophageal stricture, ulcers, and Barrett esophagus. However, the value of EGD among individuals with NCCP is low. Hsia *et al.* [15] in their endoscopic assessment of 100 consecutive NCCP patients found that 24% had esophagitis. A recent study of 3688 consecutive NCCP patients who had had EGD reported that 44.1% had a normal test, 28.3% hiatus hernia, 19.4% erosive esophagitis, 4.4% Barrett esophagus, and 3.6% esophageal stricture or stenosis [16]. Therefore, performing EGD in NCCP patients is a low-yield test, because it is unlikely to alter the management of most of these patients. However, patients with GERD-related NCCP should be checked with an endoscope at least once during their lifetime to rule out Barrett esophagus.

The PPI Test

The test is a cost-effective method of quickly diagnosing and treating simultaneously GERD-related NCCP

[17,18]. Importantly, this simple and noninvasive method is available to all physicians and specialists, and those in primary care. Studies have used variable doses of PPI for the PPI test. They included one to three PPIs per day over a period of 7 days to 4 weeks, depending on the frequency of the chest pain symptoms. An empirical trial of rabeprazole (20 mg twice daily) compared patients with either GERD-related NCCP ($n = 16$) or non-GERD-related NCCP ($n = 26$) in Korea. In addition, the study assessed the efficacy of both a 1-week and a 2-week PPI trial. All patients underwent EGD and ambulatory 24-h esophageal pH monitoring, along with baseline and prospective symptom assessment. There was no difference between GERD-related NCCP and non-GERD-related NCCP groups after the first week of PPI therapy; however, there was a significant difference after week 2 with the GERD-related NCCP group showing a better symptom response to PPI therapy than the non-GERD-related NCCP group (81% vs 27%, $p = 0.001$), respectively.

There have been two meta-analyses that have assessed the role of PPI therapy in the diagnosis of NCCP. The first, published in 2005, aimed to determine the efficacy of short-term PPIs among those with NCCP and also how useful PPIs are in diagnosing reflux-related NCCP. The analysis contained eight randomized controlled trials with either a parallel or a crossover design comparing PPI therapy with placebo. The results showed that NCCP patients taking PPIs have reduced episodes of chest pain with a relative risk (RR) of 0.54 (95% confidence interval [CI] 0.41–0.71). The number needed to treat was 3 (95% CI 2–4). Moreover, the pooled sensitivity, specificity, and diagnostic odds ratio (OR) for the PPI test compared with 24-h esophageal pH monitoring and endoscopy were 80%, 74%, and 13.83 (95% CI 5.48–34.91), respectively. Potential limitations of this study included use of crossover studies, which inflate the overall estimates, and studies with small sample sizes, and that there was evidence of publication bias. The second meta-analysis was published in 2006 and included six randomized, placebo-controlled studies with the aim of determining the efficacy of a short course of PPIs in the diagnosis of gastroesophageal reflux among patients with NCCP [19]. The analysis revealed that the PPI test had a much higher sensitivity (80%, 95% CI 71–87%) and specificity (74%, 95% CI 64 83%), compared with a sensitivity of 19% (95% CI 12–29%) and specificity of 77% (95% CI 62–87%) among the placebo group. Overall, the PPI test had greater discriminatory power, with a summary diagnostic OR of 19.35 (95% CI 8.54–43.84) compared with 0.61 (95% CI 0.20–1.86) in the placebo group.

Ambulatory 24-h Esophageal pH Monitoring

This includes both the standard catheter, ambulatory, 24-h esophageal pH monitoring and the wireless, "catheterless", Bravo pH-monitoring system, which are used to determine the level of esophageal acid exposure and the extent of chest pain symptom correlation with acid reflux events [20]. More than half of all NCCP patients are found to have abnormal esophageal acid exposure and/or a positive symptom index alone. Although the presence of an abnormal distal esophageal acid exposure during pH testing does not necessarily denote that the chest pain experienced by the patient is due to GERD, studies have demonstrated that most of these patients will respond to antireflux treatment. The pH test has several disadvantages. The catheter-based test is invasive, the wireless pH capsule is costly, and both are not widely available to physicians and inconvenient for patients. Currently, most experts reserve esophageal pH monitoring for NCCP patients who fail to respond to a course of PPI therapy.

Multichannel Intraluminal Esophageal Impedance and pH

The combination of an impedance catheter and a pH probe provides a unique opportunity to study all reflux events within the esophagus and their relationship to symptoms. In addition, the recording assembly can disclose the characteristics of the gastric refluxate (acidic, weakly acidic, alkaline, gas, liquid, and mixed gas and liquid). The specific value of the multichannel intraluminal impedance plus pH sensor and the documentation of weakly acidic reflux in patients with NCCP still need to be elucidated.

Barium Swallow

A barium swallow (esophagogram) is not useful in the diagnosis of GERD; however, the test should be considered in NCCP patients with dysphagia.

Motility Disorders

In patients with non-GERD-related NCCP, esophageal dysmotility is relatively uncommon. Studies have consistently demonstrated that approximately 70% of the patients with non-GERD-related NCCP have normal esophageal motility during esophageal manometry [21,22]. An exception to the rule is a recent study in 100 NCCP patients demonstrating that only 8% had normal esophageal manometry [23]. Overall, the relationship between non-GERD-related NCCP and esophageal dysmotility remains an area of controversy, primarily because of the common documentation of esophageal dysmotility in NCCP patients undergoing esophageal manometry without concomitant reports of chest pain symptoms. DiMarino et al. [24] suggested that esophageal dysmotility may not be the cause of patients' chest pain, but rather a proxy marker of an underlying motor disorder.

Esophageal Manometry

At present, esophageal manometry is commonly used to assess motility disorders of the esophagus [25]. The most commonly diagnosed motility disorders in NCCP patients include nutcracker esophagus, nonspecific esophageal motor disorders, and hypotensive lower esophageal sphincter (LES) [21,22]. Diffuse esophageal spasm, hypertensive LES, and achalasia are relatively uncommon in patients presenting with chest pain alone. In patients with NCCP, regardless of whether esophageal motor disorder is present or absent, except achalasia, studies have consistently demonstrated that patients are more likely to respond to a pain modulator than a muscle relaxant [26]. Achalasia requires a completely different therapeutic approach. Thus, esophageal manometry in NCCP patients is primarily performed to exclude achalasia.

Provocative Testing

An assortment of provocative tests such as the edrophonium (Tensilon) test and the Bernstein test has been used to evaluate patients with NCCP. Enthusiasm about their diagnostic role has been tempered by low sensitivity. Currently few motility laboratories are using these tests on a routine basis [27].

Esophageal Hypersensitivity

Approximately 35% of NCCP patients will demonstrate no evidence of GERD or esophageal motor disorder. These patients have been shown to have reduced perception thresholds for esophageal pain, using either balloon distension or electrical stimulation tests. Consequently, it has been hypothesized that esophageal hypersensitivity plays an important role in symptom generation of this group of patients—termed "functional chest pain of presumed esophageal origin" [28].

Balloon Distension Test

There are several tools that are used to assess the presence of esophageal hypersensitivity, mostly within the realm of investigational studies. Intraesophageal balloon distension, either by barostat or by hand-held syringe, is the sole test that is used by some motility laboratories to provoke chest pain and to assess sensory perception thresholds.

The balloon distension test is currently used primarily for research purposes to determine perception thresholds for pain in patients with functional chest pain of presumed esophageal origin, although a few laboratories continue to use this clinically.

Functional Chest Pain

Functional chest pain is one of the functional esophageal disorders. Very little is known about functional chest pain and the underlying pathophysiology remains poorly understood, diagnosis usually being based on symptoms and exclusion of organic disease. Functional chest pain can be an extremely debilitating condition that impacts greatly on quality of life, with frequent physician consultations, diagnostic tests, and use of medications (over the counter and prescription). There are guidelines as to the classification of functional chest pain, as developed by the Rome Foundation [29]. Functional chest pain (NCCP) is defined as "episodes of unexplained chest pain that usually are midline in location and of visceral quality, and therefore potentially of esophageal origin." The pain is easily confused with cardiac angina and pain from other esophageal disorders, including esophageal motor disorders and GERD.

The Rome Committee developed the following diagnostic criteria for functional chest pain of presumed esophageal origin, which must include *all* of the following:
• Midline chest pain or discomfort that is not of burning quality
• Absence of evidence that gastroesophageal reflux is the cause of the symptom
• Absence of histopathology-based esophageal motility disorders.

In addition, these criteria must be fulfilled for the last 3 months, with symptom onset at least 6 months before diagnosis. There may be benefit in using the Rome III criteria in clinical practice to define functional chest pain; however, these criteria have not been assessed in any clinical studies. Furthermore, they are not widely used by clinicians to diagnose chest pain, perhaps due to the complexity of the diagnostic criteria. Studies have found that other functional gastrointestinal (GI) disorders such as irritable bowel syndrome, functional heartburn, and functional dyspepsia may overlap with functional chest pain [30].

Psychological Evaluation

This is an important part of chest pain assessment because approximately 25% of chest pain patients with either a cardiac or a noncardiac cause of chest pain have a psychological or psychiatric disorder (depression, anxiety, neuroticism). Psychogenic chest pain hurts just as much as pain of organic origin, but it can be difficult if not impossible to determine which came first, the chest pain or the psychological state of the individual. Other patient studies have found higher rates of psychological disorders (up to 80%) among chest pain patients. Use of a screening questionnaire would be optimal, as a structured psychiatric interview is time-consuming and requires a specialized assessor for maximum efficacy.

Treatment

Treatment for NCCP should be targeted at the specific underlying mechanism responsible for a patient's symptoms.

GERD-related NCCP

Lifestyle modifications include elevation of the head of the bed, weight loss, smoking cessation, and avoidance of alcohol, coffee, fresh citrus juice, and other food products, as well as medications that can exacerbate reflux such as opiates, benzodiazepines, and calcium channel blockers [31,32].

The efficacy of H_2-receptor antagonists in controlling symptoms in patients with GERD-related NCCP has been shown to range from 42% to 52% [33].

Patients with GERD-related NCCP should be treated with at least double the standard dose of a PPI until the symptoms remit, followed by dose tapering to determine the lowest PPI dose that can control symptoms. As with other extraesophageal manifestations of GERD, NCCP patients may require more than 2 months of therapy for optimal symptom control. Long-term maintenance PPI treatment has been shown to be highly effective [34].

The value of antireflux surgery in GERD-related NCCP is unclear. Several studies have demonstrated a significant improvement in symptoms after laparoscopic fundoplication in patients with GERD-related NCCP [35,36]. In contrast, So and colleagues reported that, after laparoscopic fundoplication, relief of atypical GERD symptoms (e.g., chest pain) was less satisfactory than relief of typical GERD symptoms (e.g., heartburn) [37].

Non-GERD-related NCCP

The treatment of non-GERD-related NCCP is primarily based on esophageal pain modulation. An important development in this field was the recognition that NCCP patients with spastic esophageal motor disorders (except

achalasia), as documented by esophageal manometry, are more likely to respond to pain modulators than to muscle relaxants. Unfortunately, no large, well-designed studies to assess pain modulators in patients with non-GERD-related NCCP have been performed.

Studies that evaluated the value of nitrates in NCCP have been limited by small numbers of patients and inconsistent results with regard to drug efficacy. A placebo-controlled trial that excludes patients with GERD has yet to be performed.

As calcium plays an important role in esophageal muscle contraction, the role of calcium channel-blocking agents in patients with NCCP and esophageal spastic motility disorders has been the focus of investigation. Nifedipine (10–30 mg orally three times daily) decreases the amplitude and duration of esophageal contractions in patients with nutcracker esophagus after only 2 weeks [38]. Unfortunately, the effect of the drug disappeared after 6 weeks of treatment, with complete recurrence of symptoms. Diltiazem (60–90 mg orally four times daily) for 8 weeks significantly improved mean chest pain scores and esophageal motility studies in patients with nutcracker esophagus when compared with placebo [39,40]. However, in a study evaluating eight patients with diffuse esophageal spasm (DES), the effect of diltiazem in relieving chest pain was no different from the effect of placebo, probably due to the small number of patients who participated in the study [41]. Other calcium channel blockers have been evaluated in patients with primary esophageal motor disorders, including verapamil, fendiline, nimodipine, and nisoldipine, with various effects on LES resting pressure and esophageal amplitude contractions. Regardless, calcium channel blockers appear to have a transient esophageal motor effect that translates to a short-lived improvement in symptoms, compounded by a variety of side effects such as hypotension, bradycardia, and pedal edema.

Sildenafil is a potent selective inhibitor of cyclic GMP-specific phosphodiesterase PDE5, which inactivates the nitric oxide-stimulated GMP. Intracellular accumulation of the latter induces smooth muscle relaxation. Thus far, there have been no studies that specifically addressed NCCP patients, so the value of this compound in NCCP remains unknown. In addition, the use of this compound in NCCP will likely be limited by its cost and side effects.

The antispasmodic cimetropium bromide has been shown to be efficacious in eight NCCP patients with nutcracker esophagus when taken intravenously [42], but clinical data about the efficacy of an oral formulation are still lacking. Hydralazine, an antihypertensive compound that directly dilates peripheral vessels, was shown to improve chest pain and dysphagia by decreasing the amplitude and duration of esophageal contractions in a small study of only five patients [43]. Overall, evidence to support the therapeutic benefit of anticholinergic agents for the treatment of NCCP remains very limited.

Pain Modulators

Several drugs have been shown to have a pain-modulatory or a visceral analgesic effect, thus alleviating chest pain symptoms. These drugs include tricyclic antidepressants (TCAs), selective serotonin reuptake inhibitors (SSRIs), theophylline, and trazodone.

Several studies have demonstrated that antidepressants have a visceral analgesic effect [44], but they also appear to inhibit calcium channels and thus may have an additional muscle relaxant-like effect [45]. TCAs have both central neuromodulatory and peripheral visceral analgesic effects. Several clinical trials have found favorable TCA-related effects on esophageal pain perception in both healthy individuals and patients with NCCP.

As a result of their anticholinergic side effects, TCAs are commonly administered at night. Based on our experience, it is recommended that TCA doses be slowly titrated to a maximum of 50–75 mg daily. The incremental increase in dosing should be based on symptom improvement and development of side effects.

Trazodone (100–150 mg orally four times daily) for 6 weeks showed a significant improvement in the symptoms of patients with NCCP and esophageal dysmotility compared with placebo [46]. However, esophageal motility abnormalities remained unchanged. A small, open-label study reported symptom control and improved esophageal motility in patients with NCCP and DES after treatment with both trazodone and clomipramine [47].

A randomized trial assessing the effect of sertraline in patients with NCCP demonstrated a significant reduction in pain scores, regardless of concomitant improvement in psychological scores [48]. In addition, a recent study demonstrated that citalopram, 20 mg intravenously given in a single dose, reduced chemical and mechanical esophageal hypersensitivity without altering esophageal motility [49].

Theophylline, a xanthine derivative, has been shown to inhibit adenosine-induced angina-like chest pain and adenosine-induced pain in other regions of the body [50]. A study using an esophageal balloon distension protocol and impedance demonstrated that intravenous theophylline increased thresholds for sensation and pain in 75% of patients with functional chest pain [51]. Similar results were documented in functional chest pain patients receiving oral theophylline for a period of 3 months. In another study, the same authors showed that oral doses of theophylline 200 mg twice daily was more effective than placebo in preventing chest pain in 19 patients with functional chest pain [52].

Psychological Treatment

Several studies have demonstrated that patients with NCCP who are treated with cognitive–behavioral therapy report significant improvement in quality of life and reduction in chest pain symptoms. In addition, cognitive–behavioral therapy has been successfully used for the treatment of NCCP patients with no existing panic disorder [53]. A study evaluating patients who were treated with cognitive–behavioral therapy reported that 48% of these patients remained pain free at the 12-month follow-up, compared with only 13% of the patients in the nonintervention group. Other psychological interventions that have been suggested to be effective in patients with NCCP include reassurance, education, relaxation techniques, breathing training, and biofeedback. Biofeedback was assessed in a study that compared it with primary care visits only in patients with NCCP [54]. Patients in the biofeedback group demonstrated a significantly lower symptom frequency and severity. However, a large group of patients assigned to the biofeedback arm (52%) did not complete the study.

Hypnotherapy has been evaluated in the treatment of NCCP patients. Jones and colleagues [55] reported an 80% improvement in symptoms, with a significant reduction in pain intensity, among patients who were receiving 12 sessions of hypnotherapy, compared with only a 23% symptom improvement in the control group. The study concluded that hypnotherapy appears to have a role in treating NCCP and that further studies are needed.

Case continued

On additional questioning the patient admitted some mild intermittent dysphagia over the past few months along with some associated heartburn. EGD demonstrated an ulcerated stricture in the mid-esophagus. Biopsies were negative. On continued questioning, the patient admitted taking her son's tetracycline when her complexion was poor because it helped his acne. She usually took the tetracycline without water at bedtime. She was treated with a course of omeprazole and stopped the tetracycline. Her pain resolved and a follow-up endoscopy demonstrated resolution of the inflammatory condition of her esophagus.

Take-home points

- Chest pain need not necessarily mean pain; vague chest discomfort is common.

- Patients presenting for the first time with chest pain should be initially evaluated by a cardiologist to rule out a cardiac cause.

- A logical and systematic step-by-step approach should be used, with each individual assessed based on presenting symptoms and medical history.

- Combinations of diagnostic methods should be used to optimize the diagnosis.

- Cardiac angina and GERD are both common, and their coexistence is also common.

- High-dose PPI is an excellent first-step diagnostic/treatment for NCCP.

- The use of esophageal manometry is limited for diagnosing achalasia.

- Psychological comorbidity should be assessed in NCCP patients with signs of psychological disorder or those who are refractory to treatment.

References

1 Boie ET. Initial evaluation of chest pain. *Emerg Med Clin North Am* 2005; **23**: 937–57.

2 Eslick GD, Coulshed DS, Talley NJ. Review article: the burden of illness of non-cardiac chest pain. *Aliment Pharmacol Ther* 2002; **16**: 1217–23.

3 Wong WM, Lam KF, Cheng C, *et al.* Population based study of noncardiac chest pain in southern Chinese: prevalence, psychosocial factors and health care utilization. *World J Gastroenterol* 2004; **10**: 702–12.

4 Eslick GD, Jones MP, Talley NJ. Non-cardiac chest pain: prevalence, risk factors, impact and consulting—a population-based study. *Aliment Pharmacol Ther* 2003; **17**: 1115–24.

5 Eslick GD, Talley NJ. Natural history and predictors of outcome for non-cardiac chest pain: a prospective 4-year cohort study. *Neurogastroenterol Motil* 2008; **20**: 989–97.

6 Eslick GD. Usefulness of chest pain character and location as diagnostic indicators of an acute coronary syndrome. *Am J Cardiol* 2005; **95**: 1228–31.

7 Canto JG, Shlipak MG, Rogers WJ, *et al.* Prevalence, clinical characteristics, and mortality among patients with myocardial infarction presenting without chest pain. *JAMA* 2000; **283**: 3223–9.

8 Stern S. Angina pectoris without chest pain: clinical implications of silent ischemia. *Circulation* 2002; **106**: 1906–8.

9 Ghillebert G, Janssens J. Oesophageal pain in coronary artery disease. *Gut* 1998; **42**: 312–19.

10 Bortolotti M, Marzocchi A, Bacchelli S, *et al.* The esophagus as a possible cause of chest pain in patients with and without angina pectoris. *Hepatogastroenterology* 1990; **37**: 316–18.

11 Schofield PM, Whorwell PJ, Brooks NH, *et al.* Oesophageal function in patients with angina pectoris: a comparison of patients with normal coronary angiograms and patients with coronary artery disease. *Digestion* 1989; **42**: 70–8.

12 Makk LJ, Leesar M, Joseph A, *et al.* Cardioesophageal reflexes: an invasive human study. *Dig Dis Sci* 2000; **45**: 2451–4.

13 Gerson LB, Friday K, Triadafilopoulos G. Potential relationship between gastroesophageal reflux disease and atrial arrhythmias. *J Clin Gastroenterol* 2006; **40**: 828–32.

14 Lux G, Van Els J, The GS, *et al.* Ambulatory oesophageal pressure, pH and ECG recording in patients with normal and pathological coronary angiography and intermittent chest pain. *Neurogastroenterol Motil* 1995; **7**: 23–30.

15 Hsia PC, Maher KA, Lewis JH, *et al.* Utility of upper endoscopy in the evaluation of noncardiac chest pain. *Gastrointest Endosc* 1991; **37**: 22–6.

16 Dickman R, Mattek N, Holub J, *et al.* Prevalence of upper gastrointestinal tract findings in patients with noncardiac chest pain versus those with gastroesophageal reflux disease (GERD)-related symptoms: results from a national endoscopic database. *Am J Gastroenterol* 2007; **102**: 1173–9.

17 Fass R, Fennerty MB, Ofman JJ, *et al.* The clinical and economic value of a short course of omeprazole patients with noncardiac chest pain. *Gastroenterology* 1998; **115**: 42–9.

18 Ofman JJ, Gralnek IM, Udani J, *et al.* The cost-effectiveness of the omeprazole test in patients with noncardiac chest pain. *Am J Med* 1999; **107**: 219–27.

19 Wang W, Huang J, Zheng G, *et al.* Is proton pump inhibitor testing an effective approach to diagnose gastroesophageal

reflux disease in patients with noncardiac chest pain? *Arch Intern Med* 2005; **165**: 1222–8.

20 Prakash C, Clouse RE. Wireless pH monitoring in patients with non-cardiac chest pain. *Am J Gastroenterol* 2006; **101**: 446–52.

21 Dekel R, Pearson T, Wendel C, *et al.* Assessment of oesophageal motor function in patients with dysphagia or chest pain—the Clinical Outcomes Research Initiative experience. *Aliment Pharmacol Ther* 2003; **18**: 1083–9.

22 Katz PO, Dalton CB, Richter JE, *et al.* Esophageal testing of patients with noncardiac chest pain or dysphagia. Results of three years' experience with 1161 patients. *Ann Intern Med* 1987; **106**: 593–7.

23 Rencoret G, Csendes A, Henríquez A. Esophageal manometry in patients with non cardiac chest pain. *Rev Med Chil* 2006; **134**: 291–8.

24 DiMarino AJ Jr, Allen ML, Lynn RB, Zamani S. Clinical value of esophageal motility testing. *Dig Dis* 1998; **16**: 198–204.

25 Knippig C, Fass R, Malfertheiner P. Tests for the evaluation of functional gastrointestinal disorders. *Dig Dis* 2001; **19**: 232–9.

26 Clouse R. Managing functional bowel disorders form the top down: lessons from a well-designed treatment trial. *Gastroenterology* 2003; **125**: 249–53.

27 Eslick GD, Fass R. Non-cardiac chest pain: evaluation and treatment. *Gastroenterol Clin North Am* 2003; **32**: 531–52.

28 Fass R, Navarro-Rodriguez T. Noncardiac chest pain. *J Clin Gastroenterol* 2008; **42**: 636–46.

29 Galmiche JP, Clouse RE, Bálint A, *et al.* Functional esophageal disorders. *Gastroenterology* 2006; **130**: 1459–65.

30 Mudipalli RS, Remes-Troche JM, Andersen L, Rao SSC. Functional chest pain—esophageal or overlapping functional disorder. *J Clin Gastroenterol* 2007; **41**: 264–9.

31 Fass R, Bautista J, Janarthanan S. Treatment of gastroesophageal reflux disease. *Clin Cornerstone* 2003; **5**: 18–29.

32 Kitchin L, Castell D. Rationale and efficacy of conservative therapy for gastroesophageal reflux disease. *Arch Intern Med* 1991; **151**: 448–54.

33 Fang J, Bjorkman D. A critical approach to noncardiac chest pain: pathophysiology, diagnosis, and treatment. *Am J Gastroenterol* 2001; **96**: 958–68.

34 Fass R, Malagon I, Schmulson M. Chest pain of esophageal origin. *Curr Opin Gastroenterol* 2001; **17**: 376–80.

35 Patti M, Molena D, Perretta S, Way LW. Gastroesophageal reflux disease (GERD) and chest pain. Results of laparoscopic antireflux surgery. *Surg Endosc* 2002; **16**: 563–6.

36 Farrell TM, Richardson WS, Trus TL, *et al.* Response of atypical symptoms of gastro-oesophageal reflux to antireflux surgery. *Br J Surg* 2001; **88**: 1649–52.

37 So JB, Zeitels SM, Rattner DW. Outcomes of atypical symptoms attributed to gastroesophageal reflux treated by laparoscopic fundoplication. *Surgery* 1998; **124**: 28–32.

38 Richter JE, Dalton CG, Buice RG, Castell DO. Nifedipine: a potent inhibitor of contractions in the body of the human esophagus. Studies in healthy volunteers and patients with the nutcracker esophagus. *Gastroenterology* 1985; **89**: 549–54.

39 Richter JE, Spurling TJ, Cordova CM, Castell DO. Effects of oral calcium blocker, diltiazem, on esophageal contractions. Studies in volunteers and patients with nutcracker esophagus. *Dig Dis Sci* 1984; **29**: 649–56.

40 Cattau EL Jr, Castell DO, Johnson DA, *et al.* Diltiazem therapy for symptoms associated with nutcracker esophagus. *Am J Gastroenterol* 1991; **86**: 272–6.

41 Drenth JP, Bos LP, Engels LG. Efficacy of diltiazem in the treatment of diffuse oesophageal spasm. *Aliment Pharmacol Ther* 1990; **4**: 411–16.

42 Bassoti G, Gaburri M, Imbimbo BP, *et al.* Manometric evaluation of cimetropium bromide activity in patients with the nutcracker oesophagus. *Scand J Gastroenterol* 1988; **23**: 1079–84.

43 Mellow MH. Effect of isosorbide and hydralazine in painful primary esophageal motility disorders. *Gastroenterology* 1982; **83**: 364–70.

44 Egbunike IG, Chaffee BJ. Antidepressants in the management of chronic pain syndromes. *Pharmacotherapy* 1990; **10**: 262–70.

45 Becker B, Morel N, Vanbellinghen AM, Lebrun P. Blockade of calcium entry in smooth muscle cells by the antidepressant imipramine. *Biochem Pharmacol* 2004; **68**: 833–42.

46 Clouse RE, Lustman PJ, Eckert TC, *et al.* Low-dose trazodone for symptomatic patients with esophageal contraction abnormalities. A double-blind, placebo-controlled trial. *Gastroenterology* 1987; **92**: 1027–36.

47 Handa M, Mine K, Yamamoto H, *et al.* Antidepressant treatment of patients with diffuse esophageal spasm: a psychosomatic approach. *J Clin Gastroenterol* 1999; **28**: 228–32.

48 Varia I, Logue E, O'Connor C, *et al.* Randomized trial of sertraline in patients with unexplained chest pain of noncardiac origin. *Am Heart J* 2000; **140**: 367–72.

49 Broekaert D, Fischler B, Sifrim D, *et al.* Influence of citalopram, a selective serotonin, reuptake inhibitor, on oesophageal hypersensitivity: a double-blind, placebo-controlled study *Aliment Pharmacol Ther* 2006; **23**: 365–70.

50 Crea F, Pupita G, Galassi AR, *et al.* Role of adenosine in pathogenesis of anginal pain. *Circulation* 1990; **81**: 164–72.

51 Rao SS, Mudipalli RS, Mujica VR, *et al.* An open-label trial of theophylline for functional chest pain. *Dig Dis Sci* 2002; **47**: 2763–8.

52 Rao SS, Mudipalli RS, Remes-Troche JM, *et al.* Theophylline improves esophageal chest pain—a randomized, placebo-controlled study. *Am J Gastroenterol* 2007; **102**: 930–8.

53 van Peski-Oosterbaan AS, Spinhoven P, van Rood Y, *et al.* Cognitive–behavioral therapy for noncardiac chest pain: a randomized trial. *Am J Med* 1999; **106**: 424–9.

54 Ryan M, Gervirtz R. Biofeedback-based psychophysiological treatment in a primary care setting: an initial feasibility study. *Appl Psychophysiol Biofeedback* 2004; **29**: 79–93.

55 Jones H, Cooper P, Miller V, *et al.* Treatment of non-cardiac chest pain: a controlled trial of hypnotherapy. *Gut* 2006; **55**: 1403–8.

Other Excellent Resources

Fass R, Eslick GD. *Noncardiac Chest Pain: A Growing Medical Problem.* San Diego, CA: Plural Publishing, 2007.

Albarran J, Tagney J. *Chest Pain: Advanced Assessment and Management Skills.* Oxford: Blackwell Publishing, 2007.

CHAPTER 24

Dysphagia

Dawn L. Francis

Division of Gastroenterology and Hepatology, Mayo Clinic, Rochester, MN, USA

Summary

Dysphagia is an alarm symptom and requires further investigation. Dysphagia is typically categorized as oropharyngeal or esophageal. Patients with oropharyngeal dysphagia should have video fluoroscopic swallowing studies and evaluation by a swallowing rehabilitation expert. Patients with esophageal dysphagia require endoscopy. Patients with endoscopy-negative esophageal dysphagia should have esophageal biopsies to evaluate for eosinophilic esophagitis; if negative, they should have esophageal manometry. Treatment for all types of dysphagia is targeted at the underlying cause.

Case

A 50-year-old woman complains of "reflux." A detailed history reveals that she has frank regurgitation in the recumbent position and with bending forward, typical heartburn that is continuous and has not improved with maximum doses of acid suppressing medications. She also complains of dysphagia to both solids and liquids. Her symptoms have been present for 3 years, but have progressively worsened over the past year. She has lost 30 pounds. She has no other medical problems.

Introduction

Dysphagia refers to the subjective sensation of difficulty in swallowing. Dysphagia is a distinct symptom from other swallowing-related complaints such as odynophagia, which refers to painful swallowing, and globus sensation, the sensation of a lump in the throat.

Dysphagia is a common complaint that can occur in any age group, but is more common in the elderly population. As many as 10% of people over the age of 50 complain of dysphagia [1]. No matter the age, dysphagia is considered an alarm symptom and should prompt a diagnostic evaluation to define its etiology. A thorough

Practical Gastroenterology and Hepatology: Esophagus and Stomach, 1st edition. Edited by Nicholas J. Talley, Kenneth R. DeVault and David E. Fleischer. © 2010 Blackwell Publishing Ltd.

patient history suggests the correct etiology in as many as 85% [2] of patients. Table 24.1 lists questions to elicit the salient points of the patient's history. The differential diagnosis of dysphagia is broad and includes anatomic abnormalities, motility disorders, neuromuscular disease, and infiltrative disorders.

Pathophysiology

There are a number of potential physiologic problems that can lead to the symptom of dysphagia or odynophagia. These can be broadly categorized as infections, mucosal abnormalities, anatomic abnormalities, or functional problems of the oropharynx and esophagus.

Infections

Odynophagia is often caused by infection of the oropharynx with fungal organisms or viruses and dysphagia without odynophagia can also be due to infection. The infections that cause the symptoms of odynophagia or dysphagia are usually opportunistic infections that occur in immunosuppressed or elderly patients such as *Candida*, HSV, or CMV.

Mucosal Abnormalities

There are a number of mucosal abnormalities that can cause odynophagia, dysphagia, or both. Those associated

Table 24.1 Focused questions for patients with dysphagia.

Question	Comment
How long have you had trouble swallowing? Have your symptoms worsened with time? Is your swallowing difficulty continuous or intermittent?	Progressive dysphagia is often associated with an esophageal carcinoma, peptic stricture, or achalasia. Intermittent dysphagia may indicate the presence of a lower esophageal ring. Patients with motility disorders may have either progressive or intermittent symptoms, depending on the disorder.
Do you have trouble initiating a swallow or do you feel food getting "stuck" or "hanging up" a few seconds after swallowing?	Oropharyngeal dysphagia is often characterized by difficulty initiating a swallow and esophageal dysphagia by the onset of symptoms several seconds after the initiation of a swallow.
Do you have problems swallowing solids, liquids, or both?	Dysphagia for both solids and liquids often indicates an underlying esophageal motility disorder, whereas dysphagia for solids alone usually represents an anatomic obstruction.
Do you cough or choke after swallowing?	Coughing or choking after swallowing is often due to oropharyngeal dysphagia or a Zenker diverticulum.
Have you had unintentional weight loss?	Weight loss may be present with dysphagia of any type but is most often associated with esophageal carcinoma or achalasia.

with odynophagia are usually due to radiation injury or head and neck cancer. Those most commonly associated with dysphagia are peptic esophagitis, esophageal carcinoma, eosinophilic esophagitis, or pill esophagitis.

Anatomic Abnormalities

Anatomic abnormalities that may cause dysphagia include cricopharyngeal bar, Zenker diverticulum, esophageal webs, peptic stricture, distal esophageal rings, vascular compression of the esophagus, or compression of the esophagus by cervical osteophytes.

Functional Abnormalities

Odynophagia or oropharyngeal dysphagia may be caused by weakness of the oropharynx, cricopharyngeal hypertrophy, or by several different neuromuscular disorders. Esophageal dysphagia may be due to ineffective esophageal motility, aperistalsis, hypertensive lower esophageal sphincter (LES), nutcracker esophagus, diffuse esophageal spasm (DES), or achalasia.

Clinical Features

The most important aspect of the patient history is to define the patient's dysphagia as oropharyngeal or "transfer dysphagia" versus esophageal dysphagia. Oropharyngeal dysphagia is often characterized by the complaint of difficulty initiating a swallow, transitioning a food bolus or liquid into the esophagus, meal-induced coughing or "choking", or of food "getting stuck" immediately after swallowing. The patient will often localize the sensation to the cervical esophagus above the suprasternal notch.

The timing of the onset and worsening of symptoms of dysphagia are also important. Progressive dysphagia is often associated with an esophageal carcinoma, peptic stricture, or achalasia, whereas intermittent dysphagia may indicate the presence of a lower esophageal ring. Patients with esophageal motility disorders may have either progressive or intermittent symptoms.

An important part of the medical history is characterizing the types of food that produce symptoms, that is solids, liquids, or both. For example, dysphagia for both solids and liquids often indicates an underlying esophageal motility disorder, whereas dysphagia for solids alone usually represents an anatomic obstruction.

Oropharyngeal Dysphagia

There are many disorders that cause oropharyngeal dysphagia (Table 24.2). Generally, these include neuromuscular diseases, systemic diseases, or mechanical obstruction. When neuromuscular diseases cause oropharyngeal dysphagia, other neurological, or muscular symptoms may be present, including recurrent bouts of aspiration pneumonia from inadequate airway

Table 24.2 Causes of oropharyngeal dysphagia.

Mechanical obstruction
  Cervical osteophyte
  Cricopharyngeal bar
  Thyromegaly
  Zenker diverticulum

Neuromuscular
  Amyotrophic lateral sclerosis
  Brainstem tumors
  Cerebrovascular accident
  Multiple sclerosis
  Parkinson disease
  Peripheral neuropathy

Skeletal muscle disorders
  Myasthenia gravis
  Muscular dystrophies
  Polymyositis

Table 24.3 Causes of esophageal dysphagia.

Extraesophageal
  Cervical osteophytes
  Enlarged left atrium
  Enlarged aorta
  Enlarged or aberrant subclavian artery (dysphagia lusoria)
  Mediastinal mass

Motility disorders
  Achalasia
  Aperistalsis
  Diffuse esophageal spasm
  Hypertensive lower esophageal sphincter
  Ineffective motility
  Nutcracker esophagus

Intraesophageal
  Benign tumors or lesions
  Esophageal carcinoma
  Caustic esophagitis
  Dermatologic conditions (lichen planus, pemphigoid/ pemphigus)
  Diverticula
  Eosinophilic esophagitis
  Infection
  Radiation injury
  Rings or webs
  Stricture (benign or malignant)
  Scarring from surgery

protection, hoarseness, dysarthria, or pharyngonasal regurgitation.

Oropharyngeal dysphagia from mechanical or anatomic abnormalities may be caused by cervical osteophytes, thyromegaly, pharyngeal tonsillar enlargement, a cricopharyngeal bar (also known as hypertensive upper esophageal sphincter (UES)), or Zenker diverticulum.

Esophageal Dysphagia

Patients with esophageal dysphagia describe the onset of symptoms several seconds after the initiation of a swallow. They can sense that the food or liquid bolus has traversed the oral cavity and has entered the esophagus. They complain of food feeling "stuck" or "hung up" in transition to the stomach. They usually feel symptoms in the retrosternal area but may also feel the problem near the suprasternal notch. Retrosternal dysphagia usually corresponds to the location of the lesion, while suprasternal dysphagia is referred from below. Occasionally, patients will describe their dysphagia as regurgitation of liquid occurring during, or just after, a meal. This can be misdiagnosed as gastroesophageal reflux, especially in patients with achalasia (as in the Case presented here).

Esophageal dysphagia can be caused by a number of diseases (Table 24.3), but is most often the result of a mechanical obstruction or one of a small number of motility disorders. Esophageal dysphagia that is caused by a motility disorder is commonly characterized by dysphagia to both solids and liquids. Dysphagia that is asso-

ciated with only solid foods is more likely due to a mechanical obstruction, although mechanical obstructions may progress to the extent that there is dysphagia for both solids and liquids.

If there is episodic and non-progressive dysphagia without weight loss, then the obstruction is likely secondary to an esophageal web or a distal esophageal ring. If solid-food dysphagia is progressive, then the problem may be an esophageal stricture, carcinoma of the esophagus, or achalasia. When weight loss is present with solid-food dysphagia, concern for an esophageal carcinoma comes to the forefront.

Diagnosis

There are a limited number of tests that can be performed to evaluate dysphagia. These include: video-fluoroscopic swallowing evaluation for oropharyngeal dysphagia; and barium esophagram, esophageal manometry, and esophagogastroduodenoscopy (EGD) for esophageal dysphagia. The goal of testing is to identify structural abnormalities that can be treated endoscopi-

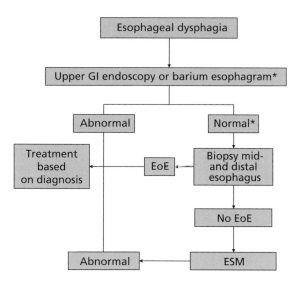

*Barium esophagram optional. It may be useful to guide endoscopic intervention in some settings.

Figure 24.1 Suggested approach to patients with clinical features of esophageal dysphagia. EoE, eosinophilic esophagitis; ESM, esophageal manometry.

cally or surgically, detect treatable underlying systemic disease, and define functional disorders.

The choice of an initial test is based on the clinical presentation and expertise that is available. If the patient has symptoms and history that are consistent with oropharyngeal dysphagia, one may elect to start the diagnostic workup with video-fluoroscopy that can identify the presence of aspiration and help in directing swallowing rehabilitation. Alternatively, if the patient has complaints that are more consistent with an esophageal anatomic abnormality, a barium esophagram, or EGD may be the best first step. For those who have an initial barium esophagram that suggests achalasia, esophageal manometry would be an appropriate next step (Figure 24.1). Many experts recommend that esophageal biopsies be obtained for patients with esophageal dysphagia if there is no endoscopic evidence of anatomic narrowing, to rule out eosinophilic esophagitis.

Therapeutics

The aims of treatment for dysphagia are to improve the mechanics of food bolus transfer, to ameliorate the sen-

Table 24.4 Treatment of oropharyngeal dysphagia.

Neuromuscular disorders
  Swallowing rehabilitation
  Medical treatment targeted at the underlying disease:
    Myasthenia gravis
    Parkinson disease
    Multiple sclerosis

Zenker diverticulum
  Botulinum toxin injection of UES
  Cricopharyngeal myotomy with diverticulectomy

Hypertensive UES/cricopharyngeal bar
  Bougie dilation
  UES botulinum toxin injection
  Cricopharyngeal myotomy

UES, upper esophageal sphincter.

Table 24.5 Treatment of esophageal dysphagia.

Mucosal disease
  Infection
    Antifungals
    Antivirals
  Eosinophilic esophagitis
    Topical or systemic corticosteroids
    Allergy testing/avoidance of allergens
  Peptic esophagitis
    Proton pump inhibitors

Motility disorders
  DES, nutcracker esophagus
    Nitrates, calcium channel blockers
    Sildenafil
    Trazadone/impramine
    Esophageal dilation
    Botulinum toxin in distal esophagus
    LES myotomy
  Achalasia
    LES myotomy for surgical candidates
    Botulinum toxin injection to LES
    Pneumatic dilation

Benign strictures, webs and rings
  Esophageal dilation
  Intralesional injection of corticosteroids
  Temporary self-expanding plastic stents
  Surgery

LES, lower esophageal sphincter; DES, diffuse esophageal spasm.

sation of dysphagia, to prevent esophageal food bolus impaction, and to prevent aspiration and its complications. The treatment strategy requires correct identification of the etiology of the patient's dysphagia for targeted interventions (Tables 24.4 and 24.5).

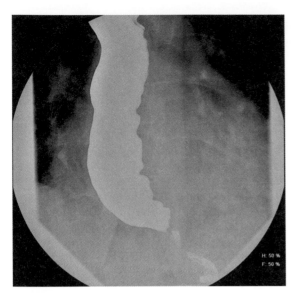

Figure 24.2 Barium esophagram showing a dilated esophagus with narrowing in the distal esophagus, consistent with achalasia.

Case continued

The symptom of dysphagia prompted an EGD. The EGD showed a dilated esophagus filled with fluid and food. There was narrowing in the distal esophagus but no associated mucosal abnormalities. A barium esophagram was performed and showed similar findings (Figure 24.2). An esophageal manometry shows a poorly relaxing LES and aperistalsis (Figure 24.3). The patient was diagnosed with achalasia based on endoscopic and manometric findings. Her symptoms of "reflux" were, in fact, due to esophageal reflux rather than gastroesophageal reflux. The patient is young and healthy and is a good surgical candidate, so was sent for a laparoscopic Heller myotomy. She was discharged from the hospital on postoperative day 2 and has had no further complaints of dysphagia. She has very mild symptoms of "heartburn" which are now well controlled with as-needed dosing of H_2 receptor antagonists. She no longer has regurgitation.

Oropharyngeal Dysphagia

Swallowing rehabilitation by a swallowing professional (in most cases a speech pathologist) is the mainstay of treatment for patients with oropharyngeal dysphagia caused by neuromuscular dysfunction and benefits most patients in this category [3,4]. Any patient with oropharyngeal dysphagia should be cautioned to chew food thoroughly and slowly and to avoid alcohol during meals. Consuming food quickly and without focused attention can lead to aspiration.

There are a number of maneuvers during swallowing that may reduce oropharyngeal dysphagia and these can be tailored to the specific defect leading to the dysphagia. Some authors believe that swallowing rehabilitation can improve oropharyngeal dysphagia even when it is caused by an anatomic abnormality. This has been demonstrated in patients with defects brought about by surgical resection of oropharyngeal tissue [5] or by caustic injury [6].

Specific pharmacologic intervention may be available for patients with oropharyngeal dysphagia that is caused by an underlying neurologic disease for which medical treatments are available, such as myasthenia gravis or Parkinson disease. However, many patients with oropharyngeal dysphagia have an underlying disease that is progressive and does not have good treatment options. For those patients, swallowing rehabilitation may prolong the time that they can meet their nutritional needs orally, but ultimately many require non-oral feeding to prevent aspiration, such as with a percutaneous gastrostomy tube.

Patients that have oropharyngeal dysphagia due to an anatomic abnormality, such as a Zenker diverticulum or cricopharyngeal bar, typically require an endoscopic or surgical intervention. Bougie dilation has been used successfully with oropharyngeal dysphagia caused by a hypertensive UES [7] or primary cricopharyngeal dysfunction [8]. Botulinum toxin injection at the UES has also been effective for hypertensive UES or Zenker diverticulum [9].

Patients with inadequate pharyngeal contraction or lack of coordination between the hypopharynx and the UES, a hypertensive UES, or Zenker diverticulum may be candidates for a cricopharyngeal myotomy. The success of this surgical intervention depends on the patient having an intact neurologic system, adequate propulsive force generated by the tongue and pharyngeal constrictors, intact initiation of swallowing, videofluorographic demonstration of obstruction to bolus flow at the level of the cricopharyngeus muscle, and manometric evidence of relatively elevated UES pressure in comparison to the pharynx [10].

Esophageal Dysphagia

Mucosal Disease

Esophageal dysphagia that is due to mucosal disease such as infections, eosinophilic esophagitis, or peptic esopha-

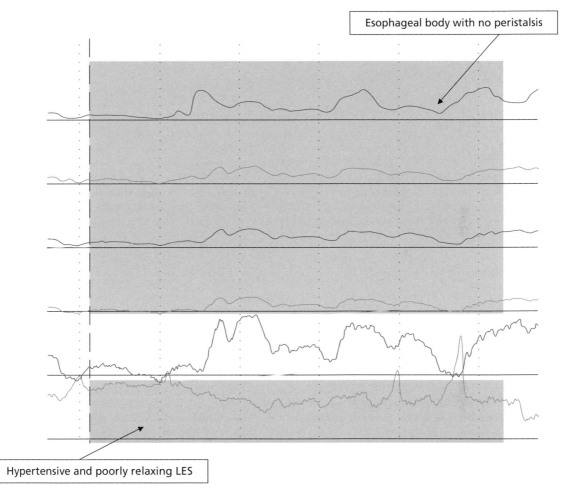

Esophageal body with no peristalsis

Hypertensive and poorly relaxing LES

Figure 24.3 Esophageal manometry with aperistalsis and hypertensive, poorly relaxing lower esophageal sphincter consistent with achalasia.

gitis can be treated with targeted medical therapy. Candida esophagitis is typically treated with fluconazole for 10–14 days. Viral esophagitis often requires 6 weeks of treatment with the appropriate antiviral. Eosinophilic esophagitis is often treated with swallowed topical corticosteroids, such as fluticasone delivered in a metered dose inhaler for 6–8 weeks. Patients with gastroesophageal reflux disease (GERD) related strictures or motility disorders will benefit from aggressive acid suppression. This is typically accomplished with proton pump inhibitors (PPI) or H_2 receptor antagonists [11,12]. PPI therapy has been shown to decrease the recurrence of esophageal strictures.

Anatomic Narrowing from Benign Disease
Esophageal narrowing that is due to esophageal webs, rings, or benign strictures is typically treated with esophageal dilation by either solid dilators (e.g., Savary, Maloney, or American) or balloon dilators. Patients with esophageal strictures that require repeated dilation may benefit from intralesional corticosteroids [13] that can be performed with standard endoscopy. In severe cases, placement of temporary self-expanding plastic esophageal stent can be helpful. Patient with refractory and severe benign esophageal strictures may require surgical resection.

Anatomic Narrowing from Malignant Disease

The reason dysphagia is an alarm symptom is because of the possibility of malignancy. Nearly 50% of patients with esophageal cancer present with disease that is already metastatic. For those patients, placement of an esophageal stent will improve their dysphagia symptoms. For those that have resectable disease, surgery is the definitive treatment.

Motility Disorders

It is known that cold foods or liquids can make some esophageal motility problems worse, so these should be avoided in patients with esophageal motility disorders, especially in those of the hypertensive category, such as nutcracker esophagus or DES.

There are medications available for some esophageal hypertensive motility disorders (i.e., DES, nutcracker esophagus, hypertensive LES). Nitrates and calcium channel blockers have been used with some effect. Sildenafil inactivates nitric oxide-stimulated cyclic guanosine monophosphate and, as a result, can relax the LES. Several investigators have studied the effect of sildenafil, at a dose of 50 mg, on the lower esophageal sphincter and have found that it was associated with symptom relief in a group of 11 patients with nutcracker esophagus or DES [14]. Trazodone and imipramine have been shown to be effective in relieving chest pain in patients with esophageal motility disorders and likely work by modifying visceral sensation.

Certain motility disorders may be improved with dilation, most notably achalasia and perhaps nutcracker esophagus. Pneumatic dilation with large diameter balloons (30–40 mm) has been used with some success in patients with achalasia, but the perforation risk is significant and, as a result, many clinicians have moved away from dilation as a first-line treatment for achalasia.

Botulinum toxin has been used with variable success in patients with achalasia. The effect is shorter lasting than with myotomy, but appears to be a safe alternative to pneumatic dilation for patients that are not surgical candidates [15]. Botulinum toxin has been reported to be effective in diffuse esophageal spasm and other non-specific motility disorders in small, uncontrolled studies.

LES myotomy is primarily for achalasia and, in severe cases, diffuse esophageal spasm. The most common approach is the modified Heller approach. The Heller myotomy relieves symptoms associated with achalasia in up to 90% of patients and the mortality rate is similar to pneumatic dilation for achalasia (0.3%). The response seems to be more durable than that of pneumatic dilation [16]. As laparoscopic myotomy is becoming more common, this surgery has become a more common treatment for achalasia.

Prognosis

Most patients with esophageal dysphagia do well with treatment focused on the underlying etiology. Patients with oropharyngeal dysphagia fare less well as the cause of the oropharyngeal dysphagia is usually a progressive and untreatable neuromuscular disease. Though swallowing rehabilitation can help, patients may ultimately require non-oral feeding to prevent aspiration.

Take-home points

Diagnosis:
- Dysphagia can be categorized as "esophageal" or "oropharyngeal."
- Esophageal dysphagia is an "alarm symptom" that must be investigated, typically with endoscopy.
- Oropharyngeal dysphagia is due to mucosal or motor abnormalities of the oropharynx. Diagnosis requires functional evaluation with a video fluoroscopic swallowing study.
- Patients with endoscopy-negative dysphagia should have further investigation to identify the etiology of the symptom. Appropriate studies may include mid-esophageal biopsies, video-fluoroscopic swallowing study, or esophageal manometry.

Treatment:
- Treatment for dysphagia is targeted at the underlying disease.
- Patients with oropharyngeal dysphagia should be treated with swallowing rehabilitation.
- Patients with anatomic narrowing of the distal esophagus can be treated with endoscopy-directed dilation, intralesional injection of corticosteroids, temporary plastic stent placement, or surgery.
- Patients with hypertensive esophageal motility disorders can be treated with medications, botulinum toxin injection in the distal esophagus and, in severe cases, with surgery.
- Achalasia should be treated surgically unless the patient is not a surgical candidate because of other significant co-morbidities.

References

1 Lindgren S, Janzon L. Prevalence of swallowing complaints and clinical findings among 50-79-year-old men and women in an urban population. *Dysphagia* 1991; **6**: 187–92.

2 Edwards DA. Discriminative information in the diagnosis of dysphagia. *J R Coll Physicians London* 1975; **9**:257–63.

3 Neuman S. Swallowing therapy with neurologic patients: results of direct and indirect therapy methods in 66 patients suffering from neurological disorders. *Dysphagia* 1993; **8**: 150–3.

4 Huckabee ML, Cannito MP. Outcomes of swallowing rehabilitation in chronic brainstem dysphagia: a retrospective evaluation. *Dysphagia* 1999; **14**: 93–109.

5 Zuydam AC, Rogers SN, Brown JS, *et al.* Swallowing rehabilitation after oro-pharyngeal resection for squamous cell carcinoma. *Br J Oral Max Surg* 2000; **38**: 513–8.

6 Shikowitz MJ, Levy J, Villano D, *et al.* Speech and swallowing rehabilitation following devastating caustic ingestion: Techniques and indicators for success. *Laryngoscope* 1996; **106** (Suppl. 78): 1–12.

7 Hatlebakk J, Castell J, Spiegel J, *et al.* Dilatation therapy for dysphagia in patients with upper esophageal sphincter dysfunction—manometric and symptomatic response. *Dis Esophagus* 1998; **11**: 254–9.

8 Solt J, Bajor J, Moizs M, *et al.* Primary cricopharyngeal dysfunction: treatment with balloon catheter dilatation. *Gastrointest Endosc* 2001; **54**: 767–71.

9 Yokoyama T, Asai M, Kumada M, *et al.* Botulinum toxin injection into the cricopharyngeal muscle for dysphagia: report of 2 successful cases. *J Oto-Rhino-Laryngolog Soc Japan* 2003; **106**: 754–7.

10 Buchholz DW. Cricopharyngeal myotomy may be effective treatment for selected patients with neurogenic oropharyngeal dysphagia. *Dysphagia* 1995; **10**: 255.

11 Stal JM, Gregor JC, Preiksaitis HG, *et al.* A cost-utility analysis comparing omeprazole with ranitidine in the maintenance therapy of peptic esophageal stricture. *Can J Gastroenterol* 1998; **12**: 43–9.

12 Marks RD, Richter JE, Rizzo J, *et al.* Omeprazole versus H2-receptor antagonists in treating patients with peptic stricture and esophagitis. *Gastroenterology* 1994; **106**: 907–15.

13 Kochhar R, Makharia G. Usefulness of intralesional triamcinolone in treatment of benign esophageal strictures. *Gastrointest Endosc* 2002; **56**: 829–34.

14 Eherer AJ, Schwetz I, Hammer HF, *et al.* Effect of sildenafil on oesophageal motor function in healthy subjects and patients with oesophageal motor disorders. *Gut* 2002; **50**: 758.

15 Pasricha PJ, Ravich WJ, Hendrix TR, *et al.* Intrasphincteric botulinum toxin for the treatment of achalasia. *N Engl J Med* 1995; **332**: 774–8.

16 Vela MF, Richter JE, Khandwala F, *et al.* The long-term efficacy of pneumatic dilatation and Heller myotomy for the treatment of achalasia. *Clin Gastroenterol Hepatol* 2006; **4**: 580–7.

CHAPTER 25
Rumination

H. Jae Kim

Divisions of Gastroenterology and Hepatology, Mayo Clinic, Scottsdale, AZ, USA

Summary

Rumination syndrome is a functional gastroduodenal disorder characterized by the repetitive, effortless regurgitation of recently ingested food into the mouth followed by rechewing and reswallowing or expulsion. Initially described in infants and children, it is now widely recognized that this occurs in people of all ages. Recognition of the clinical features of rumination syndrome is essential to make the diagnosis. A timely diagnosis, reassurance, and behavioral therapy are crucial to avoid continued deterioration, inappropriate tests, and unnecessary treatments.

Case

An 18-year-old female presents with daily regurgitation with meals for 1 year. This occurs only when she is eating or shortly after eating. She has made a habit of rechewing and reswallowing the regurgitated food but will spit it out when the regurgitant is bitter or sour. Persistent symptoms have led to reduced oral intake and 9 kg (20 lb) weight loss. She was given the diagnosis of gastroesophageal reflux disease (GERD) and told to start daily proton pump inhibitor. This failed to help her and she returns for a further opinion.

Definition and Epidemiology

Rumination is a clinical syndrome characterized by frequent (often daily), effortless regurgitation of recently ingested food into the mouth without forceful retching followed by remastication and reswallowing or expectorating of food. This syndrome has been described in almost equal prevalence among disabled infants (6–10% [1,2]) and in institutionalized adults (8–10% [3–5]). The syndrome is also recognized as a cause of postprandial

regurgitation in children, adolescents, and adults with normal development [6–9]. The Rome III consensus criteria used to diagnose in these age groups is summarized in Table 25.1 [10–12]. The prevalence in the normal development group is unknown because of the secretive nature of this condition in many patients and lack of awareness of this entity among physicians. In general, rumination is more common in females.

Clinical Features, Pathophysiology, and Diagnosis

Repetitive regurgitation usually begins within minutes of starting a meal and may persist for more than 30 min after completing a meal. A sensation of belching may precede regurgitation, and the regurgitant consists of recognizable food, which has the pleasant taste of the recently ingested food. Symptoms often cease when regurgitated food becomes acidic to taste. Weight loss may be considerable and is not uncommon in female adolescent patients. Many patients describe their regurgitation as "vomiting" but close questioning can distinguish their problems.

Although the etiology and pathophysiology of rumination syndrome remain unclear, it appears that abdominal

Practical Gastroenterology and Hepatology: Esophagus and Stomach, 1st edition. Edited by Nicholas J. Talley, Kenneth R. DeVault and David E. Fleischer. © 2010 Blackwell Publishing Ltd.

Table 25.1 Rome III Consensus Criteria for Rumination Syndrome. (Adapted from [10–12].)

Neonate/toddler

Must include all of the following for at least 3 months:

1 Repetitive contractions of the abdominal muscles, diaphragm, and tongue

2 Regurgitation of gastric content into the mouth, which is either expectorated or rechewed and reswallowed

3 Three or more of the following:
   a Onset between 3 and 8 months
   b Does not respond to management for GERD or to anticholinergic drugs, hand restraints, formula changes, and gavage or gastrostomy feedings
   c Unaccompanied by signs of nausea or distress
   d Does not occur during sleep and when the infant is interacting with individuals in the environment

Child/adolescent

Must include all of the following:

1 Repeated painless regurgitation and rechewing or expulsion of food that
   a Begin soon after ingestion of a meal
   b Do not occur during sleep
   c Do not respond to standard treatment for gastroesophageal reflux

2 No retching

3 No evidence of an inflammatory, anatomic, metabolic, or neoplastic process that explains the subject's symptoms

Adult

Must include both of the following:

1 Persistent or recurrent regurgitation of recently ingested food into the mouth with subsequent spitting or remastication and swallowing

2 Regurgitation is not preceded by retching

Supportive criteria:

1 Regurgitation events are usually not preceded by nausea

2 Cessation of the process when the regurgitated material becomes acidic

3 Regurgitant contains recognizable food with a pleasant taste

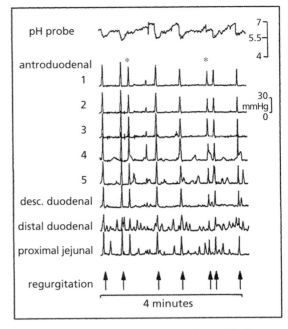

Figure 25.1 Gastrointestinal manometric tracing and distal esophageal pH in rumination patient. Note concurrence of regurgitation (arrows) with decreases in pH and R or simultaneous waves consistent with increased intra-abdominal pressure. * Two R waves that are not associated with regurgitation or decrease in intraesophageal pH. (Reprinted from [13].)

muscle contraction together with relaxation of the lower esophageal sphincter (LES) in the early postprandial period is responsible for the regurgitation. Gastroduodenal manometry demonstrates characteristic, brief, simultaneous increases in gastric and small bowel pressure (rumination or "r" waves) seen in all abdominal recording ports during the postprandial period (Figure 25.1 [13]). These represent abdominal wall contractions and if performed with esophageal pH monitoring, they are associated with a decrease in distal esophageal pH.

Although the "r" waves may be characteristic of rumination syndrome, the diagnostic utility of gastroduodenal manometry is low as up to 50% of patients will not exhibit these waves.

Others have documented the importance of LES relaxation as a prerequisite to regurgitation of gastric contents [14,15] suggesting an adaptation of the belch reflex that overcomes or changes the function of the LES. The belch reflex involves a vagally mediated, prolonged relaxation of the LES, which is thought to be induced by gastric distension with air [16]. For example in health, LES pressure increases with increased intra-abdominal pressure; however, in rumination, transient LES relaxations occur during the abdominal straining events.

Rumination is frequently confused with anorexia nervosa, bulimia, GERD, and gastrointestinal motility disorder, such as gastroparesis, or functional vomiting. Patients often undergo extensive and costly testing before diagnosis. A careful interpretation of each test result is necessary in these patients. For example, abnormal esophageal pH testing may be a consequence of rumination, rather than from true GERD. In these patients, a careful analysis may show that acid reflux occurs with a meal only, and minimal or no acid reflux is noted with non-meal or at night time in the supine position. Gastric emptying study may be difficult to perform in these patients due to the necessity of a radiolabeled meal ingestion. The potential for expectoration of the meal is high, and when the majority of the meal is expelled, the study cannot be completed. For those whom the expectoration is minimal, a 4-h scintigraphy is recommended over a 90-min study with data extrapolation.

In summary, lack of awareness of the clinical features, female predominance, and considerable weight loss on presentation contribute to the underdiagnosis and misdiagnosis of rumination syndrome. Often a good history, recognition of the clinical features, and observation are sufficient to make the diagnosis of rumination.

Treatment

Treatment is best accomplished with behavioral modification and biofeedback therapy administered in a formal eating-regulation program. The behavioral approach focuses on diaphragmatic breathing as a means to create a competing behavior and break the cycle of food regurgitation [17,18]. This helps teach patients to relax abdominal muscles during and after eating. In a retrospective review of 46 patients who received behavioral therapy, complete disappearance of the behavior was seen in 30% and partial improvement in 55% of patients [19]. The use of oral medications such as antidepressants, antiemetics, proton pump inhibitors, prokinetics, and anticholinergics has been disappointing [13]. Surgery (Nissen fundoplication, gastric pacer, etc.) is neither recommended nor effective in rumination syndrome and in fact may worsen symptoms due to the patient's loss of ability to engage in this behavior in the absence of an effective psychological intervention.

> - Weight loss is not uncommon and may be considerable.
> - Gastroduodenal manometry is not necessary to make the diagnosis.
> - Timely diagnosis, reassurance, and behavioral therapy are crucial to avoid continued deterioration, inappropriate tests, and unnecessary treatments.
> - Behavioral modification and biofeedback therapy are the mainstay of rumination treatment.

References

1 Chatoor J, Dickson L, Einhorn A. Rumination: etiology and treatment. *Pediatr Ann* 1984; **13**: 924–9.

2 Winton A, Singh NN. Rumination in pediatric populations: a behavioral analysis. *J Am Acad Child Adolesc Psychiatry* 1983; **22**: 269–75.

3 Rast J, Ellinger-Alien JA, Johnston JM. Dietary management of rumination: four case studies. *Am J Clin Nutr* 1985; **42**: 95–101.

4 Rogers B, Stratton P, Victor J, *et al.* Chronic regurgitation among persons with mental retardation: a need for combined medical and interdisciplinary strategies. *Am J Ment Retard* 1992; **96**: 522–7.

5 Singh NN. Rumination. In: Ellis NR, ed. *International Review of Research in Mental Retardation*, Vol. **10**. New York: Academic, 1981: 139–82.

6 Amarnath R, Abell TL, Malagelada JR. The rumination syndrome in adults. *Ann Intern Med* 1986; **105**, 513–18.

7 Brown WR. Rumination in the adult: a study of two cases. *Gastroenterology* 1968; **54**: 933–9.

8 LaRocca FEF, Della-Fera MA. Rumination: its significance in adults with bulimia nervosa. *Psychosomatics* 1986; **27**: 209–12.

9 Levine DF, Wingate DL, Pfeffer JM, Butcher P. Habitual rumination: a benign disorder. *BMJ* 1983; **287**: 255–6.

10 Hyman PE, Milla PJ, Benninga MA. Childhood functional gastrointestinal disorders: neonate/toddler. *Gastroenterology* 2006; **130**: 1519–26.

11 Rasquin A, Di Lorenzo C, Forbes D. Childhood functional gastrointestinal disorders: child/adolescent. *Gastroenterology* 2006; **130**: 1527–37.

12 Tack J, Talley NJ, Camilleri M. Functional gastroduodenal disorders. *Gastroenterology* 2006; **130**: 1466–79.

13 O'Brien M, Bruce BK, Camilleri M. The rumination syndrome: clinical features rather than manometric diagnosis. *Gastroenterology* 1995; **108**: 1024–9.

14 Breumelhof R, Smout AJPM, Depler ACTM. A. The rumination syndrome in an adult patient. *J Clin Gastroenterol* 1990; **12**: 232–4.

Take-home points

- Rumination can be recognized in children, adolescents, and adults, and must be distinguished from vomiting.
- A sufficient clinical history and observation are adequate to make the diagnosis.

15 Smout A, Breumelhof R. Voluntary induction of transient lower esophageal sphincter relaxation in an adult patient with the rumination syndrome. *Am J Gastroenterol* 1990; **85**: 1621–5.

16 Wyman JB, Dent J, Heddle R, *et al*. Control of belching by the lower esophageal sphincter. *Gut* 1990; **31**: 639–46.

17 Wagaman JR, Williams DE, Camilleri M. Behavioral intervention for the treatment of rumination. *J Pediatr Gastroenterol Nutr* 1998; **27**: 596–8.

18 Chitkara DK, Van Tilburg M, Whitehead WE, Talley NJ. Teaching diaphragmatic breathing for rumination syndrome. *Am J Gastroenterology* 2006; **101**: 2449–52.

19 Chial HJ, Camilleri M, Williams DE. Rumination syndrome in children and adolescents: diagnosis, treatment, and prognosis. *Pediatrics* 2003; **111**: 158–62.

CHAPTER 26
Halitosis

Ganesh R. Veerappan[1] *and James H. Lewis*[2]

[1] Gastroenterology Service, Walter Reed Army Medical Center, Washington, DC, USA
[2] Division of Gastroenterology, Georgetown University Medical Center, Washington, DC, USA

Summary

The majority of cases of halitosis originate from the oral cavity. Less commonly halitosis is due to a systemic disease (e.g., liver failure), esophageal, or gastric disease. Initial evaluation may lead to an oral source such as poor dentition, periodontal disease, or an abscess. Mouthwash can reduce oral bacteria and neutralize odor. On very rare occasions, gas chromatography is useful to distinguish the offending gas. Since the tongue may be a source, tongue cleaning is warranted.

Case

A 48-year-old female comes to the physician stating that the last two social relationships in which she had been involved ended with the man saying that he didn't enjoy kissing her because she had bad breath. She had gone to the dentist and he had told her that she had no dental or periodontal problems. She had tried six different mouthwashes which had been advertised on TV but they didn't work for her like they did with the lady in the commercial who smiled and kissed her husband with relief. She said she had read in a magazine that there was some stomach infection that could cause halitosis and she wanted to be tested for that. She also had symptoms of reflux but taking antacids or over the counter acid suppressants hadn't made a difference. The gastroenterologist reluctantly scheduled her for an endoscopy which was normal except for a small hiatal hernia. Biopsies from the antrum and body were taken and both revealed *H. pylori*. The patient was placed on a 14-day course of proton pump inhibitor and two antibiotics and reported that her breath had improved. A urea breath test for *H. pylori* 3 months later showed no evidence of infection. She contacted one of the men whom had been offended by her breath and they had a few more dates, but eventually he broke up with her saying he didn't like her personality. She met another man 6 months later over the Internet and they were eventually married in Aruba.

Practical Gastroenterology and Hepatology: Esophagus and Stomach, 1st edition. Edited by Nicholas J. Talley, Kenneth R. DeVault and David E. Fleischer. © 2010 Blackwell Publishing Ltd.

Definition and Epidemiology

Halitosis describes an unpleasant or offensive odor in the breath. This condition has been associated with psychosocial embarrassment and may impact personal relationships [1]. The exact incidence of bad breath is not known although it is common and affects people of all ages. The prevalence of bad breath according to a few population studies in various countries ranges from 15 to 30% [2–4].

Bad breath is worse or at maximal prevalence upon awakening, and due to the common nature of this it has been termed "morning halitosis" [1]. This has no clinical consequence and results from increased microbial metabolic activity during sleep and decreased salivary flow [5].

Halitophobics are those that fear they have bad breath when indeed they don't and they make up 25% of individuals seeking professional counsel for bad breath [6]. These people wrongly interpret actions of others as indication of offensive breath and often become fixated with teeth cleaning, gum chewing, and mouthwash [1].

Etiology and Pathophysiology

Halitosis originates from either the oral cavity, nasal passages, tonsils, and systemic or respiratory causes for halitosis (Table 26.1) [7]. Eighty to ninety percent of all cases originate from the oral cavity [8]. The tongue is the

Table 26.1 Causes of halitosis.

Oral disease: tongue, food particles, gingivitis, peridontitis, pericoronitis, xerostomia, oral ulceration, oral malignancy, peri-implant disease, deep carious lesions, exposed necrotic tooth pulp, oral wounds, imperfect dental restorations, unclean dentures

Nasal passages: sinusitis, nasal polyps, history of cleft palate or craniofacial anomalies, foreign bodies

Oropharynx/respiratory: tonsiliths, foreign body, bronchial or lung infections

Systemic: liver failure, chronic kidney disease, various carcinomas (oral cavity, pharynx, tonsils, tongue, nasopharynx), medications, metabolic dysfunction (diabetes), biochemical disorders (trimethylaminuria)

Gastrointestinal: *Helicobacter pylori*, gastroesophageal reflux disease

Lifestyle: cigarette smoking, alcohol, garlic, onions, spices, cabbage, cauliflower, radish

major source of halitosis and periodontal disease seems only a fraction of the overall problem [9,10]. The oral malodor arises from microbial degradation of organic substrates present in saliva, oral soft tissues, and retained debris. Microbial degradation products are volatile sulfur-containing compounds [11].

There are many Gram-positive and negative bacteria that have been implicated. These bacterial interactions are most likely to occur when food debris collects in between teeth, in the gingival crevices, and at the posterior portion of tongue. The dorsal aspect of tongue may retain large amounts of desquamated cells, leukocytes, and microorganisms [1]. Oral pathology such as advanced gingivitis and periodontal disease also contribute to halitosis. Other dental problems and poor oral hygiene have been associated with halitosis including peri-implant disease, deep carious lesions, exposed necrotic tooth pulp, oral wounds, imperfect dental restorations, and unclean dentures [12]. Lack of oral cleansing due to xerostomia also has potential to cause or enhance malodor.

The nasal passages are the second most common cause of halitosis [8]. Nasal malodour is "cheesy", which differs from other forms of bad breath [13]. Causes include sinusitis, polyps affecting airflow, or a history of cleft palate or other craniofacial anomalies. Foreign bodies placed in nostrils are a common cause of halitosis in children [14]. The tonsils are a minor cause of halitosis, and not common enough to be a reason to get a tonsillectomy.

Often odor is created from tonsilloliths that form in the crypts of the tonsils. Halitosis may be caused by respiratory, bronchial, or lung infections, which may result in nasal or sinus secretions passing into the oropharynx.

Some systemic causes of bad breath include kidney failure, liver failure, various carcinomas, medications, metabolic dysfunction, and biochemical disorders [15]. Classically, acetone breath has been associated with uncontrolled diabetes, but is not very common. All these presentations are uncommon and usually present in the later stages of these disease processes. Carcinomas in the oral cavity, pharynx, tonsils, base of tongue, and nasopharynx are potential causes of halitosis in a patient with significant risk factors.

Trimethylaminuria ("fish odor syndrome") is a rare disorder characterized by oral and body malodor. This genetic disorder involves the inability to breakdown trimethylamine-N-oxide, resulting in excess trimethylamine that produces a pungent ammoniacal odor, similar to rotten fish. Management includes reducing or eliminating precursors of trimethylamine in the diet, such as rapeseed oil, carnitine, certain legumes and sulfur-containing foods including eggs

Halitosis is rarely associated with diseases of the esophagus, stomach, and intestines and is not an indication for endoscopy. Recently, there has been an association described between halitosis and gastroesophageal reflux disease (GERD), but still a relatively new idea [16,17]. *Helicobacter pylori* has been shown to produce sulfur compounds, and has been considered as a possible cause of halitosis [18–20].

Some halitosis is purely due to lifestyle. Certain habits such as cigarette smoking and alcohol are common causes of bad breath and are only transient. Bad breath is also associated with ingestion of certain foods such as garlic, onions, spices, cabbage, cauliflower, and radish [5]. Halitosis associated with garlic may remain in the mouth several hours after meticulous oral hygiene. This odor has been attributed to a gas (allyl methyl sulfide) that is absorbed into systemic circulation and excreted through the lungs for hours after ingestion [21].

Diagnosis

Before halitosis may be managed effectively, an accurate diagnosis must be achieved. A detailed history including medical and dental history, diet, and a detailed oral and periodontal exam is a necessary part of the evaluation. However, it is difficult for a patient to self-assess the extent of their disorder and it is recommended that these individuals bring a confidant to the visit to provide more accurate data [22].

Physical exam includes a detailed oral and periodontal examination, preferably by a dentist or someone invested in oral hygiene. Ultimate assessment is done by smelling the exhaled air of the mouth and nose and comparing the two [23]. Odor from the mouth but not nose is likely to be an oral source. Odor from nose and alone is likely to be coming from the nose or sinuses [24]. If odor from nose and mouth are similar then it is likely from a systemic cause of halitosis.

More objective measurements of halitosis are available, but are not used clinically because of expense and time constraints [5]. There are instruments to detect volatile sulfur compounds, but cannot detect other classes of volatile compounds and so are not very sensitive [5]. Gas chromatography is the method of choice for distinguishing gas mixture of bad breath, and less cumbersome, less expensive gas chromatographs are being developed [5].

Therapeutics

Management of halitosis depends largely on the cause identified. The majority of patients have an oral source and management will focus on managing oral halitosis primarily (Figure 26.1). Treatment focuses on educating the patient as to the common causes of halitosis and tools to prevent this, which include good oral hygiene with brushing and flossing. Avoiding smoking, drugs, and food that may contribute to halitosis may be reasonable. In addition, chewing gum, mints, or fennel seeds may mask the bad breath. Treatment is also directed at reducing accumulation of food debris and malodor-producing bacteria. This requires treating oral/dental disease, improving oral hygiene, and reducing tongue coating.

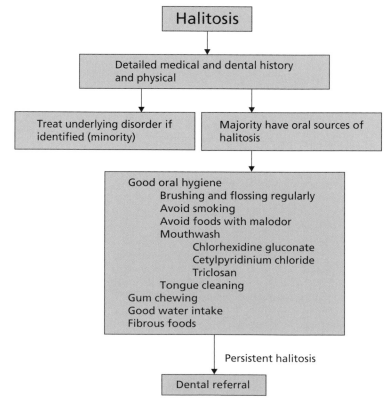

Figure 26.1 Treatment algorithm for halitosis.

Oral hygiene involves tooth brushing, flossing, and the use of mouthwashes. Rinsing and gargling with mouthwash have also been used to reduce oral bacteria and neutralize odoriferous compounds exhaled [25]. Mouthwashes containing chlorhexidine gluconate, cetylpyridinium chloride, or triclosan have shown some benefit [26–28]. A recent Cochrane Review pooled five randomized controlled trials and concluded that mouth rinses may play an effective role in reducing halitosis, but a few of the trials had incomplete data [29].

If oral hygiene is already good, the tongue is the likely source and hence tongue cleaning is indicated. The aim is to dislodge trapped food, cells, and bacteria from between the filiform papillae to decrease concentration of volatile sulfur compounds. Tongue cleaning may be done with a tongue scraper or toothbrush. Studies have shown a limited benefit of prolonged tongue scraping, but many still recommend this be done regularly [30].

Other therapies include eating fibrous foods, brief gum chewing, and sufficient water intake. Antibiotics have been used by multiple physicians, but often only result in a transient relief of halitosis and is not advisable. Treatment of *H. pylori* with triple therapy in patients with functional dyspepsia resulted in resolution of halitosis in one study [31]. Dental referrals for patients with persistent halitosis is reasonable, when odor is deemed to be originating from an oral source. If the cause of halitosis is identified (periodontal disease, gingivitis, postnasal drip, systemic illness), the treatment involves treating the patient's underlying condition.

Take-home points

Diagnosis:

- In 80–90% of cases of halitosis originate from the oral cavity with the tongue being the major source.
- Halitosis is rarely associated with diseases of the esophagus, stomach, and intestines and is not an indication for endoscopy.
- A detailed history, including medical and dental history, diet, and a detailed oral and periodontal exam are important parts of the evaluation.

Therapy:

- Treatment focuses on educating patient as to the common causes of halitosis and tools to prevent this, which include good oral hygiene with brushing and flossing.
- Mouthwash can reduce oral bacteria and neutralize odoriferous compounds.

- Studies have shown limited benefit of prolonged tongue scraping, but this is still recommended in patients with halitosis.
- Dental referral for patients with persistent halitosis is reasonable.

References

1 Porter SR, Scully C. Oral malodour (halitosis). *BMJ* 2006; **333**: 632–5.

2 Rosenberg M, Knaan T, Cohen D. Association among bad breath, body mass index, and alcohol intake. *J Dent Res* 2007; **86**: 997–1000.

3 Liu XN, Shinada K, Chen XC, *et al.* Oral malodor-related parameters in the Chinese general population. *J Clin Periodontol* 2006; **33**: 31–6.

4 Nadanovsky P, Carvalho LB, Ponce de Leon A. Oral malodour and its association with age and sex in a general population in Brazil. *Oral Dis* 2007; **13**: 105–9.

5 Scully C, Greenman J. Halitosis (breath odor). *Periodontol 2000* 2008; **48**: 66–75.

6 Seemann R, Bizhang M, Djamchidi C, *et al.* The proportion of pseudo-halitosis patients in a multidisciplinary breath malodour consultation. *Int Dent J* 2006; **56**: 77–81.

7 Tangerman A. Halitosis in medicine: a review. *Int Dent J* 2002; **52** (Suppl. 3): 201–6.

8 Delanghe G, Ghyselen J, van Steenberghe D, Feenstra L. Multidisciplinary breath-odour clinic. *Lancet* 1997; **350**: 187.

9 Bosy A, Kulkarni GV, Rosenberg M, McCulloch CA. Relationship of oral malodor to periodontitis: evidence of independence in discrete subpopulations. *J Periodontol* 1994; **65**: 37–46.

10 Rosenberg M. Bad breath and periodontal disease: how related are they? *J Clin Periodontol* 2006; **33**: 29–30.

11 Tonzetich J. Production and origin of oral malodor: a review of mechanisms and methods of analysis. *J Periodontol* 1977; **48**: 13–20.

12 van den Broek AM, Feenstra L, de Baat C. A review of the current literature on aetiology and measurement methods of halitosis. *J Dent* 2007; **35**: 627–35.

13 Rosenberg M. Clinical assessment of bad breath: current concepts. *J Am Dent Assoc* 1996; **127**: 475–82.

14 Katz HP, Katz JR, Bernstein M, Marcin J. Unusual presentation of nasal foreign bodies in children. *JAMA* 1979; **241**: 1496.

15 Durham TM, Malloy T, Hodges ED. Halitosis: knowing when 'bad breath' signals systemic disease. *Geriatrics* 1993; **48**: 55–9.

16 Moshkowitz M, Horowitz N, Leshno M, Halpern Z. Halitosis and gastroesophageal reflux disease: a possible association. *Oral Dis* 2007; **13**: 581–5.

17 Struch F, Schwahn C, Wallaschofski H, *et al*. Self-reported halitosis and gastro-esophageal reflux disease in the general population. *J Gen Intern Med* 2008; **23**: 260–6.

18 Adler I, Denninghoff VC, Alvarez MI, *et al*. *Helicobacter pylori* associated with glossitis and halitosis. *Helicobacter* 2005; **10**: 312–7.

19 Hoshi K, Yamano Y, Mitsunaga A, *et al*. Gastrointestinal diseases and halitosis: association of gastric Helicobacter pylori infection. *Int Dent J* 2002; **52** (Suppl. 3): 207–11.

20 Lee H, Kho HS, Chung JW, *et al*. Volatile sulfur compounds produced by *Helicobacter pylori*. *J Clin Gastroenterol* 2006; **40**: 421–6.

21 Suarez F, Springfield J, Furne J, Levitt M. Differentiation of mouth versus gut as site of origin of odoriferous breath gases after garlic ingestion. *Am J Physiol* 1999; **276**: G425–30.

22 Rosenberg M, Kozlovsky A, Gelernter I, *et al*. Self-estimation of oral malodor. *J Dent Res* 1995; **74**: 1577–82.

23 Donaldson AC, Riggio MP, Rolph HJ, *et al*. Clinical examination of subjects with halitosis. *Oral Dis* 2007; **13**: 63–70.

24 Rosenberg M, McCulloch CA. Measurement of oral malodor: current methods and future prospects. *J Periodontol* 1992; **63**: 776–82.

25 Porter SR, Scully C. Oral malodour (halitosis). *BMJ* 2006; **333**: 632–5.

26 Roldan S, Herrera D, O'Connor A, *et al*. A combined therapeutic approach to manage oral halitosis: a 3-month prospective case series. *J Periodontol* 2005; **76**: 1025–33.

27 Roldan S, Herrera D, Santa-Cruz I, *et al*. Comparative effects of different chlorhexidine mouth-rinse formulations on volatile sulphur compounds and salivary bacterial counts. *J Clin Periodontol* 2004; **31**: 1128–34.

28 Roldan S, Winkel EG, Herrera D, *et al*. The effects of a new mouthrinse containing chlorhexidine, cetylpyridinium chloride and zinc lactate on the microflora of oral halitosis patients: a dual-centre, double-blind placebo-controlled study. *J Clin Periodontol* 2003; **30**: 427–34.

29 Fedorowicz Z, Aljufairi H, Nasser M, *et al*. Mouthrinses for the treatment of halitosis. *Cochrane Database Syst Rev* 2008; **4**: CD006701.

30 Outhouse TL, Al-Alawi R, Fedorowicz Z, Keenan JV. Tongue scraping for treating halitosis. *Cochrane Database Syst Rev* 2006; **19**(2): CD005519.

31 Katsinelos P, Tziomalos K, Chatzimavroudis G, *et al*. Eradication therapy in *Helicobacter pylori*-positive patients with halitosis: long-term outcome. *Med Princ Pract* 2007; **16**: 119–23.

CHAPTER 27

Hiccups

Ganesh R. Veerappan[1] and James H. Lewis[2]

[1] Gastroenterology Service, Walter Reed Army Medical Center, Washington, DC, USA
[2] Division of Gastroenterology, Georgetown University Medical Center, Washington, DC, USA

Summary

Most instances of transient hiccups are of little clinical significance. If hiccups last for more than 48h that often implies an underlying structural, physical, or neoplastic disorder, which necessitates an evaluation for a cause. The afferent limb of the hiccup arc is via the vagus and phrenic nerves and the efferent limb is via the phrenic nerve. More than 100 conditions have been associated with hiccups. Men are more likely to have an underlying cause discovered than women. Hiccups are commonly seen with medications used for endoscopy but the explanation is not clear. Among the gastrointestinal causes of hiccups are gastroesophageal reflux disease, infectious esophagitis, achalasia, and carcinomatosis. Chlorpromazine is the only FDA approved drug for hiccups. Baclofen has emerged as the most successful pharmacologic treatment for hiccups.

Case

A 54-year-old male was hospitalized for persistent vomiting, dehydration, abdominal pain, and hiccups of one week's duration. He had been receiving outpatient external beam radiation therapy for retroperitoneal sarcoma that had initially been treated with local resection 10 months earlier, but was admitted from the Radiation Oncology Clinic after a recent abdominal CT scan revealed progression of his disease with studding of the peritoneum consistent with carcinomatosis and dilated small bowel loops with air/fluid levels consistent with obstruction. The stomach was also found to be dilated, but his abdomen was only minimally distended. He refused nasogastric decompression, preferring to be made nothing by mouth (NPO) and given intravenous fluids. His hiccups had increased in frequency to about 12 times per minute and were now occurring around the clock and interfering with his ability to sleep. Chlorpromazine was administered at a dose of 25mg IV every 8h but this produced unwanted somnolence and hypotension and was discontinued in favor of metoclopramide 10mg IV every 6h. However, the hiccups still failed to respond after another 72h and he was evaluated by the Gastroenterology Service who recommended consideration of a percutaneous endoscopic gastrostomy (PEG) for decompression since the

patient was adamant that he did not want a nasogastric tube, but the PEG was also refused. It was recommended that baclofen 10mg every 6h be tried. Over the course of the next 48h the hiccups decreased in frequency and disappeared 2 days later. He was able to tolerate small amounts of liquids and was discharged on baclofen.

Definition and Epidemiology

Hiccups have long been considered a medical curiosity. Although most hiccups occur as brief, self-limited episodes lasting up to a few minutes, persistent hiccups that last longer than 48h or recur at frequent intervals often imply an underlying physical, structural, metabolic, neoplastic, or infectious cause. Occasionally, hiccups are intractable, occurring continuously for months or years, and can result in significant morbidity [1]. Intractable hiccups are responsible for approximately 4000 hospitalizations per year in the United States [2]. Interestingly, hiccups affect men more than women [3].

The term "hiccup" refers to the onomatopoeic attempt to vocalize the sound produced by the abrupt closure of the glottis after the sudden contraction of the inspiratory muscles [4]. "Hiccough" was used in the older literature and likely represented the previously held belief that

Practical Gastroenterology and Hepatology: Esophagus and Stomach, 1st edition. Edited by Nicholas J. Talley, Kenneth R. DeVault and David E. Fleischer. © 2010 Blackwell Publishing Ltd.

hiccups occur as a result of abnormal respiratory reflex. The medical term for hiccups, singultus, is derived from the Latin root *singult*, meaning the act of catching one's breath during sobbing [1].

Pathophysiology/Clinical Features

Hiccups do not appear to serve any particularly useful or protective function. However, because they may occur during fetal and neonatal life and are seen in other mammals, they may represent a primitive or vestigial reflex whose functional or behavioral significance has been lost [5,6]. One theory speculates that intrauterine hiccups permit training of the diaphragm without aspiration of amniotic fluid [7].

A relationship between hiccups and the phrenic nerve was recognized by an Edinburgh physician in 1833 [8]. Current theories developed further by Bailey and colleagues described the concept of a hiccup reflex arc [9,10]. In current theory, the afferent limb of hiccup reflex is composed of the vagus and phrenic nerves, and the sympathetic chain arising from T6–T12, with a hiccup center located in the upper spinal cord in (C3–5). The efferent limb remains primarily the phrenic nerve, although nerves to the glottis and accessory muscles of the respiration are also involved, as patients are reported to continue to hiccup even after transection of both phrenic nerves [1,11]. This reflex pathway is similar to those that produce coughing, sneezing, swallowing, and vomiting [4] (Figure 27.1).

More than 100 conditions have been associated with hiccups, including a variety of structural, metabolic, inflammatory, neoplastic, infectious, and drug-related causes (Table 27.1). For many, a relationship with one or more limbs of the reflex arc can be demonstrated, whereas for others, the association is more obscure [1].

Benign Transient Causes

Transient hiccups are benign and occur nearly universally in all individuals from time to time. Such hiccups are often due to overdistension of stomach, commonly caused by overeating, drinking carbonated beverages, aerophagia, alcohol use, and sudden excitement or emotional stress [1]. The mechanism is presumed to be gastric distension stimulating gastric branches of vagus nerve or via direct irritation of the diaphragm by an overinflated stomach [1,4]. Alcohol-induced hiccups are also likely from gastric distension and/or the central effects of alcohol on the cerebral cortex, which remove inhibitions normally serving to dampen the hiccup reflex [12]. Sudden excitement, emotional stress, smoking, and change in food/body temperature have also been associated with temporary hiccups [4].

Intraoperative hiccups may occur for a number of reasons including: extension of neck with stretching of the roots of the phrenic nerve; the use of short-acting barbiturates; inadequate ventilation during anesthesia; gastric distension or ileus. A light plane of anesthesia may suppress inhibitory influences that normally function to prevent hiccups. Postoperative hiccups account for as many as 25% of hiccups in men, usually appearing within 4 days of surgery. A majority of these episodes follow intra-abdominal surgery, with the remainder resulting from urinary tract, central nervous system, and chest surgery procedures [4]. Hiccups are also commonly seen

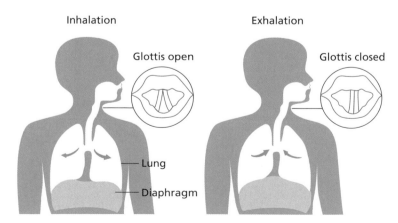

Figure 27.1 Anatomic representation of the diaphragm, lungs, and glottis in inhalation and exhalation during hiccups.

during endoscopy, either from the use of opioids or midazolam used for sedation, or from gastric distension from air insufflation.

Persistent Hiccups

The longer the duration of a hiccup bout, the more likely an organic cause exists. The etiopathogenic causes of persistent and intractable hiccups can be broadly categorized as central nervous system disorders, toxic–metabolic causes, diseases affecting the diaphragm or vagus nerve, drugs, general anesthesia, postoperative causes, inflammatory, neoplastic, and infectious causes (Table 27.1).

All these causes stimulate one or more limbs of the hiccup reflex arc.

Of particular interest to gastroenterologists are the gastrointestinal (GI) and hepatic causes of hiccups. Conditions such as gastroesophageal reflux disease (GERD), infectious esophagitis, esophageal obstruction (stricture, cancer, rings), achalasia, abdominal carcinomatosis, or widespread surgical adhesions have been associated with hiccups [4]. Significant morbidity has been associated with intractable hiccups. Inability to eat, significant weight loss, exhaustion, insomnia, cardiac arrhythmias, and even death have all been associated with persistent hiccups [1].

Table 27.1 Causes of hiccups (after ref [4]).

Central nervous system
  Structural lesions: intracranial neoplasms, hydrocephalus, multiple sclerosis, brainstem tumors, syringomyelia, ventriculi–peritoneal shunt, glaucoma, Parkinson disease
  Vascular lesions: vascular insufficiency, arteriovenous malformation, intracranial hemorrhage, temporal arteritis
  Trauma: skull fracture, epilepsy
  Infectious: meningitis, encephalitis, neurosyphilis, brain abscess

Toxic–metabolic causes
  Chronic kidney disease, diabetes mellitus, alcohol, gout, hyponatremia, hypokalemia, hypocalcemia, hypocarbia, fever, insulin shock therapy

Diaphragmatic irritation
  Diaphragmatic tumors, eventration, myocardial infarction, pericarditis, hiatus hernia, splenomegaly, hepatomegaly, subphrenic abscess, perihepatitis, esophageal cancer, aberrant cardiac pacemaker electrode

Vagus nerve irritation
  Meningeal branches: meningitis
  Pharyngeal branches pharyngitis, laryngitis
  Auricular branches: hair, insect, foreign body
  Recurrent laryngeal nerve: goiter, neck cyst, tumors, scrofula
  Thoracic branches: pneumonia, empyema, bronchitis, asthma, pleuritis, achalasia, sarcoidosis, esophageal obstruction, esophagitis, thoracic aortic aneurysm, tuberculosis, myocardial infarction, pericarditis, mediastinitis, cor pulmonale, herpes zoster, lung cancer, mediastinal hematoma
  Abdominal branches: gastric distension, gastric cancer, gastritis, peptic ulcer, gastric ulcer, pancreatic cancer, pancreatitis, pseudocyst, intra-abdominal abscess, bowel obstruction, cholelithiasis, cholecystitis, abdominal aortic aneurysm, ulcerative colitis, Crohn disease, gastrointestinal hemorrhage, prostatic disorders, parasitic infestation, appendicitis, hepatitis

Drugs
  Methyldopa, short-acting barbiturates, dexamethasone, methylprednisolone, diazepam, chlordiazepoxide

General anesthesia
  Inadequate ventilation, suppression of normal inhibitory influences, intubation, recovery period, traction of viscera, hyperextension of neck, gastric distension or ileus

Postoperative
  Manipulation of diaphragm, prostatic and urinary tract surgery, craniotomy, thoractomy, laparotomy

Infectious
  Meningitis, encephalitis, typhoid fever, cholera, *Candida* esophagitis, malaria, herpes zoster, acute rheumatic fever, influenza, tuberculosis

Psychogenic
  Hysterical neurosis, conversion reaction, sudden shock, grief reaction, malingering, personality disorders, anorexia nervosa, enuresis

Evaluation

Brief hiccup bouts are common and do not require medical intervention. However, persistent and intractable hiccups necessitate a thorough evaluation in order to find the underlying etiology and guide successful treatment. The extent of the work up should reflect the degree of morbidity. An underlying organic cause is discovered in 90% of men with persistent hiccups, whereas women are less likely to have a specific cause identified [1]. A complete history including duration of the hiccups, alcohol and drug use, and medications should be sought. Physical examination should be focused on eliciting structural or neurological abnormalities, mass lesions, tenderness, or inflammation. Hiccups have been attributed to foreign bodies in the ear canal, prompting a thorough aural exam.

Initial laboratory tests should include a complete blood count (CBC), chemistry panel, urinanalysis, and chest X-ray. Liver associated enzymes, thyroid tests, electrocardiogram (ECG), and imaging of the abdomen, pelvis, thorax, and head are often performed routinely. In cases where the likely cause of hiccups remains obscure, additional testing can be pursued, including lumbar puncture, panendoscopy, esophageal manometry, pulmonary function tests, bronchoscopy, and electricoencephalogram. Exploratory laparotomy or other surgery is occasionally required.

Therapeutics

Numerous therapies have been proposed for the control or elimination of hiccups [13]. However, most of these are based on a small number of isolated case reports and many of the better-known hiccup "cures" are mostly anecdotal. Whenever possible, treatment should be directed at the specific illness causing the hiccups (Figure 27.2).

Non-pharmalogic Therapy

Many of the original "hiccup cures" can be traced back hundreds or thousands of years. Plato is credited with being the first to recommend a sudden slap on the back as a means of scaring away hiccups. This probably worked by inducing a sudden gasp in the person being struck, thereby breaking the hiccup cycle, giving rise to other therapies aimed at disrupting the respiratory rhythm [1,14]. These included breath holding, gargling with water, and tickling the patient's nose to induce sneezing [15,16]. Other physical and mechanical cures attempt to disrupt the diaphragmatic contractions that occur during hiccupping. Pulling the knees up to chest or leaning forward to compress the diaphragm [1] may increase positive airway pressure and hyperinflate the lungs, which stimulates the Hering–Breuer reflex, and disrupts the abnormal hiccup pattern [17]. Performing a Valsalva maneuver, hyperventilating, involuntary gasping using smelling salts, and inhaling 5% carbon dioxide also have been described [4]. Counter-stimulating the vagal branches of the pharynx have been accomplished by swallowing a teaspoon of sugar in a single "gulp."

Relief of gastric distension with emetics, gastric lavage, or nasogastric aspiration may be an effective way to relieve hiccups when the stomach is overdistended with air, food, or liquid. Stimulation of the oropharynx is often cited as a way to terminate hiccups. This can be achieved by placing traction on the tongue, lifting the uvula with a spoon, manipulating the pharynx with a rubber tube or cotton swab, or by swallowing granulated sugar, honey, or peanut butter. Each method has anecdotal success, suggesting that irritation of the soft palate or pharynx may inhibit afferent impulses transmitted by the vagus nerve [4].

Hypnotherapy and acupuncture have been reportedly used to cure hiccups in patients due to a number of different causes. While acupuncture for hiccups has been traditionally practiced in the Far East [16], it is becoming a more commonplace therapy in western centers as well, especially when no specific cause of hiccups can be identified.

Pharmacotherapy

Several pharmacologic agents have been used for the treatment of persistent or intractable hiccups, although there are few controlled trials to confirm what is largely anecdotal evidence of their success. The following agents have been the most frequently employed for hiccups of various causes. Doses and routes of administration are provided in Figure 27.2.

• **Baclofen**, an analogue of the inhibitory neurotransmitter gamma-aminobutyric acid (GABA), has emerged as the most successful general hiccup therapy, with multiple studies showing successful treatment of hiccups

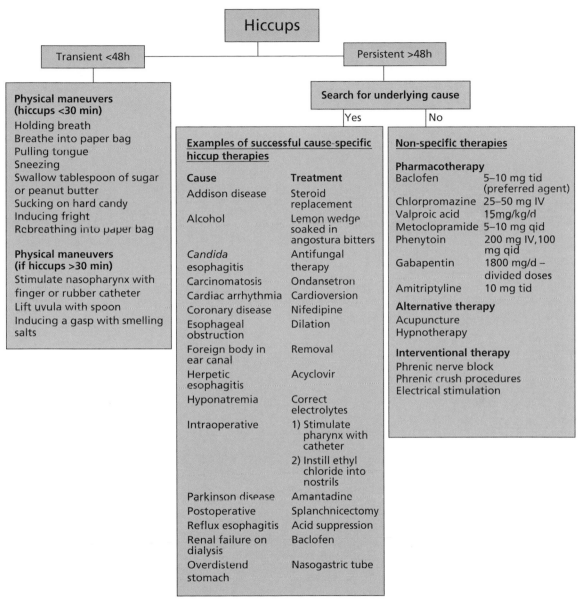

Figure 27.2 Algorithm for treating hiccups.

[18–21]. Baclofen is believed to reduce excitability and depress reflex hiccup activity, as demonstrated in animal studies. It also blocks esophageal and gastric distension. Baclofen is relatively fast acting with a half-life of 3–4 h and is cleared by the kidneys. Side effects include drowsiness, insomnia, weakness, ataxia, dizziness, and confusion, and may be poorly tolerated by elderly patients. The

drug should be used cautiously in patients with renal failure [22].

• **Chlorpromazine**, a phenothiazine antipsychotic, is the only medication specifically approved by the Food and Drug Administration for the treatment of hiccups. Its use was first described in the 1950s with an 80% success rate [23]. Intravenous administration is considered to be most effective, although the drug must be infused slowly to prevent hypotension. Oral doses (25–50 mg three times per day) have been used successfully for treatment of hiccups as an alternative therapy [2]. Chlorpromazine tends to be more poorly tolerated in the elderly, causing dizziness and orthostatic hypotension.

• **Metoclopramide**, a dopamine antagonist and gastric motility agent, is often used in the treatment of hiccups although it is not as effective as chloropromazine [24]. It has terminated hiccups in patients with gastric distension caused by diabetic gastroparesis.

• **Anticonvulsants**, such as phenytoin, valproic acid, carbamazepine, gabapentin, and the benzodiazepenes have had limited success in terminating hiccups [25–28]. Gabapentin has been shown to treat hiccups in patients with cancer and central nervous system disorders (Guillain–Barré and stroke) [2,29–31].

Anesthesia-related hiccups have been stopped with methylphenidate, ethyl chloride spray, ephedrine, and catheter stimulation of the pharynx [32–34]. Postoperative hiccups have been cured with amphetamine and ketamine [35–37]. Marijuana has even been used in patients with AIDS [38]. Amantadine, a dopaminergic agonist, has had anecdotal success in treating hiccups in patients with Parkinson disease. Chronic hiccups associated with esophageal disorders (e.g., gastroesophageal reflux disease, achalasia, esophagitis) have been relieved with treatment of underlying condition.

anesthetic, are reserved for refractory cases. Unfortunately, results have been variable, and such procedures may result in impaired respiratory function. Electrical stimulation of the phrenic nerve has seen limited use to treat refractory hiccups [39].

Take-home points

Evaluation:

• Transient hiccups are benign, last seconds to minutes, and do not require evaluation.

• Bouts lasting more than 48 h often imply an underlying physical, infectious, structural, neoplastic, or metabolic disorder.

• Persistent hiccups necessitate a thorough evaluation in order to find the underlying etiology and guide successful treatment.

• The extent of the work-up should reflect the degree of morbidity of the hiccups; even an extensive evaluation may at times fail to uncover a specific or readily treatable cause.

Treatment:

• Begins with various physical and mechanical maneuvers for transient hiccups.

• Treat the specific underlying cause when one is identified e.g., GERD.

• Baclofen remains the only pharmacologic therapy proven effective in the controlled clinical trial setting.

• Acupuncture, hypnosis and surgical therapies to crush or transect phrenic nerves have been used in refractory cases.

Conclusions

While the majority of hiccups are either socially amusing, embarrassing, or annoying, they are self limited and rarely require treatment other than simple physical maneuvers such as holding your breath, pulling on tongue, sneezing, sucking on hard candy, or swallowing some sugar or peanut butter. Persistent or intractable hiccups can be associated with significant morbidity and often require an extensive evaluation to find the cause. If an underlying condition cannot be treated specifically or effectively (e.g., carcinomatosis), pharmacologic therapy may be tried. If this proves unsuccessful, alternative therapeutic approaches, including acupuncture or hypnosis, can be attempted.

Surgical approaches, including phrenic nerve crushing or transection, or use of phrenic nerve block with a local

References

1 Lewis JH. Hiccups: Causes and cures. *J Clin Gastroenterol* 1985; **7**: 539–52.

2 Schuchmann JA, Browne BA. Persistent hiccups during rehabilitation hospitalization: three case reports and review of the literature. *Am J Phys Med Rehabil* 2007; **86**: 1013–8.

3 Fisher CM. Protracted hiccup—a male malady. *Trans Am Neurol Assoc* 1967; **92**: 231–3.

4 Lewis JH. Hiccups: reasons and remedies. In: Lewis JH, ed. *A Pharmalogic Approach to Gastrointestinal Disorders.* Baltimore: Williams & Wilkins, 1995: 209–27.

5 Dunn PM. Fetal hiccups. *Lancet* 1977; **2**: 505.

6 Miller FC, Gonzales F, Mueller E, McCart D. Fetal hiccups: an associated fetal heart rate pattern. *Obstet Gynecol* 1983; **62**: 253–5.

7 Fuller GN. Hiccups and human purpose. *Nature* 1990; **343**: 420.

8 Shortt T. Hiccup, its causes and cure. *Med Surg J (Edinburgh)* 1833; **39**: 305.

9 Samuels L. Hiccup; a ten year review of anatomy, etiology, and treatment. *Can Med Assoc J* 1952; **67**: 315–22.

10 Bailey H. Persistent hiccup. *Practitioner* 1943; **150**: 173–7.

11 Salem MR. An effective method for the treatment of hiccups during anesthesia. *Anesthesiology* 1967; **28**: 463–4.

12 Hulbert NG. Hiccoughing (hiccup or singultus). *Practitioner* 1951; **167**: 286–9.

13 Friedman NL. Hiccups: a treatment review. *Pharmacotherapy* 1996; **16**: 986–95.

14 Obis P, Jr. Remedies for hiccups. *Nursing* 1974; **4**: 88.

15 Engleman EG, Lankton J, Lankton B. Granulated sugar as treatment for hiccups in conscious patients. *N Engl J Med* 1971; **285**: 1489.

16 Bendersky G, Baren M. Hypnosis in the termination of hiccups unresponsive to conventional treatment. *Arch Intern Med* 1959; **104**: 417–20.

17 Baraka A. Inhibition of hiccup by pulmonary inflation. *Anesthesiology* 1970; **32**: 271–3.

18 Ramirez FC, Graham DY. Treatment of intractable hiccup with baclofen: results of a double-blind randomized, controlled, cross-over study. *Am J Gastroenterol* 1992; **87**: 1789–91.

19 Guelaud C, Similowski T, Bizec JL, *et al.* Baclofen therapy for chronic hiccup. *Eur Respir J* 1995; **8**: 235–7.

20 Burke AM, White AB, Brill N. Baclofen for intractable hiccups. *N Engl J Med* 1988; **319**: 1354.

21 Turkyilmaz A, Eroglu A. Use of baclofen in the treatment of esophageal stent-related hiccups. *Ann Thorac Surg* 2008; **85**: 328–30.

22 Chou CL, Chen CA, Lin SH, Huang HH. Baclofen-induced neurotoxicity in chronic renal failure patients with intractable hiccups. *South Med J* 2006; **99**: 1308–9.

23 Friedgood CE, Ripstein CB. Chlorpromazine (thorazine) in the treatment of intractable hiccups. *J Am Med Assoc* 1955; **157**: 309–10.

24 Madanagopolan N. Metoclopramide in hiccup. *Curr Med Res Opin* 1975; **3**: 371–4.

25 Petroski D, Patel AN. Letter: Diphenylhydantoin for intractable hiccups. *Lancet* 1974; **1**: 739.

26 Jacobson PL, Messenheimer JA, Farmer TW. Treatment of intractable hiccups with valproic acid. *Neurology* 1981; **31**: 1458–60.

27 McFarling DA, Susac JO. Letter: Carbamazepine for hiccoughs. *JAMA* 1974; **230**: 962.

28 Fariello RG, Mutani R. Letter: Treatment of hiccup. *Lancet* 1974; **2**: 1201.

29 Hernandez JL, Pajaron M, Garcia-Regata O, *et al.* Gabapentin for intractable hiccup. *Am J Med* 2004; **117**: 279–81.

30 Porzio G, Aielli F, Narducci F, *et al.* Hiccup in patients with advanced cancer successfully treated with gabapentin: report of three cases. *N Z Med J* 2003; **116**: U605.

31 Tegeler ML, Baumrucker SJ. Gabapentin for intractable hiccups in palliative care. *Am J Hosp Palliat Care* 2008; **25**: 52–4.

32 Macris SG, Gregory GA, Way WL. Methylphenidate for hiccups. *Anesthesiology* 1971; **34**: 200–1.

33 Vasiloff N, Cohen DD, Dillon JB. Effective treatment of hiccup with intravenous methylphenidate. *Can Anaesth Soc J* 1965; **12**: 306–10.

34 Sohn YZ, Conrad LJ, Katz RL. Hiccup and ephedrine. *Can Anaesth Soc J* 1978; **25**: 431–2.

35 Shantha TR. Ketamine for the treatment of hiccups during and following anesthesia: a preliminary report. *Anesth Analg* 1973; **52**: 822–4.

36 Tavakoli M, Corssen G. Control of hiccups by ketamine: a preliminary report. *ALA J Med Sci* 1974; **11**: 229–30.

37 Teodorowicz J, Zimny M. The effect of ketamine in patients with refractory hiccup in the postoperative period. Preliminary report. *Anaesth Resusc Intensive Ther* 1975; **3**: 271–2.

38 Gilson I, Busalacchi M. Marijuana for intractable hiccups. *Lancet* 1998; **351**: 267.

39 Okuda Y, Kitajima T, Asai T. Use of a nerve stimulator for phrenic nerve block in treatment of hiccups. *Anesthesiology* 1998; **88**: 525–7.

CHAPTER 28

Dyspepsia and Indigestion

Neelendu Dey[1] and Kenneth McQuaid[2]

[1] University of California San Francisco, San Francisco, CA, USA
[2] University of California San Francisco *and* GI Section, San Francisco VA Medical Center, San Francisco, CA, USA

Summary

Dyspepsia is a symptom of postprandial distress, early satiation, or epigastric discomfort that is described by patients by various terms, including "indigestion." The etiology is suspected by the clinician to arise from the upper gastrointestinal tract, though additional etiologies must be considered. Most patients with these symptoms have functional dyspepsia. The most common organic etiologies include peptic ulcer, gastroesophageal reflux disease, and medication side effect. In patients less than 55 years of age who have no alarm features, the most cost-effective approach is an initial test-and-treat strategy for *H. pylori*, followed by empiric proton pump inhibitor therapy and, ultimately, EGD if symptoms persist.

Case

A 57-year-old man with a 1-year history of gout, hypertension, diabetes, and previous alcohol abuse presents with the complaint of "indigestion," describing frequent "fullness" after meals. He denies heartburn, epigastric burning or pain, nausea, vomiting, or weight loss. The primary-care physician obtained an *H. pylori* serology, which is negative, and prescribed once-daily proton pump inhibitor without benefit. What is the differential diagnosis? What is the next step in management?

Definition and Epidemiology

"Dyspepsia" is a medical term used by clinicians to refer to upper abdominal symptoms that patients may describe as "indigestion", "discomfort", "burning", "pain", "fullness", or "bloating". "Dyspepsia" has an extensive differential diagnosis and is not a diagnosis in and of itself (Table 28.1). A diagnosis of "functional dyspepsia" is made in patients with chronic dyspepsia who after evaluation (including endoscopy) have no evidence of structural disease. Although "indigestion" is synonymous with

Practical Gastroenterology and Hepatology: Esophagus and Stomach, 1st edition. Edited by Nicholas J. Talley, Kenneth R. DeVault and David E. Fleischer. © 2010 Blackwell Publishing Ltd.

dyspepsia, it is used informally by patients and in advertisements to refer to intermittent, self-limited postprandial upper abdominal symptoms, often caused by dietary excesses or alcohol.

An international committee of clinical investigators (Rome III Committee) defines dyspepsia as one of more of the following symptoms: postprandial distress, early satiation, or epigastric pain or burning. There is controversy as to whether heartburn (substernal burning) should be included as a dyspepsia symptom. The Rome III group recognizes that heartburn may coexist with dyspepsia but believes it should be considered a separate entity. In clinical practice, it is sometimes difficult to distinguish these symptoms.

Dyspepsia occurs in up to 30% of adults per year, although less than half seek medical evaluation. It accounts for 2–5% of primary care visits, up to 30% of gastroenterology referrals, and impacts significantly on quality of life, productivity, and health-care costs [1].

Definitions

• Dyspepsia: one or more upper abdominal symptoms described by patients as discomfort, burning, pain, postprandial fullness, indigestion, or bloating. Its definition has changed over time, and its connotations among clinicians are varied.

Table 28.1 Differential diagnosis.

Most common
  Functional dyspepsia
  Peptic ulcer disease (usually secondary to *H. pylori* and/or
    non-steroidal anti-inflammatory drugs)
  Gastroesophageal reflux disease
  Medication side effect

Less common
  Carbohydrate malabsorption (e.g., lactose intolerance, sorbitol in
    "sugar-free" foods)
  Malignancy: stomach, esophagus, pancreas, hepatobiliary
  Irritable bowel syndrome
  Gastroparesis (diabetes, vagotomy)
  Small bowel bacterial overgrowth (consider: diabetes, prior
    surgery)
  Biliary pain (cholelithiasis, cholecholithiasis)
  Chronic pancreatitis (especially if history of alcohol abuse)
  Chronic mesenteric ischemia
  Infection: viral, parasitic (*Giardia, Strongyloides, Anisakiasis*),
    bacterial (syphilis)
  Crohn disease
  Infiltrative disease (e.g., sarcoidosis)
  Metabolic disturbances (e.g., thyroid disease,
    hyperparathyroidism)
  Pregnancy

• The Rome III Committee definition of dyspepsia: the presence of bothersome postprandial fullness, early satiation, and/or epigastric pain or burning. These symptoms are suggestive of a gastroduodenal disorder.
• Rome III Committee definition of functional dyspepsia: at least 3 months of dyspepsia in the absence of any apparent organic, systemic, or metabolic disease likely to explain the symptoms.
• Epigastric pain syndrome: a subgroup of functional dyspepsia characterized by intermittent pain or burning of at least moderate severity that is localized to the epigastrium and is not be related to meals [2].
• Postprandial distress syndrome: a subgroup of functional dyspepsia characterized by frequent meal-induced symptoms defined as either (i) post-prandial fullness after ordinary-sized meals or (ii) early satiation that prevents finishing a regular meal [2].

Pathophysiology

Dyspepsia has a wide differential diagnosis, and the pathophysiology depends on the etiology. In one-third of

patients, symptoms can be attributed to an organic etiology such as gastroesophageal reflux (GERD), peptic ulcer disease (PUD; >90% caused by *H. pylori* and/or non-steroidal anti-inflammatory drugs (NSAIDs)), or gastric cancer. Most other patients have functional dyspepsia, an entity for which the pathophysiology is poorly understood.

A large overlap exists between functional dyspepsia and other functional gastrointestinal disorders such as irritable bowel syndrome (IBS). The pathophysiology of functional dyspepsia involves an interplay of psychosocial factors and abnormal gastrointestinal physiology along the "brain–gut axis." Identified pathophysiologic pathways include delayed gastric emptying, impaired fundic accommodation, myoelectric disturbance, and visceral hypersensitivity; however, no single pathway accounts for symptoms in all patients. Psychiatric diagnoses (predominantly anxiety disturbances) are more prevalent in patients with functional dyspepsia than with dyspepsia of organic origin [3].

Clinical Features

Patients describe dyspepsia symptoms using vague terms. It is important to elucidate the most bothersome symptom, its abdominal location, and whether it is induced by meals. Common symptoms include burning, pain, discomfort, postprandial distress, and early satiation. Dyspepsia is located in the epigastrium or upper abdomen and is mild-to-moderate in severity. The presence of predominant heartburn in conjunction with other dyspepsia symptoms strongly suggests GERD. Predominant symptoms of nausea, vomiting, belching, or bloating that is unrelated to meals are not consistent with dyspepsia. Severe upper abdominal pain suggests other ominous diagnoses such as perforated ulcer, acute pancreatitis, or acute hepatobiliary disorders.

Clinicians typically diagnose "dyspepsia" when they suspect an underlying gastroduodenal disorder. However, similar symptoms sometimes are caused by intestinal, pancreatic, and hepatobiliary disorders (Table 28.1). Small intestinal disorders (such as lactose intolerance, celiac disease, or *Giardia* infection) more commonly present with periumbilical cramps, bloating, and altered bowel habits. Biliary pain caused by cholelithiasis or choledocholithiasis is characterized by severe, episodic pain in the epigastrium or right upper quadrant that last one to several hours. Chronic pancreatitis is associated with moderate to severe epigastric or periumbilical pain lasting hours to weeks that may radiate to the back.

Suspicion for structural disorders (e.g., malignancy) causing dyspepsia is increased in patients who are older (greater than age 55), have a family history of upper gastrointestinal malignancy, or have other "alarm" features. These include dysphagia, persistent nausea and/or vomiting, weight loss, overt symptoms of gastrointestinal bleeding, or iron-deficiency anemia. Functional dyspepsia is suspected in patients with chronic symptoms (more than 6 months), especially if they are younger (less than age 55), have no "alarm" features, or have concomitant altered bowel habits suggestive of IBS. Major gastroenterology societies have published extensive guidelines on the diagnosis and treatment of dyspepsia [4,5]. A review of those approaches is presented in the following sections.

Diagnosis

Initial evaluation consists of a careful history and physical examination followed by supplemental testing or an initial course of empirical therapy. The nature, location, chronicity, and severity of the symptoms should be elucidated. Past medical history should document disorders that may affect gastrointestinal motility (diabetes, vagotomy) or cause malabsorption (chronic pancreatitis, celiac sprue). It is important to elicit medications that cause dyspepsia (Table 28.2), especially NSAIDs (an important cause of ulcer disease). Questioning should review dietary precipitants such as lactose, "sugar-free" products, caffeinated beverages, and alcohol ingestion. In patients with chronic symptoms, a preliminary psychosocial history should be obtained, including the reason for seeking medical evaluation at this time, current stressors, and childhood trauma.

If patients are *older than* 55 years of age or have alarm features, a diagnostic esophagogastroduodenoscopy (EGD) is warranted to exclude upper GI malignancy. Unfortunately, the sensitivity and specificity of alarm features for upper GI malignancy is limited (about 67%); however, their negative predictive value is high (99%) due in large part to the low prevalence of upper GI malignancy among young patients [6].

Table 28.2 Common culprit drugs.

NSAIDs

Anti-inflammatory/immunomodulators: prednisone, azathioprine, methotrexate

Minerals: potassium, iron

Oral antibiotics: penicillins, cephalosporins, macrolides

HIV protease inhibitors

Digoxin

Nitrates

Loop diuretics

Antihypertensive medications: ACE inhibitors, angiotensin-receptor blockers

Cholesterol-lowering agents: niacin, fibric acid derivatives (gemfibrozil, fenofibrate)

Narcotics

Colchicine

Estrogens: oral contraceptives, hormonal replacement

Parkinson drugs: levodopa, dopamine agonists, MAO B inhibitors

Diabetes medications: metformin, acarbose, exenatide

Neuropsychiatric medications: cholinesterase inhibitors (donepezil, rivastigmine); SSRIs (e.g., fluoxetine, sertraline); serotonin-norepinephrine-reuptake inhibitors (e.g., venlafaxine, duloxetine)

Alcohol

NSAID, non-steroidal anti-inflammatory drug; ACE, angiotensin-converting enzyme; MAO, monoamine oxidase; SSRI, selective serotonin reuptake inhibitor.

If no alarm features are present, the most cost-effective approach is a non-invasive test for *H. pylori* (urea breath test, fecal antigen test or, less preferred, IgG serology). Patients who are *H. pylori*-positive should be empirically treated with standard therapy whereas *H. pylori*-negative patients may be given an empiric proton pump inhibitor for 4–8 weeks. Patients whose symptoms persist after 1–3 months of empiric anti-*H. pylori* therapy and/or empiric proton pump inhibitor therapy should undergo EGD with gastric biopsy (to assess for *H. pylori*).

Further work-up is not recommended for most patients with chronic dyspepsia. Abdominal ultrasonography or CT imaging may be warranted for symptoms suggestive of pancreaticobiliary disorders. For presumed functional dyspepsia, testing for pathophysiologic disturbances with gastric emptying study, barostat, or electrogastrography is not recommended outside of tertiary centers.

Case continued

A careful medication and dietary history is obtained. He has been taking metformin for 1 year and recently started exenatide. He also consumes many "sugar-free" products containing sorbitol. Despite the absence of alarm features, EGD is performed because of the patient's age.

Treatment

Offending medicine or food should be eliminated. Dyspepsia secondary to other organic etiologies such as *H. pylori* , GERD, or PUD should be treated appropriately. Functional dyspepsia is best treated with a conservative approach. Initial management involves acknowledgement and validation of symptoms. A therapeutic alliance may be forged by reassurance, establishment of a treatment plan, and regular meetings. Auxiliary measures may include a diary (to document diet, stress, and activities) and psychology evaluation. Therapies such as meditation, yoga, or exercise are logical but are of unproven efficacy.

Medical therapy should be reserved for symptoms refractory to conservative measures. Systematic reviews document limited efficacy of pharmacotherapy in functional dyspepsia with a high placebo response rate. Safety and tolerability therefore should be the foremost concern. Eradication of *H. pylori* results in a small but significant relative risk reduction in functional dyspepsia (8%; number need to treat: 18). Therefore, testing (and treating) for *H. pylori* should be pursued, if not done previously. Patients with persistent symptoms after initial anti-*H. pylori* therapy should be tested after 4 weeks with a urea breath test or fecal antigen test to confirm eradication. Acid suppression is a safe first-line therapy that may be efficacious, particularly in those with epigastric pain or burning. Proton pump inhibitors appear to have modest superiority compared to placebo, although study results are heterogeneous. Proton pump inhibitors lead to a 14% risk reduction in functional dyspepsia with an estimated number needed to treat of 7–9. Other therapies, such as antidepressants and psychotherapy, appear promising but their value is not well established. The prokinetic agents cisapride and domperidone appeared

effective in studies of low methodologic quality. Cisapride was withdrawn from the market; however, domperidone is available in many countries worldwide. Metoclopramide is widely available and may be effective for short-term use; chronic therapy is not recommended due to risk of neuropsychiatric side effects, especially in older patients [7].

Case continued

An EGD is normal. The patient is reassured and advised to avoid "sugar-free" foods. He is given a trial of exenatide with rapid improvement in symptoms.

Take-home points

- Dyspepsia is a symptom of postprandial distress, early satiation, or epigastric pain that is referred to by patients by various terms, including "indigestion."

- The majority of patients with these symptoms have functional dyspepsia.

- The most common organic etiologies include peptic ulcer (*H. pylori*-related or NSAID-related), GERD, *H. pylori*-related gastritis, and medication side effect.

- A diagnostic EGD is warranted in patients ≥55 years or who have alarm features.

- In young patients (<55 years) without alarm features, the most cost-effective approach is an test-and-treat strategy for *H. pylori*, followed by empiric proton pump inhibitor therapy, if needed. Patients with persistent symptoms after 4–8 weeks of empirical treatment should undergo EGD. Further work-up is not advised in most patients with presumed functional dyspepsia.

- The initial management of functional dyspepsia should involve acknowledgement and validation of symptoms followed by reassurance.

- The efficacy of medical therapy for functional dyspepsia is limited. Acid suppression is a safe first-line measure.

References

1 El-Serag HB, Talley NJ. Systemic review: the prevalence and clinical course of functional dyspepsia. *Aliment Pharm Therap* 2004; **19**: 643–54.

2 Geeraerts B, Tack J. Functional dyspepsia: past, present, and future. *J Gastroenterol* 2008; **43**: 251–5.

3 Tack J, Talley NJ, Camilleri M, *et al.* Functional gastroduodenal disorders. *Gastroenterology* 2006; **130**: 1466–79.

4 Talley NJ, Vakil NB, Moayyedi P. American Gastroenterological Association technical review on the evaluation of dyspepsia. *Gastroenterology* 2005; **129**: 1756–80.

5 Talley NJ, Vakil N. Practice Parameters Committee of the American College of Gastroenterology. *Am J Gastroenterol* 2005; **100**: 2324–37.

6 Vakil N, Moayyedi P, Fennerty MB, Talley NJ. Limited value of alarm features in the diagnosis of upper gastrointestinal malignancy: systematic review and meta-analysis. *Gastroenterology* 2006; **131**: 390–401.

7 Moayyedi P, Soo S, Deeks J, *et al.* Pharmacological interventions for non-ulcer dyspepsia. *Cochrane Database Syst Rev* 2006; **4**: CD001960.

29

CHAPTER 29
Nausea and Vomiting

John K. DiBaise

Divisions of Gastroenterology and Hepatology, Mayo Clinic, Scottsdale, AZ, USA

Summary

Nausea and vomiting are common, frequently distressing and occasionally disabling symptoms that can occur due to a variety of causes. Although a diagnosis is possible in most cases of acute nausea and vomiting after completing a thorough history and examination, for those whose symptoms persist or are chronic and the diagnosis remains uncertain, further testing guided by the clinical presentation is generally indicated. Additional testing may include laboratory studies, radiologic and endoscopic imaging studies, and, occasionally, an assessment of gastrointestinal motor activity. The standard approach to the management of nausea and vomiting includes correction of fluid, electrolyte, and nutritional deficiencies, treatment of the underlying cause if known, and suppression of the symptoms using dietary, pharmacological, and, sometimes, surgical interventions. Importantly, correction of clinical consequences of vomiting such as dehydration, electrolyte abnormalities, and malnutrition, and suppression of symptoms should be initiated either before or concurrently with the diagnostic evaluation.

Case

A 27-year-old man presented for evaluation of gastroparesis. He had been previously healthy until approximately 3 months ago when he developed an insidious onset of nausea and vomiting. His prior evaluation, consisting of routine laboratory studies, abdominal ultrasound, and cholecystokinin-cholescintigraphy, was normal, leading to the eventual performance of a gastric emptying test that demonstrated delayed emptying of a solid meal. A trial of metoclopramide and promethazine did not result in improvement of his symptoms. Presently, he has constant nausea, feels full with eating small portions, and about every other day will vomit items he had eaten several hours previously. He denies abdominal pain, but has noticed a decrease in appetite, frequent pyrosis, and a slight increase in frequency of his bowel movements. He has lost about 15 kg. Physical examination revealed an overweight young man but was otherwise unremarkable.

Definition and Epidemiology

Nausea and vomiting are common, frequently distressing, and occasionally disabling symptoms that can occur due to a variety of causes. Nausea is the painless, unpleasant, subjective feeling of an impending need to vomit. In contrast, vomiting is the rapid, forceful expulsion of upper gastrointestinal contents from the mouth. Nausea is frequently not followed by vomiting; however, vomiting is usually preceded by nausea. Retching refers to the repetitive contractions of the abdominal musculature and labored, rhythmic respirations that usually precede vomiting but may also occur without subsequent vomiting (i.e., 'dry heaves'). Vomiting must be differentiated from regurgitation, which describes the effortless flow of gastroesophageal contents into the mouth, and rumination, whereby an effortless regurgitation of recently ingested food into the mouth occurs, followed by rechewing and reswallowing or spitting out. Both regurgitation and rumination are usually not preceded by nausea or, by definition, retching.

While difficult to accurately assess the economic burden related to nausea and vomiting, when

Practical Gastroenterology and Hepatology: Esophagus and Stomach, 1st edition. Edited by Nicholas J. Talley, Kenneth R. DeVault and David E. Fleischer. © 2010 Blackwell Publishing Ltd.

considering only the more common causes of acute nausea and vomiting such as acute gastroenteritis, postoperative, pregnancy and chemotherapy, it is apparent that the socioeconomic burden to affected patients and society (i.e., employers, health-care industry) is significant, related at least in part to restricted activities and social functioning, lost work productivity, increased length of hospitalization, and home nursing support [1].

Pathophysiology

Much is known about the pathophysiology of vomiting due to its stereotypical behavior and relative ease of study using experimental models. In contrast, much less is known about nausea as it cannot be readily studied in animals. During the retching phase of vomiting, diaphragmatic, respiratory, and abdominal muscles simultaneously contract or relax and the glottis closes. With expulsion, prolonged contraction of several groups of muscles including the abdominal, intercostal, and laryngeal and pharyngeal muscles occurs in the absence of diaphragmatic contraction and the glottis opens. Heart and respiratory rates increase, sweating occurs, giant retrograde contractions develop in the small bowel, and both the gastric fundus and lower esophageal sphincter relax. Thus, it is important to realize that expulsion results not from a primary change in gut function but instead occurs because of changes in intra-abdominal and intrathoracic pressure generated by the muscles of respiration.

Coordination of this combination of events takes place at the level of the medulla oblongata [2]. The major components of this neural circuitry include the area postrema in the floor of the fourth ventricle, which lies outside the blood–brain barrier and contains a "chemoreceptor trigger zone" that detects emetic agents in the blood and cerebrospinal fluid and transmits this information to the nucleus tractus solitarius (NTS). Vagal afferent nerves from the gut that detect noxious luminal contents and changes in tone also terminate in the NTS. Neurons from the NTS project to a central pattern generator which then coordinates the previously described behaviors by projecting information to the various nuclei involved. The neurotransmitters involved in these processes are incompletely understood. Importantly, this central pattern generator is not a discrete site (i.e., "vom-

iting center") but instead consists of groups of loosely organized neurons throughout the medulla that must be activated in the appropriate sequence.

Clinical Features

A thorough history detailing the temporal features of the nausea and vomiting, the presence of associated symptoms and the characteristics of the emesis along with a careful physical examination are crucial elements in determining the cause and consequences of nausea and vomiting [3]. Determining whether the symptoms are acute or chronic is the first step. Most episodes of acute nausea and vomiting have a recognized primary cause and resolve spontaneously or can be readily resolved. In contrast, chronic nausea and vomiting, defined as the persistence of nausea and vomiting for over a month, frequently presents more of a clinical challenge because of an inability to identify the underlying cause or adequately control the symptoms. Table 29.1 lists some clinical features that may help in the identification of the diagnosis.

Table 29.1 Clinical features that may aid in the diagnosis of nausea and vomiting.

Clinical feature	Examples
Associated symptom(s)	
Abdominal pain	Pancreatitis, intestinal obstruction
Altered menses	Pregnancy
Chest pain	Myocardial infarction
Depression, anxiety	Psychiatric cause
Diarrhea, fever	Gastroenteritis
Headache, neck stiffness, altered mental status, focal neurological signs	Brain tumor, meningitis
Tinnitus, vertigo	Meniere disease
Weight loss	Neoplasm
Characteristics of the emesis	
Bloody or coffee-ground	Ulcer, Mallory–Weiss tear
Bilious	Obstruction distal to major papilla
Continuous	Conversion disorder
Episodic	Cyclic vomiting syndrome
Feculent	Intestinal obstruction
Food eaten >1 hour previously	Gastroparesis
Food eaten <1 hour previously	Bulimia/rumination
Morning vomiting	Pregnancy
Projectile	Gastric outlet obstruction

Findings on physical examination that may both aid in the diagnosis and assess consequences of nausea and vomiting include resting tachycardia, orthostasis, poor skin turgor, and dry mucus membranes which suggest the presence of significant dehydration. A general examination may detect changes associated with systemic conditions like scleroderma, Addison disease and hypo- or hyperthyroid disease. Lanugo-like hair, parotid gland enlargement, loss of dental enamel, and calluses on the dorsal aspect of the hand are associated with eating disorders. The presence of generalized lymphadenopathy, occult blood in the stool and cachexia raise the possibility of an underlying neoplasm. Jaundice, conjunctival icterus and/or hepatomegaly suggest the presence of benign or malignant hepatic disease. Focal neurologic signs, papilledema, nystagmus, nuchal rigidity, altered mentation, abnormal deep tendon reflexes, and the presence of asterixis suggest central, labyrinthine, infectious, or metabolic origins of nausea and vomiting. The abdominal examination is of particular importance in the evaluation of nausea and vomiting. Hypo- or hyperactive bowel sounds suggest the presence of an ileus or bowel obstruction, respectively. Abdominal distension also raises the possibility of bowel obstruction. A succussion splash may be present in gastric outlet obstruction or gastroparesis. Abdominal tenderness or peritoneal signs suggest the presence of an intra-abdominal inflammatory or infectious process. An abdominal mass may reflect either a benign or malignant process.

Diagnosis

Although a diagnosis is possible in most cases of acute nausea and vomiting after completing a thorough history and examination, for those whose symptoms persist or are chronic and the diagnosis remains uncertain, further testing guided by the clinical presentation is generally indicated (Figure 29.1). Additional testing may include laboratory studies, radiologic and endoscopic imaging studies, and, occasionally, an assessment of gastrointestinal motor activity. Unfortunately, no controlled trials exist to guide this diagnostic evaluation; therefore, recommendations are typically based upon expert consensus and opinion [3]. Importantly, correction of clinical consequences of vomiting such as dehydration, electrolyte abnormalities, and malnutrition, and suppression of

symptoms using empiric antiemetic and/or prokinetic treatment should be initiated either before or concurrently with the diagnostic evaluation.

Laboratory Testing

As most cases of acute nausea and vomiting are self-limited, testing may not be needed. In cases where the symptoms are more significant or particularly concerning signs or symptoms or potential complications are present, initial laboratory studies may include electrolytes, renal function, glucose, hemogram, liver tests, and pancreatic enzymes. Pregnancy testing should be performed in women of childbearing potential when symptoms persist or imaging studies are being considered. When the symptoms are more persistent or become chronic, additional blood tests to consider include thyroid studies, cortisol level, C-reactive protein or erythrocyte sedimentation rate, and celiac disease antibodies. Serum drug levels should be considered in individuals taking drugs such as digoxin and theophylline. Additional serologic testing may be indicated when the initial tests are abnormal or the history is suggestive.

Radiologic and Endoscopic Imaging

When the diagnosis remains unclear, an evaluation of the gastrointestinal tract by radiologic and endoscopic means should be considered. While recognizing that they are imperfect in terms of both sensitivity and specificity, due to their ease and cost, supine and upright plain films of the abdomen should be considered initially to exclude intestinal obstruction. If inconclusive for small bowel obstruction and clinical suspicion persists, further evaluation using barium contrast small bowel series or a more detailed enteroclysis should be considered, although in the present day, computerized tomography (CT) enterography seems to be replacing barium studies as the preferred modality [4]. CT enterography has the advantage of not only providing images of the small bowel lumen but also images the small bowel wall, other structures within the abdomen and retroperitoneum, and allows for a determination of the patency of the mesenteric vessels. Magnetic resonance (MR) enterography has similar capabilities and has the advantage of no radiation exposure but is more costly than CT and oftentimes provides a claustrophobic experience for the patient [5]. Ultrasonography is another method to image the gall bladder and hepatobiliary system without the need for radiation

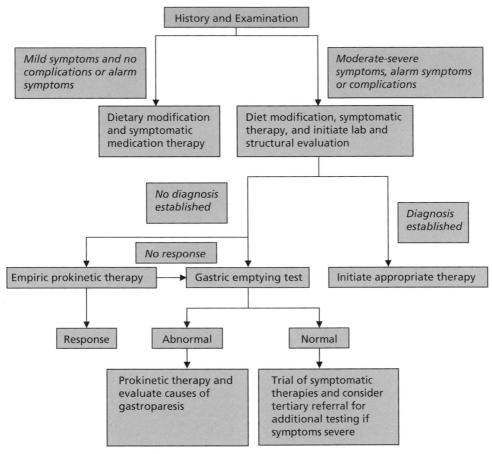

Figure 29.1 Management algorithm. (Adapted from Hasler and Chey [13], with permission from Elsevier.)

but tends to be less useful for visualizing the pancreas and is more operator-dependent. CT or MR imaging of the brain may be indicated in those with severe, unexplained nausea and vomiting but is generally most useful when a headache or neurologic signs are present. Although more costly and with increased risk, esophagogastroduodenoscopy is more useful than a barium contrast study of the upper gut for detecting mucosal lesions and allows for mucosal biopsies to be taken and treatment of gastric outlet obstruction when present. If colonic obstruction is suspected, a contrast enema, typically using gastrograffin, or CT imaging should be performed before considering colonoscopy.

Gastrointestinal Motility Testing

Routine laboratory testing and radiologic and endoscopic imaging studies are often normal in individuals with chronic nausea and vomiting. In this setting, testing of gastrointestinal motility may be appropriate. The most common test used to screen for gastric motor dysfunction measures the rate of gastric emptying following the ingestion of a standardized meal. In the United States, this is most commonly accomplished clinically using a meal labeled with a radionuclide; however, gastric emptying can also be measured using ultrasonography, MR imaging and a stable-isotope breath test, which while benefiting from a lack of need for radiation, suffer from limitations related to availability, operator-dependence, meal content, and cost [6]. Unfortunately, regardless of the method used, inconsistencies in test methodologies and generally poor correlation between the test results and the clinical response to prokinetic medications has led to frustration over the clinical utility of this test. Furthermore, an abnormal test does not prove that the symptoms are caused by abnormal gastric emptying. As a consequence, empiric treatment with a course of a prokinetic and/or an antiemetic may be worthwhile before ordering a test of gastric emptying.

Other tests that have been advocated as alternatives or complementary to the gastric emptying test include electrogastrography (EGG) and gastroduodenal or small bowel manometry. EGG uses cutaneous electrodes to record the gastric slow wave activity while manometry involves the direct recording of intraluminal pressure activity via a catheter incorporating pressure sensors positioned in the distal stomach, duodenum, and/or jejunum. Unfortunately, similar problems exist regarding the clinical relevance of the test results and they are further limited by general lack of availability and expertise in their interpretation [6]. Therefore, the place of these tests in the evaluation of the individual with chronic unexplained nausea and vomiting remains poorly defined [3].

Psychological Assessment

An evaluation of psychological causes should be considered in those individuals with chronic unexplained nausea and vomiting after common organic causes and gut dysmotility have been excluded.

Differential Diagnosis

A diverse array of disorders can produce acute or chronic nausea with or without vomiting (Table 29.2). In the acute setting, these symptoms most often arise to protect the individual from toxic insults. A pathophysiological explanation is usually less clear in the setting of chronic nausea and vomiting but most certainly depends upon the underlying etiology.

Therapeutics

The standard approach to the management of nausea and vomiting as illustrated in Figure 29.1 is three-fold [3]: (i) correction or fluid, electrolyte and nutritional deficiencies; (ii) treatment of the underlying cause if known; and (iii) suppression of the symptoms using dietary, pharmacological, and, sometimes, surgical interventions.

Table 29.2 Acute and chronic causes of nausea and vomiting.

Medications
  Antiarrhythmics, antibiotics, anticonvulsants, antiparkinsonian drugs, cancer chemotherapy, digoxin, exenatide, hypervitaminosis A, lubiprostone, metformin, narcotics, nicotine patch, non-steroidal anti-inflammatory drugs, sulfasalazine, theophylline

Drugs
  Alcohol, marijuana (cannabinoid-hyperemesis syndrome), opiates

Toxin exposures
  Arsenic poisoning, food poisoning, heavy metals

Radiation therapy

Infections
  Gastrointestinal, non-gastrointestinal

Organic gastrointestinal conditions
  Celiac disease, cholecystitis, cholelithiasis, Crohn disease, eosinophilic gastroenteritis, food allergy, gastroesophageal reflux disease, hepatitis, hepatic failure, mechanical bowel obstruction, mesenteric ischemia, pancreatic cancer, pancreatitis, peptic ulcer disease, postoperative

Functional gastrointestinal conditions
  Chronic intestinal pseudo-obstruction, cyclic vomiting syndrome, functional dyspepsia, chronic idiopathic nausea, functional vomiting, gastroparesis

Non-gastrointestinal conditions
  Addison disease, angioedema, acute intermittent porphyria, brain tumor, congestive heart failure, diabetic ketoacidosis, hypercalcemia, hyper/hypothyroidism, increased intracranial pressure, Meniere disease, migraine, motion sickness, myocardial infarction, nephrolithiasis, occult malignancy, pregnancy, severe pain, uremia

Psychiatric conditions
  Anxiety, conversion disorder, depression, eating disorder, panic disorder

In the acute setting, once medical and surgical emergencies have been excluded and the individual assessed for complications of nausea and vomiting (e.g., dehydration, malnutrition), a decision needs to be made whether hospitalization is needed. Fortunately, most cases are self-limited and not severe enough to require hospitalization; however, hospitalization should be considered in cases of severe dehydration or electrolyte abnormalities, when age or medical comorbidities increase the likelihood of complications, and when outpatient management has failed. Rehydration with oral fluids is generally sufficient for most cases of acute nausea and vomiting along with short-term antiemetic therapy generally administered orally or rectally and plans for follow-up if symptoms worsen or do not improve.

Dietary Modification

The treatment of chronic nausea and vomiting, while similar tends to be more challenging particularly when a specific cause has not been identified—an all-too-common situation. Furthermore, nutritional problems tend to be more of an issue than in the acute setting. Because of the limitations of pharmacological therapies in this situation, dietary modification tends to play a more important role in terms of not only nutritional replenishment but also symptom relief. Ingestion of a liquid diet when symptoms are most severe with gradual advancement to a more solid diet when symptoms lessen is generally recommended [7]. Other commonly utilized strategies include the ingestion of small portion meals and a restriction of fat and fiber intake. The use of oral nutritional supplements is often recommended and, when nutrition is severely compromised and symptoms persistent, enteral or parenteral nutrition support may be needed.

Pharmacological Options

Acute and chronic nausea and vomiting is often relieved, at least partially, with the use of antiemetic and prokinetic medications; however, there are no controlled trials of therapies outside the setting of surgery, chemotherapy and radiation therapy supporting any specific medical therapy and the issue of which drug is preferable in which patients remains poorly defined. Antiemetics suppress nausea and vomiting through actions primarily within the central nervous system, although newer agents appear to work at least in part to block receptors in the peripheral endings of vagal afferents [2]. Prokinetics act peripherally to alter gastrointestinal motor function primarily via cholinergic agonism, motilin agonism, and/or dopamine antagonism [7]. There are a number of classes of antiemetic agents (Table 29.3) and side effects tend to vary based on the class. Antiemetics are available in a variety of formulations (e.g., oral, rectal, parenteral) and may be used in combination. Prokinetic agents are typically used when gastrointestinal dysmotility is suspected or proven. Unfortunately, the few agents that are currently readily available in the United States (e.g., metoclopramide, erythromycin) are limited by side effects,

Table 29.3 Classes of antiemetic agents.

Class	Examples
Anticholinergic	Scopolamine
Antihistamine	Meclizine, hydroxyzine
Phenothiazine	Prochlorperazine, promethazine
Benzamide	Trimethobenzamide, metoclopramide
Butyrophenone	Droperidol
Serotonin (5-HT$_3$) antagonist	Ondansetron, granisetron
Neurokinin-1 antagonist	Aprepitant
Corticosteroid	Dexamethasone
Benzodiazepine	Lorazepam, diazepam
Cannabinoid	Dronabinol

modest efficacy, and tolerance to long-term use. Combination antiemetic and prokinetic therapy is often used with variable success to manage chronic nausea and vomiting related to gut dysmotility syndromes.

Low-dose tricyclic antidepressants (e.g., amitriptyline, nortriptyline, doxepin) at a median dose of about 50 mg/day for 3 to 6 months appear to be used fairly commonly in clinical practice to treat chronic nausea and vomiting, usually of a functional etiology based mostly on small, uncontrolled trials [8]. Antimigraine drugs, including tricyclic antidepressants, are commonly used to prevent attacks of cyclic vomiting syndrome, while antiseizure medications have recently also been suggested to be useful [9].

Surgical Options

While infrequently utilized, surgical treatments may be helpful and/or necessary in both acute and chronic nausea and vomiting. Those with chronic severe nausea and vomiting, particularly those with severe gastroparesis, may benefit from a gastrostomy and/or jejunostomy tube for the purpose of supplementing oral nutrition, decompressing the gut, or both [10]. Completion gastrectomy may be worthwhile in the patient with severe postsurgical gastroparesis [11]. High-frequency gastric electrical stimulation via serosally implanted electrodes is a new therapeutic approach for patients with medically-refractory gastroparesis and a recent report suggests it may be effective for treating chronic severe nausea and vomiting regardless of whether gastric emptying is delayed or not [7,12].

Psychological, Behavioral, and Integrative Options

Integrative management approaches such as ginger, pyridoxine, hypnotherapy, and acupuncture/acupressure have been suggested to be useful. Psychological therapies, biofeedback therapy, and relaxation techniques may also be of benefit to some individuals.

Case continued

On the basis of the patient's lack of previous medical problems and the diversity of his gastrointestinal symptoms, celiac disease was suspected and, indeed, IgA tissue transglutaminase antibodies were highly positive as were antiendomysial antibodies. Subsequent esophagogastroduodenoscopy (EGD) confirmed the diagnosis, demonstrating scalloping of the duodenal folds with marked villous atrophy histologically. Los Angeles classification Grade B esophagitis was also noted. Treatment with a gluten-free diet and daily proton pump inhibitor was initiated and led to a near complete resolution of his symptoms and an improvement in his weight when seen in follow-up.

Take-home points

- A wide variety of disorders can produce acute or chronic nausea with or without vomiting. Most cases of nausea and vomiting are self-limited with infectious gastroenteritis and food poisoning accounting for the majority.

- In most cases of nausea and vomiting, a diagnosis is possible following the completion of a thorough history and a careful physical examination and additional testing is not needed. Pregnancy should always be considered in women of childbearing age.

- For those whose symptoms are severe, associated with complications or are chronic and the diagnosis remains uncertain, further testing guided by the clinical presentation is generally indicated to enable a diagnosis and allow targeted treatment. Additional testing may include laboratory studies, a structural evaluation of the gastrointestinal tract, and, occasionally, an assessment of gastrointestinal motor activity.

- Correction of clinical consequences of vomiting such as dehydration, electrolyte abnormalities, and malnutrition, and suppression of symptoms using empiric antiemetic and/or prokinetic treatment should generally be initiated either before or concurrently with the diagnostic evaluation.

- Hospitalization should be considered when severe dehydration, electrolyte abnormalities, or malnutrition are present, when age or medical comorbidities increase the likelihood of complications, and when outpatient management has failed.

- The standard approach to managing nausea and vomiting includes correction of fluid, electrolyte and nutritional deficiencies, treatment of the underlying cause if known, and suppression of the symptoms using dietary, pharmacological, and, sometimes, surgical interventions.

References

1 Sandler RS, Everhart JE, Donowitz M, *et al.* The burden of selected digestive diseases in the United States. *Gastroenterology* 2002; **122**: 1500–11.

2 Hornby PJ. Central neurocircuitry associated with emesis. *Am J Med* 2001; **111**: 106S–12S.

3 Quigley EMM, Hasler WL, Parkman HP. AGA technical review on nausea and vomiting. *Gastroenterology* 2001; **120**: 263–86.

4 Fletcher JG, Huprich J, Loftus Jr EV, *et al.* Computerized tomography enterography and its role in small-bowel imaging. *Clin Gastroenterol Hepatol* 2008; **6**: 283–9.

5 Gonçalves Neto JA, Elazzazi M, Altun E, Semelka RC. When should abdominal magnetic resonance imaging be used? *Clin Gastroenterol Hepatol* 2008; **6**: 610–15.

6 Camilleri M, Hasler WL, Parkman HP, *et al.* Measurement of gastroduodenal motility in the GI laboratory. *Gastroenterology* 1998; **115**: 747–62.

7 Abell TL, Bernstein RK, Cutts T, *et al.* Treatment of gastroparesis: a multidisciplinary clinical review. *Neurogastroenterol Motil* 2006; **18**: 263–83.

8 Prakash C, Lustman PJ, Freedland KE, Clouse RE. Tricyclic antidepressants for functional nausea and vomiting: clinical outcome in 37 patients. *Dig Dis Sci* 1998; **43**: 1951–6.

9 Clouse RE, Sayuk GS, Lustman PJ, Prakash C. Zonisamide or levetiracetam for adults with cyclic vomiting syndrome: a case series. *Clin Gastroenterol Hepatol* 2007; **5**: 44–8.

10 DiBaise JK, Decker GA. Enteral access options and management in the patient with intestinal failure. *J Clin Gastroenterol* 2007; **41**: 647–56.

11 Jones MP, Maganti K. A systematic review of surgical therapy for gastroparesis. *Am J Gastroenterol* 2003; **98**: 2122–9.

12 Gourcerol G, Leblanc I, Leroi AM, *et al.* Gastric electrical stimulation in medically refractory nausea and vomiting. *Eur J Gastroenterol Hepatol* 2007; **19**: 29–35.

13 Hasler WL, Chey WD. Nausea and Vomiting. *Gastroenterology* 2003; **125**: 1860–7.

CHAPTER 30

Hematemesis

Thomas O.G. Kovacs and Dennis M. Jensen

Department of Medicine, David Geffen School of Medicine at UCLA, Los Angeles, CA, USA

Summary

The initial approach to the patient with hematemesis should combine an evaluation of the severity of upper gastrointestinal (UGI) hemorrhage, based on a focused history and physical examination, with prompt and vigorous resuscitation. An early decision should be made on whether hospitalization is required and intensive care unit (ICU) admission indicated. All patients with acute severe UGI bleeding should be admitted to an ICU or monitored bed, because, in almost all hospitals, the major causes of morbidity and mortality, such as continued bleeding, associated illness, or postoperative complications, are better managed on an ICU than on a regular ward. Medical therapy with an intravenous proton pump inhibitor (PPI) should be initiated before endoscopy in patients with suspected ulcers. In cirrhotic patients with UGI hemorrhage, intravenous octreotide is recommended if variceal bleeding is suspected, and prophylactic antibiotics administered for 7 days. After resuscitation and initiation of medical therapy, urgent endoscopy is recommended for diagnosis and treatment.

Case

A 81-year-old man is brought to the emergency room from a nursing home. An aide states that the patient "coughed up" some maroon-colored blood and then passed out "for awhile." The nurse on duty reports that the patient has been in the facility for rehabilitation for a broken hip and that he has a complex history. He had an ulcer operation 40 years ago and "part of his stomach was removed." He also had an aortic aneurysm and they had to operate for that about 10 years ago.

He has bad arthritis and takes ibuprofen each day for that. When he was hospitalized for the broken hip he had a "blood clot" and has been on coumadin. He was supposed to have his INR checked last week but he refused the blood draw because he had "too many bruises already." He was never a drinker but had gotten hepatitis from the blood transfusion for the ulcer and the doctors told him that he had cirrhosis. He noticed recently that his legs and belly got "swelled up."

In the emergency room, his BP is 100/78 mmHg lying and 82/60 mmHg sitting. His corresponding pulse is 100 and 110 beats/min. His oxygen saturation is 88%. An ECG shows a right bundle-branch block. He responds to questions appropriately and complains of a headache. His hemoglobin is 7.2 g/dL and hematocrit 26%; at the time of hip surgery they were 11.4 g/dL and 34%, respectively. His INR is 4.5. He refuses to have a nasogastric tube placed. Two large-bore intravenous cannulae have been placed and a blood transfusion is ordered. He is started on an intravenous proton pump inhibitor and intravenous octreotide. The gastroenterology doctor on call is notified and he orders him admitted to the ICU. He also asks that intravenous erythromycin be given in anticipation of an esophagogastroduodenoscopy (EGD) when he is stabilized. The gastroenterologist tells the patient's primary care doctor that the differential diagnosis is broad but includes variceal bleeding, a Mallory–Weiss tear, a bleeding ulcer, and an aortoenteric fistula, and that the prolonged prothrombin time is making the bleeding worse.

Introduction

Upper gastrointestinal (UGI) bleeding, which is defined as hemorrhage proximal to the ligament of Treitz, occurs frequently and is a common cause of hospitalization or inpatient bleeding, resulting in substantial patient morbidity, mortality, and medical care expense [1–4]. Hematemesis, which consists of vomiting either

Practical Gastroenterology and Hepatology: Esophagus and Stomach, 1st edition. Edited by Nicholas J. Talley, Kenneth R. DeVault and David E. Fleischer. © 2010 Blackwell Publishing Ltd.

Table 30.1 causes of hematemesis and prevalence of causes of upper gastrointestinal (UGI) hemorrhage.

Etiology	CURE data (%) [3]	Others [11] (%)
Peptic ulcer disease	45	35–50
Varices (esophageal or gastric)	15	10–15
Gastric or duodenal erosions	10	5–15
Angioectasias	7	5–10 (including gastric antral vascular ectasia— watermelon stomach)
Mallory–Weiss tear	7	5–10
Esophagitis	5	3–7
Upper gastrointestinal tumor	5	2–5
Portal hypertension gastropathy	2	1–3
Large hiatus hernia—Cameron lesions	2	1–2
Dieulafoy lesion	2	0.5–1
Aortoenteric fistula	<1	<1

bright-red blood, suggestive of recent and/or continued hemorrhage, or darker, "coffee-ground" liquid, suggestive of older or quiescent bleeding, is one of the most common manifestations of acute UGI hemorrhage. About 40–50% of cases of UGI bleeding are caused by peptic ulcer disease (duodenal, gastric, and marginal) [3]. Variceal hemorrhage occurs in 14–20% [3]. Other, less common but important potential etiologies are listed in Table 30.1.

Initial Approach to the Patient

The initial approach to the patient with UGI bleeding includes evaluation of severity of the hemorrhage, patient resuscitation, a medical history and physical examination, and consideration of possible interventions. The initial clinical assessment should focus on the patient's hemodynamic state, which has a higher initial priority than other considerations including localization of the bleeding source. Patient resuscitation should begin early. Important determinants of resuscitation include adequate intravenous (IV) access, accurate assessment of blood loss, and appropriate fluid and blood product infusion [1]. The initial aim of therapy is to restore blood volume through fluid replacement to ensure that tissue perfusion and oxygen delivery are not compromised.

Large-bore (14–18 gauge) intravenous catheters are recommended to infuse physiological or 0.9% saline and maintain systolic blood pressure >100 mmHg and pulse <100 beats/min. Packed red blood cell transfusions are given to maintain the hematocrit >24–30%, depending on the patient's age and comorbidities. Supplemental oxygen provides adequate oxygen-carrying capacity in elderly people or those with associated cardiopulmonary conditions.

Airway protection is also important, especially with severe UGI hemorrhage. Endotracheal intubation should be strongly considered in patients with ongoing hematemesis or altered mental status, to prevent aspiration and to prepare for emergency endoscopy. Aspiration is a common cause of endoscopy-associated hypoxia and a leading cause of the morbidity and mortality related to severe UGI bleeding, especially in patients with cirrhosis. For example, in a non-randomized study, respiratory complications occurred in 22% of patients with severe acute UGI bleeding. Risk factors for respiratory complications included advanced liver disease, esophageal bleeding, and age >70 years. Patients with respiratory complications had a much higher mortality rate than patients without these complications (70% vs 4%) [3].

If present, an associated coagulopathy should be corrected with a fresh frozen plasma (FFP) infusion to lower a prolonged prothrombin time to <15 s (or reduce an elevated international normalized ratio [INR] to <1.5), and, with platelet transfusion, to provide a platelet count >50 000/mm³.

History

In a patient with acute UGI bleeding, the initial history should be brief and focused on determining the symptoms of severity and the potential etiologies of the hemorrhage. Recurrent or ongoing hematemesis, melena or hematochezia, syncope, dizziness, and chest pain are all markers of severity and acuity. Essential history includes prior episodes of UGI bleeding and their cause, past history of chronic liver disease or peptic ulcer, and use of aspirin, nonsteroidal antiinflammatory drugs (NSAIDs), or anticoagulants such as warfarin or clopidogrel. The presence of symptoms of gastroesophageal reflux disease, prior vomiting or retching, past UGI surgery, and past abdominal aortic aneurysm repair should also be quickly determined.

Physical Examination

In a patient with acute UGI bleeding, the patient's pulse, blood pressure, and orthostatic changes may help determine the degree of hypovolemia and guide resuscitation. Resting tachycardia (pulse ≥100 beats/min) suggests mild-to-moderate hypovolemia, whereas hypotension (systolic blood pressure <100 mmHg) represents an approximate 40% loss of blood volume. Orthostatic hypotension (pulse increase of ≥20 beats/min or decrease in systolic pressure ≥20 mmHg on standing) suggests a ≥15% loss of blood volume [6]. Other important physical findings include abdominal surgical scars, tenderness or a mass, or features of chronic liver disease, especially those associated with portal hypertension such as ascites, splenomegaly, and ecchymoses or petechiae.

Laboratory Studies

Important laboratory studies should include complete blood count (CBC) with platelet count, coagulation profiles, and serum chemistry, especially blood urea nitrogen (BUN), creatinine, and liver function tests. Patients with acute UGI bleeding will usually have an elevated BUN level secondary to an increased intestinal absorption of degraded blood urea and hypovolemia leading to prerenal azotemia. An elevated BUN/creatinine ratio >20:1 suggests a UGI rather than a lower GI source for the bleed. Blood should also be sent for type and crossmatch for packed red blood cells and other blood products (platelets or FFP), if these are low.

Nasogastric Aspiration

Nasogastric (NG) or orogastric tube placement for aspiration and lavage may be useful to detect the presence of intragastric blood, either large-volume red blood or coffee grounds, to empty the stomach before endoscopy, and to lessen the likelihood of aspiration. The finding of a bloody NG aspirate predicted high-risk endoscopic stigmata in a study of patients with acute UGI bleeding [7]. However, in this same study, the NG aspirate was most useful in hemodynamically stable patients without hematemesis, but with either melena or hematochezia. High-risk endoscopic findings occurred in about 15% of patients without coffee grounds or blood in their NG aspirates [7].

A bilious, nonbloody, NG aspirate in a patient with GI bleeding implies that the bleeding is distal to the ligament of Treitz or stopped several hours previously. There is no role for guaiac testing of NG tube aspirates for the presence of occult blood because NG tube insertion is likely to produce trauma with minor bleeding and a false-positive result. Patients with witnessed hematemesis do not need NG tube placement for diagnostic evaluation. Further, there is no therapeutic value in iced saline lavage. If lavage is performed, lukewarm water is just as effective and cheaper than saline. However, a randomized trial of gastric lavage before endoscopy showed an improvement only in endoscopic visualization of the gastric fundus, without any additional beneficial outcome [8].

Intravenous erythromycin (a motilin receptor agonist that stimulates gastrointestinal motility) may improve the quality of endoscopic examination in patients with UGI hemorrhage by promoting the emptying of intragastric blood. A recent cost-effectiveness study confirmed that giving IV erythromycin before endoscopy for UGI bleeding resulted in cost savings and an increase in quality-adjusted life-years [9]. As a result of these benefits, IV erythromycin 250 mg or IV metoclopramide 10 mg, 30–60 min before endoscopy, is recommended for selected patients with severe UGI hemorrhage to potentially improve UGI visualization.

Triage

Patients with severe UGI hemorrhage should be hospitalized. If they are hemodynamically unstable, have active ongoing hematemesis, or large-volume bright blood per NG tube or rectum (e.g. hematochezia), and have associated medical comorbidities that may be aggravated by the bleeding, patients should be admitted to an ICU for continuous monitoring [1]. Selected patients with self-limited UGI bleeding, stable vital signs, absence of liver disease or coagulopathy, and who are dependable and have help at home can be considered for outpatient management, rather than hospitalization [10].

Clinical and laboratory parameters have been used to guide risk stratification of patients with UGI bleeding. Both the Blatchford score and the clinical Rockall score have been used before EGD in patients with acute UGI bleeding to predict those at high risk versus those at low risk. In a recent study, patients with a low-risk clinical score had a decreased chance of having high-risk endoscopic stigmata and a very low risk of adverse outcomes, suggesting that this clinical scoring system may be applied in the future to reduce the need for urgent endoscopy [10].

Medical Therapy

After initial resuscitation and evaluation, medical therapy should be started. Several studies and meta-analyses of proton pump inhibitor (PPI) use in peptic ulcer bleeding have confirmed that PPIs reduce rebleeding, surgery, transfusion requirements, and duration of hospitalization, without decreasing mortality [5,11]. These reports suggest that an IV PPI infusion was most beneficial after endoscopic hemostasis of high-risk ulcer stigmata, but not as a stand-alone therapy. These stigmata of ulcer hemorrhage include active bleeding, nonbleeding visible vessel, or adherent clot, but not oozing bleeding (without other stigmata), clean ulcer base, or flat spots [5]. The recommended dose of PPIs for these high-risk ulcer stigmata, based on published randomized trials, is the equivalent of omeprazole 80 mg by IV bolus, followed by an 8 mg/h infusion for 72 h [1,5]. However, PPIs are not approved by the US Food and Drug Administration for such medical therapy of either UGI or peptic ulcer bleeding. An early, pre-endoscopy IV PPI bolus and infusion in patients with UGI hemorrhage is controversial. In one report, this pre-endoscopy PPI infusion decreased the need for endoscopic therapy, the number of actively bleeding peptic ulcers, and duration of hospitalization, but did not change other clinical outcomes [12]. Other studies have not shown any significant benefit in important clinical outcomes such as mortality, rebleeding, or

surgery [13], or cost-effectiveness in North America [14]. In patients with UGI hemorrhage presumed to be from ulcers, IV PPI therapy in some dosage schedules before endoscopy appears reasonable in view of its potential benefits and negligible risks [1,5].

In patients with UGI bleeding and associated liver disease, pharmacologic therapy with octreotide should be started as soon as a variceal hemorrhage is suspected and continued for 3–5 days after the diagnosis is confirmed [5,15]. Octreotide is safe and can be given continuously for 5 days or longer. Octreotide should be administered as an initial IV bolus of 50 µg, followed by a continuous infusion of 50 µg/h. Clinical trials suggest that octreotide is particularly useful as an adjunct to endoscopic therapy. In addition, patients with cirrhosis and GI hemorrhage should receive short-term (7 days maximum) antibiotic prophylaxis. Oral norfloxacin (400 mg twice daily) or IV ciprofloxacin, if oral administration is not possible, is recommended, except in patients with advanced cirrhosis in whom IV ceftriaxone (1 g/day) may be preferable [5,15].

After the patient has been stabilized and medical treatment instituted, urgent endoscopy is recommended for diagnosis and therapy, because of its high accuracy and low complication rate [5,16]. Endoscopy, using large single-channel or double-channel therapeutic endoscopes, is diagnostic in about 95% of UGI hemorrhage patients [5]. Endoscopy may also reveal stigmata of hemorrhage on ulcers or varices with important prognostic value, assisting in the triage of patients into high or low risk [5,16]. (These specific findings are discussed further in Chapter 47.)

The timing of endoscopy may depend on several variables including available resources, but patients with active bleeding should undergo endoscopy soon after resuscitation [5]. Urgent endoscopy (within 6 h) should be considered, particularly in patients with cirrhosis, in patients with recurrent inpatient bleeding, or in the rare patient with a suspected aortoenteric fistula. For other hemodynamically stable, UGI bleed patients, urgent endoscopy should be performed within 12 h.

Take-home points

Diagnosis
- Of UGI bleeds 40–50% are caused by peptic ulcer disease.

- The initial assessment should focus on the patient's hemodynamic state.
- An essential history includes information about previous UGI bleeding, history of liver disease, and use of nonsteroidals or other medications.
- Physical examination should assess for orthostatic hypotension which implies >15% blood loss.
- Nasogastric aspiration is useful for determining whether there is blood in the UGI tract and what the color is.

Management
- For UGI bleed presenting as hematemesis, assess for pulse, blood pressure, and orthostasis; obtain a brief focused history and lab results, and start resuscitation.
- Admit to ICU vs monitored bed.
- Endotracheal intubation if hematemesis persists or if there is altered mental status.
- Start IV proton pump inhibitor.
- Start IV octreotide infusion and antibiotics, if cirrhotic.
- Consider IV erythromycin or metoclopramide.
- EGD for diagnosis and therapy within 12 h.

Acknowledgments

Dr Jensen's research in GI bleeding is supported by NIH-NIDDK.K24 DK02650 and NIH-NIDDK.AM 41301 CURE CORE Grant (Human Studies Core).

References

1 Kovacs TOG. Management of upper gastrointestinal bleeding. *Curr Gastroenterol Rep* 2008; **10**: 535–42.

2 Kovacs TOG, Jensen DM. The short-term medical management of non-variceal upper gastrointestinal bleeding. *Drugs* 2008; **68**: 2105–11.

3 Kovacs TOG, Jensen DM. Recent advances in the endoscopic diagnosis and therapy of upper gastrointestinal, small intestinal, and colonic bleeding. *Med Clin North Am* 2002; **86**: 1319–56.

4 Gralnek IM, Barkun AN, Bardou M. Management of acute bleeding from a peptic ulcer. *N Engl J Med* 2008; **359**: 928–37.

5 Savides TS, Jensen DM. GI bleeding. In: Feldman M, Friedman LS, Brandt LJ (eds), *Sleisenger and Fordtran's Gastrointestinal and Liver Disease Pathophysiology/Diagnosis/Management*, 8th edn. Philadelphia: Saunders/Elsevier, 2010: in press.

6 Kupfer Y, Cappell MS, Tessler S. Acute gastrointestinal bleeding in the intensive care unit. The internist's perspective. *Gastroenterol Clin North Am* 2000; **29**: 275–307.

7 Aljebreen AM, Fallone CA, Barkun AN. Nasogastric aspirate predicts high-risk endoscopic lesions in patients with acute upper-GI bleeding. *Gastrointest Endosc* 2004; **59**: 172–8.

8 Lee SD, Kearney DJ. A randomized, controlled trial of gastric lavage prior to endoscopy for acute upper gastrointestinal bleeding. *J Clin Gastroenterol* 2004; **38**: 861–5.

9 Winstead NS, Wilcox CM. Erythromycin prior to endoscopy for acute upper gastrointestinal hemorrhage: a cost-effectiveness analysis. *Aliment Pharmacol Ther* 2007; **26**: 1371–7.

10 Romagnuolo J, Barkun AN, Armstrong D, *et al.* Simple clinical predictors may obviate urgent endoscopy in selected patients with non-variceal upper gastrointestinal tract bleeding. *Arch Intern Med* 2007; **167**: 265–70.

11 Bardou M, Toubouti Y, Benhaberou-Brun D, *et al.* Meta-analysis: proton-pump inhibition in high-risk patients with peptic ulcer bleeding. *Aliment Pharmacol Ther* 2005; **21**: 677–86.

12 Lau JY, Leung WK, Wu JCY, *et al.* Omeprazole before endoscopy in patients with gastrointestinal bleeding. *N Engl J Med* 2007; **356**: 1631–40.

13 Dorward S, Sreedharan A, Leontiadis GI, *et al.* Proton pump inhibitor treatment initiated prior to endoscopic diagnosis in upper gastrointestinal bleeding. *Cochrane Database Syst Rev* 2006; (4): CD005415.

14 Al-Sobah S, Burkun AN, Herba K, *et al.* Cost-effectiveness of proton-pump inhibition before endoscopy in upper gastrointestinal bleeding. *Clin Gastroenterol Hepatol* 2008; **6**: 418–25.

15 Garcia-Tsao G, Sanyal AJ, Grace ND, *et al.* Prevention and management of gastroesophageal varices and variceal hemorrhage in cirrhosis. *Hepatology* 2007; **46**: 922–38.

16 Kovacs TOG, Jensen DM. Endoscopic treatment of peptic ulcer bleeding. *Curr Treat Opt Gastroenterol* 2007; **10**: 143–8.

V PART 5

Diseases of the Esophagus

31

CHAPTER 31

Gastroesophageal Reflux Disease

Kenneth R. DeVault

Division of Gastroenterology and Hepatology, Mayo Clinic, Jacksonville, FL, USA

Summary

Gastroesophageal reflux disease (GERD) is one of the most common disorders in both primary care and in gastroenterology consultation. The pathophysiology of GERD is primarily related to failure of the lower esophageal sphinter's antireflux mechanism, but other factors may contribute in selected patients. While erosive esophagitis is the most specific sign of GERD, the majority of patients with GERD will have a relatively normal endoscopic appearance to their esophagus. Ambulatory reflux monitoring and therapeutic trials are often used to confirm the disease in patients where that confirmation is critical. Acid suppression, usually with proton pump inhibitors, remains the mainstay of GERD treatment both in the acute and chronic environments. Surgery for GERD is an option for selected patients and there is hope that an endoscopic approach may be developed and confirmed as an additional therapeutic option.

Case

A 63-year-old male presents with a history of heartburn and regurgitation for at least 15 years. These symptoms are worse after a large or late meal and tend to wake him up two or three nights per week. He has awakened with a cough on occasion. He has no dysphagia, odynophagia, symptoms or signs of blood loss, or weight loss. In fact he has gained about 12 kg in the past 10 years. Antacids provided partial, short-term symptom relief. His primary physician started him on omeprazole 20 mg daily, which improved, but did not relieve his symptoms. Due to the long duration of his symptoms, an endoscopy is performed, which shows a 5-cm hiatal hernia, but no evidence of esophagitis or Barrett esophagus.

Definition and Epidemiology

Gastroesophageal reflux disease (GERD) is defined as symptoms or mucosa damage resulting from the reflux of gastric content into the esophagus. GERD is one of the most common disorders in the Western world, affecting up to 20% the US population on at least a weekly basis. The classic symptoms of GERD are heartburn and regurgitation, but there have been other symptoms and diseases associated with this condition including non-cardiac chest pain, chronic cough, asthma, sleep disturbances, and many others. Mucosa damage can vary from none, to mild esophagitis, to more severe esophagitis, and less commonly, Barrett esophagus and esophageal carcinoma. The goal of therapy is to control both symptoms and mucosal damage. GERD is commonly a chronic condition, requiring chronic, often life-long treatment. GERD is also a very costly condition, for example in the USA it has been estimated to cost up to $10 billion annually, $6 billion of which are drug costs. In addition, there are substantial indirect costs of decreased work productivity as well as significant GERD-related impairments in the quality of life.

Pathophysiology

Lower Esophageal Sphincter Abnormalities

Although the symptoms and mucosal damage caused by GERD are almost universally related to acid, the disorder

Practical Gastroenterology and Hepatology: Esophagus and Stomach, 1st edition. Edited by Nicholas J. Talley, Kenneth R. DeVault and David E. Fleischer. © 2010 Blackwell Publishing Ltd.

itself is primarily a motility disorder. The lower esophageal sphincter (LES) is a 2–4 cm segment of smooth muscle that connects the distal esophagus to the stomach. This muscle has intrinsic muscular activity and is contracted in the "resting" state. While this circular, smooth muscle is the actual LES, some of the pressure and function of this organ is provided by the diaphragmatic hiatus. Finally, the sphincter normally extends into the abdominal cavity and additional positive pressure from that cavity contributes to the functional LES. The normal pressure at the esophagogastric junction varies with the method used to obtain measurement, but resting pressures below 5–15 mm Hg are almost always considered hypotensive. Abnormalities at the lower esophageal sphincter underlie the majority of reflux episodes. The most obvious abnormality is a weak and incompetent lower esophageal sphincter; for example, when patients with GERD and either normal esophagogastroduodenoscopy (EGD), lower LES pressure, and worsening acid exposure were associated with more severe esophageal mucosal disease [1] (Figure 31.1).

Only a minority of GERD patients will be found to have a resting LES pressure below normal and the more common abnormality appears to be inappropriate relaxation of the LES with normal, or at times elevated, resting pressures. The physiology of inappropriate LES relaxation is not clear, but accounts for up to 75% of reflux episodes in normal controls and in patients without severe esophagitis. These relaxations are more common during upright, daytime reflux episodes and may be triggered by hormonal changes, perhaps related to dietary factors. Since physiologic relaxation of the LES occurs with each swallow (dry or wet), perhaps the mechanism

relates to a pathologic aberrance in this physiologic relaxation. In addition, gastric distension (as with a large meal) has been suggested to increase the rate of transient relaxations. Other factors suggested to increase these events include: stress, pharyngeal stimulation, sleep difficulties, and general anesthesia.

Hiatal Hernia

Hiatal hernias are one mechanism by which the sphincter mechanism may be weakened. This lesion results in the disassociation of the smooth muscle LES and the striated muscle contribution from the hiatus. The presence of a hiatal hernia is neither sensitive nor specific for significant reflux but weak sphincter pressures and more severe mucosal disease (including Barrett esophagus) are often correlated with large, fixed hernias. A hernia on EGD provides support, but not proof, for the diagnosis in patients with a history of GERD symptoms.

Motility-induced Esophageal Acid Clearance

The increased use of esophageal manometry in patients with GERD has lead to the recognition of frequent peristaltic dysfunction in the esophageal body. This concept has received new emphasis as more patients are referred for antireflux surgery and the manometric findings are used to guide antireflux surgery. It is important to recognize that the loss of peristalsis in GERD may reverse after a course of acid suppression although the response has varied between studies. In addition to changes in primary peristalsis, patients with GERD often have a decrease in secondary peristalsis, which may result in longer acid contact times. Direct inflammation or perhaps an indirect process mediated by the release of some local substances by the inflamed mucosa seems to "stun" the esophageal smooth muscle. Interrupting acid exposure with medications or surgery may break this feedback loop and allow the motility to recover. Most patients with GERD have normal gastric emptying, but there is a subset where problems in this area complicate their disease. Several of the factors related to the pathophysiology of GERD are presented in Figure 31.2.

Salivary Neutralization

Swallowed saliva is an important protective factor in GERD. Saliva may protect the esophagus by both diluting and neutralizing esophageal acid (with bicarbonate), ini-

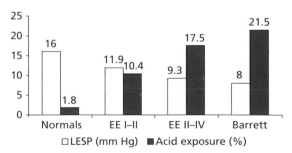

Figure 31.1 Lower esophageal sphincter pressure (LESP) and acid exposure in Barrett esophagus. (Reproduced from Coenraad *et al.* [1].)

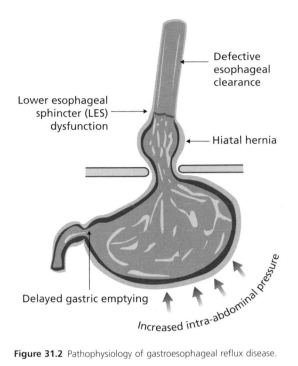

Figure 31.2 Pathophysiology of gastroesophageal reflux disease.

tiate swallowing, and primary peristaltic clearance of refluxed acid, and by possibly promoting esophageal healing through epidermal growth factors. Acid reflux into the esophagus results in a reflex increase in salivary flow that may be perceived by the patient as "water brash". Any agent that decreases salivary flow may worsen reflux. This is especially important with medications with anticholinergic side effects.

Epithelial Resistance to Injury

The distal esophagus is exposed to acid for up to 5% of a 24 h period in normal controls. It also may take at least twice this much exposure to result in esophagitis. Unlike the stomach, the esophagus does not have a well-developed pre-epithelial defense and the majority of resistance comes from the epithelium itself. The lining of the esophagus is composed of a stratified squamous epithelium. The more luminal layers of this epithelium are exposed to the highest concentrations of acid and protect the deeper layers. The junctions between cells are "tight" and limit the diffusion of hydrogen ions. Postepithelial defense is provided by factors derived from the blood supply to the esophageal mucosa. This blood flow both

carries nutrients to the esophageal lining and carries away and neutralizes harmful factors.

Non-acid Reflux

Reflux of non-acidic material may occasionally contribute to symptoms and mucosal disease, but it is clear that acid is the main culprit in both patients with partial gastrectomies and in those with an intact pylorus. On the other hand it is also clear that some material from the duodenum will occasionally reflux into the stomach and, if in the stomach, may potentially reflux into the esophagus. Animal studies indicate that this material may produce esophageal damage and even predispose to cancer. The finding of bile-stained gastric mucosa is neither specific nor sensitive for duodenogastroesophageal reflux. Attempts to document this disorder with biliary scintigraphy has also been less than successful. If bile or the misnamed "alkaline" reflux is to be diagnosed, evaluation of esophageal bile acid using an ambulatory monitor is more accurate than attempting to quantify esophageal alkalinization using a pH probe. Acid suppression with an agent such as omeprazole not only controls acid reflux, but also decreases the measurable reflux of bilirubin-containing material. In summary, bile or non-acid reflux may contribute to symptoms and mucosal damage in some patients with GERD, but the vast majority of patients have acid-related disease.

Clinical Features

Erosive Esophagitis

When acid refluxes into the esophagus, in sufficient amounts for sufficient duration, the mucosa begins to break down resulting in the most specific sign of GERD, erosive esophagitis. Esophagitis can vary from mild erosions to severe circumferential ulcerations. Patients most likely to get esophagitis (particularly severe esophagitis) are those with the most disordered esophageal physiology (low LES pressure, large hiatal hernias, weak peristalsis, etc.). Unfortunately, the symptom severity in GERD patients is not highly predictive of the presence or absence of esophagitis. Esophagitis can only be diagnosed with endoscopy and the severity should be graded (see below and Chapter 6). Patients with the most severe forms of esophagitis may develop strictures either coexistent with the esophagitis or as a residual after healing (Chapter 37).

Non-erosive Reflux Disease and Functional Heartburn

When patients with typical reflux symptoms of heartburn, regurgitation, or both undergo endoscopy up to 75% will have neither esophagitis nor evidence of Barrett esophagus [2]. These patients have been described as having endoscopic negative or, more commonly, non-erosive reflux disease (NERD). Certainly, patients without esophagitis and with a positive pH test can be diagnosed with GERD. Patients with normal acid exposure, but who report symptoms with a majority of their reflux episodes documented during an ambulatory pH study have also been considered to have NERD, although others have labeled them as having "functional heartburn." Whether these patients are part of the spectrum of GERD or have another diagnosis, such as dyspepsia, is not clear. It seems that the most respected definition of functional heartburn (the Rome III criteria) would include these patients as functional heartburn since it was defined as "burning retrosternal discomfort or pain without evidence that gastroesophageal acid reflux is the cause of the symptoms in the absence of histopathology based esophageal motility disorders" [3].

In a study of nearly 1000 patients presenting with typical reflux symptoms, only 32% had erosive esophagitis [4]. More importantly, neither physician evaluation nor a validated questionnaire that segregated patient into mild, moderate, or severe symptoms were predictive of esophagitis. When studied with ambulatory pH, NERD patients have lower esophageal acid exposures on average and are more likely to have normal acid exposure. For example, over 90% of patients with Barrett esophagus and more than 75% of esophagitis patients were demonstrated to have pathologic acid exposure compared to only 45% of symptomatic patients without esophageal damage [5]. In addition to lower acid exposures, the esophageal exposure to other gastric substances including bile is less common in NERD patients compared to those with esophagitis and more complicated reflux disease. All that having been said, NERD patients may require as aggressive and perhaps more aggressive therapy than patients with erosive esophagitis.

Diagnosis

Endoscopy

Endoscopy is indicated mainly in two situations; when the so-called warning symptoms (dysphagia, odynophagia, weight loss, signs of GI blood loss) are present and in patients thought to be at risk for Barrett esophagus. The former patients should be easily identified with a carefully obtained history, but who to screen for Barrett esophagus is more problematic. Current guidelines would suggest that patients who are at least 40–50 years old with a history of symptoms for at least 5–10 years might benefit most from screening [6]. Other groups that may benefit from endoscopy include those who develop new symptoms at an older age and those with severe symptoms that do not respond to medical therapy. Recent studies suggest that endoscopy in GERD patients with refractory symptoms may reveal eosinophilic esophagitis in a subset (see Chapter 34). Endoscopic techniques are extensively discussed elsewhere (Chapter 6), but deserves additional mention here. An endoscopy for GERD should clearly describe the esophageal mucosa, the esophagogastric junction, and biopsy any area of concern. The entire length of the esophagus should be carefully viewed and biopsies obtained if the endoscopic or clinical picture suggests eosinophilic esophagitis or other non-GERD diagnoses. Esophagitis is only diagnosed if there are breaks in the mucosa of the esophagus and should be graded using an accepted scale, preferable the Los Angeles Classification or another well-validated scale. The extent of columnar replacement of esophageal mucosa should be clearly described and measured. The distance from the teeth to the esophagogastric junction should be recorded. A retroflexed view is obtained and any hernia should be described and measured (see Table 31.1 for indications for endoscopy).

The ability to image the esophagus in a less-invasive and perhaps less-expensive manner remains a goal of several research programs. A disposable esophageal pill camera has been developed and marketed. In early, very small studies, this device had impressive sensitivity and specificity when compared to routine endoscopy (see Chapter 19) [7]. Recently, there have been several studies challenging these early findings and an additional study is underway. Unsedated, small-caliber endoscopy through the mouth or nose has also been studied and

Table 31.1 Gastroesophageal reflux disease symptoms leading to early testing.

Endoscopy
  Dysphagia
  Odynophagia
  Gastrointestinal blood loss
  Unintended weight loss
  Refractory symptoms (?)
  Patients at risk for Barrett esophagus

Ambulatory pH testing
  Symptoms refractory to therapeutic trial
  Option as initial approach in patients with atypical symptoms
  Confirm disease prior to endoscopic or surgical therapy

Cardiac testing
  Chest pain
  Refractory heartburn in patient at risk for cardiac disease

may allow screening of the esophagus in a less-expensive environment.

Ambulatory Reflux Monitoring

There have been several methods developed to test for reflux from the stomach to the esophagus. Traditionally, these have consisted of a tube with an electrode that measure pH passed through the nose into the esophagus. Recently, both a tubeless pH monitoring device and impedance-based devices (to evaluate non-acid reflux) have been developed. Ambulatory reflux tests are most useful in patients with GERD symptoms that have not responded to empiric therapy and to confirm GERD in patients under evaluation for endoscopic or surgical therapy (see Chapter 17 and Figure 31.1) [8].

Other Tests

Barium studies do not provide accurate data in the evaluation of GERD and should not be routinely used outside of patients with dysphagia and in some selected patients prior to endoscopic or surgical therapy. While esophageal motility testing will reveal abnormalities in LES pressure and esophageal peristalsis in many GERD patients, the use of this test is restricted to finding the location of the LES to facilitate accurate placement of reflux monitoring probes and perhaps to help guide antireflux surgery. Likewise, some patients with GERD will have evidence of

delayed gastric emptying with nuclear medicine testing, but testing for this is not routinely recommended. Patients who are at risk for cardiac disease may need additional testing to rule out coronary artery disease.

Therapeutic Trials as Diagnostic Tools

There is no "gold-standard" test to confirm the diagnosis and most experts believe a trial of medication to be the best diagnostic and therapeutic approach to the majority of patients with symptoms suggestive of GERD. For patients with heartburn or regurgitation, response to high-dose proton pump inhibitors (PPIs) has a sensitivity of 75% and specificity of 55% when compared with ambulatory pH testing [9]. Though using response to acid suppression is not a perfect strategy to diagnose GERD, it is cost-effective and has become the preferred initial approach to patients with GERD-related symptoms. That having been said, although most experts would continue to use empiric acid suppression when an untested patient responds, they would also require confirmatory testing (usually with ambulatory reflux testing) prior to a more invasive approach endoscopic or surgical approach. While generally acceptable, many experts believe that this approach has resulted in the exponential growth in GERD related prescriptions some of which may be inappropriate given the low specificity.

Therapeutics

Lifestyle Changes

Education of the patient about factors that may precipitate reflux remains reasonable. Numerous studies have indicated that elevation of the head of the bed, decreased fat intake, cessation of smoking, and avoiding recumbency for 3 h postprandially all decrease distal esophageal acid exposure, although data reflecting the true efficacy of these maneuvers in patients is almost completely lacking. Certain foods (chocolate, alcohol, peppermint, coffee, and perhaps onions and garlic) have been noted to lower LES pressure, although randomized trials are also not available to test the efficacy of these maneuvers. Many authors assume the 20–30% placebo response rate seen in most randomized trials is due to lifestyle changes, but this has not been rigorously tested. The potential negative effect of lifestyle changes on a patient's quality of life has also not been examined.

Antacids and Antirefluxants

Antacids are better than placebo in achieving relief of heartburn. In certain circumstances, antacids may be preferred to other acid-suppressing medications. They are inexpensive and have a very rapid onset. Alginate-based formulations have been available for the past 30 years and have been marketed under a variety of brand names, the most common of which is Gaviscon®. Alginates act by a unique mechanism in which the alginate precipitates in the presence of gastric acid forming a gel. The gel then traps carbon dioxide creating foam that floats on the surface of gastric contents like a raft on water.

Acid Suppression

Acid suppression is the mainstay of GERD therapy. This has evolved quickly over the past few decades. The histamine type-2 receptor antagonists (H_2RA) were introduced in the 1980s and, for the first time, provided a specific pharmacological approach to control acid secretion. Eventually, four of these agents were marketed in the USA (cimetidine, ranitidine, famotidine, and nizatidine). H_2RAs are relatively effective in treating heartburn symptoms with a rapid onset of action. Though H_2RAs offer an improvement over placebo for healing of mild esophagitis, they have limited utility, regardless of dose, in healing more severe esophagitis. Patients who continue to have heartburn after 6 weeks of treatment with H_2RAs are unlikely to respond to prolonged courses or increased dosages. These agents have various approved doses and there are small differences in side effects, but overall, their efficacy is quite similar.

In the 1989, the first proton pump inhibitor (omeprazole) was developed. This was followed by the introduction of three additional agents (lansoprazole, pantoprazole, and rabeprazole) with similar efficacies. A review of 33 randomized trials including over 3000 patients showed that symptomatic relief can be expected in 27% of patients treated with placebo, 60% treated with H_2RAs, and 83% treated with PPIs [10]. Of those patients with esophagitis, 24% treated with placebo, 50% treated with H_2RAs, and 78% treated with PPI had mucosal healing. The best dose timing for maximum serum concentration and efficacy is when the largest numbers of proton pumps are active. Meals stimulate proton pumps, so dosing the drug 15–60 min prior to a meal produces the most effective acid suppression. It has been suggested that patients on once-daily PPIs take the dose prior to breakfast. However, a recent study has shown that nighttime acid is better controlled if the PPI is taken prior to the evening meal [11].

PPI therapy does have some limitations. Once-daily PPI therapy suppresses gastric acid for 11.2 to 15.3 h during a 24-h day [12]. Recently, an optically pure preparation of omeprazole was tested and approved as a different agent (esomeprazole). Esomeprazole has shown some increased efficacy when compared to omeprazole, lansoprazole, and pantoprazole in certain subsets of patients, although huge studies were required in order to achieve statistical significance. Finally, omeprazole was combined with an antacid in a new formulation that may have some advantages over the parent compound including the ability to be taken without meals and perhaps more rapid onset of action. Several other agents are under development in attempts to address both rapidity of onset and duration of action. A common approach to symptoms that are not responding to once daily PPI is to increase the PPI dose to twice daily (properly taken prior to meals), although this still leaves the stomach with a pH below 4.0 for at least 20% of the time, with the majority of this acidity occurring at night. The currently available acid suppressants are listed in Table 31.2.

Prokinetic (Motility) Therapy

Prokinetic drugs are appealing in the treatment of GERD as they may increase gastric emptying, improve peristalsis, and increase LES pressure. Unfortunately, these agents are typically not effective as monotherapy and their side-effect profiles often limit their use. The prokinetic drugs that have been used in GERD include bethanecol, metoclopramide, cisapride, domperidone, baclofen, and tegaserod. Bethanecol and metoclopramide have poor efficacy, common side-effects and are not recommend for routine use in GERD. Domperidone is a promotility agent with efficacy in gastric motility disorders, but was disappointing when tested in GERD and has not come to the US market. Cisapride has been associated with fatal cardiac arrhythmias and significant cardiotoxicity, especially when taken together with protease inhibitors, macrolide antibiotics, and imidazoles and has resulted in its withdrawal from routine availability in the USA. Baclofen is a GABA receptor agonist. It appears to

Table 31.2 Currently available acid suppressants and usual dose.

Class	Generic name	US trade name	Usual GERD dose
PPI	Omeprazole*	Prilosec, Zegerid†	20–40 mg once daily
	Lansoprazole	Prevacid	30 mg once daily
	Rabeprazole	Aciphex	20 mg once daily
	Pantoprazole	Protonix	40 mg once daily
	Esomeprazole	Nexium	20–40 mg once daily
	Dexlansoprazole DDR	Kapidex	30–60 mg once daily
H₂RA	Cimetidine*	Tagamet	300–400 mg twice daily
	Ranitidine*	Zantac	150 mg twice daily
	Famotidine*	Pepcid, Pepcid Complete†	20–40 mg twice daily
	Nizatidine*	Axid	150 mg twice daily

* OTC and generics available.
† Combination of agent with antacid.
PPI, proton pump inhibitor; H₂RA, histamine type-2 receptor antagonist.

suppress transient LES relaxation and, therefore, reduces the number of reflux episodes and the amount of esophageal acid exposure with a single dose (40 mg). Unfortunately, baclofen has a limiting side effect profile (e.g., nausea, vomiting, somnolence, seizures, death upon withdrawal). There is much ongoing research attempting to design a reflux inhibitor with the efficacy of baclofen, yet without side effects. Tegaserod is a 5HT-4 receptor agonist with promotility effects. It has been shown to reduce esophageal acid exposure, but it does not appear to be an effective monotherapy in the treatment of GERD symptoms. Reports of increased cardiovascular events with the medication have resulted in its withdrawal from the US market.

Long-term (Maintenance) Therapy

Many patients with GERD require long-term, possibly life-long, therapy; therefore maintenance therapy to keep symptoms comfortably under control and prevent complications is a major concern. This will vary in each patient and may require only antacids and lifestyle modifications in up to 20% of patients. Patients whose disease has required proton pump inhibitors for control often will have symptomatic relapses and failure of healing of esophagitis on standard dose, or even higher-dose H₂RA and/or prokinetic therapy. A full dose of H₂RA given once daily, although effective for peptic ulcer disease, is not appropriate for GERD. There does not appear to be a safety advantage with using a lower PPI dose for maintenance, but the indication for some PPIs do suggest a

lower maintenance dose (esomeprazole 20 mg and lansoprazole 15 mg are examples). Ultimately, whatever dose of medication is needed to control symptoms is the dose that should be used and may include full or even increased dose PPI in many patients.

There are clear data that full-dose proton pump inhibitors lengthen the interval between symptomatic relapses in patients with esophageal strictures requiring dilation [13]. There are no similar data in regards to the prevention or prevention of progression of Barrett esophagus. It does not appear that Barrett esophagus will regress with either medical or surgical therapy. There have been reports of occasional "islands" of squamous epithelium appearing with chronic proton pump inhibitor therapy, but the significance of this is not known. There is one retrospective study suggesting less dysplasia in patients with Barrett who take PPI [14], but this needs confirmation in a large, properly designed trial.

Since many patients will be treated with PPI on a long-term basis, safety is a prominent concern. Effective gastric acid suppression produces varying degrees of hypergastrinemia although there are no significant, documented adverse effects of elevated gastrin in PPI treated patients. Several retrospective studies have recently suggested small but significant increases in community acquired pneumonia [15], *Clostridium difficile* infection [16] and hip fractures [17] in patients on PPI (particularly higher than indicated doses). Atrophic gastritis in chronic omeprazole users is common, but it seems to occur predominantly in patients who are infected with *H. pylori*. No patients have developed PPI-induced gastric dysplasia or cancer. Patients on long-term omeprazole may develop vitamin B_{12} malabsorption and should have vitamin B_{12} levels periodically assessed. Drugs that require acid for absorption that are potentially altered with PPI therapy include ketoconazole, iron salts, and digoxin. When PPI therapy is initiated, the International Normalized Ratio (INR) and prothrombin time may be altered in patients on warfarin. An adverse interaction between proton pump inhibitors and the antiplatelet drug clopidogrel has been recently reported, leading to a general warning suggesting careful consideration before using these agents together.

On-demand Therapy

Intermittent therapy with an H_2RA or PPI is most likely to be successful in patients without esophagitis and with mild to moderate heartburn. There are very few data to support any one approach for "on-demand" therapy. H_2RA taken on an as-needed basis provides acceptable control in patients with mild, intermittent symptoms. PPI do not seem to be a good choice for on-demand therapy since their onset of action does not maximize for a few days. That having been said, there are data and experience to suggest this approach may be beneficial in some patients. A more reasonable use of PPI is on an intermittent basis, where, rather than taking one pill, the patient may take a few day courses when their symptoms are bothering them more. This approach has not been approved as an indication in the USA (with the exception of the label for OTC Prilosec), but is a more accepted approach in Europe.

Endoscopic and Surgical Approaches

The vast majority of GERD patients will have mucosal disease and the majority of symptoms controlled with medical therapy. There is a small subset with symptoms that either are, or appear to be, refractory to medical therapy. Of these symptoms, regurgitation seems the most reasonable, since current therapy addresses the acid content of the refluxate but probably allows continued reflux of neutralized material in a subset of patients. A trial that randomized 310 patients between surgery and PPIs found surgery to be slightly superior to omeprazole at the end of 7 years in regards to control of GERD symptoms, although there were more bothersome

side effects in the surgical group [18]. Proper selection and preoperative evaluation of patients is very important. In a study of 100 patients, the best predictors of a good outcome were; age less than 50 years and typical reflux symptoms that had completely resolved on medical therapy [19]. It is also clear that these typical reflux symptoms are more likely to resolve after surgery than the other atypical and supraesophageal symptoms. If typical reflux esophagitis is not present endoscopically, ambulatory pH testing should be performed to confirm the disease (see Chapter 17 for additional details).

A great deal of excitement had been generated by the introduction of techniques designed to control reflux endoscopically, although some of that excitement has recently waned (see Chapter 41 for additional details). All of these techniques seem to produce an improvement in reflux symptoms, although significant changes in lower esophageal sphincter pressure have not been documented and less than 35% of patients have been demonstrated to have normalization of intraesophageal acid exposure (measured with ambulatory pH testing). When the results of the available studies (both published manuscripts and abstracts) are critically examined, many issues remain unresolved including long-term durability and safety, efficacy of these procedures performed outside of clinical trials, and efficacy in atypical presentations of GERD, among others.

Case continued

On additional questioning you find that the patient has been taking his omeprazole at bedtime since he assumed that would be the best way to control his symptoms. You suggest that he would be better served by taking the medication prior to a meal and since his symptoms are primarily at night, prior to dinner would be best. You also suggest that he lower the size of his meals, avoid eating late at night, and decrease fat and alcohol. The patient returns 6 weeks later and has noted a marked improvement in his symptoms. He still will experience mild heartburn when he overeats, but overall is very pleased with his current level of symptom control. You review maintenance options for GERD including the risks and benefits of chronic PPI therapy and reflux surgery. You agree on continued PPI therapy on a long-term basis. A suggested approach to patients with GERD is shown in Figure 31.3.

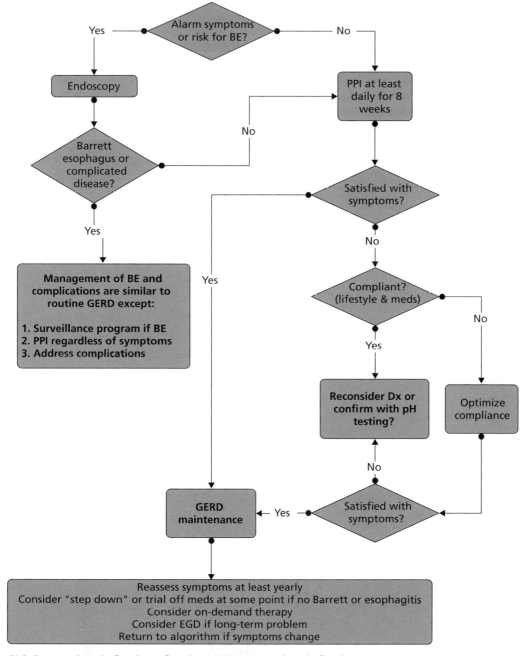

Figure 31.3 Gastroesophageal reflux disease flow chart. GERD, gastroesophageal reflux disease; PPI, proton pump inhibitor; BE, Barrett esophagus; Dx, diagnosis.

Take-home points

Diagnosis:

- Empiric therapy (usually with a PPI) is indicated in the majority of GERD patients.

- Endoscopy is indicated in patients with warning symptoms and in some patients with chronic disease to screen for Barrett esophagus.

- Barium testing is generally not helpful in GERD.

- Ambulatory reflux testing is indicated in patients who do not respond to empiric therapy in whom GERD is still a concern and to confirm the disease prior to endoscopic or surgical therapy.

Therapy:

- Lifestyle modifications may help some patients, but the majority of patients will require additional therapy for symptom control.

- Acid suppression remains the mainstay of GERD therapy in the majority of patients.

- Proton pump inhibitors provide outstanding acid suppression given once daily.

- There are no currently available promotility agents with acceptable efficacy and side-effect profile to make them viable agents for the majority of GERD patients.

- Surgical therapy, performed by an experienced surgeon, is a maintenance option for the patient with well-documented GERD.

- Research is ongoing into less-invasive, endoscopic therapies for GERD, but most of the currently available methods should remain in investigational environments.

References

1 Coenraad M, Masclee AA, Straathof JW, *et al.* Is Barrett's esophagus characterized by more pronounced acid reflux than severe esophagitis? *Am J Gastroenterol* 1998; **93**: 1068–72.

2 Chey WD. Endoscopy-negative reflux disease: concepts and clinical practice. *Am J Med* 2004; **117**: 36S–43S.

3 Galmiche JP, Clouse RE, Balint A, *et al.* Functional esophageal disorders. In: Drossman DA *et al. Rome III: The Functional Gastrointestinal Disorders*, 3rd edn. McLean, VA, USA: Degnon Associates, Inc, 2006: 369–418.

4 Venables TL, Newland RD, Patel AC, *et al.* Omeprazole 10 milligrams once daily, omeprazole 20 milligrams once daily or ranitidine 150 milligrams twice daily, evaluated as initial therapy for the relief of symptoms of gastro-oesophageal reflux disease in general practice. *Scand J Gastroenterol* 1997; **32**: 965–73.

5 Martinez SD, Malagon IB, Garewal HS, *et al.* Non-erosive reflux disease (NERD)-acid reflux and symptom patterns. *Aliment Pharmacol Therap* 2003; **17**: 537–45.

6 Sampliner RE. Updated guidelines for the diagnosis, surveillance and therapy of Barrett's esophagus. *Am J Gastroenterol* 2002; **97**: 1888–95.

7 Eliakim R, Sharma VK, Yassin K, *et al.* A prospective study of the diagnostic accuracy of Pill Cam ESO esophageal capsule endoscopy versus conventional upper endoscopy in patients with chronic gastroesophageal reflux disease. *J Clin Gastroenterol* 2005; **39**: 572–8.

8 DeVault KR, Castell DO. Updated guidelines for the diagnosis and treatment of Gastroesophageal reflux disease. *Am J Gastroenterol* 2005; **100**: 190–200.

9 Johnsson F, Weywadt L, Solhaug JH, *et al.* One-week omeprazole treatment in the diagnosis of gastro-oesophageal reflux disease. *Scand J Gastroenterol* 1998; **33**: 15–20.

10 DeVault KR, Castell DO. Guidelines for the diagnosis and treatment of gastroesophageal reflux disease. Practice Parameters Committee of the American College of Gastroenterology. *Arch Intern Med* 1995; **155**: 2165–73.

11 Hatlebakk JG, Katz PO, Kuo B, Castell DO. Nocturnal gastric acidity and acid breakthrough on different regimens of omeprazole 40 mg daily. *Aliment Pharmacol Ther* 1998; **12**: 1235–40.

12 Miner P, Katz PO, Chen Y, Sostek M. Gastric acid control with esomeprazole, lansoprazole, omeprazole, pantoprazole and rabeprazole: a five-way crossover trial. *Am J Gastroenterol* 2003; **98**: 2616–20.

13 Marks RD, Richter JE, Rizzo J, *et al.* Omeprazole versus H2-receptor antagonists in treating patients with peptic stricture and esophagitis. *Gastroenterology* 1994; **106**: 907–15.

14 El-Serag HB, Aguirre TV, Davis S, *et al.* Proton pump inhibitors are associated with reduced incidence of dysplasia in Barrett's esophagus. *Am J Gastroenterol* 2004; **99**: 1877–83.

15 Laheij RJF, Sturkenboom MCJM, Hassing J-H, *et al.* Risk of community-acquired pneumonia and use of gastric acid–suppressive drugs. *JAMA* 2004; **292**: 1995–60.

16 Dial S, Delaney JA, Barkun AN, Suissa S. Use of gastric acid-suppressive agents and the risk of community-acquired Clostridium difficile-associated disease. *JAMA* 2005; **294**: 2989–95.

17 Yang YX, Lewis JD, Epstein S, Metz DC. Long-term proton pump inhibitor therapy and risk of hip fracture. *JAMA* 2006; **296**: 2947–53.

18 Lundell L, Miettinen P, Myrvold HE, *et al.* Seven-year follow-up o a randomized clinical trial comparing proton-pump inhibition with surgical therapy for reflux oesophagitis. *Br J Surg* 2007; **94**: 198–203.

19 Jackson PG, Cleiber MA, Askari R, Evans SRT. Predictors of outcome in 100 consecutive laparoscopic antireflux procedures. *Am J Surg* 2001; **181**: 231–5.

CHAPTER 32

Extraesophageal Gastroesophageal Reflux Disease

Christen Klochan[1] and Michael F. Vaezi[2]

[1] Department of Internal Medicine, Vanderbilt University, Nashville, TN, USA
[2] Division of Gastroenterology, Hepatology and Nutrition, Vanderbilt University Medical Center
Nashville, TN, USA

Summary

Gastroesophageal reflux disease commonly presents with heartburn and regurgitation. However, due to unknown mechanisms some patients with gastroesophageal reflux disease (GERD) present with extraesophageal symptoms such as dental erosions, laryngitis, asthma, cough, or non-cardiac chest pain. Diagnostic tests in extraesophageal reflux are usually not helpful to establish cause and effect association between GERD and the extraesophageal symptoms or signs. Thus, empiric therapy with aggressive acid suppression, usually twice-daily dosing of PPIs, is currently recommended. In those who improve with such therapy, it is likely that GERD was the cause of the extraesophageal presentation. In those who are unresponsive to such therapy, diagnostic testing with impedance/pH monitoring may be reasonable to exclude continued acid or weakly acid reflux. However, PPI-unresponsive patients usually have other causes for the extraesophageal symptoms and signs than GERD. Surgical fundoplication is an appropriate alternative to PPI therapy in those who either do not wish to take this medication long term, cannot afford them, or have side effects with their use. Fundoplication is currently not recommended in those who are unresponsive to PPI therapy.

Case

A 46-year-old female presents on referral from her ENT physician for evaluation and treatment of her throat clearing and chronic cough. She has a history of asthma and postnasal drip from seasonal allergies and has been treated aggressively by her pulmonary and allergy physician for the past 3 years. She has undergone laryngoscopy by her ENT physician, which showed laryngeal irritation that suggested "GERD". The patient is on once-daily proton pump inhibitor intermittently which has only minimally helped her symptom. She does have heartburn and occasional regurgitation, especially at nights when in the supine position.

Practical Gastroenterology and Hepatology: Esophagus and Stomach, 1st edition. Edited by Nicholas J. Talley, Kenneth R. DeVault and David E. Fleischer. © 2010 Blackwell Publishing Ltd.

Definition and Epidemiology

Definition

Gastroesophageal reflux disease (GERD) is implicated as the causative agent in the development of many extraesophageal symptoms [1]. GERD is a common medical condition affecting approximately 35–40% of the adult population in the Western world with 36% having at least once-monthly symptoms. The role of GERD in causing extraesophageal symptoms, including laryngitis, asthma, cough, chest pain, and dental erosions, is increasingly recognized [2]. Chronic laryngeal signs and symptoms associated with GERD are often referred to as reflux laryngitis or laryngopharyngeal reflux. It is estimated that nearly 10% of ear, nose, and throat (ENT) patient visits are possible due to GERD-related laryngeal complaints. These patients often complain of sore throat, hoarseness, throat clearing as well as dysphagia and cough. Classic reflux symptoms (heartburn and regurgitation) which are referred to as "typical GERD" may be absent in more than half the patients presenting with extraesophageal symptoms [3].

A recent consensus (the Montreal Consensus) defined GERD as "a condition which develops when the reflux of stomach contents causes troublesome symptoms and/or complications" [4]. The Montreal definition of GERD recognizes two categories of symptoms, esophageal and extraesophageal. Within the extraesophageal syndromes the "established" associations include those with GERD and chronic cough syndrome, reflux laryngitis syndrome, reflux asthma syndrome, and reflux dental erosion syndrome (Table 32.1). The symptoms not as well established include pharyngitis, sinusitis, idiopathic pulmonary fibrosis, and recurrent otitis media. The definition stipulates that the symptoms should be sufficiently bothersome to affect an individual's well being, and that the patient should be the one to determine whether the symptoms are bothersome.

Table 32.1 Extraesophageal manifestations of gastroesophageal reflux disease.

ENT
  Laryngitis
  Sinusitis
  Otitis media
  Laryngeal ulcers
  Granuloma
  Polyps/vocal cord nodules
  Laryngeal cancer
  Chronic sore throat
  Globus pharyngeus
  Roenke edema
  Subglottic stenosis
  Dysphonia
  Dysgeusia

Pulmonary
  Asthma
  Chronic cough
  Pneumonia
  Bronchitis
  Interstitial fibrosis

Cardiac
  Chest pain
  Sinus arrhythmia

Other
  Dental erosions
  Halitosis
  Sandifer syndrome

Key Terms

• Microaspiration: non-overt entrance of gastroduodenal contents into the larynx or airways due to a problem with protective mechanisms
• Regurgitation: the perception of flow of refluxed gastric content into the mouth or hypopharynx
• Globus sensation: a feeling of choking or a lump in the throat more prominent between meals and generally disappearing at night
• Non-cardiac chest pain: crushing chest pain identical to angina, where after a thorough workup, no evidence of ischemia is found
• Dysphagia: a perceived impassage of food from the mouth into the stomach

Epidemiology

The exact prevalence of the various extraesophageal manifestations is unknown. Estimates vary due to differences in definitions and methods used to establish the diagnosis. However, the prevalence of GERD may be different depending on each extraesophageal manifestation (Table 32.2). Classic reflux symptoms are absent in 40–60% of asthmatics, in 57–94% of patients with ENT complaints, and in 43–75% of patients with chronic cough. Up to 78% of patients with chronic sore throat have GERD. Of patients who present to otolaryngologists, 4–10% do so because of complaints related to GERD. Thus, GERD should be included in the differential diagnosis of patients presenting with extraesophageal symptoms, especially when alternative diagnoses are excluded [2,6].

In a study of 101 366 patients with erosive esophagitis or strictures discharged from a Veteran Affairs hospital between 1981 and 1994, these GERD patients were

Table 32.2 Prevalence of various conditions in patients with gastroesophageal reflux disease and the general population. Data from Garcia-Campean et al. [5].

	GERD (%)	General population (%)
Chest pain	69	31
Chronic cough	75	25
Asthma	45–80	10
Dental erosions	20–55	2–19

found to be at increased risk of extraesophageal syndromes [7]. In this study, erosive esophagitis and stricture were associated with laryngitis (OR 2.01, CI 1.53–2.63), asthma (OR 1.51, CI 1.43–1.59), pneumonia (OR 1.15, CI 1.12–1.18). A recent systematic review of studies assessing the prevalence of GERD in patients with asthma concluded that there is a significant association between GERD and asthma [8]. This study evaluated 28 publications and reported pooled odds ratio of 5.5 (95%CI 1.9–15.8) for studies reporting the prevalence of GERD symptoms in asthmatics and 2.3 (95%CI 1.8–2.8) for those studies measuring the prevalence of asthma in GERD.

Pathophysiology, Clinical Features, and Differential Diagnosis

Two mechanisms have been proposed to explain extraesophageal symptoms of GERD: microaspiration (reflux) and vagal stimulation (reflex) (Table 32.3) [9]. Microaspiration involves the entrance of gastroduodenal contents into the larynx or airways due to a failure of normal protective mechanisms. These chemicals can include acid, pepsin, bile, and pancreatic enzymes. Chronic irritation causes laryngitis, chronic cough, or asthma. In the second mechanism, the presence of acid within the distal esophagus causes stimulation of acid-sensitive receptors innervated by the vagus nerve. Because the esophagus and bronchial tree share innervation by the vagal nerve, this stimulation may result in non-cardiac chest pain, cough, or asthma.

Laryngopharyngeal Reflux

The mechanism of laryngopharyngeal reflux may involve a primary defect in the upper esophageal sphincter. However, defects in the lower esophageal sphincter or in esophageal motility may also have a role. The mechanism relates to direct contact of pepsin and bile acids on the laryngeal tissues in an acidic pH; exposures without an acidic environment do not appear to cause tissue injury [10]. The presence of noxious irritants in the tracheobronchial tree causes paralysis of cilia with resultant mucus stasis. This can lead to accumulation of mucus, chronic throat clearing, and pneumonia.

Delahunty, in 1972, was the first to suggested that proliferative changes in the laryngeal epithelium may be due to acid reflux. Symptoms may include hoarseness, throat clearing, cough, sore or burning throat, dysphagia, and globus sensation. Chronic laryngitis and difficult-to-treat sore throat are associated with acid reflux in as many as 60% of patients [2]. Most patients with laryngeal findings from GERD will respond to aggressive therapy with PPIs. However, the current dilemma in this field is what the likelihood of association between GERD and laryngeal symptoms may be in those unresponsive to PPI therapy. Most recent data suggest that GERD is likely not the cause of persistent symptoms in this group. The issue of "silent" reflux causing laryngeal irritation or symptoms in this group is currently controversial. Failure to diagnose early symptoms of laryngopharyngeal reflux may result in progression to the more serious complications of contact ulcers, granuloma, subglottic stenosis, and lower airway disease [11]. However, prospective controlled data in this area are lacking.

Symptoms of laryngopharyngeal reflux may be due to smoking, toxic inhalants, allergies, postnasal drip, alcohol, chronic cough and infections, vocal cord dysfunction, or muscle tension dysphonia in those with hoarseness. In patients with structural laryngeal pathology it is important that an otolaryngologist with experience continues with patient follow up as individual causes are explored and treated.

Asthma

Asthma has a strong correlation with GERD. The relationship is complicated by the fact that both conditions

Table 32.3 Extraesophageal manifestations of gastroesophageal reflux disease and their proposed mechanisms.

Symptom	Mechanism
Chest pain	Visceral hypersensitivity, vagal stimulation
Chronic cough	Microaspiration, vagal stimulation
Asthma	Microaspiration, vagal stimulation
Laryngitis	Laryngopharyngeal reflux, chronic cough
Otitis media	Reflux into middle ear cavity
Obstructive sleep apnea	May cause gastroesophageal reflux disease through negative intrathoracic pressure and traction on phrenoesophageal ligament
Dental erosions	Chemical erosion

seem to induce the other. GERD can induce asthma by the vagally-mediated or microaspiration mechanisms described above. Wright *et al.* showed that acid in the esophagus caused decreased air flow in asthmatic patients, and that atropine prevented this effect, suggesting that esophagobronchial reflexes through the vagus nerve were present [12]. Asthma can induce GERD by several mechanisms. First, an asthma exacerbation results in negative intrathoracic pressure, which may overcome the tension in the lower esophageal sphincter and cause reflux. Second, medications used to treat asthma (theophylline, β-agonists, steroids) can affect the protective mechanisms against GERD.

Patients with asthma whose symptoms are worse after meals, or those who do not respond to traditional asthma medications, should be suspected of having GERD. Additionally, patients who experience heartburn and regurgitation before the onset of asthma symptoms may have GERD as a potential cause for worsening asthma symptoms. Patients often present with adult-onset symptoms that are only partially responsive to aggressive asthma therapies. Most will report presence of heartburn and occasionally regurgitation. Aggressive therapy of *both* GERD and asthma are indicated in this group of patients in order to provide symptomatic relief for these difficult to treat patients.

Chronic Cough

GERD is one of the three most common causes of chronic cough (asthma and postnasal drip being the other two) [13,14]. Similar to asthma, GERD and chronic cough can induce each other. GERD can induce chronic cough through both laryngeal and tracheobronchial irritation by refluxed material, and by vagal stimulation. Chronic cough increases the negative intrathoracic pressure for short times, making reflux events more likely.

GERD-related chronic cough typically occurs during the day, in the upright position, and is non-productive. GERD should be suspected in patients with cough whose symptoms have been chronic, not smokers, not on any cough-inducing medications (such as angiotensin-converting enzyme (ACE) inhibitors), with normal chest X-ray, and in those in whom there is no evidence of asthma or postnasal drip. The American College of Chest Physicians have named the above clinical criteria for suspecting GERD-related cough, and they concur with

the treatment recommendations below [15]. Presence of regurgitation, especially when in the supine position or when symptoms worsen after meals, may be useful clues.

The differential for chronic cough includes asthma, postnasal drip, GERD, chronic lung disease (including chronic bronchitis, restrictive lung diseases and infiltrative lung diseases), toxic inhalants, and tic disorders. However, it is imperative that patients are initially investigated for malignancy and medication-related causes.

Non-cardiac Chest Pain

In approximately one-third of patients with angina-type symptoms, ischemia is excluded and no etiology for the pain is found; 25–50% of those patients will have abnormal reflux events on pH monitoring, suggesting that GERD may have a role in causing the chest pain. Direct contact of the esophageal mucosa with gastroduodenal agents such as acid and pepsin, leading to vagal stimulation, is the most likely cause of these symptoms [16,17]. Other GI etiologies may include esophageal motility disorders such as nutcracker esophagus or diffuse esophageal spasm.

Data suggest that GERD may account for symptoms in 25–55% of patients with non-cardiac chest pain [16]. The differentiation of angina versus non-cardiac chest pain can be difficult, as GERD and coronary artery disease (CAD) often co-exist. Some studies have found correlations between ST segment changes on Holter monitoring with reflux events. Furthermore, reflux can be worsened with exercise, particularly running, and can cause non-cardiac chest pain mimicking exertional angina. Long-term follow up of patients diagnosed with non-cardiac chest pain do not show increased mortality compared to the general population, so the classification of non-cardiac chest pain does not represent a failure to diagnose cardiac chest pain. Medications such as nitroglycerin and calcium channel blockers used to treat angina may also relieve symptoms caused by esophageal spasm. However, these medications also relax the lower esophageal sphincter, possibly leading to increased reflux events.

GERD-related chest pain may be indistinguishable from angina. Other causes of chest pain may include esophageal motility disorders, gastritis, peptic ulcer disease, or chronic pancreatitis. Because of the difficulty in distinguishing the two and the implications of making the incorrect diagnosis, cardiac chest pain should always be ruled out before diagnosing GERD or embarking on a search for gastrointestinal causes for chest pain.

Dental Erosions

Acid reflux in the oral cavity causes chemical erosion of the coronal tooth structure. This differs from dental caries in that the process does not involve bacteria. However, both processes ultimately result in the loss of the tooth. Schroeder *et al.* found a relationship between reflux events on ambulatory pH monitoring and dental erosions [18]. They took 12 patients identified by dentists as having dental erosions and performed 24-h pH monitoring. Ten out of these 12 patients were found to have GERD on pH monitoring. They also looked at 30 patients who had undergone pH monitoring for GERD and referred them for dental evaluation. Seven out of those 10 patients who had proximal reflux events on pH monitoring were found to have dental erosions, compared to four out of 10 with distal reflux and one out of 10 without reflux. Other processes that can contribute to erosion include impaired saliva production, altered buffering capacity, and frequent vomiting.

Obstructive Sleep Apnea

Obstructive sleep apnea may be a cause rather than a result of nocturnal reflux events. This may be due to episodes of significant negative intrathoracic pressure and traction on the phrenoesophageal ligament. However, as for asthma, prevalence studies suggest an association while the causal relationship remains elusive.

Otitis Media

Small-scale, observational studies suggest that otitis media may be related to GERD. Tasker *et al.* have found pepsin and pepsinogen in fluid taken from the middle ear cavity [19]. They sampled fluid taken from the middle ear cavity of 65 children undergoing myringotomy and found that 59/65 samples contained pepsinogen or pepsin, 29% of which were active. They concluded that refluxate can reach the middle ear and that treatment of GERD should be considered in patients with otitis media with effusion. This may be more important in children.

Diagnostic Approach

Given the non-specific nature of the extraesophageal symptoms and the poor sensitivity and specificity of diagnostic tests such as pH monitoring, laryngoscopy, or endoscopy for establishing a GERD etiology, empiric therapy with PPIs has become common practice. Testing is usually indicated in patients with persistent symptoms despite therapy, those with warning signs (i.e., dysphagia, weight loss, bleeding), prior to fundoplication, or in those patients with long-standing GERD in order to rule out Barrett esophagus. Common tests include endoscopy, and 24-h pH monitoring.

Endoscopy

Esophagitis is uncommonly seen in extraesophageal GERD patients. In contrast to typical GERD patients, in whom esophagitis is seen in 50% of endoscopies, esophagitis is found in extraesophageal GERD patients only 10–30% of the time. Therefore, it is neither a sensitive nor specific tool for diagnosing extraesophageal GERD. However, if a patient has warning signs or is considering surgery, endoscopy is indicated. In most patients presenting with continued symptoms, endoscopy is performed not to rule in GERD but to rule out other upper GI structural causes for patients' symptoms.

Laryngoscopy

Patients with laryngeal symptoms are often referred to ENT for laryngoscopy. Findings on laryngoscopy do not necessarily implicate gastric contents as the causative irritants. The initial endoscopic lesions associated with GERD were erosions and lesions such as vocal cord ulcerations. However, erythema and edema are now considered by many in the ENT community to suggest GERD [20]. The identifying findings in reflux laryngitis include erythematous arytenoids and a gray appearance of the interarytenoid region. Additionally, patients with GERD may exhibit abnormalities such as erythema and edema of the posterior larynx, vocal cord polyps granuloma, subglottic stenosis, ulcerations, vocal cord nodules, leukoplakia, and cancer. These findings are not specific for GERD; other causes of these findings may include smoking, alcohol, postnasal drip, viral illness, voice overuse, or environmental allergens. Studies suggest that laryngeal abnormalities involving the vocal cords and medial arytenoid walls may be more specific for GERD

[2]. Laryngoscopy in patients with throat symptoms is not to rule in GERD but to rule out cancer and causes other than GERD. The suspicion of GERD in this group is not based on specific laryngeal findings but more on a lack of more serious condition and uncertainty for the role of other factors.

pH Monitoring

Twenty-four hour pH monitoring has been used by some to diagnose reflux, but its utility is hampered by poor sensitivity (70–80%) and frequent false negatives (20–50%). Studies are conflicting as to the usefulness of pH monitoring in diagnosing extraesophageal GERD. This may be due to several factors, including variable probe position, the definition of abnormal reflux, day-to-day variability of reflux events, and the intermittent nature of reflux events. The presence of acid in the upper esophagus and hypopharynx may be seen in up to 10% of asymptomatic volunteers. Therefore, 24-h pH monitoring can neither definitively diagnose nor exclude extraesophageal reflux as the cause of patients' symptoms. Wireless pH monitoring may increase the sensitivity of pH monitoring by capturing rare events during prolonged monitoring. However, since most patients in whom this test is utilized are symptomatic despite therapy the unresolved question is whether to perform pH monitoring on or off PPI therapy. Recent data suggest on-therapy testing with impedance monitoring may be the single best test [21]. However, this point is controversial and some suggest off-therapy testing as the initial diagnostic approach [22]. Impedance/pH monitoring increases the sensitivity of the traditional ambulatory pH testing by detecting non-acid liquid (decreased impedance) or gas reflux (increased impedance). The most recent AGA guidelines suggest empiric therapy followed by pH monitoring for those unresponsive [23].

Therapeutic Approach

Given the non-specific nature of the extraesophageal symptoms and the poor sensitivity and specificity of diagnostic tests such as pH monitoring, laryngoscopy, or endoscopy for establishing a GERD etiology, empiric therapy with PPIs has become common practice (Figure 32.1). Most therapeutic trials of these syndromes have used twice-daily dosing of PPIs for treatment periods of 3 to 4 months. The rationale for this dosing comes from pH monitoring data demonstrating that the likelihood of normalizing esophageal acid exposure with twice daily PPIs in GERD patients is 93–99%; the logic then being that lesser dosing does not exclude the possibility of a poor response because of inadequate acid suppression. Having said that, there are no controlled studies investi-

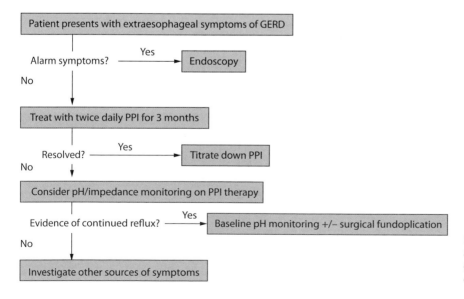

Figure 32.1 Management algorithm for extraesophageal gastroesophageal reflux disease.

gating the optimal dosage or duration of PPI therapy in extraesophageal GERD syndromes. The only supportive data for twice-daily PPI dosing are uncontrolled open-label studies of suspected reflux laryngitis or asthma. Patients are difficult to treat and may not respond to traditional therapy, perhaps because of the over-diagnosis of extraesophageal GERD.

The fact that placebo-controlled trials in patients with extraesophageal symptoms [24,25] show a limited or no benefit from PPIs compared to placebo, is probably due to several reasons: (i) An overlap in extra-esophageal symptoms and signs between GERD and other causes which leads to over-diagnosis of GERD; (ii) multifactorial nature of the presenting extraesophageal symptoms, with GERD as only one of the causes; and (iii) the possibility of weakly acidic or non-acid reflux as the etiology for persistent symptoms in some patients unresponsive to PPI therapy.

"Step-down therapy" is recommended for patients with extraesophageal GERD (Figure 32.1). Initial therapy with twice daily PPI dosing should be limited with an endpoint of titration to the lowest dose of acid suppression with controlled symptoms or to no acid suppression if symptoms do not improve after 2 months of therapy. pH/impedance monitoring on therapy could be considered to help identify that small subgroup that continues to have abnormal esophageal acid or non-acid exposure. However, in most non-responders search for other potential etiologies for patients' symptoms should be explored.

Surgical Treatment

Surgery does not seem to benefit patients who do not respond to PPI therapy. Allen and Anvari studied surgical treatment of GERD in chronic cough. In their 42 patients, 51% had resolution of cough and 31% had improvement [26]. They later determined that response to PPI predicted surgical outcome. Similarly, in a concurrent controlled study of non-responders to PPIs, Swoger *et al.* established that surgical fundoplication is of limited clinical utility after 1 year follow up of symptoms and objective parameters [27]. A recent study in 17 patients with positive symptom index on impedance monitoring found that surgical fundoplication was successful in 94% of cases [28]. However, the lack of a control group and multiple study biases limit the conclusions from this study. Thus, at this point, surgical fundoplication cannot

be recommended to those unresponsive to PPI therapy unless symptoms such as regurgitation are accompanied by endoscopic findings of hiatal hernia and baseline abnormal acid reflux parameters.

Case continued

Our patient had no warning signs that necessitated endoscopy. She had not had an adequate trial of PPI therapy, since she had only been intermittently on a once-daily PPI. Therefore, she was initiated on a 2-month trial of twice-daily PPI without any further testing. She had complete resolution of her heartburn, and her throat clearing and cough had improved. She did not notice a difference in her asthma symptoms. Impedance pH monitoring on therapy suggested control of acid and non-acid reflux. pH monitoring off therapy suggested only mild reflux at baseline in the upright position and the PPI dose was reduced to once daily to be taken prior to breakfast. The patient continued to show symptomatic improvement of her heartburn and throat clearing.

Take-home points

- Extraesophageal reflux disease is an increasingly recognized complication of reflux of gastric contents presenting with different symptomatic manifestations.

- The mechanism of extraesophageal GERD involves both a reflex (vagal stimulation) and reflux (microaspiration, chemical irritation) pathway.

- Endoscopy and pH monitoring are poorly sensitive and are not required for the diagnosis of extraesophageal GERD but indicated in the presence of alarm symptoms.

- GERD should be suspected in patients with cough whose symptoms have been chronic, non-smokers, not on any cough-inducing medications (such as ACE inhibitors), with normal chest X-ray, and in those in whom there is no evidence of asthma or postnasal drip.

- Reflux into the larynx can cause laryngeal irritation which can cause voice symptoms.

- Dual impedance/pH monitoring may improve the sensitivity and specificity of diagnostic testing; however, outcome data are needed to better understand its role in this group of patients.

References

1 Vaezi MF. Therapy insight: gastroesophageal reflux disease and laryngopharyngeal reflux. *Nat Clin Pract Gastroenterol Hepatol* 2005; **2**: 595–603.

2 Vaezi MF, Hicks DM, Abelson TI, Richter JE. Laryngeal signs and symptoms and gastroesophageal reflux disease: a critical assessment of cause and effect association. *Clin Gastroenterol Hepatol* 2003; **1**: 333–44.

3 Koufman JA. The otolaryngologic manifestations of gastro-esophageal reflux disease (GERD): a clinical investigation of 225 patients using ambulatory 24-hour pH monitoring and an experimental investigation of the role of acid and pepsin in the development of laryngeal injury. *Laryngoscope* 1991; **101** (Suppl. 53): 1–78.

4 Vakil N, van Zanten SV, Kahrilas P, *et al.* and the Global Consensus Group. The Montreal definition and classification of gastroesophageal reflux disease: a global evidence-based consensus. *Am J Gastroenterol* 2006; **101**: 1900–20.

5 Garcia-Campean D, Gonzalez MV, Galindo G, *et al.* Prevalence of gastroesophageal reflux disease in patients with extraesophageal symptoms referred from Otolaryngology, Allergy and Cardiology practices: A prospective study. *Dig Dis* 2000; **18**: 178–82.

6 Shaker R. Protective mechanisms against supraesophageal GERD. *Clin Gastroenterol* 2000; **30**: S3–S8.

7 el-Serag HB, Sonnenberg A. Comorbid occurrence of laryngeal or pulmonary disease with esophagitis in United States military veterans. *Gastroenterology* 1997; **113**: 755–60.

8 Havemann BD, Henderson CA, El-Serag HB. The association between gastro-oesophageal reflux disease and asthma: a systematic review. *Gut* 2007; **56**: 1654–64.

9 Vakil N. The frontiers of reflux disease. *Dig Dis Sci* 2006; **51**: 1887–95.

10 Adhami T, Goldblum JR, Richter JE, Vaezi MF. The role of gastric and duodenal agents in laryngeal injury: an experimental canine model. *Am J Gastroenterol* 2004; **99**: 2098–106.

11 el-Serag HB, Hepworth EJ, Lee P, *et al.* Gastroesophageal reflux disease is a risk factor for laryngeal and pharyngeal cancer. *Am J Gastroenterol* 2001; **96**: 2013–8.

12 Wright RA, Miller SA, Corsello BF. Acid-induced esophago-bronchial-cardiac reflexes in humans. *Gastroenterology* 1990; **99**: 71–3.

13 Irwin RS, Richter JE. Gastroesophageal reflux and chronic cough. *Am J Med* 2000; **95**: S9–S14.

14 Irwin RS, Curley FJ, French CL. Chronic cough. *Am Rev Respir Dis* 1990; **141**: 640–7.

15 Irwin R. Chronic cough due to gastroesophageal reflux disease: ACCP evidence-based clinical practice guidelines. *Chest* 2006; **129**: 80–94.

16 Richter J. Chest pain and gastroesophageal reflux disease. *J Clin Gastroenterol* 2000; **30**: S39–S41.

17 Ockene MS. Unexplained chest pain in patients with normal coronary arteriograms: A follow-up study of functional status. *N Engl J Med* 1980; **30**: 1249–52.

18 Schroeder PL, Filler SJ, Ramirez B, *et al.* Dental erosion and acid reflux disease. *Ann Intern Med* 1995; **122**: 809–15.

19 Tasker A, Dettmar PW, Panetti M, *et al.* Is gastric reflux a cause of otitis media with effusion in children? *Laryngoscope* 2002; **112**: 1930–4.

20 Ahmed T, Khandwala F, Abelson TI, *et al.* Chronic Laryngitis associated with GERD: prospective assessment of differences in practice patterns between gastroenterologists and ENT physicians. *Am J Gastroenterol* 2006; **101**: 470–8.

21 Pritchett JM, Slaughter JC, Vaezi MF. Is esophageal impedance monitoring detecting something new? A case-control study assessing predictive nature of non-acid reflux. *Gastroenterology* 2008; **134**: 711 (A-101).

22 Hemmink GJ, Bredenoord AJ, Weusten BL, *et al.* Esophageal pH-impedance monitoring in patients with therapy-resistant reflux symptoms: "on" or "off" proton pump inhibitor? *Am J Gastroenterol* 2008; **103**: 1–8.

23 Kahrilas P, Shaheen N, Vaezi MF. American Gastroenterologic Association Medical position statement on the management of gastroesophageal reflux disease. *Gastroenterology* 2008; **135**: 1383–91.

24 Littner MR, Leung FW, Ballard ED, *et al.* Effects of 24 weeks of lansoprazole therapy on asthma symptoms, exacerbations, quality of life, and pulmonary function in adult asthmatic patients with acid reflux symptoms. *Chest* 2005; **128**: 1128–35.

25 Qadeer MA, 1Department of Gastroenterology and HepatologyPhillips CO, 2Department of General Internal Medicine3Department of Quantitative Health Sciences, Cleveland Clinic Foundation, Cleveland, OhioLopez AR,3Department of Quantitative Health Sciences, Cleveland Clinic Foundation, Cleveland, Ohio *et al.* Proton pump inhibitor therapy for suspected GERD-related laryngitis: a meta analysis of randomized controlled trials. *Am J Gastroenterol* 2006; **101**: 2646–54.

26 Allen CJ, Anvari M. Gastro-oesophageal reflux related cough and its response to laparoscopic fundoplication. *Thorax* 1998; **53**: 963–8.

27 Swoger J, Ponsky J, Hicks DM, *et al.* Surgical fundoplication in laryngopharyngeal reflux unresponsive to aggressive acid suppression: a controlled study. *Clin Gastroenterology Hepatol* 2006; **4**: 433–41.

28 Mainie I, Tutuian R, Agrawal A, *et al.* Combined multichannel intraluminal impedance-pH monitoring to select patients with persistent gastro-oesophageal reflux for laparoscopic Nissen fundoplication. *Br J Surg* 2006; **93**: 1483–7.

CHAPTER 33
Barrett Esophagus

Yvonne Romero, Vikneswaran Namasivayam, and Kee Wook Jung

Division of Gastroenterology and Hepatology, Department of Medicine, Mayo Clinic, Rochester, MN, USA

Summary

In the USA, esophageal cancer is uncommon with approximately 14 000 new cases diagnosed annually. Squamous cell carcinoma and adenocarcinoma are the two important histologic types of esophageal cancer. Thirty years ago, squamous cell cancer was by far the most common type of esophageal cancer in the USA, and adenocarcinoma of the esophagus has been increasing in frequency over the last few decades to the point that it is now the most common type of esophageal cancer. Gastroesophageal reflux disease and Barrett esophagus are the major known risk factors for esophageal adenocarcinoma. Specific endoscopic and pathologic criteria must be met before diagnosing a patient with Barrett esophagus, which is considered a premalignant condition. A false-positive diagnosis can have serious psychological and financial consequences. This review summarizes the criteria for the diagnosis of Barrett esophagus, which should be distinguished from intestinal metaplasia of the cardia, as this carries far less neoplastic risk. Surveillance recommendations for patients with Barrett esophagus are summarized, and practical treatment options for patients with dysplasia in Barrett esophagus are also presented.

Case

One year ago, during an endoscopic examination for the evaluation of abdominal pain, a 66-year-old white man who had no history of heartburn or acid regurgitation was diagnosed with Barrett esophagus by his family physician. He had never used acid-suppressing medications. Last year's endoscopy report described "an irregular Z-line." The pathology report reads: "Barrett's cells present without dysplasia." The pathology slides are sent to your office for review and your pathologist agrees that there is intestinal metaplasia with goblet cells without dysplasia. At his first surveillance endoscopy the Z-line (the squamocolumnar junction) is located at the top of the gastric folds. There is a small 2-cm hiatus hernia. Due to the previous diagnosis of Barrett esophagus, biopsies are collected from the normal appearing and normally located Z-line, and show focal intestinal metaplasia with goblet cells, without dysplasia. Surveillance is no longer advised. As a result of this disparity in diagnosis the patient requests another appointment with you. He is told that at the most recent endoscopy no changes of Barrett esophagus were seen in the "tubular esophagus" and it is probable that the first set of biopsies was taken from the "top of the stomach."

Practical Gastroenterology and Hepatology: Esophagus and Stomach, 1st edition. Edited by Nicholas J. Talley, Kenneth R. DeVault and David E. Fleischer. © 2010 Blackwell Publishing Ltd.

Barrett Esophagus

Definition and Epidemiology

Barrett esophagus is the condition in which the lining of the esophagus changes from stratified squamous epithelium to an abnormal columnar epithelium that has both gastric and intestinal features [1]. The condition is judged to be a consequence of chronic gastroesophageal reflux disease (GERD). Barrett metaplasia predisposes to the development of esophageal adenocarcinoma, a malignancy with an incidence that has increased by more than 500% over the past three decades in Western countries [2].

Diagnosis

The diagnosis of Barrett esophagus is established by endoscopic examination and esophageal biopsy. To diagnose Barrett esophagus, the endoscopist must ascertain that columnar epithelium extends proximal to the gastroesophageal junction, and biopsy specimens of that esophageal columnar lining must show metaplasia [3]. The gastroesophageal junction is the level at which the esophagus joins the stomach, and is defined endoscopically as the top of the gastric folds. This region can be

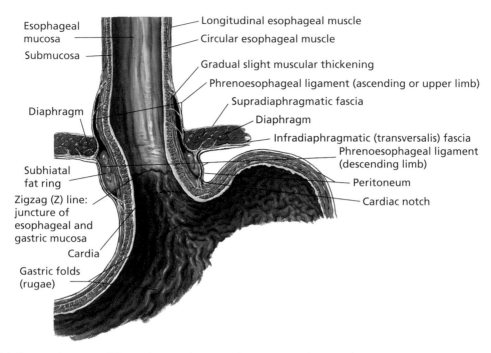

Esophageal mucosa
Submucosa
Diaphragm
Subhiatal fat ring
Zigzag (Z) line: juncture of esophageal and gastric mucosa
Cardia
Gastric folds (rugae)

Longitudinal esophageal muscle
Circular esophageal muscle
Gradual slight muscular thickening
Phrenoesophageal ligament (ascending or upper limb)
Supradiaphragmatic fascia
Diaphragm
Infradiaphragmatic (transversalis) fascia
Phrenoesophageal ligament (descending limb)
Peritoneum
Cardiac notch

Figure 33.1 The normal anatomy of the esophagus and gastroesophageal junction. (Reprinted from Netter's Gastroenterology © Elsevier Inc. All rights reserved)

difficult to localize with precision, however. Normally, the pale-pink stratified squamous epithelium that lines the esophagus can be distinguished easily from the red-colored columnar epithelium of the stomach (Figure 33.1). These two epithelial types normally meet at the top of the gastric folds. This squamocolumnar junction, which is commonly saw-toothed or zigzag in distribution, is often called the Z-line (Figure 33.1). Commonly, the squamocolumnar junction (Z-line) and the gastroesophageal junction (top of the gastric folds) coincide.

The endoscopist suspects Barrett esophagus when salmon-colored epithelium, similar in appearance to that of the stomach, extends above the gastroesophageal junction into the distal esophagus (Figure 33.2). The diagnosis is confirmed when biopsy specimens of the esophageal columnar lining reveal intestinal metaplasia with goblet cells (Figure 33.3), also known as specialized intestinal metaplasia. The term "long-segment Barrett esophagus" has been used when specialized intestinal metaplasia lines at least 3 cm of the distal esophagus (Figure 33.4). The term "short-segment Barrett esophagus" refers to segments of specialized intestinal metaplasia that line <3 cm

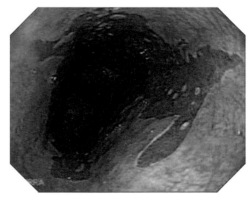

Figure 33.2 Barrett esophagus at endoscopy. (Courtesy of Joseph A. Murray, MD.)

of the esophagus. The existence of short-segment Barrett esophagus was not widely appreciated until 1985. Reports published before that time include primarily cases of long-segment Barrett esophagus. Although the 3 cm cut-off measurement is arbitrary, its continued use is helpful in genetic studies in which clarity of the phenotype is imperative to distinguish Barrett esophagus from intestinal metaplasia of the cardia.

Prevalence

The prevalence of Barrett esophagus among white people of European decent in developed countries does not appear to have changed significantly over the past two decades [4]. Two landmark population-based studies conducted in enumerated cohorts of predominantly Scandinavian and German descent have shown the age- and sex-adjusted prevalence of Barrett segments >3 cm

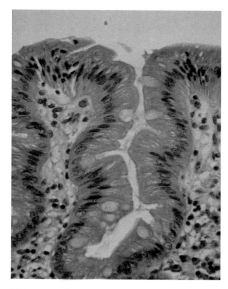

Figure 33.3 Intestinal metaplasia with goblet cells. (From Romero [4], with permission of the Mayo Foundation for Medical Education and Research and courtesy of Dr Thomas C. Smyrk.)

length to have been 0.34% in 1990 [5], compared with 0.5% in 2005 for Barrett segments >2 cm in length [6]. The 2005 study did not report the number of cases with classic long-segment Barrett esophagus and hence a direct comparison in prevalence between the two points in time cannot be made. Trends in the diagnosis of Barrett esophagus over time have been difficult to measure accurately because of substantial increases in access to endoscopy, and improvement in physician recognition of short-segment disease.

Risk Factors

Risk factors for Barrett esophagus include advanced age, male sex, white ethnicity, and GERD symptoms of prolonged (>5 years) duration [7]. Alcohol use, particularly beer and spirits, may be weakly associated with Barrett esophagus, but to a far lesser extent. Red wine may have a mildly protective effect [8]. Tobacco use also has a weak association with Barrett esophagus [9]. The role of genetics and obesity is currently under investigation. Families with multiple members with Barrett esophagus or esophageal cancer have been reported [10–12]. Obesity is a strong risk factor for esophageal adenocarcinoma [13–15]; its role in Barrett esophagus is less certain. It is not known if being overweight or obese increases the risk of neoplastic progression in patients with Barrett esophagus or whether weight loss can reduce the risk.

Barrett esophagus is an acquired disorder thought to develop in genetically predisposed individuals in response to chronic reflux. The mean age at time of diagnosis is

Figure 33.4 Patients with long-segment Barrett esophagus (image on the right-hand side of the figure) or short-segment Barrett esophagus (middle image) have salmon-colored mucosa extending proximally into the tubular esophagus. Biopsy specimens show intestinal metaplasia with goblet cells. When intestinal metaplasia with goblet cells is found on biopsy of a normal appearing and normally located Z-line, the patient meets the criteria for intestinal metaplasia of the cardia (image on left-hand side of the figure). (From Romero [4], with permission of the Mayo Foundation for Medical Education and Research. Courtesy of Alan Cameron, MD.)

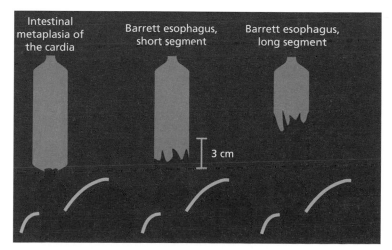

63 years. This is not meant to imply that Barrett esophagus develops at age 63; it may have been present for decades before diagnosis. Age as a risk factor is biased by the presence of GERD symptoms, individual healthcare-seeking behavior, the availability of open-access endoscopy, and physician threshold in requesting endoscopy. Barrett esophagus is rarely diagnosed in children, and most documented cases in children are associated with altered mental status (such as with Down syndrome) or with a disorder that predisposes to severe reflux (such as cerebral palsy). Large cohort and population-based studies have shown men to have a 1.5- to 2.6-fold higher risk of Barrett esophagus compared with women [7,16]. Long-segment Barrett esophagus is frequently described in Western countries but appears to be far less common in Asia. The prevalence of Barrett esophagus in a recent report of a Chinese population undergoing endoscopy was 0.06%, most with short-segment disease [17]. The disease is uncommon in Korea [18]. In multiracial Malaysia, Barrett esophagus is more often diagnosed in Indians than in other ethnic groups [19]. Within the USA, a single tertiary care center located in a major multiracial metropolis published a retrospective cross-sectional cohort report of 2100 people endoscoped between 2005 and 2006. White individuals (6.1%) were far more likely to have Barrett esophagus of any length compared with black (1.6%, $p = 0.004$) and Hispanic individuals (1.7%, $p = 0.0002$) [20].

Heartburn, defined as a burning pain or discomfort behind the breastbone in the chest, and acid regurgitation, a bitter or sour-tasting fluid coming up into the throat, are classic GERD symptoms. Among white adults, 3.5–7% with GERD symptoms have long-segment Barrett esophagus [21]. However, even some asymptomatic white adults have been found to have long-segment Barrett esophagus on endoscopic examinations. Only 0.2% of African Americans with GERD symptoms have Barrett esophagus. The role of genetics, lifestyle, diet, medications, supplements, socioeconomic status, perception of reflux, healthcare-seeking behavior, and access to healthcare, and their relative contributions to the development and diagnosis of Barrett esophagus have yet to be clarified. What is known is that patients who are newly diagnosed with Barrett esophagus overestimate their risk of cancer [22] and face increased insurance premiums [23].

Cancer Risk

As a group, individuals with Barrett esophagus have a 30- to 50-fold higher risk of esophageal adenocarcinoma compared with those without Barrett esophagus (relative risk) [3]. The annual absolute risk of malignant transformation is approximately 0.005, i.e., 1 cancer develops per 200 patient-years [24]. It has been estimated that a 50-year-old man with Barrett esophagus and otherwise normal life expectancy has a 3–10% lifetime risk (cumulative incidence) of developing esophageal adenocarcinoma. Thus, more than 90% of Barrett esophagus patients will not develop cancer. Most people will die with Barrett esophagus rather than from its complications. An individual's risk is best estimated by the degree of dysplasia found in esophageal biopsy specimens.

Genetic instability precedes the development of dysplasia, which develops as a consequence of genetic abnormalities and mutations that give cells growth advantages. For patients without dysplasia, the cancer risk is <0.5% per year. The cancer risk for patients with low-grade dysplasia is 8–10% over 5 years (Figure 33.5) and, for

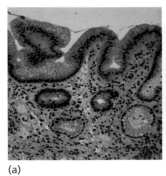
(a)

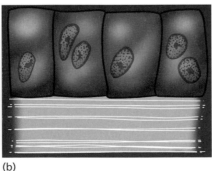
(b)

Figure 33.5 Low-grade dysplasia. (Part (a) is courtesy of Thomas C. Smyrk, MD.)

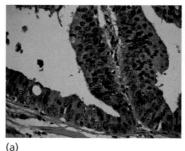
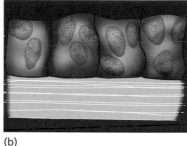

Figure 33.6 High-grade dysplasia. (Part (a) is courtesy of Thomas C. Smyrk, MD.)

(a)   (b)

Table 33.1 The 2008 American College of Gastroenterology surveillance recommendations based on the degree of dysplasia.

Most severe degree of dysplasia	Documentation	Follow-up
No dysplasia	Two EGDs with biopsy *within* 1 year	EGD every 3 years
Low-grade dysplasia	Expert pathologist confirmation Next EGD *within* 6 months	EGD every year until no dysplasia × 2, then can return to no dysplasia algorithm
High-grade dysplasia	Mucosal irregularity Repeat EGD with biopsies to rule out adenocarcinoma within 3 months Expert pathologist confirmation	Endoscopic resection Continued 3-monthly surveillance or intervention based on results and patient

EGD, esophagogastroduodenoscopy.

patients with high-grade dysplasia, the risk of cancer is 28–36% over 5 years (Figure 33.6). These varying risks of neoplastic progression have resulted in surveillance and management guidelines based on the most severe degree of dysplasia detected at endoscopy. Updated guidelines were published in 2008 [25] (Table 33.1).

Surveillance Intervals

If at initial endoscopy no dysplasia is detected, the recommendation is to repeat endoscopy within 1 year to exclude prevalent cancer. If dysplasia is not present at the second endoscopic procedure, the surveillance interval can be increased to every 3 years.

Upon identification of low-grade dysplasia, the recommendation is to repeat endoscopy within 6 months. If the repeat examination confirms low-grade dysplasia, annual endoscopy is recommended. However, it appears that low-grade dysplasia may regress. If no dysplasia is seen on annual surveillance examinations for 2 years in a row, the recommendation is to repeat endoscopy at 3 years.

If endoscopy shows high-grade dysplasia, a number of management options are available (see Treatment below).

The American College of Gastroenterology recommends consideration of endoscopic resection of any focal lesion to obtain more tissue for more accurate staging of disease.

There is considerable interobserver variation among pathologists in the grading of dysplasia. Therefore, the American College of Gastroenterology recommends that the esophageal biopsy specimens of patients initially deemed to have low- or high-grade dysplasia be reviewed by an expert gastrointestinal pathologist before acting on the results. Inflammation commonly causes reactive atypia, a cellular response to inflammation that can be mistaken for dysplasia. Therefore, one should attempt to optimize medical management of GERD with aggressive acid suppression before endoscopic examination for patients with Barrett esophagus to minimize the effects of reflux esophagitis on the interpretation of dysplasia.

Surveillance Technique

The recommendations listed above are predicated on the assumption that an adequate number of surveillance biopsies has been collected. Although various surveillance biopsy strategies have been proposed, the minimal criteria, from both medical and legal perspectives, are as follows:

• Inspect the Barrett esophagus segment carefully

• Biopsy any unusual areas, such as ulcers or nodules, first

• In separate bottles, place four-quadrant biopsies collected at 2-cm intervals.

For example, a bland 5-cm segment of Barrett esophagus should result in a minimum of 12 biopsy specimens placed in 3 pathology bottles (Figure 33.7). Even with this time-consuming process, less than 5% of the surface area of the esophagus is sampled. The logic behind this recommendation is the patchy nature of dysplasia best demonstrated in the work of Cameron and Carpenter in 1997 (Figure 33.8) [26]. In their project, the esophagectomy specimens of patients who underwent surgery for high-grade dysplasia were mapped for degree of dysplasia. In Figure 33.8, in the third specimen on the right, an early

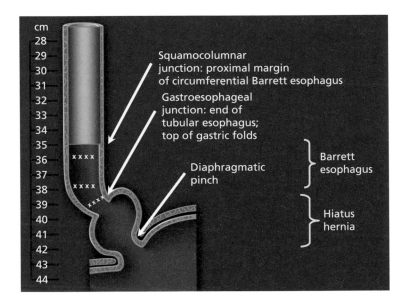

Figure 33.7 Surveillance biopsies for Barrett esophagus.

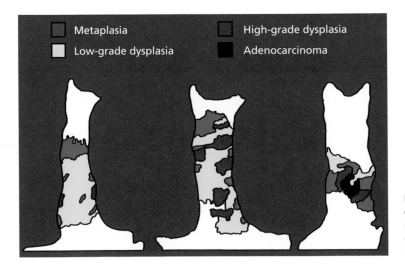

Figure 33.8 Mapping dysplasia in three esophagectomy specimen from patients who proceeded to surgery for high-grade dysplasia. (From Cameron and Carpenter [26], with permission.)

cancer was present, but was not appreciated by the endoscopist. The purpose of collecting randomly distributed biopsies is to detect dysplasia or early cancer that is not apparent to the naked eye. Sampling error is one of the greatest limitations of the management of patients with Barrett esophagus.

Treatment

The management of Barrett esophagus consists of medical therapy to control GERD symptoms and heal reflux esophagitis, and periodic surveillance endoscopy to identify high-grade dysplasia, the threshold for intervention.

Medical Therapy

There is no convincing evidence that medical therapy causes complete regression of Barrett esophagus. Medical therapy is important in resolving heartburn and acid regurgitation, and in healing reflux esophagitis. Although considerable indirect evidence suggests that reduction of gastric acid secretion with proton pump inhibitors (PPIs) may have a cancer-preventive role in Barrett esophagus, there is no definitive evidence that PPI therapy diminishes the risk of cancer. Some authorities have even proposed that PPI therapy may increase neoplastic risk, but this has not been demonstrated in population-based studies.

Surgery

There is no definitive evidence that fundoplication to limit reflux of gastric contents into the esophagus diminishes the risk of neoplastic progression in patients with Barrett esophagus.

Until recently, the standard of care for patients with Barrett esophagus with high-grade dysplasia or early superficial stage I esophageal adenocarcinoma had been esophagectomy because, in retrospective series, 11–43% of patients undergoing resection were found to harbor occult carcinoma [27]. More recent data suggest that this risk may be lower [28]. Esophagectomy should still be considered for younger and physically fit patients with high-grade dysplasia because it is the only modality that removes locoregional lymph nodes. Patients interested in pursuing esophagectomy should be referred to high-volume centers, as perioperative mortality rates vary from 3% to 20%, depending on the experience of the center [29].

Endoscopic Approaches

Endoscopic approaches that can be used to remove or ablate dysplastic epithelium include endoscopic mucosal resection, photodynamic therapy, radiofrequency ablation, and cryotherapy [30–33]. These techniques are discussed in detail in Chapters 10 and 11. These methods are always combined with acid suppression therapy, based on the observation that re-injury to metaplastic epithelium followed by healing in a low acid environment can lead to re-epithelialization with neosquamous mucosa. All endoscopic approaches carry the risk of recurrence or neoplastic progression, because residual columnar cells that escape destruction may still possesses neoplastic potential, and none of the endoscopic approaches can remove cancers that have metastasized to periesophageal lymph nodes. Hence, continued clinical and endoscopic surveillance is required. The risk of stricture formation for each technique is linearly related to depth of injury.

Observation: Intense Surveillance

The initial 1998 recommendations of the American College of Gastroenterology included the option of intense (four quadrant biopsies every 1 cm) surveillance (every 3 months), especially for patients with high-grade dysplasia who are too old or infirm to undergo esophagectomy. If the high-grade dysplasia were to progress to cancer, then the patient and physician would have to decide whether to accept the higher risk of mortality from esophagectomy, or to consider other forms of palliative therapy. This scenario prompted many discussions about terminating surveillance in patients with Barrett esophagus with concomitant severe co-morbidities. The option to offer intense surveillance to patients with high-grade dysplasia remains in the updated 2008 guidelines, although the recent publication of high-quality studies showing the efficacy of endoscopic ablative techniques such as photodynamic therapy and radiofrequency ablation has diminished enthusiasm for the surveillance option in patients with high-grade dysplasia.

Although high-grade dysplasia is the strongest predictor of neoplastic progression to cancer at 5 years (up to 38%), this figure also implies that 60% of patients diagnosed with high-grade dysplasia will *not* develop cancer within 5 years. This may be due to a number of factors such as removal of the neoplastic cells with surveillance biopsies and over-interpretation of inflammation as dysplasia. With the advent of endoscopic mucosal resection and radiofrequency ablation, it has become more challenging to decide when to terminate surveillance.

Impact of Surveillance on Survival

The goal of endoscopic surveillance for patients with Barrett esophagus is to decrease mortality from esophageal adenocarcinoma. To achieve this goal, two major obstacles must be overcome. First, individuals at risk, meaning those with Barrett esophagus, must be identified. Second, a minimally invasive, easily accessible, and inexpensive treatment must be available that will permanently eradicate the premalignant lining. As described above, with the advent of endoscopic treatment, progress is being made on the last issue.

To date, surveillance has not been shown to increase survival for patients with Barrett esophagus or to decrease deaths from adenocarcinoma in the general population. One reason might be that most cases of Barrett esophagus in the community go undiagnosed. In a large cohort study, few (4%) patients with both Barrett esophagus and esophageal adenocarcinoma had been diagnosed with Barrett esophagus before the diagnosis of cancer [34]. In a prospective cohort study in Olmsted County, Minnesota, conducted in 1987, for every 16 people with long-segment Barrett esophagus, only one person was aware of his or her disease. In a follow-up study in the same population in 1998, this had improved to one in seven people. Assuming that radiofrequency ablation or a similar technique eventually demonstrates the favorable characteristics listed above, reducing the risk of cancer in one in seven people at risk is unlikely to substantially impact the population's mortality from esophageal cancer. Only when most people at risk have been diagnosed will surveillance have the possibility of demonstrating a survival advantage. Case series have shown that patients with Barrett esophagus who are diagnosed with esophageal adenocarcinoma during routine surveillance are usually found to have earlier stage disease and longer survival than patients simultaneously diagnosed with Barrett esophagus and cancer. These reports cannot be used to support the benefit of surveillance due to the issue of lead-time bias.

Screening for Barrett Esophagus

Screening implies testing a large population to identify those with Barrett esophagus. Screening aims to identify people with Barrett esophagus who will then undergo surveillance to identify the dysplastic changes that herald the development of carcinoma. Given that surveillance of patients with Barrett esophagus has not definitively shown a survival advantage, and due to the risk of overdiagnosis of intestinal metaplasia of the cardia as Barrett esophagus, the role of screening for Barrett esophagus remains unproved [25]. Nevertheless screening is commonly practiced and frequently employed when a physician sees a patient who has long-standing GERD and is at risk of Barrett esophagus.

Intestinal Metaplasia of the Cardia

Definition and Epidemiology

Intestinal metaplasia of the cardia is defined as the histologic finding of intestinal metaplasia with goblet cells at a normally located and normal-appearing squamocolumnar junction (the Z-line) [3,35]. Before 1994, biopsies collected from the Z-line were uncommon. Currently, intestinal metaplasia of the cardia is not classified as Barrett esophagus; 6–36% of US adults are found to have intestinal metaplasia of the cardia when endoscoped for any indication. Its prevalence increases with age, suggesting that it is an acquired condition. However, unlike Barrett esophagus, intestinal metaplasia of the cardia is found equally in men and women, white and black individuals, and those with or without GERD symptoms. The role of *Helicobacter pylori* in the development of intestinal metaplasia of the cardia is under investigation. As the risk of cancer is low and virtually the same as that of the general population, approximately 3–4 individuals/100 000 persons per year, surveillance is not specifically recommended by any professional gastrointestinal society. Two international expert work groups have advised that "the normal appearing and normally located squamocolumnar junction should not be biopsied" [3,35]. Some have even called for pathologists to avoid the temptation to describe their histologic interpretation as "Barrett cells present" in favor of "intestinal metaplasia with goblet cells present. In the right endoscopic setting, this might represent Barrett esophagus." This is especially key in the era of the internet when patients review their medical records and investigate key words, only to learn that Barrett esophagus has neoplastic potential, which may result in unnecessary psychological distress. Long-term, population-based, follow-up studies of cohorts with intestinal metaplasia of the cardia are not available, but the practical conclusion seems clear. If one in five adults has intestinal metaplasia of the cardia, and 7000 of 300 million US citizens develop esophageal adenocarcinoma annually, the risk that a single person with intestinal metaplasia of the cardia will develop adenocarcinoma must be extremely small.

Take-home points

Diagnosis

- The diagnosis of Barrett esophagus requires endoscopic recognition of columnar epithelium extending above the gastroesophageal junction into the esophagus, and histologic confirmation that the esophageal epithelium is metaplastic.

- The normal appearing and normally located squamocolumnar junction (Z-line) should not be biopsied.

- The cancer risk of Barrett esophagus without dysplasia is approximately 0.5% per year.

- The cancer risk for intestinal metaplasia of the cardia does not appear to differ substantially from that for individuals in the general population, and hence is extremely low.

Surveillance

- Guidelines delineating a recommended surveillance algorithm for Barrett esophagus are provided by national gastrointestinal societies.

- The timing of surveillance depends on the most severe degree of dysplasia within a segment of Barrett esophagus mucosa.

Therapy

- Neither acid-suppressing medications nor surgery has been proved to diminish the risk of esophageal cancer in patients with Barrett esophagus.

- Endoscopic surveillance programs have not been shown to increase survival for patients with Barrett esophagus.

- Photodynamic therapy, with or without endoscopic mucosal resection, and esophagectomy are techniques that have ≥5-year follow-up data and, in excellent hands, have similar outcomes in patients with high-grade dysplasia or early cancer in Barrett esophagus.

- Enthusiasm for the use of photodynamic therapy is tempered by its high frequency of complications, including esophageal stricture formation and photosensitivity reactions.

- Radiofrequency ablation holds great promise in eradicating dysplasia and reducing the risk of progression to cancer in patients with dysplasia in Barrett esophagus.

References

1 Spechler SJ. Clinical practice. Barrett's esophagus. *N Engl J Med* 2002; **346**: 836–42.

2 Pohl H, Welch HG. The role of overdiagnosis and reclassification in the marked increase of esophageal adenocarcinoma incidence. *J Natl Cancer Inst* 2005; **97**: 142–6.

3 Sharma P, McQuaid K, Dent J, *et al.* A critical review of the diagnosis and management of Barrett's esophagus: the AGA Chicago Workshop. *Gastroenterology* 2004; **127**: 310–30.

4 Romero Y. Barrett's esophagus and esophageal cancer. In: Hauser SC, Pardi DS, Poterucha JJ (eds), *Mayo Clinic Gastroenterology and Hepatology Board Review*, 3rd edn. Rochester: Mayo Clinic Scientific Press; 2008: 21–32.

5 Cameron AJ, Zinsmeister AR, Ballard DJ, Carney JA. Prevalence of columnar-lined (Barrett's) esophagus. Comparison of population-based clinical and autopsy findings. *Gastroenterology* 1990; **99**: 918–22.

6 Ronkainen J, Aro P, Storskrubb T, *et al.* Prevalence of Barrett's esophagus in the general population: an endoscopic study. *Gastroenterology* 2005; **129**: 1825–31.

7 Holmes RS, Vaughan TL. Epidemiology and pathogenesis of esophageal cancer. *Semin Radiat Oncol* 2007; **17**: 2–9.

8 Kubo A, Levin TR, Block G, *et al.* Alcohol types and sociodemographic characteristics as risk factors for Barrett's esophagus. *Gastroenterology* 2009; **136**: 806–15.

9 Kubo A, Levin TR, Block G, *et al.* Cigarette smoking and the risk of Barrett's esophagus. *Cancer Causes Control* 2009; **20**: 303–11.

10 Crabb DW, Berk MA, Hall TR, Conneally PM, Biegel AA, Lehman GA. Familial gastroesophageal reflux and development of Barrett's esophagus. *Ann Intern Med* 1985; **103**: 52–4.

11 Jochem VJ, Fuerst PA, Fromkes JJ. Familial Barrett's esophagus associated with adenocarcinoma. *Gastroenterology* 1992; **102**: 1400–2.

12 Fahmy N, King JF. Barrett's esophagus: an acquired condition with genetic predisposition. *Am J Gastroenterol* 1993; **88**: 1262–5.

13 Chow WH, Blot WJ, Vaughan TL, *et al.* Body mass index and risk of adenocarcinomas of the esophagus and gastric cardia. *J Natl Cancer Inst* 1998; **90**: 150–5.

14 Lagergren J, Bergstrom R, Lindgren A, Nyren O. Symptomatic gastroesophageal reflux as a risk factor for esophageal adenocarcinoma. *N Engl J Med* 1999; **340**: 825–31.

15 Anderson LA, Watson RG, Murphy SJ, *et al.* Risk factors for Barrett's oesophagus and oesophageal adenocarcinoma: results from the FINBAR study. *World J Gastroenterol* 2007; **13**: 1585–94.

16 Blot WJ, McLaughlin JK. The changing epidemiology of esophageal cancer. *Semin Oncol* 1999; **26**: 2–8.

17 Tseng PH, Lee YC, Chiu HM, *et al*. Prevalence and clinical characteristics of Barrett's esophagus in a Chinese general population. *J Clin Gastroenterol* 2008; **42**: 1074–9.

18 Kim JH, Rhee PL, Lee JH, *et al*. Prevalence and risk factors of Barrett's esophagus in Korea. *J Gastroenterol Hepatol* 2007; **22**: 908–12.

19 Rajendra S, Kutty K, Karim N. Ethnic differences in the prevalence of endoscopic esophagitis and Barrett's esophagus: the long and short of it all. *Dig Dis Sci* 2004; **49**: 237–42.

20 Abrams JA, Fields S, Lightdale CJ, Neugut AI. Racial and ethnic disparities in the prevalence of Barrett's esophagus among patients who undergo upper endoscopy. *Clin Gastroenterol Hepatol* 2008; **6**: 30–4.

21 Winters C Jr, Spurling TJ, Chobanian SJ, *et al*. Barrett's esophagus. A prevalent, occult complication of gastroesophageal reflux disease. *Gastroenterology* 1987; **92**: 118–24.

22 Shaheen NJ, Green B, Medapalli RK, *et al*. The perception of cancer risk in patients with prevalent Barrett's esophagus enrolled in an endoscopic surveillance program. *Gastroenterology* 2005; **129**: 429–36.

23 Shaheen NJ, Dulai GS, Ascher B, Mitchell KL, Schmitz SM. Effect of a new diagnosis of Barrett's esophagus on insurance status. *Am J Gastroenterol* 2005; **100**: 577–80.

24 Shaheen NJ, Crosby MA, Bozymski EM, Sandler RS. Is there publication bias in the reporting of cancer risk in Barrett's esophagus? *Gastroenterology* 2000; **119**: 333–8.

25 Wang KK, Sampliner RE. Updated guidelines 2008 for the diagnosis, surveillance and therapy of Barrett's esophagus. *Am J Gastroenterol* 2008; **103**: 788–97.

26 Cameron AJ, Carpenter HA. Barrett's esophagus, high-grade dysplasia, and early adenocarcinoma: a pathological study. *Am J Gastroenterol* 1997; **92**: 586–91.

27 Nigro JJ, Hagen JA, DeMeester TR, *et al*. Occult esophageal adenocarcinoma: extent of disease and implications for effective therapy. *Ann Surg* 1999; **230**: 433–8; discussion 8–40.

28 Wang VS, Hornick JL, Sepulveda JA, Mauer R, Poneros JM. Low prevalence of submucosal invasive carcinoma at esophagectomy for high-grade dysplasia or intramucosal adenocarcinoma in Barrett's esophagus: a 20-year experience. *Gastrointest Endosc* 2009; **69**: 777–83.

29 Birkmeyer JD, Siewers AE, Finlayson EV, *et al*. Hospital volume and surgical mortality in the United States. *N Engl J Med* 2002; **346**: 1128–37.

30 Prasad GA, Wang KK, Buttar NS, *et al*. Long-term survival following endoscopic and surgical treatment of high-grade dysplasia in Barrett's esophagus. *Gastroenterology* 2007; **132**: 1226–33.

31 Overholt BF, Lightdale CJ, Wang KK, Canto MI. Photodynamic therapy with porfimer sodium for ablation of high-grade dysplasia in Barrett's esophagus: international, partially blinded, randomized phase III trial. *Gastrointest Endosc* 2005; **62**: 488.

32 Shaheen NJ, Sharma P, Overholt BF, *et al*. Radiofrequency ablation in Barrett's esophagus with dysplasia. *N Engl J Med* 2009; **360**: 2277–88.

33 Dumot JA, Vargo JJ 2nd, Falk GW, Frey L, Lopez R, Rice TW. An open-label, prospective trial of cryospray ablation for Barrett's esophagus high-grade dysplasia and early esophageal cancer in high-risk patients. *Gastrointest Endosc* 2009; **70**: 635–44.

34 Corley DA, Levin TR, Habel LA, Weiss NS, Buffler PA. Surveillance and survival in Barrett's adenocarcinomas: a population-based study. *Gastroenterology* 2002; **122**: 633–40.

35 Vakil N, van Zanten SV, Kahrilas P, Dent J, Jones R. The Montreal definition and classification of gastroesophageal reflux disease: a global evidence-based consensus. *Am J Gastroenterol* 2006; **101**: 1900–20; quiz 43.

CHAPTER 34
Eosinophilic Esophagitis

Jeffrey A. Alexander

Department of Gastroenterology and Hepatology, Division of Internal Medicine, Mayo Clinic, Rochester, MN, USA

Summary

It is not clear why eosinophilic esophagitis is now seen commonly when it was not described before 1978. It should be suspected in patients that present with dysphagia and food impaction. Patients may present as children or as adults. About 50% of the patients have allergies or asthma. The typical endoscopic findings are concentric rings, furrows, or white spots in the esophagus. The diagnosis is made by an esophageal biopsy showing 15 or more eosinophils/hpf (and exclusion of gastroesophageal reflux disease). Medication and/or esophageal dilations are used to treat the acute disease. Maintenance therapy may be required.

Case

A 38-year-old male presents with 8 years of solid-food dysphagia. He eats slowly, chews well, and takes liquid with each swallow. He particularly has trouble with dry meats and bread. Once a week, he has food stick for several minutes before passing. Six years ago he had a meat impaction removed endoscopically. He has heartburn once a week and takes antacids about once a month. He has a history of seasonal allergies and mild asthma. His physical exam is normal, showing good dentition and moist mucus membranes.

Definition and Epidemiology

The first case of eosinophilic esophagitis (EoE) was described by Landres *et al.* in 1978 [1]. EoE is a clinical–pathologic syndrome and was recently defined by a consensus group of experts to require three conditions: (i) esophageal symptoms; (ii) 15 or more eosinophils/high power field (hpf) on esophageal biopsy; and (iii) the exclusion of gastroesophageal reflux disease (GERD) (Table 34.1) [2].

EoE in adults and children behaves somewhat differently. The primary symptom in adults is solid-food dys-

phagia and food impaction. This chapter will focus on adult EoE, commenting on pediatric EoE where appropriate.

About 70% of EoE patients are males, and this disease has been reported in whites, African Americans, Latins, and Asians [2]. EoE has been reported in Europe, Asia, Australia, North and South America, and the Middle East. To date, there has been no proven geographic, ethnic, or socioeconomic predilection for EoE, but details in these reports are minimal. However, the majority of the reports have come from the westernized developed countries, raising the possibility of predisposing geographic or socioeconomic factors. Some studies have suggested a seasonal variation in EoE with more activity during the higher aeroallergen seasons [4], but this has not been a universal finding.

Four population studies have shown an increased prevalence of the disease over time with prevalence rates reported from 8.9 to 120/100 000 people. However, one study found a prevalence of 7.3/100 000 and found this prevalence unchanged over a 9-year period. Two population studies have suggested a true increased incidence of EoE over time. The incidence in Hamilton County, Ohio increased approximately twofold from 9.1 to 15.9/100 000 from 2000 to 2007 [3]. The incidence in Olmsted County, Minnesota has increased almost 30-fold over the last 15 years from 0.35 to 9.45/100 000 [4]. Interestingly, two studies have shown the percentage of esophageal biopsies

Practical Gastroenterology and Hepatology: Esophagus and Stomach, 1st edition. Edited by Nicholas J. Talley, Kenneth R. DeVault and David E. Fleischer. © 2010 Blackwell Publishing Ltd.

Table 34.1 Definition of eosinophilic esophagitis.

1 Esophageal symptoms
   Adults: dysphagia, food impaction, heartburn, regurgitation,
     chest pain
   Children: dysphagia, food impaction, feeding disorder, vomiting
     abdominal pain, heartburn, regurgitation, diarrhea

2 Histology
   Greater than or equal to 15 eosinophils/hpf on any one biopsy
     specimen
   Normal gastric and duodenal biopsies

3 Exclusion of GERD by pH testing or high-dose PPI treatment
   failure

GERD: gastroesophageal reflux disease; PPI: proton pump inhibitor.

with EoE has remained constant over time, though the total number of biopsies per year has increased dramatically over the last decade. It remains uncertain if this represents a true increased incidence or merely increased recognition; it is likely to be some of both. Physicians have dilated the normal-appearing esophagus without biopsies in patients with solid-food dysphagia with success for years; it is likely many of these patients had unrecognized EoE. It is very plausible, as well, that the increase in this disease is related to the increase in allergic disease in our society over the last several decades.

EoE is not rare; the incidence of EoE appears similar to that of Crohn disease, which has an annual incidence of 12.9/100 000 in Olmsted County, Minnesota. Interestingly, 15 or greater eosinophils/hpf were found histologically in 1.1% of 1000 randomly selected people in northern Sweden. This is 50–100 times the prevalence of EoE we have recognized clinically, suggesting that the majority of patients with esophageal eosinophilia may well be minimally symptomatic [5].

Pathophysiology

Our understanding of this newly recognized disease is only in its infancy; the pathophysiology of EoE is only beginning to be unraveled. The leading hypothesis suggests that antigenic exposure to a food or aeroallergen, in a genetically predisposed host, leads to esophageal eosinophilia. This process involves a Th2 cytokine response and is mediated by interleukin-4 (IL-4), IL-5, and IL-13.

The role of food allergens is supported by the dramatic response of esophageal eosinophilia and symptoms in children to an elemental diet [6]. The possible role of aeroallergens is supported by the increased proximal esophageal eosinophil counts and, in some series, clustering of new cases during the aeroallergen season [4].

Familial clustering of EoE has been reported [7]. A positive family history of EoE in a first-degree relative is seen in about 5–10% of pediatric EoE patients, suggesting a genetic predisposition to the disease.

Genetic studies have demonstrated dysregulation of 1% of the human genome in children with EoE [8]. This genetic footprint is clearly different than in GERD patients and can resolve with dietary therapy in children. Interestingly, in these studies the gene encoding eotaxin-3, a potent chemoattractant, was increased 53-fold. Moreover, a single nucleotide polymorphism in the eotaxin-3 gene was found to be associated with susceptibility to EoE and may be the genetic link.

There is likely a complex interaction of eosinophils and mast cells in EoE. Eosinophil products likely lead to remodeling at the cellular level once released from degranulated eosinophils. This process involves angiogenesis and leads to subepithelial fibrosis [9]. The pathogenesis of dysphagia in EoE can be due to stricture formation related to this fibrosis. However, the rapid response to topical steroid therapy suggests there is likely a non-fibrotic mechanism delaying the transport of solid food as well, which is not well understood at this time. The mechanism of symptoms in children is poorly understood, though some of the symptoms may be related to under-appreciated food impaction.

GERD can cause esophageal eosinophilia; the frequency of GERD in patients with esophageal eosinophilia and dysphagia is significant [10,11]. It is likely these two diseases are interrelated but the actual mechanism of this relationship needs to be elucidated [12].

Clinical Features

EoE in adults presents with the primary symptom of solid-food dysphagia and food impaction beginning in early adulthood. Commonly, symptoms of dysphagia will have been present for years before the diagnosis is made. EoE has been reported to be present in 25–55% of patients presenting with food impaction [13,14]. The symptoms of EoE in children can be considerably different compared to adults. As children age, dysphagia becomes more prominent, but, at a very young age, the presentation can vary considerably [3]. Young children may present with symptoms of heartburn and regurgitation, emesis, vomiting, failure to thrive, abdominal pain, chest pain, or diarrhea. It is uncertain what role dysphagia and food impaction play in these symptoms in young children, who may have a difficult time expressing their symptomatology.

EoE is frequently associated with other atopic diseases including allergic rhinitis, asthma, and atopic dermatitis. One of these atopic diseases is present in 52–70% of adults and 53% of children with EoE. About 30% of adults and 50% of children have elevated blood eosinophilia counts but generally less than twice normal. Serum IgE levels have been reported elevated in about 70% of EoE patients [2].

The endoscopic findings of EoE are suggestive but not specific for the disease. The most common endoscopic findings are horizontal circular rings and linear vertical furrows (Videos 14 and 15). White spots, seen less frequently, are felt to represent eosinophilic abscesses. Strictures may be present throughout the esophagus with EoE but are most common in the proximal and midesophagus. The mucosal fragility or "crepe paper esophagus" can lead to linear mucosal shearing after passing an endoscope or dilator (Figure 34.1). Of note, a normal-appearing esophagus can be present in one-third of EoE patients. Fifteen percent of adult patients undergoing endoscopy for solid-food dysphagia and 10% of those with solid-food dysphagia and a normal-appearing esophagus at endoscopy have been shown to have EoE [10].

Esophageal manometry has been abnormal in about half of adult EoE patients studied [15]. Various abnormalities have been reported including hypo- and hyper-contraction and incomplete lower esophageal sphincter relaxation. However, non-specific uncoordinated contractions have been the most common motility pattern reported. Prior to the establishment of the current definition of EoE, which excludes GERD, ambulatory pH testing had been reported to be abnormal in 18% of the 91 adult patients tested [2]. Endoscopic ultrasound was reported in one pediatric series to show thickening of the mucosa, submucosa, and muscularis propria in EoE [16].

Esophageal intraepithelial eosinophils are the hallmark

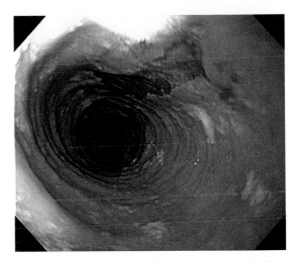

Figure 34.1 Mucosal tear postdilation in eosinophilic esophagitis.

of EoE. There are no specific histopathologic findings that clearly separate EoE from other etiologies of esophageal eosinophilia. However, certain features have been found to be suggestive of EoE and have been reported to appear more frequently or more prominently in EoE than in GERD patients [17]:

1 Superficial layering of eosinophils in the upper half of the squamous epithelium

2 Eosinophilic abscesses defined as clusters of four or more eosinophils

3 Basal zone hyperplasia and papillary lengthening.

Diagnosis

The diagnosis of EoE is made by the typical history, endoscopy with biopsy, and the exclusion of GERD. As previously mentioned, the typical endoscopic findings support but are not required for the diagnosis. The preferred level of the esophagus to biopsy for EoE is uncertain. Biopsies from the distal esophagus may have a slightly greater eosinophil density than the more proximal esophagus but eosinophilia is usually detectable at all levels [18]. Five biopsies have been shown to have 100% sensitivity for EoE, using the current cut off of 15 eosinophils per any one hpf [18]. Patients should have at least five biopsy specimens obtained, including samples from the distal and more proximal esophagus [2].

Case continued

The primary differential diagnosis of non-progressive solid-food dysphagia in a young adult is EoE, esophageal ring, extrinsic vascular esophageal compression, achalasia, and GERD with a peptic stricture. The history of food impaction, mild GERD symptoms, and atopy bring EoE, peptic stricture, or a ring to the top of the list. A barium swallow is always a reasonable first test for the evaluation of dysphagia. However, with no history to suggest oropharyngeal dysphagia and no liquid dysphagia we chose to start the evaluation with a complete blood count (CBC) and esophagogastroduodenoscopy (EGD) with esophageal biopsy.

His CBC was only remarkable for a normal absolute eosinophil count of 320.

His EGD showed concentric rings and furrows in the upper two-thirds of the esophagus. Midesophageal biopsies showed hyperplastic squamous mucosa with up to 60 eosinophils/hpf.

These findings were felt to be consistent with EoE, but an esophageal ambulatory pH study or diagnostic treatment trial of twice-daily proton pump inhibitor (PPI) therapy is required to clinically exclude GERD and confirm the EoE diagnosis.

Differential Diagnosis

The differential diagnosis of solid-food dysphagia is displayed in Table 34.2. Eosinophils in esophageal mucosa are a non-specific finding. Esophageal eosinophilia has been seen in many conditions including GERD, Crohn disease, connective tissue disease, drug hypersensitivity reactions, infection, and the eosinophilic diseases of hypereosinophilic syndrome, eosinophilic gastroenteritis, and primary EoE. Eosinophilic gastroenteritis can have mucosal, submucosal, or serosal eosinophilic infiltration, can involve any area of the gastrointestinal tract, and can present with a multitude of GI symptoms. In EoE, the esophageal infiltration is limited to the esophageal mucosa.

Esophageal eosinophilia can be seen not uncommonly in GERD. It was believed for many years that the eosinophilic infiltrates in GERD were generally mild with a density of fewer than 10 eosinophils/hpf. Resolution of esophageal symptoms and marked histologic esophageal eosinophilia has been well documented with PPI therapy, suggesting an etiologic role of acid reflux [19]. Although, significant esophageal eosinophilia can be seen with

Table 34.2 Differential diagnosis of solid-food dysphagia.

Condition	Comment
Esophageal rings/webs	Some Schatzki rings EoE related
Peptic stricture	GERD symptoms may or may not be present
Achalasia	Progresses to solid and liquid dysphagia over time
GERD	Likely overlap with EoE
Pill-induced stricture	Odynophagia common, more acute onset
Extrinsic vascular compression	Aorta, subclavian artery, thoracic aneurysm
Extrinsic malignant compression	Shorter duration and progressive symptoms
Esophageal malignancy	Shorter duration and progressive symptoms
Infection	Shorter duration of symptoms *Candida*, HSV, CMV, HIV; odynophagia often present
Distal esophageal spasm	Liquid dysphagia and pain unassociated with food impaction more common
Connective tissue disease	Often solid and liquid dysphagia
Neuromuscular diseases	Primarily oropharyngeal symptoms with transfer and liquid dysphagia with aspiration
Cricopharyngeal narrowing ± Zenker diverticulum	Primarily oropharyngeal symptoms

EoE: eosinophilic esophagitis; GERD: gastroesophageal reflux disease.

GERD it is uncommon. Eosinophil counts of more than 20 eosinophils/hpf were reported in only 1.1% of 3648 patients referred to a thoracic surgery group, over 98% of which had GERD [20].

Therapeutics

Treatment of Active Disease

PPI

There have been rare reports of complete histologic and clinical remission of esophageal symptoms and esophageal eosinophilia with PPI therapy even with very high esophageal eosinophil counts [18]. Early studies suggested that children with lower level esophageal eosinophil counts were more likely to respond to acid-blocking medication and were more likely to have abnormal 24-h esophageal pH studies than those children with higher esophageal eosinophil counts [21,22]. Currently, all patients require a negative pH study or a failure to respond to high-dose PPI therapy before establishing a diagnosis of EoE [2]. Therefore, by definition, PPI treatment is ineffective in EoE. However, in reality the issue is likely more complex. PPI therapy is likely effective in treating esophageal eosinophilia associated with GERD and may be effective in treating GERD associated with EoE, which is not an uncommon situation.

Steroids

Swallowed aerosolized topical steroid is the first-line therapy for EoE. Several open-label trials have shown 95% clinical response rates with complete resolution of symptoms in 75% of patients treated for 4–6 weeks [23]. Fluticasone, in doses of 440–880 μg (two to four puffs of 220 μg/puff inhaler) twice daily, has been the most studied topical steroid. Swallowed aerosolized fluticasone is given without a spacer and patients should not eat for 1 h post administration. Budesonide mixed with sucralose or ricinol, a mucosal adherent, has also been reported to be effective [24]. These swallowed solutions may potentially deliver the medication more effectively to the esophagus. In the only controlled treatment trial in EoE, swallowed aerosolized fluticasone in a dose of 440 μg twice daily in children led to a complete histologic response in 50% of patients treated compared to 9% of the placebo group [25]. The major side effect of oral topical steroid therapy is oral candidiasis, seen in about 15% of cases. This complication can potentially be minimized by rinsing the mouth with water and expectorating after drug administration. There is some potential toxicity from long-term use of this high dose of topical steroid, but this has not been evaluated in EoE.

Systemic steroid therapy has shown to be effective in EoE in doses up to 60 mg or 1–2 mg/kg in children in early studies. In a trial of previously untreated patients, compared to topical fluticasone, the histologic healing was better with oral prednisone but the symptomatic response and time to recurrence post-treatment between both agents was similar [26]. Due to its toxicity, systemic steroid therapy is rarely used in EoE and only if topical

steroid therapy failures. How effective it is in treating patients with topical steroid failure is unclear. Currently, topical steroid therapy is the first-line treatment for adults and children.

Other Agents

The leukotriene receptor antagonist montelukast used in high dose, up to 100 mg/day, has been shown to lead to symptomatic remission and maintenance of remission in a small open-label experience in eight patients [27]. Oral cromolyn sodium did not seem to be effective in 14 pediatric patients treated. Antihistamines (H_1 blockers with or without H_2 blockers) have not been formally studied though would be of theoretic benefit.

An anti-IL-5 monoclonal antibody, mepolizumab, has been shown to be effective and well tolerated in the treatment of esophageal symptoms and eosinophilia in eight patients with hypereosinophilic syndrome in two reports. However, in a recent trial of steroid-dependant or refractory EoE patients, mepolizumab was only modestly effective. The anti-IL-5 therapy did show some effects on decreasing esophageal and systemic eosinophilia, but did not lead to histologic remission. Partial symptom relief was seen in a minority of patients [28].

Esophageal Dilation

Esophageal dilation is an effective therapy for EoE and is the primary therapy for fibrotic stricturing disease [23]. However, esophageal perforation has been reported in EoE associated with food impaction, as well as mere passage of an endoscope. Esophageal dilation in EoE frequently is associated with esophageal mucosal tears (Figure 34.1) and pain, as well as anecdotal reports of perforation. Esophageal perforation was seen in 8% of 38 patients dilate in one series [29]. However, a large series found no perforations in 152 dilation procedures suggesting that dilation can be performed safely in EoE [30]. One-half of the patients required repeat dilation in that series.

Esophageal dilation as the initial therapy for EoE is supported by some, but, in light of the potential risk, dilation should be reserved for adults that have failed medical therapy and children that have failed medical and dietary therapy. Dilation is particularly necessary in patients with fibrotic strictures and little active inflammatory disease, reflected in low or no eosinophilic infiltration. Dilation in EoE should be done with caution and generally not progressing more than 3 mm in size per session.

Dietary Therapy

Elimination diets have been dramatically successful in children with EoE. Liacoros has found a 97% histologic and clinical response in 164 children treated with an elemental diet with average time to response of 8.5 days [6]. These diets are expensive and unpalatable requiring nasal gastric tube placement in 80% of the patients. A six-food elimination diet avoiding cow's milk, eggs, soy, nuts, wheat, and fish has lead to a clinical and histologic response in 74% of children [31]. A preliminary report on dietary therapy in 18 adults with the six-food elimination diet found a significant histologic response in one-third of patients [32].

Dietary therapy directed by allergy testing in children has had mixed results. The largest study showed a 77% response rate to a food elimination diet directed by skin prick testing (immediate hypersensitivity) and skin patch testing (delayed hypersensitivity) [33]. Milk allergy testing has a low negative predictive value and most pediatric allergists will restrict cow's milk regardless of allergy testing. Patch testing had a small incremental yield over skin prick testing alone.

In children, a six-food or allergy testing directed diet should be attempted. If successful, foods may be reintroduced every few weeks. Vitamin and micronutrient deficiencies can develop and patients should be followed by a dietician with expertise in this area. Elemental diets should be reserved for refractory patients. The role of dietary therapy in adults is uncertain at this time.

Maintenance Therapy

Since recurrence of symptoms post-therapy is nearly universal in EoE, effective maintenance therapy is critically needed in this disease. Outside of the eight adult patients mentioned above treated with montelukast, and dietary therapy in children, there are no reports of maintenance therapy in EoE. Since esophageal eosinophilia can lead to fibrosis, one wonders about the potential long-term risks of untreated EoE in asymptomatic patients [9]. However, with the frequency of this disease and the rarity of adults with refractory esophageal strictures of uncertain etiology or related to EoE, maintenance therapy in asymptomatic adults can not be routinely recommended at this time until further data are available.

Therapeutic Endpoint

The endpoint of therapy in adults is controversial: should we shoot for symptomatic response or histologic remission? Since recurrent esophageal eosinophilic infiltration is common, severe long-term sequela infrequent, and maintenance therapy uncertain, the current clinical endpoint should be resolution of symptoms. The length of therapy is uncertain. Most studies have treated patients for 4–8 weeks, though the dysphagia usually resolves within the first 2 weeks of therapy. As mentioned above, greater histologic improvement has not been associated with a longer time to relapse [26]. In adults, repeat endoscopy is not routinely performed if dysphagia resolves. In younger children, repeat endoscopy and biopsy is often needed since symptom response can be more difficult to assess and dietary therapy difficult to maintain.

With the little controlled data available, it is not possible to make definite evidence-based recommendations for management; a possible management algorithm is displayed in Figure 34.2.

Case continued

The patient was treated for 4 weeks with omeprazole 20 mg twice daily. His heartburn resolved, but there was no response of his dysphagia. He was then treated with swallowed fluticasone 880 μg twice daily for 6 weeks with complete resolution of his dysphagia after 1 week of therapy. His symptoms recurred in 6 months time and he responded again to topical steroid therapy.

Prognosis

Straumann *et al.* have followed 30 adult patients for a mean follow-up time of 7.2 years [7]. The disease course was variable but only resolved in 10% of patients. The disease did cause dysphagia requiring eating and dietary adjustment, but did not significantly affect the quality of life or longevity. The eosinophilic infiltrates remained confined to the esophagus. Gross endoscopic abnormalities and elevated plasma eosinophil counts were associated with more severe symptomatology. Interestingly six of the seven patients from whom subepithelial tissue was available had evidence of fibrosis present.

Recurrence of EoE post-treatment may be essentially universal. We found symptomatic recurrence in 91% of

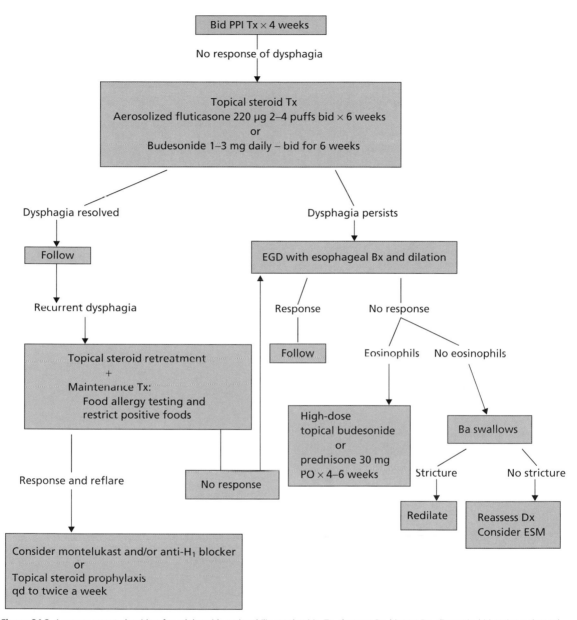

Figure 34.2 A management algorithm for adults with eosinophilic esophagitis. Tx, therapy; Bx, biopsy; Dx, diagnosis; bid, twice a day; qd, every day; PPI, proton pump inhibitor; Ba, barium; EGD, esophagogastroduodenoscopy; ESM, esophageal motility testing.

our adult patients within 13 months of stopping steroid therapy [34]. Liacouras *et al.* similarly reported almost universal recurrence in 381 pediatric patients after dietary or steroid therapy [6]. This very high recurrence rate highlights the need for better maintenance therapy in EoE.

Take-home points

- EoE in adult patients presents with solid-food dysphagia and food impaction.
- One-half of the patients have a history of seasonal allergies, asthma, or allergic dermatitis.

- Typical endoscopic findings of concentric rings, furrows, white spots, or mucosal fragility are present in the majority of patients.

- The diagnosis is made by esophageal biopsy showing 15 or more eosinophils/hpf and the exclusion of GERD.

- All patients with solid-food dysphagia require esophageal biopsy.

- Most patients respond to topical steroid therapy but recurrent dysphagia after stopping therapy is extremely common.

- Esophageal dilation can be performed and is effective but may be associated with some increased risk of perforation.

- Our understanding of the pathophysiology, treatment, and potential prevention are still in their infancy.

- We have numerous questions to answer regarding the etiology and pathogenesis, natural history, and treatment including endpoints of therapy, maintenance therapy, and role of treatment in the asymptomatic patient.

References

1 Landres RT, Kuster GG, Strum WB. Eosinophilic esophagitis in a patient with vigorous achalasia. *Gastroenterol* 1978; **74**: 1298–301.

2 Furuta GT, Liacouras CA, Collins MH, *et al.* Eosinophilic esophagitis in children and adults: a systematic review and consensus recommendations for diagnosis and treatment. *Gastroenterol* 2007; **133**: 1342–63

3 Noel RJ, Putnam PE, Rothenberg ME. Eosinophilic esophagitis. *N Engl J Med* 2004; **351**: 940–1.

4 Prasad G, Smyrk T, Schleck C, *et al.* Secular trends in the epidemiology and outcomes of eosinophilic esophagitis in Olmsted County, Minnesota (1976–2007). *Gastroenterology* 2008; **134**: S1976.

5 Ronkainen J, Talley NJ, *et al.* Prevalence of oesophageal eosinophils and eosinophilic oesophagitis in adults: the population-based Kalixanda study. *Gut* 2007; **56**: 615–20.

6 Liacouras CA, Spergel JM, Ruchelli E, *et al.* Eosinophilic esophagitis: a 10-year experience in 381 children. *Clin Gastroenterol Hepatol* 2005; **3**: 1198–206.

7 Straumann A, Spichtin HP, Grize L, *et al.* Natural history of primary eosinophilic esophagitis: a follow-up of 30 adult patients for up to 11.5 years. *Gastroenterology* 2003; **125**: 1660–9.

8 Blanchard C, Wang N, Rothenberg ME. Eosinophilic esophagitis: pathogenesis, genetics, and therapy. *J Allergy Clin Immunol* 2006; **118**: 1054–9.

9 Aceves SS, Newbury RO, Dohil R, *et al.* Esophageal remodeling in pediatric eosinophilic esophagitis. *J Allergy Clin Immunol* 2007; **119**: 206–12.

10 Prasad GA, Talley NJ, Romero Y, *et al.* Prevalence and predictive factors of eosinophilic esophagitis in patients presenting with dysphagia: a prospective study. *Am J Gastroenterol* 2007; **102**: 2627–32.

11 Peterson A, Thomas K, Hilden K, *et al.* Comparison of esomeprazole to aerosolized swallowed fluticasone for eosinophilic esophagitis. *Dig Dis Sci* 2009, in press.

12 Spechler SJ, Genta RM, Souza RF. Thoughts on the complex relationship between gastroesophageal reflux disease and eosinophilic esophagitis. *Am J Gastroenterol* 2007; **102**: 1301–06.

13 Desai TK, Stecevic V, Chang CH, *et al.* Association of eosinophilic inflammation with esophageal food impaction in adults. *Gastrointest Endosc* 2005; **61**: 795–801.

14 Prasad G, Reddy J, Enders F, *et al.* Predictors of recurrent esophageal food impaction: a population-based case-controlled study. *J Clin Gastroenterol Hepatol* 2008; **42**: 771–5.

15 Sgouros SN, Bergele C, Mantides A. Eosinophilic esophagitis in adults: a systematic review. *Eur J Gastroenterol Hepatol* 2006; **18**: 211–17.

16 Fox VL, Nurko S, Teitelbaum JE, *et al.* High-resolution EUS in children with eosinophilic "allergic" esophagitis. *Gastrointest Endosc* 2003; **57**: 30–6.

17 Parfitt JR, Gregor JC, Suskin NG, *et al.* Eosinophilic esophagitis in adults: distinguishing features from gastroesophageal reflux disease: a study of 41 patients. *Mod Pathol* 2006; **19**: 90–6.

18 Gonsalves N, Policarpio-Nicolas M, Zhang Q, *et al.* Histopathologic variability and endoscopic correlates in adults with eosinophilic esophagitis. *Gastrointest Endosc* 2006; **64**: 313–19.

19 Ngo P, Furuta GT, Antonioli DA, Fox VL. Eosinophils in the esophagus--peptic or allergic eosinophilic esophagitis? Case series of three patients with esophageal eosinophilia. *Am J Gastroenterol* 2006; **101**: 1666–70.

20 Rodrigo S, Abboud G, Oh D, *et al.* High intraepithelial eosinophil counts in esophageal squamous epithelium are not specific for eosinophilic esophagitis in adults. *Am J Gastroenterol* 2008; **103**: 435–42.

21 Ruchelli E, Wenner W, Voytek T, *et al.* Severity of esophageal eosinophilia predicts response to conventional gastroesophageal reflux therapy. *Pediatr Dev Pathol* 1999; **2**: 15–18.

22 Steiner SJ, Gupta SK, *et al.* Correlation between number of eosinophils and reflux index on same day esophageal biopsy and 24 hour esophageal pH monitoring. *Am J Gastroenterol* 2004; **99**: 801–5.

23 Bohm M, Richter JE. Treatment of eosinophilic esophagitis: overview, current limitations, and future direction. *Am J Gastroenterol* 2008; **103**: 2635–44.

24 Aceves SS, Bastian JF, Newbury RO, Dohil R. Oral viscous budesonide: a potential new therapy for eosinophilic esophagitis in children. *Am J Gastroenterol* 2007; **102**: 2271–9; quiz 2280.

25 Konikoff MR, Noel RJ, Blanchard C, *et al.* A randomized, double-blind, placebo-controlled trial of fluticasone propionate for pediatric eosinophilic esophagitis. *Gastroenterology* 2006; **131**: 1381–91.

26 Schaefer ET, Fitzgerald JF, Molleston JP, *et al.* Comparison of oral prednisone and topical fluticasone in the treatment of eosinophilic esophagitis: a randomized trial in children. *Clin Gastroenterol Hepatol* 2008; **6**: 165–73.

27 Attwood SE, Lewis CJ, Bronder CS, *et al.* Eosinophilic oesophagitis: a novel treatment using Montelukast. *Gut* 2003; **52**: 181–5.

28 Straumann A, Conus S, Kita H, *et al.* Mepolizumab, a monoclonal antibody to IL-5, for severe eosinophilic esophagitis in adults: a randomized placebo-controlled double-blind trial. *J Allergy Clin Immunol* 2008; **121**: 171, S44.

29 Cohen MS, Kaufman A, DiMarino AJ, Jr, Cohen S. Eosinophilic esophagitis presenting as spontaneous esophageal rupture (Boerhaave's syndrome). *Clin Gastroenterol Hepatol* 2007; **5**: A24.

30 Gonsalves N, Karmali K, Hirano I. Safety and response of esophageal dilation in adults with eosinophilic esophagitis (EE): a single center experience of 81 patients. *Gastroenterology* 2007; **132**: T2034, A-607.

31 Kagalwalla AF, Sentongo TA, Ritz S, *et al.* Effect of six-food elimination diet on clinical and histologic outcomes in eosinophilic esophagitis. *Clin Gastroenterol Hepatol* 2006; **4**: 1097–102.

32 Gonsalves N, Yang G, Doerfler B *et al.* A prospective clinical trial of the six-food elimination diet and reintroduction of causative agents in adults with eosinophilic esophagitis. *Gastroenterology* 2008; **134**: 727.

33 Spergel JM, Andrews T, Brown-Whitehorn TF, *et al.* Treatment of eosinophilic esophagitis with specific food elimination diet directed by a combination of skin prick and patch tests. *Ann Allergy Asthma Immunol* 2005; **95**: 336–43.

34 Helou E, Simonson J, Arora A. Three-year follow up of topical corticosteroid treatment for eosinophilic esophagitis in adults. *Am J Gastroenterol* 2008; **103**: 2194–9.

CHAPTER 35
Esophageal Motility Disorders

Kenneth R. DeVault

Division of Gastroenterology and Hepatology, Mayo Clinic, Jacksonville, FL, USA

Summary

Esophageal motility can become abnormal by either becoming "spastic" with disordered and sometimes high-pressure contractions or becoming weak with no contractions or weakly ineffective contractions. Achalasia is the best characterized motility disorder, yet the etiologic agent behind the disorder is unknown. Diffuse esophageal spasm (DES) is a motility disorder characterized by simultaneous esophageal contractions intermixed with more normal sequences. High-pressure or "nutcracker" esophagus is characterized by normally transmitted peristaltic waves with higher than expected amplitudes. Treatment of these disorders focuses on lowering the lower esophageal sphincter pressure and may include medications (nitrates and calcium blockers), injectables (botox), endoscopic dilation, and surgical myotomy. There is another set of disorders characterized by absent or weak (ineffective) motility. Scleroderma is the classic disorder in this category, but more patients have gastroesophageal reflux disease (GERD) and other conditions affecting esophageal muscles or nerves. GERD is perhaps the most common etiology of a "weak" esophagus. There is no specific treatment for ineffective peristalsis, but, as many of these patients have coexisting GERD, acid suppression is reasonable.

Case

A 45-year-old man presents with complaints of heartburn and chest pain. These symptoms have been present for at least 10 years and are becoming more severe. He states that the symptoms almost always happen after a meal and, when he gets the symptoms, he produces a good bit of saliva. He occasionally regurgitates the meal that he has just ingested with relief of the symptoms. His weight has been stable over the years, but he has lost about 5 kg in the past 3 months. He has been on a proton pump inhibitor (PPI) for 10 years at increasing doses and currently is on esomeprazole 40 mg twice daily and ranitidine 300 mg at bedtime. He recently had a persistent cough and his internist obtained a chest radiograph that showed clear lung fields, but an air–fluid level behind the chest.

Introduction

The normal physiology associated with esophageal peristalsis is described in Chapter 1.2. This physiology can

Practical Gastroenterology and Hepatology: Esophagus and Stomach, 1st edition. Edited by Nicholas J. Talley, Kenneth R. DeVault and David E. Fleischer. © 2010 Blackwell Publishing Ltd.

become disordered in several ways. There can be a loss of coordination or development of high-pressure contractions that may produce dysphagia, chest pain, or both (spastic dysmotility). There can also be disorders with weak or ineffective peristalsis. This dysfunction may be either primary (idiopathic) or secondary to many different systemic diseases. The pathophysiology, diagnosis, and therapy of these disorders are discussed in this chapter.

Spastic Motility Disorders

Normal esophageal peristalsis requires a balance of excitatory neurologic input (usually cholinergic) and inhibitory input (non-adrenergic, non-cholinergic—NANC) [1]. When these forces become imbalanced, the esophageal peristaltic sequence may become disordered and produce symptoms. Achalasia is the best-described esophageal motility disorder and some senior authors have challenged whether the other "disorders" are truly disorders or better termed as "manometric abnormalities" [2].

Achalasia

Achalasia is characterized by a lower esophageal sphincter (LES) that does not relax appropriately with swallowing, which can have either a normal or an elevated resting pressure. In addition, the esophageal body shows no evidence of organized peristalsis. It appears that loss of the inhibitory, NANC nerves (especially those containing vasoactive intestinal polypeptide [VIP] and nitric oxide [NO]) in the lower esophagus brings about this disorder [3]. The factor that causes this loss of innervation is not clear. Theories have included genetics, viral infections, autoimmune disease, and neurodegeneration similar to Parkinson disease, but none of these has been confirmed. In fact, it is not clear whether the loss of neurons begins centrally or at the level of the LES. These neurologic changes result in muscular changes with almost uniform thickening of the LES muscle. Chagas disease is a multisystem infectious disease caused by the protozoan *Trypanosoma cruzi* which is endemic in certain Central and South American countries. It has a similar esophageal presentation to achalasia, but, unlike achalasia, affects other organs including the small bowel, colon, rectum, and heart [4]. Reference laboratories now have antibody tests for this disease, which should be considered in an achalasia patient presenting from an endemic area. Many other conditions can mimic idiopathic achalasia, including the following:

- Chagas disease
- Tumors in the area of the LES
  - Esophageal malignancies:
    adenocarcinoma
    squamous cell carcinoma
    lymphoma
  - Other malignancies:
    liver
    gastric
    lung
    peritoneal
    kidney
  - Benign stromal tumors (e.g., gastrointestinal stromal tumor)
- Distant malignancy (paraneoplastic)
- Sarcoidosis
- Amyloidosis
- Sphingolipidosis (Anderson–Fabry disease)
- Postoperative after fundoplication or bariatric surgery
- Neurofibromatosis.

Malignancy can produce achalasia by three potential mechanisms: direct obstruction at the esophagogastric junction (EGJ) from the tumor itself, infiltration of the myenteric plexus producing a more typical "neurogenic" achalasia, or by the production of autoantibodies by a distant malignancy such as a small-cell carcinoma [5].

Patients with achalasia typically present with several months to many years of dysphagia and may occur in any age group. It is often progressive, starting as intermittent dysphagia to solids and progressing to dysphagia to liquids and solids. Patients often learn to stand up and move about when dysphagia occurs, which may force the bolus into the stomach. Frank regurgitation, nocturnal aspiration, and pulmonary compromise complicate advanced cases. Chest pain is another common symptom of achalasia and may be the only symptom in some cases. These symptoms can occasionally be confused with heartburn and many achalasia patients are mistakenly given trials of acid blockers at some point in the course of their illness. Weight loss often occurs later in the course and actually is frequently the reason for a more detailed evaluation leading to the diagnosis. Another potential complication of achalasia is the development of esophageal carcinoma, although many authors now believe that most of those patients do not have idiopathic achalasia and actually have pseudoachalasia due to the malignancy itself [6]. As a result of the low incidence of this problem, endoscopic surveillance programs are not indicated in patients with achalasia.

Clinical suspicion, barium testing, manometry, and endoscopy combine to make this diagnosis, which may be delayed for years when clinical suspicion is insufficient. Barium testing almost always suggests the diagnosis. The typical finding is a dilated esophagus with a smoothly tapered, narrowed lower portion, which has been described as a "bird-beak" appearance (Figure 35.1). Advanced cases may develop large epiphrenic diverticula. When the esophagus becomes so dilated that a portion extends inferior to the LES, treatment becomes very difficult. Not all patients have profound changes, so giving a solid bolus and demonstrating the bolus to "hang up" at the EGJ may aid in the diagnosis. Manometry is required to confirm achalasia. The classic finding is of a poorly relaxing LES and an aperistaltic esophageal body (Figure 35.2). LES pressure is elevated in most untreated patients, but this is not a required finding for diagnosis.

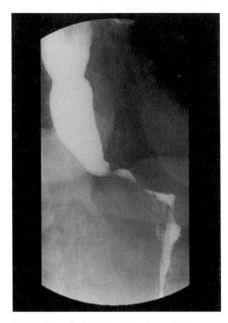

Figure 35.1 Barium of achalasia: this is the typical appearance of achalasia on a barium esophagogram. The esophagus is usually, but not always, dilated with a smooth tapering into what has been described as a "bird-beak" appearance. Secondary achalasia due to a malignancy at the esophagogastric junction may have an appearance identical to idiopathic achalasia and must be excluded with endoscopic visualization.

The proximal smooth muscle portion usually maintains peristaltic function. Passing the catheter through the LES into the stomach may present a challenge and the combination of a manometrically aperistaltic esophageal body and a compatible barium study is sufficient for diagnosis in most cases. If LES evaluation is needed for confirmation, the catheter may be placed across the sphincter endoscopically or fluoroscopically in the difficult patient. Normally, the manometric pressure in the stomach is higher than in the esophagus, but in achalasia this can be reversed due to the pressure of the retained esophageal fluid column. The LES does not relax completely in almost all cases of achalasia, although false relaxation can be seen if the monitoring site migrates out of the sphincter during swallowing. Endoscopy is neither sensitive nor specific as a diagnostic tool in achalasia, but is still an important part of the evaluation. Tumors at the EGJ may produce a radiographic and manometric appearance identical to idiopathic achalasia and are more common in older patients. Endoscopy, with a careful

retroflexed view of the EGJ, can usually (but not always) exclude a mucosal lesion producing secondary achalasia. At times, the LES is quite tight, requiring some pressure on the endoscope in order to enter the stomach. The mucosa of the esophagus is frequently thickened due to chronic stasis, but achalasia may be complicated by *Candida albicans* infection in some cases. Some centers add endoscopic ultrasonography to rule out a submucosal process, but, although possible, these lesions are very rare and most do not consider this a mandatory part of the evaluation.

Achalasia is not usually a "curable" illness. There have been reports of a return of peristalsis after treatment, but this is probably the exception rather than the rule [7]. Treatment has focused on relieving the obstruction at the EGJ and hence allowing the still aperistaltic esophagus to essentially empty by a combination of gravity and the force generated by the proximal striated muscle components. As the pathophysiology of the disorder centers around loss of NO-containing neurons, nitrates and similar agents would seem to be a reasonable approach. Unfortunately, most studies have failed to demonstrate long-term efficacy with either nitrates or other smooth muscle relaxants, including calcium channel blockers and anticholinergics, leading most experts to use these therapies only in patients unfit for or unwilling to undergo more definitive therapy. If used, they should be given in a rapidly absorbed form (sublingual nifedipine or nitrates) before meals. Recently, sildenafil (a phosphodiesterase blocker) has been suggested to lower LES pressure in achalasia and may be a reasonable trial, although somewhat limited by the high cost of this medication [8]. Injection of botulinum toxin A (botox) has been used in the treatment of many disorders characterized by spastic muscle function. This leads to the introduction of intrasphincteric botox as a treatment for achalasia. Initial studies were promising [9], but longer-term trials have been more discouraging [10]. Some have advocated this as a diagnostic test for achalasia, but there is suggestion that botox injection may lead to fibrosis at the EGJ, making later, more definitive therapy more difficult [11]. When patients respond to botox, but develop recurrent symptoms, many will respond to a second injection, but those who do not initially respond are rarely helped with repeated injections. Due to concerns about the long-term efficacy of this approach, most experts now limit their use of botox to those either needing palliation while

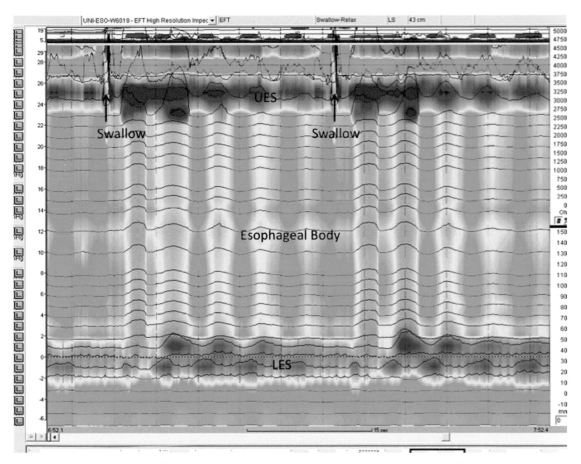

Figure 35.2 Manometry of achalasia: this is a high-resolution manometry tracing from a patient with achalasia. The two swallows can be seen to begin normally in the upper esophageal sphincter area, but the esophageal body has all simultaneous, repetitive, low-pressure contractions and there is minimal evidence of relaxation of the lower esophageal sphincter.

waiting for, or who would not tolerate, other endoscopic or surgical therapy. The technique for botox injection is simple: 100 units of the agent are gently reconstituted with 5 mL *preservative-free* saline. The botox is then injected in 1-mL (20-unit) boluses around the LES using a standard sclerotherapy needle. Initial studies used a total dose of 80 units, but many go ahead and administer the entire 100 units.

Mechanical disruption of the LES has been the traditional treatment for achalasia and can be accomplished in one of two ways: forceful pneumatic dilation or surgical myotomy. Traditional (20 mm or less) dilation provides minimal benefit in patients with achalasia. Forceful, pneumatic dilation with 30–40 mm balloons is more

effective. These balloons do not fit through the endoscope, so they are placed under fluoroscopic control after endoscopic localization of the LES. The exact method of pneumatic dilation varies among experts, but modern studies suggest starting with a smaller balloon (30 mm) and working up to a larger balloon if symptoms persist. Traditionally the balloon was left inflated for up to 60 s, but most now limit the inflation time to approximately 15 s with similar results [12]. A contrast study should be obtained immediately after the dilation to evaluate for a possible perforation, which has been reported in up to 3% of cases. Late perforation is possible, so patients should be observed closely for up to 24 h. Interestingly some (perhaps most) limited perforations can be managed conservatively with antibiotics and nil-by-mouth status. If surgery is required for a perforation, a simultaneous myotomy should be performed if technically possible. Some authors advocate a timed barium study after dilation as a way to determine if the dilation was sufficient [13]. They then advocate an additional dilation with a larger balloon when emptying remains poor independent of symptom response. Interestingly, younger patients do not seem to respond as well to pneumatic dilation [14].

The most common surgical approach to achalasia is the so-called modified Heller myotomy which has been performed since the early part of the 20th century. This procedure divides the muscle fibers of the distal esophagus and proximal stomach down to the level of the mucosa, which reliably produces a drop in LES pressure into the normal or even hypotensive range [15].

Traditionally, Heller procedures were performed through an open thoracotomy with all of the perioperative risk and discomfort associated with that procedure. This led many centers to favor pneumatic dilation as first-line therapy. The approach to achalasia has recently been altered by less invasive approaches to myotomy. The surgery can now be performed via either a laparoscopic or a thoracoscopic approach [16]. Most centers are favoring the laparoscopic approach where a very loose, partial (Toupet) fundoplication is performed after the myotomy, with results comparable to the older, open approach [17]. Although most patients respond to this surgery, some do not. Postoperative dysphagia may be due to an incomplete myotomy, scaring at the myotomy site, obstruction from the fundoplication, paraesophageal hernias, diverticula, or massive esophageal dilation. If it appears that the problem is an incomplete myotomy or fundoplication, pneumatic dilation may be attempted, but some patients will need a surgical revision to either loosen the fundoplication or extend the myotomy, or both. In refractory cases and in those with a massively dilated esophagus, esophagectomy may be the only option for symptomatic improvement, especially in patients experiencing pulmonary or nutritional compromise [18].

Diffuse Esophageal Spasm

DES is another well-characterized motility disorder. It has traditionally been described manometrically, although there are radiographic findings associated with the disorder. Similar to achalasia, the underlying etiology of the disorder is poorly understood, but is likely related to loss of inhibitory innervation of the esophagus. There have been reports of DES progressing to achalasia [19], but most cases seem either to be stable over time or to vary in severity (both improvement and deterioration have been reported). Some pathologic studies have suggested a thickening in the esophageal wall in these patients with confirmation provided by endoscopic ultrasonography [20].

Patients with DES usually present with chest pain, dysphagia, or both, but up to 20% will have heartburn as their primary complaint [21]. A barium study can suggest the diagnosis with the classic finding being a segmented or "corkscrew" esophagus. Other patients will have a normal study and a solid bolus may or may not become lodged. DES has been defined by a manometric profile of some simultaneous contractions (at least 30%) intermixed with some normal peristaltic sequences (Figure 35.3) [22]. There is a wide variety of findings with some patients having only the minimal number of simultaneous contractions, whereas others are much closer to achalasia with minimal peristaltic contractions. Some patients will have triple peaked contractions and repetitive contractions lasting several seconds. Patients with a weak esophagus may have low-pressure (<30 mmHg), simultaneous contractions, which are different from DES

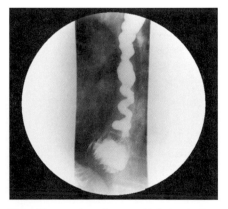

Figure 35.3 Diffuse esophageal spasm: this is the classic appearance of esophageal spasm on barium testing. The diagnosis of diffuse esophageal spasm cannot be made on barium alone and must be confirmed with manometry, showing a mixture of 20% or more simultaneous contractions with some normally propagated contractions.

and probably should be considered as ineffective motility (see below). Esophageal impedance testing has demonstrated normal bolus transit in some sequences that appear to be simultaneous by manometric criteria. The LES can be normal, hypotensive, or poorly relaxing in DES. Symptoms, manometric, and radiographic findings are often discordant. There are data to suggest a psychological basis for symptoms even in patients with a definable manometric disorder such as DES [23].

The treatment of DES is similar to that of achalasia, although, as its symptoms are usually less severe, medical therapy is more commonly used. Nitrates, calcium channel blockers, and sildenafil have all been used with moderate success. Cold liquids seem to be more likely to produce symptoms and warm water swallows have been used as therapy in DES [24]. In patients with pain and less dysphagia, a trial of a low-dose antidepressant may be reasonable (trazodone 50–150 mg at bedtime [25] and imipramine 50 mg at bedtime [26] have been best studied). Botox injection at the LES has been used in an open-label trial with promising results but has not been subjected to an adequately controlled trial [27]. Others will try to inject botox into the parts of the esophagus with more of a "spastic" appearance, but this has not been tested. Pneumatic dilation [28] and even long myotomy [29] are options in refractory cases. GERD can coexist with DES and a trial of acid suppression or an ambulatory reflux test is also reasonable.

High-pressure "Nutcracker" Esophagus

The widespread use of manometry for patients with chest pain and dysphagia in the 1980s led to the observation that there is a group of patients (particularly chest pain patients) who have higher than expected pressures in an otherwise normally peristaltic esophagus. These were initially described as "super squeezers", but the term "nutcracker esophagus" was later coined and became the standard label for these patients [30]. There is some controversy over whether this manometrically defined condition is a true disorder or a statistical aberration, because it is based on the distal esophageal pressure being outside two standard deviations of the mean (>180 mmHg with most systems). It has been suggested that this disorder is often related to increased stress and anxiety rather than innate esophageal pathology. In fact, under stress, normal individuals may develop esophageal pressures in the nutcracker range [31]. We tend to segregate these patients into "statistical nutcrackers" where the pressure is moderately elevated and "true nutcrackers" where there is very high pressure (up to 500 mmHg) with frequent prolonged or bizarre-appearing contractions (Figure 35.4). It would seem that the former are more likely stress related, whereas the latter have some problem with neurologic input to the esophagus.

The treatment of symptoms associated with nutcracker esophagus has used agents that lower esophageal pressure (nitrates and calcium channel blockers) with variable success. As in DES, patients with chest pain and nutcracker esophagus may respond to agents that lower visceral sensitivity, such as antidepressants. A botox injection may also be attempted, although not well studied. A long surgical myotomy has been used in a handful of patients with variable results.

Spastic Disorders of the LES

Manometrically, the LES can be abnormal in resting pressure, relaxation, or both. Correlation of these findings with symptoms is challenging. It is possible that some of these patients are actually in the earliest stage of achalasia, although prospective data are lacking. Overall, it is often difficult to attribute symptoms to this finding, but, if the complaint is dysphagia, use of agents that lower LES pressure, performance of dilations, or injection of botox may be considered.

Disorders with Weak or Ineffective Peristalsis

Aperistalsis Associated with Rheumatologic and other Systemic Disorders

The classic disorder associated with severe loss of peristalsis is scleroderma or systemic sclerosis. Patients with these disorders are found to have an aperistaltic (or nearly so) esophagus and, in contrast to achalasia, a very-low-pressure LES. The pathophysiology was originally felt to be due to fibrosis of esophageal muscle, but recent data suggest that the initial and perhaps primary problem is a loss of innervation [32]. Patients often present with dysphagia and usually have other symptoms and findings, which makes the diagnosis evident. The absence of peristalsis and LES pressure predispose to particularly severe gastroesophageal reflux and patients frequently

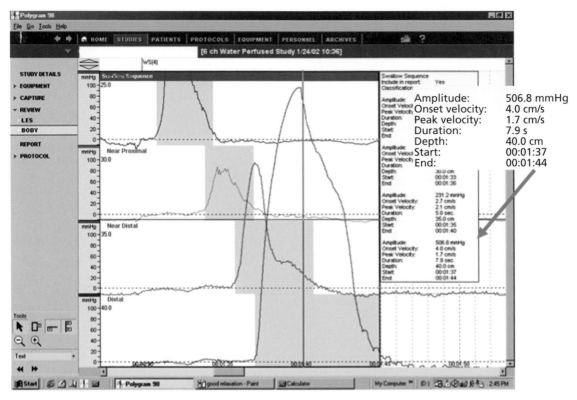

Figure 35.4 Nutcracker esophagus is defined as a statistically determined increase in peristaltic pressures in the distal esophagus (>180 mmHg). Many feel this "diagnosis" to be more a marker of anxiety than anything else, but an occasional patient has very high pressures that seem to be a marker of underlying neuropathy. This example shows a distal pressure of >500 mmHg in a patient with severe chest pain with swallowing.

develop strictures and Barrett esophagus. In recent years, it has been suggested that some of the lung disease associated with scleroderma may in fact be due to reflux and aspiration [33]. Patients are occasionally diagnosed in error with achalasia when they have a distal stricture or tumor that makes their esophagus appear more consistent with that diagnosis. Esophageal involvement may be the only gastrointestinal manifestation of disease, but other patients will have small bowel and colon symptoms as well as the most severe cases losing the ability to maintain oral nutrition.

Although scleroderma is the classic disorder, peristaltic dysfunction has been associated with almost all of the connective tissue disorders and the potential etiologies of hypotensive esophageal dysmotility include:
• GERD
• Rheumatologic disease
  ◦ Scleroderma
  ◦ Mixed connective tissue disease
  ◦ Rheumatoid arthritis
  ◦ Systemic lupus erythematosus
• Endocrine disease
  ◦ Diabetes
  ◦ Hypothyroidism
• Miscellaneous
  ◦ Alcoholism
  ◦ Amyloidosis
  ◦ Intestinal pseudo-obstruction
  ◦ Steroid myopathy
  ◦ Multiple sclerosis
• Drugs
  ◦ Opiates
  ◦ Anticholinergics
• Idiopathic.

Most series suggest that 40% or more of patients with manometry consistent with "scleroderma esophagus" do not actually have scleroderma or a similar rheumatologic disorder [34]. In addition to these disorders, any systemic disease that produces a gastrointestinal neuropathy or myopathy may lead to esophageal dysfunction (see list above). This dysfunction is particularly common in diabetes with 60% of those with long-term diabetes demonstrating manometric changes, although those changes do not always correlate with symptoms [35].

Diagnosis relies on the examiner having sufficient clinical suspicion based on the patient's underlying non-esophageal conditions, e.g., patients with scleroderma are diagnosed based on their cutaneous findings and patients with diabetes by their history or with simple blood tests. Generally, a barium swallow will suggest an esophageal disorder but confirmation is obtained with manometry. In difficult cases, the LES pressure (or lack thereof) is the deciding factor between achalasia and a scleroderma-like condition. An esophagogastroduodenoscopy (EGD) is important to screen for Barrett esophagus and to dilate strictures if present, both of which are common in scleroderma and similar disorders.

There is no specific treatment for severe hypotensive esophageal dysmotility, but patients may have severe acid reflux and most benefit from proton pump inhibitor therapy. Their reflux may be particularly difficult to treat and require dosing more than once daily. Although somewhat controversial, severe reflux cases, particularly if there is fear of aspiration, may benefit from a carefully performed, very loose, partial fundoplication [36]. If there is associated gastric dysmotility, promotility agents may be of benefit. Rarely, patients will develop enough nutritional compromise that tube-based enteral nutrition will be needed.

GERD-related Dysmotility

The widespread availability of motility testing and the increase in reflux surgery brought about by the laparoscopic technique has led to more patients with GERD undergoing manometry. These studies have revealed that GERD patients commonly have a variety of motility issues ranging from mild, non-specific changes to aperistalsis that is identical to that seen with scleroderma. The vast majority of GERD patients do not require motility testing, nor is there a clinical indication to search for a motility disorder. On the other hand, patients with dysphagia and GERD who do not have a stricture and those being considered for reflux surgery should be studied. There is controversy over whether these disorders improve with medical or surgical therapy [37]. Most surgeons continue to "tailor" their surgery based on motility, and limit the fundoplication to a partial repair in patients with severe dysmotility, although modern data seem to refute the assumption that this approach decreases postoperative dysphagia [38]. Nevertheless, preoperative manometry remains reasonable to exclude the occasional achalasia patient presenting with GERD-like symptoms (somewhere between 1% and 3% of patients referred for reflux surgery may have achalasia). Dysphagia in patients with severe hypomotility who have undergone fundoplication is particularly difficult to diagnose and treat. Dysphagia may require pneumatic dilation or take down of the fundoplication in some patients who do not respond to traditional dilation (up to 20 mm) [39].

Aging-related Dysmotility

A decrease in esophageal amplitude pressures with aging has been reported in the eighth and ninth decades [40]. This has resulted in the identification of a group of older patients who have aperistalsis, but whose manometry and radiographic studies do not support the diagnosis of either achalasia or "scleroderma" esophagus. These disorders appear to be more than a simple manometric curiosity, because radiological studies have demonstrated poor bolus clearance from the esophagus in older patients [41].

Although the effect of aging on the esophagus remains unclear, some data from pathology studies are available. In the human esophagus, the number of myenteric neurons decrease with aging, which could result in dysmotility related to relative deinnervation. Pathologic changes seen in the esophagus with aging are very similar to the changes seen in patients with spastic esophageal motility disorders such as achalasia and diffuse esophageal spasm [42]. Gastrointestinal amyloid deposition was found in 38 of 110 (38%) autopsies in patients over the age of 85 without known amyloidosis, although only 11 of the cases had esophageal deposition [43]. It is unclear if any of these patients had premorbid esophageal conditions or complaints, but these are very provocative data because many diseases related to aging, including Alzheimer's disease, are thought to be related to abnormal amyloid deposition.

An increase in the number of disordered "tertiary" contractions on barium examination has not correlated well with esophagus symptoms, although there is some correlation with manometric changes. Esophageal manometry may uncover a primary motility disorder such as achalasia, diffuse esophageal spasm, or scleroderma-like esophagus. Finally, most of these patients should have an endoscopy to exclude Barrett esophagus and other mucosal or obstructive lesions, all of which tend to be more common in older patients.

Non-specific Disorders of Ineffective Motility

The term "non-specific esophageal motility disorder" (NEMD) has recently been supplanted by the term "ineffective esophageal motility" (IEM) [44]. IEM may be due to systemic disease, GERD, or perhaps aging, but there are patients who have this finding without an identifiable underlying etiology. Findings include distal esophageal amplitudes of <30 mmHg, low-pressure simultaneous contractions, isolated areas of failed peristalsis, and absent peristalsis in patients without achalasia. Interestingly, the new technique of combined impedance/manometry has suggested that many of these seemingly ineffective contractions actually are effective in clearing a bolus (at least a liquid bolus) from the esophagus. It is important to have a careful approach when manometry has the type of changes that do not meet the criteria for the better-defined disorders. A clear explanation of how common and "severe" abnormal sequences are in an individual patient will provide much more information than attempting to label them an IEM, NEMD, or even mild DES.

Case continued

The patient underwent a barium swallow that demonstrated a dilated esophagus with a smoothly tapered narrowing at the esophagogastric junction. Achalasia was confirmed manometrically. Botox injection, laparoscopic myotomy, and pneumatic dilation were all discussed with the patient and he chose pneumatic dilation. The endoscopic appearance was also consistent with achalasia, including a carefully performed retroflexed view of the cardia. A 30-mm pneumatic dilator was confirmed to be across the LES fluoroscopically and then inflated to 12 lb/in^2 for 15 s. There was a moderate amount of blood on the dilator. A water-soluble contrast swallow was performed and no perforation noted. At 6-week follow-up, the patient was swallowing much better and had gained back all 5 kg of the weight lost.

Take-home points

- Achalasia is the prototypical esophageal motility disorder characterized by aperistalsis of the esophageal body and a poorly relaxing LES.
- Achalasia is treated by improving LES relaxation with medications, injectables, dilation, and/or surgery.
- Other spastic motility disorders include diffuse esophageal spasm, nutcracker esophagus, and spastic disorders of the LES.
- Scleroderma (systemic sclerosis) produces an aperistaltic esophagus with a very weak LES and predisposes to severe reflux complications.
- Most patients with a weak esophagus actually do not have scleroderma and may have other rheumatologic conditions or, perhaps most commonly, severe GERD.
- Dysmotility may occur with other systemic illnesses such as diabetes and may also occur with aging.

References

1 Devault KR, Rattan S. Physiological role of neuropeptides in the gastrointestinal smooth muscle sphincters: neuropeptide and VIP-oxide interactions. In: Walsh J, Dockray G (eds), *Gut Peptides: Biochemistry and Physiology.* New York: Raven Press; 1994: 715–48.

2 Spechler SJ, Castell DO. Non-achalasia esophageal motility abnormalities. In: Castell DO, Richter HE (eds), *The Esophagus,* 4th edn. Philadelphia: Lippincott, Williams & Wilkins; 2004: 262–74.

3 Csendes A, Smok G, Braghetto I, *et al.* Gastroesophageal sphincter pressure and histological changes in distal esophagus in patients with achalasia of the esophagus. *Dig Dis Sci* 1985; **30**: 941–5.

4 Oliveira RB, Filho FJ, Dantas RO, *et al.* The spectrum of esophageal motor disorders in Chagas' disease. *Am J Gastroenterol* 1995; **90**: 119–24.

5 Liu W, Fackler W, Rice TW, *et al.* The pathogenesis of pseudoachalasia: A clinicopathologic study of 13 cases of a rare entity. *Am J Surg Pathol* 2002; **26**: 784–8.

6 Dunaway PM, Wong RKH. Risk and surveillance intervals for squamous cell carcinoma in achalasia. *Gastrointest Endosc Clin North Am* 2001; **11**: 425–34.

7 Bianco A, Cagossi M, Scrimieri D, Greco AV. Appearance of esophageal peristalsis in treated idiopathic achalasia. *Dig Dis Sci* 1986; **31**: 40–8.

8 Bortolotti M, Mari C, Lopilator C, *et al.* Effects of sildenafil on esophageal motility of patients with idiopathic achalasia. *Gastroenterology* 2000; **118**; 253–7.

9 Pasricha PJ, Ravich WJ, Hendrix TR, *et al.* Intrasphincteric botulinum toxin for the treatment of achalasia. *N Engl J Med* 1995; **322**: 774–8.

10 Vaezi MF, Richter JE, Wilcox CM, *et al.* Botulinum toxin versus pneumatic dilatation in the treatment of achalasia: A randomized trial. *Gut* 1999; **44**: 231–9.

11 Horgan S, Hudda K, Eubanks T, *et al.* Does botulinum toxin injection make esophagomyotomy a more difficult operation? *Surg Endosc* 1999; **13**: 576–9.

12 Gideon RM, Castell DO, Yarze J. Prospective randomized comparison of pneumatic dilatation technique in patients with idiopathic achalasia. *Dig Dis Sci* 1999; **44**: 1853–7.

13 Vaezi MF, Baker ME, Richter JE. Assessment of esophageal emptying post-pneumatic dilation: Use of the timed barium esophagram. *Am J Gastroenterol* 1999; **94**: 1802–7.

14 Clouse RE, Abramson BK, Todorczuk JR. Achalasia in the elderly: Effects of aging on clinical presentation and outcome. *Dig Dis Sci* 1991; **36**: 225–8.

15 Csendes A, Velasco N, Braghetto I, Henriquez A. A prospective randomized study comparing forceful dilatation and esophagomyotomy in patients with achalasia of the esophagus. *Gastroenterology* 1981; **80**: 789–95.

16 Pellegrini C, Wetter LA, Patti M, *et al.* Thoracoscopic esophagomyotomy: Initial experience with a new approach for the treatment of achalasia. *Ann Surg* 1992; **216**: 291–6.

17 Zaninotto G, Costantini M, Molena D, *et al.* Treatment of esophageal achalasia with laparoscopic Heller myotomy and Dor partial anterior fundoplication: Prospective evaluation of 100 consecutive patients. *J Gastrointest Surg* 2000; **4**: 282–9.

18 Banbury MK, Rice TW, Goldblum JR, *et al.* Esophagectomy with gastric reconstruction for achalasia. *J Thorac Cardiovasc Surg* 1999; **117**: 1077–84.

19 Vantrappen G, Janssens J, Hellemans J, Coremans G. Achalasia, diffuse esophageal spasm, and related motility disorders. *Gastroenterology* 1979; **76**: 450–7.

20 Pehlivanov N, Liu J, Kassab GS, *et al.* Relationship between esophageal muscle thickness and intraluminal pressure in patients with esophageal spasm. *Am J Physiol Gastrointest Liver Physiol* 2002; **282**: G1016–23.

21 Reidel WL, Clouse RE. Variations in clinical presentation of patients with esophageal contraction abnormalities. *Dig Dis Sci* 1985; **30**: 1065–71.

22 Pandolfino JE, Kahrilas PJ. American Gastroenterological Association medical position statement: Clinical use of esophageal manometry. *Gastroenterology* 2005; **128**: 207–8

23 Song CW, Lee SJ, Jeen YT, *et al.* Inconsistent association of esophageal symptoms, psychometric abnormalities and dysmotility. *Am J Gastroenterol* 2001; **96**: 2312–16.

24 Triadafilopoulos G, Tsang HP, Segall GM. Hot water swallows improve symptoms and accelerate esophageal clearance in esophageal motility disorders. *J Clin Gastroenterol* 1998; **26**: 239–44.

25 Clouse RE, Lustman PJ, Eckert TC, *et al.* Low-dose trazodone for symptomatic patients with esophageal contraction abnormalities: A double-blind, placebo-controlled trial. *Gastroenterology* 1987; **92**: 1027–36.

26 Cannon RO, Quyyumi AA, Mincemoyer R, *et al.* Imipramine in patients with chest pain despite normal coronary angiograms. *N Engl J Med* 1994; **330**: 1411–17.

27 Storr M, Allescher HD, Rosch T, *et al.* Treatment of symptomatic diffuse esophageal spasm by endoscopic injections of botulinum toxin: A prospective study with long term follow up. *Gastrointest Endosc* 2001; **54**: 754–9.

28 Ebert EC, Ouyang A, Wright SH, *et al.* Pneumatic dilatation in patients with symptomatic diffuse esophageal spasm and lower esophageal sphincter dysfunction. *Dig Dis Sci* 1983; **28**: 481–5.

29 Ellis FH Jr. Long esophagomyotomy for diffuse esophageal spasm and related disorders: An historical overview. *Dis Esophagus* 1998; **11**: 210–14.

30 Benjamin SB, Gerhardt DC, Castell DO. High amplitude, peristaltic esophageal contractions associated with chest pain and/or dysphagia. *Gastroenterology* 1979; **77**: 478–83.

31 Anderson KO, Dalton CB, Bradley LA, Richer JE. Stress induces alterations of esophageal pressures in healthy volunteers and non-cardiac chest pain patients. *Dig Dis Sci* 1989; **34**: 83–91.

32 Cohen S, Fisher R, Lipshutz W, *et al.* The pathogenesis of esophageal dysfunction in scleroderma and Raynaud's disease. *J Clin Invest* 1972; **51**: 2663–8.

33 Ebert EC. Esophageal disease in scleroderma. *J Clin Gastroenterol* 2006; **40**: 769–75.

34 Schneider HA, Yonker RA, Longley S, *et al.* Scleroderma esophagus: A nonspecific entity. *Ann Intern Med* 1984; **100**: 848–50.

35 Clouse RE, Lustman PJ, Reidel WL. Correlation of esophageal motility abnormalities with neuropsychiatric status in diabetics. *Gastroenterology* 1986; **90**: 1146–54.

36 Orringer MB. Surgical management of scleroderma reflux esophagitis. *Surg Clin North Am* 1983; **63**: 859–67.

37 Hunter JG, Trus TL, Branum GD, *et al.* A physiologic approach to laparoscopic fundoplication for gastroesophageal reflux disease. *Ann Surg* 1996; **223**: 673–85.

38 Varin O, Velstra B, DeSutter S, Ceelen W. Total vs partial fundoplication in the treatment of gastroesophageal reflux: a meta-analysis. *Arch Surg* 2009; **144**: 273–8.

39 Hui JM, Hunt DR, de Carle DJ, *et al.* Esophageal pneumatic dilation for postfundoplication dysphagia: safety, efficacy, and predictors of outcome. *Am J Gastroenterol* 2002; **97**: 2986–91.

40 Bloem BR, Lagaay AM, van Beek W, *et al.* Prevalence of subjective dysphagia in community residents aged over 87. *BMJ* 1990; **300**: 721–2.

41 Aviv JE, Martin JH, Jones ME, *et al.* Age-related changes in pharyngeal and supraglottic sensation. *Ann Otol Rhinol Laryngol* 1994; **103**: 749–52.

42 Eckhardt VF, LeCompte PM. Esophageal ganglia and smooth muscle in the elderly. *Am J Dig Dis* 1978; **23**: 443

43 Adams CW, Brain RH, Trounce JR. Ganglion cells in achalasia of the cardia. *Virchows Arch A Pathol Anat Histol* 1976; **372**: 75–9.

44 Leite LP, Johnston BT, Barrett J, *et al.* Ineffective esophageal motility (IEM). The primary finding in patients with non-specific esophageal motility disorder. *Dig Dis Sci* 1997; **42**: 1859–65.

CHAPTER 36

Infections in the Immunocompetent and Immunocompromised Patient

Colin Brown and C. Mel Wilcox

Division of Gastroenterology and Hepatology, University of Alabama, Birmingham, AL, USA

Summary

Esophageal symptoms such as odynophagia and dysphagia are suggestive of esophageal infection in immunocompromised patients. Common causes of immunocompromise include neutropenia (usually iatrogenic), HIV, transplantation, and immunomodulator therapy (including high-dose steroids). The most common infections include *Candida* species, herpes simplex virus (HSV), and cytomegalovirus (CMV), each of which have suggestive endoscopic findings, can be confirmed with biopsy and/or brushings, and have effective therapies. These therapies most often include fluconazole for *Candida* spp., acyclovir for HSV, and ganciclovir or foscarnet for CMV. Other rare infections include mycobacteria, other bacteria, actinomycosis, and other viral, fungal, and protozoal infections.

Case

You are consulted on the care of a 47 year old with a 2-week history of odynophagia. The patient received a kidney transplant 8 months ago, for long-standing diabetes mellitus. Corticosteroids were tapered off 2 months ago and mycophenolate is continued for immunosuppression. A 1-week empirical trial of fluconazole failed to relieve the symptoms. The patient has no evidence of oropharyngeal disease on physical examination.

Given the lack of response to empirical fluconazole, esophagogastroduodenoscopy is performed, demonstrating shallow ulceration of the mid-esophagus and one solitary lesion distally. Multiple biopsies of the mid and distal ulceration were performed. Histopathologic examination shows viral cytopathic effect typical of cytomegalovirus esophagitis. Intravenous ganciclovir is instituted resulting in a symptomatic improvement.

Introduction

A variety of pathogens can infect the esophagus in both the immunocompetent and the immunocompromised

Practical Gastroenterology and Hepatology: Esophagus and Stomach, 1st edition. Edited by Nicholas J. Talley, Kenneth R. DeVault and David E. Fleischer. © 2010 Blackwell Publishing Ltd.

patient. Although there is no standard definition for an immunocompromised patient, a practical list of conditions includes the following:

- Neutropenia (absolute neutrophil count <500/mm^3)
- HIV with CD4 count <200
- Solid organ transplantation
- Bone marrow transplantation
- Leukemia/lymphoma
- Cytotoxic chemotherapy
- High-dose steroids (40 mg prednisone or equivalent) for 2 weeks
- Immunomodulator therapy, i.e., azathioprine, methotrexate
- Asplenism
- Any inherited immune deficiency.

Many other medical conditions can render patients immunocompromised such as diabetes, cirrhosis, restrictive and obstructive lung disease, malnutrition, prolonged hospitalization, and exposure to broad-spectrum antibiotics. With an aging population exposed to an increasing number of medical and procedural therapies, the line between the immunocompromised and the immunocompetent patient will continue to blur.

Overview of the Immune System

The two major pathways for the body's immune response are cellular and humoral. Humoral immunity comes from the production of antibodies whereas cellular immunity comes from the direct interaction between antigens and lymphocytes.

A brief review of the native immune response is as follows: an antigen is processed by an antigen-presenting cell (APC) by either phagocytosis or endocytosis. The processed antigen is then presented on the class II MHC (major histocompatibility complex) molecule to a resting T-helper (CD4-positive) cell. The interaction between the APC and the T-helper cell generates the release of interleukins which further stimulate the T-helper cell.

Once the T-helper cell has been activated, it produces a variety of cytokines that exert an influence on cytotoxic T (CD8-positive) cells, macrophages, neutrophils, B lymphocytes, and natural killer cells. Cytotoxic T cells are induced to attack native cells expressing antigen on the class I MHC molecule and kill the target cell, with the release of lytic enzymes and perforins. Macrophages become larger and more phagocytic, and express more class II MHC molecules on their surface, which perpetuates the immune response. Neutrophils are recruited to the site of infection where they ingest and kill the offending agent. Natural killer cells are lymphocytes that express neither CD4 nor CD8, but when activated they recognize antigens (usually viral or tumor proteins) on the class I MHC molecule or portions of antibodies that adhere to the compromised cell. B cells are induced to proliferate as well as to differentiate into antibody-secreting plasma cells. Although this description only approximates the more complex immune response that occurs in vivo, it gives an idea of the major factors and points of disruption in the immunosuppressed patient [1].

As mentioned above, many pharmacologic agents can hamper the body's immune response. This has become an increasing problem with the advent of transplantation medicine and increased therapeutics for a spectrum of autoimmune disorders. Table 36.1 illustrates how these different agents work.

Candida Esophagitis

Candida esophagitis is primarily caused by *Candida albicans*—an organism that can colonize the esophagus in up to 25% of normal individuals, although more recent data

Table 36.1 Mechanisms of immune suppression and the target cells based on agent.

Drug	Mechanism	Effect on Immune System
Corticosteroids	Blocks transcription mediated by NF-κB	Decreased production of cytokines
Azathioprine/ mercaptopurine	Antagonizes purine metabolism	Reduces B-cell and T-cell proliferation
Cyclosporine/ tacrolimus	Calcineurin inhibition	Reduces interleukin production
Sirolimus	Binds to FKBP-12 intracellular protein	Inhibits T-cell proliferation by arresting the cell cycle
Infliximab/ adalumimab	Antibody to tumor necrosis factor	Inhibits cytokine induction and leukocytic migration
Mycophenolate	Prevents guanosine monophosphate production	Reduces B-cell and T-cell proliferation

suggest a much lower prevalence of 7.5% [2]. Other species that can involve the esophagus include *Candida glabrata*, *C. krusei*, and *C. tropicalis*. Infection occurs when the immune system can no longer prevent the fungus from invading the epithelium [1].

Candida esophagitis is one of the more prevalent infections in immunocompromised patients. It is an AIDS-defining illness for HIV-infected patients but its presence is not solely limited to them. The cases of 51 consecutive non-HIV patients diagnosed with candida esophagitis were reported, and concurrent carcinoma, uncontrolled diabetes, and recent steroid or antibiotic use increased the odds ratio (from 4.55 to 8.05) for infection. Renal transplant recipients are also at high risk and studies have shown that infection can occur despite nystatin prophylaxis. A later study of 265 renal allograft patients taking one of 3 different immunosuppressant regimens revealed an incidence of 10.5% [3].

With respect to HIV infection, the incidence of candida esophagitis escalates with declining CD4 counts. A review of two cohorts of French HIV-infected patients totaling 2664 found an incidence ratio of candida esophagitis from 0.3 cases/100 person-years in patients with CD4 counts >500 to 11 cases/100 person-years for those with CD4 counts <50. Another American cohort of HIV patients with CD4 counts <300 (mean 117) revealed a higher incidence of 13.3/100 patient-years with a 30% probability of developing infection over a course of 3 years [4].

Immunocompetent patients with esophageal motility disorders are also susceptible to candida esophagitis. An incidence of 44% has been reported in scleroderma patients without acid suppression and in 89% taking a proton pump inhibitor (PPI) or an H_2-receptor blocker. Persistent candidal infections have been described in postmyotomy achalasia patients.

The typical presentation of candida esophagitis is dysphagia or odynophagia. In a small study of 18 patients, 13 (72%) presented with dysphagia and 2 (11%) odynophagia. Patients may be asymptomatic. In one of the earlier case studies, only 14 of 27 patients with the disease had esophageal symptoms. In a later series looking specifically at HIV-infected patients with oral and esophageal candidiasis, 43% of those with an infected esophagus were asymptomatic [5]. Conversely, patients can have such advanced disease that they present with luminal impingement.

The diagnosis is typically made endoscopically, followed by biopsy or brushing. A whitish plaque or exudate, which can be circumferential or patchy, is the most common endoscopic finding; however, other findings include mucosal friability and erythema (Figure 36.1a). This plaque is typically adherent to the mucosa and cannot be washed off but can be removed with the endoscope (Figure 36.1b). Ulcers are very rare and when identified they should be attributed to a different etiology [6]. Infiltration of the plaque by the fungus confirms the diagnosis pathologically. Rarely, the fungus can be found invading muscularis propria and adventitia. Typical endoscopic findings are highly accurate. Physical findings on oral examination can be indicative of esophageal infection as the positive and negative predictive values for oral candidiasis have been measured at 90% and 82%, respectively [7]. The administration of barium can support the diagnosis. A "foamy esophagus" manifested by tiny bubbles resting on top of the barium column has been described in scleroderma patients diagnosed with candida esophagitis. Other findings on barium swallow include the plaques, altered motility, and a "shaggy

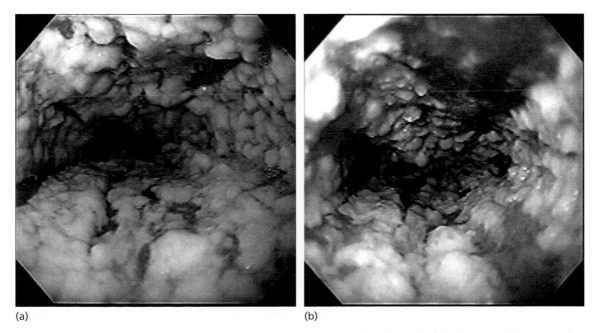

(a)   (b)

Figure 36.1 Candida esophagitis: (a) multiple plaques coat the esophageal mucosa; (b) with removal of the plaque material, no mucosal lesions are evident.

contour" that is associated with advanced disease. Retrospective studies report the sensitivity of barium esophageal studies at 80%.*

The high prevalence of candida esophagitis in HIV-infected patients raises the possibility of empirical therapy for certain patient populations with typical signs and symptoms (thrush, dysphagia, odynophagia). It appears that such an approach can be economical with regard to HIV-infected patients with low CD4 counts. However, failure to respond to therapy within a week should lower the threshold for a diagnostic procedure [8].

Fluconazole is the mainstay of therapy for candida esophagitis. This triazole medication inhibits the cytochrome P450 enzyme and the production of sterols necessary for membrane integrity. The drug has been studied in comparison to many other antifungals and trials have reported clinical response rates ranging from 80% to 90% [9]. Treatment courses range anywhere from 7 days to 14 days, although some protocols have extended therapy to 8 weeks based on symptom response. The dose usually consists of 200 mg for the first day and 100 mg daily for the duration of treatment.

The drug is generally well tolerated and the prolonged half-life of 30 h allows for once-daily dosing. Reported side effects include nausea, gastrointestinal upset, and skin rash. Severe hepatotoxicity has been reported but one series of liver transplant recipients receiving prophylactic fluconazole showed no incidence of liver injury. Transplant recipients may require increased monitoring as the drug increases the level of common immunosuppressants, including cyclosporine and tacrolimus.

Other -azoles have been studied. In a large Italian study consisting of HIV patients, itraconazole was less efficacious than fluconazole, but led to a clinical response in 75% and an endoscopic response in 66% of the patients [10]. Fluconazole has also been shown to be superior to ketoconazole, which had a clinical response rate of 65% and an endoscopic response rate of 52% when compared with fluconazole (85% and 91%, respectively). The difference in efficacy may be related to better absorption of fluconazole, which is independent of gastric pH, whereas the other -azole therapies do not achieve the same plasma concentration in the setting of

gastric hyposecretion [10]. The oral solution form of itraconazole may be better absorbed and is as efficacious as fluconazole tablets.

Other agents have been used in the treatment of candidal infections. One study compared the fungal wall inhibitor caspofungin (50 mg i.v. daily) to fluconazole (200 mg i.v. daily) in patients with candida esophagitis, yielding similar response rates and no significant adverse events [11]. The fluorinated pyrimidine analog flucytosine has been shown to be inferior to fluconazole (endoscopic cure of 33% compared with 70%), but can be more effective when combined with itraconazole (clinical cure rate of 97%). Amphotericin can be used with success, but its significant side-effect profile makes it a less desirable agent for treating candida esophagitis.

Herpes Simplex Virus

Although herpes simplex virus type 1 (HSV-1) virus is a common cause of oral pharyngeal symptoms, it can present as esophagitis in both immunocompromised and occasionally immunocompetent patients. In an autopsy study of 1307 patients, a prevalence of 1.5% was found with 18 patients having an underlying malignancy, and the 6 other patients separate causes [12]. A consecutive series of 221 renal transplant recipients identified 5 cases of HSV esophagitis, all occurring after treatment for acute cellular rejection. Although HSV esophagitis is an AIDS-defining illness, it is relatively uncommon compared with other causes of esophageal pathology in HIV-infected patients. An 18-month prospective study of 154 HIV patients with gastrointestinal symptoms led to the diagnosis of HSV esophagitis in 4 patients [13]. Another review of 100 AIDS patients with esophageal ulcers (median CD4 count 15) reported only 5 HSV cases and another 4 with both HSV and cytomegalovirus (CMV) [14]. Odynophagia is the typical presentation of HSV esophagitis. In a study of 38 patients odynophagia was a presenting symptom in 29 patients [15]. Fever, nausea, vomiting, dysphagia, heartburn, abdominal pain, and weight loss are other features of HSV infection [14–16]. Less common presentations include bleeding, fistula formation, strictures, and even perforation [14,15]. Physical exam leads to the concomitant finding of oropharyngeal lesions 20–30% of the time [14,15].

The diagnosis is established by endoscopy and biopsy. Fluid-filled vesicles similar to the oral lesions are present early in the course of disease [13]. The more common

---

*Levine MS, Macones AJ Jr, Laufer I. Candida esophagitis: accuracy of radiographic diagnosis. *Radiology*, 1985; **154**(3): 581–7.

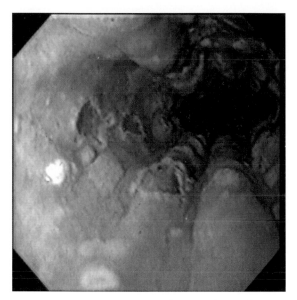

Figure 36.2 Herpes simplex virus esophagitis: multiple well-circumscribed ulcerations are present in the mid-esophagus.

finding is the presence of multiple, well-circumscribed ulcers (Figure 36.2). The ulcers can be either shallow with a whitish exudate or "punched out" in appearance, with a yellow base and raised margins ("volcano ulcers"). The ulcers tend to be smaller (1–5 mm) than ulcers caused by CMV. The ulcers are interspersed throughout otherwise normal mucosa, but advanced disease can lead to diffuse mucosal injury and a "pseudomembranous" appearance. The entire esophagus can be involved, and typically the lesions settle in the mid- to distal esophagus. Isolated upper esophageal lesions are rare [14]. Barium radiography may support this diagnosis. Typical findings include discrete ulcers scattered throughout normal mucosa or plaques without ulceration. The sensitivity of double-contrast barium swallow has been reported at 56% [17].

The optimal site for biopsy is the interface between the ulcer and the squamous epithelium. Histopathologic changes include multinucleated giant cells, intranuclear inclusion bodies, macrophage proliferation, and balloon degeneration of the epithelium. Cytologic specimens obtained by brushings subjected to immunohistochemical stains can make the diagnosis, but are rarely necessary [18]. The virus can be cultured in a variety of media (rabbit kidney cells, embryonic lung fibroblasts); however, DNA hybridization techniques can be employed when histopathology is indeterminate.

For immunocompetent patients, the infection is self-limiting, requiring only supportive care [15]. Immunocompromised patients, however, should be treated with acyclovir as the standard of care. Acyclovir is a nucleoside analog that inhibits viral DNA polymerase. It is generally well tolerated but adequate volume resuscitation is required when given intravenously to prevent crystallization in the kidneys. In the setting of esophagitis, the medication can be given either parentally or orally at a dose of 15–30 mg/kg per day, in divided doses. Treatment regimens are usually 10 days to 2 weeks. The treatment is generally efficacious—the above series of 34 HSV-infected HIV patients reported only 1 treatment failure and 5 relapses. As the virus is not eradicated, long-term maintenance therapy may be required, especially in those who relapse. Prophylaxis for transplant recipients has also been used with success [16]. In the case of acyclovir resistance, the DNA/RNA polymerase inhibitor foscarnet can be employed. However, this medication has a more significant side-effect profile, including renal failure, electrolyte disturbances, and genital ulceration.

Cytomegalovirus

CMV is a common pathogen in immunosuppressed patients and causes an AIDS-defining illness. CMV disease presents most frequently as retinitis, but also as encephalitis, pneumonia, viremia, colitis, and esophagitis. A multicenter prospective study of 8500 HIV-infected patients and 2778 AIDS patients found that, over a 2-year period, 14.6% developed CMV disease and 65 (2.3%) developed esophagitis. The median CD4 count of those who developed disease was 21/mm³. Of 1227 patients with AIDS identified over a 10-year period [19], 304 patients (24.8%) were diagnosed with CMV and 16 of those patients (1.3%) had esophagitis. CMV infection is a frequent complication in the transplant setting as the incidence of gastrointestinal CMV disease ranges from 2.5% to as high as 16% in certain transplant recipients.

Odynophagia and dysphagia are the most common clinical manifestations of CMV infection of the esophagus, but patients can also present with substernal chest pain, nausea and vomiting, weight loss, and fever [20]. Unusual manifestations include esophageal strictures, upper gastrointestinal bleeding, and bronchoesophageal fistulas.

Endoscopic evaluation with biopsy is the gold standard for diagnosis. The disease causes esophageal ulceration,

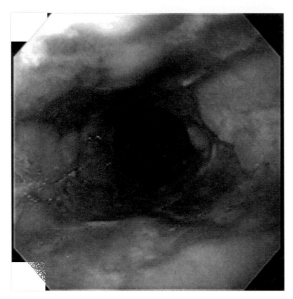

Figure 36.3 Cytomegalovirus esophagitis: several large ulcerations are present with surrounding normal mucosa.

the appearance of which can be varied [21]. In HIV patients, the virus is the most common etiology of ulceration—in one series 50 of 100 patients with ulcerative esophagitis had CMV as the cause [14]. In contrast to HSV esophagitis, the ulcers are often larger than 1 cm, but smaller ulcers can also be present. A patient can have either solitary or multiple ulcers ranging in depth (Figure 36.3). Similar to HSV, the ulcers are localized in the mid- to distal esophagus and are interspersed throughout normal mucosa, although concomitant candidal infection is often present [20]. As expected the radiographic features of CMV esophagitis are also varied. In one series of 16 patients with CMV esophagitis, barium esophagograms revealed a range of findings from superficial esophagitis to multiple deep ulcerations that resembled esophageal tumors [22]. These ulcers were often oval in shape and ranged in size from 0.5 cm to 5 cm [22].

A biopsy of the ulcer is the best way to establish the diagnosis and brushings are often not sufficient [18]. Biopsies taken at the interface between the ulcer and normal tissue will yield the highest number of infected cells, although biopsies of the ulcer base are recommended [16,18]. Deep biopsies are indicated because infected cells are found in the lamina propria and granulation tissue, and not the squamous epithelium. To maximize diagnostic yield, a total of 10 biopsies should be

taken [23]. Histologic examination is usually sufficient for diagnosis and findings include the presence of large cells with multiple small intracytoplasmic inclusion bodies, and a "halo" around the nucleus, with nuclear inclusions as well [16,18]. Viral culture, while specific, does little to add to the sensitivity of the sampling. In one series of 16 patients with CMV esophagitis, only 5 viral cultures were positive [18]. *In situ* hybridization is another technique that can identify the virus.

Once the diagnosis is established, treatment with a variety of systemic antivirals is employed. Ganciclovir and foscarnet are the two primary agents for treatment of CMV esophagitis. Ganciclovir, because of its more favorable side-effect profile, has been the first-line agent. It is a DNA polymerase inhibitor that is given intravenously at a dose of 5 mg/kg every 12 h for 14–21 days. Response rates for therapy ranges from 70% to 80% [24]. In the setting of a partial response, therapy can be protracted to 6 weeks. Severe neutropenia is what has led to the discontinuation of the drug in the literature [24], and other side effects include central nervous system effects, hepatotoxicity, fever, and rash. Foscarnet has also been used with success, often in the setting of treatment failures with ganciclovir [14,24]. This drug, which inhibits DNA and RNA polymerase—and may be effective in vivo against HIV—is given at a dose of 90 mg/kg twice daily for a period of 14–21 days. When compared directly with ganciclovir, the two medications had similar efficacy rates. Reported side effects of the medication include renal impairment and electrolyte disturbances, and adequate hydration needs to be maintained. For both treatments, relapse rates are reported to be as high as 40% in the setting of continued immunosuppression, with relapse occurring an average of 9 months after treatment [24].

Mycobacterial Infections

Mycobacterial disease places an enormous burden on the health of the population worldwide, with immunosuppressed individuals being disproportionately at risk. *Mycobacterium avium* complex (MAC) has shown affinity for hosts who are transplant recipients and have advanced AIDS. Mycobacterial tuberculosis can infect transplant recipients, but has a major impact on patients with advanced HIV disease. Mycobacterial disease of the esophagus is a rare manifestation of infection. Tuberculous esophagitis has been reported to occur in only 0.15%

of cases of patients afflicted with the mycobacterium [25]. Of 2176 patients at an Indian hospital with persistent dysphagia (>6 weeks), 12 cases (0.55%) of tuberculous esophagitis were diagnosed [26]. Esophageal disease has traditionally been thought to be a consequence of mediastinal spread, but Jain *et al.* [26] found that the majority of the disease was limited to the esophagus. The incidence of MAC esophagitis has not been studied systematically, and the organism's involvement in the esophagus is limited to case reports.

The presentation of esophageal disease is variable. One such series looked at 11 patients with tuberculous esophagitis, 9 of whom had dysphagia and 2 bleeding. In another series of 12 patients, all complained of dysphagia and other manifestations included weight loss, fever, retrosternal pain, and cough [26]. Other reported manifestations include odynophagia esophagomediastinal, or esophagotracheal fistula and perforation [27]. Few cases of MAC esophagitis have been reported. There was one case report of a fistula and one case of odynophagia and dysphagia. When found in the gastrointestinal tract, MAC preferentially resides in the duodenum where it is associated with diarrhea, fever, weight loss, and abdominal pain.

Endoscopic findings demonstrate that most of the lesions in tuberculous esophagitis are located in the mid-esophagus [26,27]. Findings are variable and include ulcers (multiple or single), infiltrative growths resembling tumors, strictures, and fistulae [26,27]. Ulcers associated with tuberculous esophagitis have been described as irregular in shape, gray at the base, and friable. They can range in size from small punctate lesions. Radiographic findings usually include a normal chest radiograph and computed tomography of the chest if the esophagus is the primary site, but these films are non-specifically abnormal in the setting of a secondary infection [26,28]. Pulmonary lesions, mediastinal adenopathy, or even a mediastinal mass can appear on these films [28]. A barium swallow can demonstrate ulcerations, strictures, pseudotumors, and fistula formations [26,28]. Ulcerations can be present in the setting of MAC esophagitis.

Biopsy is required for diagnosis and the presence of caseating granulomas, with the presence of acid-fast bacilli (AFB; stain or culture) confirming the presence of tuberculous disease. In the series by Jain *et al.* [26] granulomas (caseating or non-caseating) were found in all 12

cytology specimens and 4 biopsy specimens, and, in the 11 specimens that underwent AFB staining, 7 were positive [26]. Polymerase chain reaction (PCR) testing is another method used with success. At times, confirmatory diagnosis is not achieved, and determination of the disease is by response to empirical therapy [27].

Therapy for tuberculous esophagitis consists of a multidrug regimen for a protracted course of 6–9 months. Standard therapy consists of rifampin, isoniazid, pyrazinamide, and ethambutol, although multidrug-resistant strains have emerged as a global health problem. Successful treatment can lead to fistula closure, although surgery may be ultimately necessary. MAC is treated with clarithromycin and ethambutol, and patients with continued immunosuppression may require life-long therapy.

Other Infections

Bacterial Infections

Bacterial infections of the esophagus are rare complications of the immunocompromised state. One case series of 23 patients noted that 14 had an underlying malignancy and 10 were neutropenic [29]. The entity is rare in HIV disease, but there have been recorded cases as well as a case in a patient with chronic obstructive pulmonary disease and a depressed CD4 T-cell count in the setting of steroid use. The infections consist of oral flora and, in the series by Walsh *et al.* [29], a mixture of Gram-positive cocci and Gram-negative bacilli were found. The endoscopic appearance is usually non-specific esophagitis, potentially exhibiting friability, pseudomembranes, or ulcerations. Diagnosis is made by the presence of bacteria invading the esophageal mucosa. Treatment is usually with a broad-spectrum β-lactam antibiotic.

Actinomycosis has been reported as an esophageal pathogen. Patients are also afflicted with either HIV or malignancy [30]. Patients typically have dysphagia or odynophagia and endoscopy usually reveals ulcers that can be as big as 12 cm. One additional bacterium of note is *Treponema pallidum* which can present as esophageal ulceration and strictures in the setting of tertiary syphilis [16].

Protozoal Infections

Protozoal infections of the esophagus are rare. One patient with advanced HIV with symptoms of odynophagia and ulcerations on endoscopy was diagnosed with trichomonas esophagitis. Leishmaniasis and cryptosporidial disease have also been reported [25]. Immunocompetent patients in endemic areas can present with achalasia as a sequela from Chagas disease mediated by *Trypanosoma cruzi*.

Other Fungal Infections

Aspergillus and *Histoplasma* spp. can involve the esophagus. Aspergillus esophagitis has been seen in bone marrow transplant recipients and patients with blood-borne malignancies [31]. Patients present with dysphagia and findings include esophagitis and shallow ulceration. Treatment is accomplished with amphotericin or caspofungin. Histoplasmosis can present as dysphagia in immunosuppressed patients. Nodular ulcerations can be found on endoscopy [32]. Treatment can be accomplished with ketoconazole, itraconazole, or amphotericin.

Other Viral Infections

Varicella-zoster virus has been reported in the setting of esophagitis [33]. It can present as either vesicles or ulcers in the setting of concurrent skin findings. Papillomavirus has been associated with squamous cell papillomas in the esophagus and may be a potential etiologic agent in squamous cell cancer of the esophagus. Epstein–Barr virus has also been debated as an oncogenic agent in the esophagus. This virus has been associated with deep linear ulcers in the mid-esophagus [34].

Take-home points

Diagnosis

- Odynophagia and dysphagia in an immunocompromised patient should alert the clinician to the possibility of an esophageal infection.
- Empirical antifungal therapy is appropriate in selected patients, but failure to respond within 1 week warrants endoscopic investigation.
- HSV esophagitis typically presents endoscopically with multiple, small, well-circumscribed ulcers.
- The endoscopic appearance of CMV esophagitis is variable, although ulcers tend to be large and deep.

Therapy

- A 1- to 2-week course of fluconazole is the standard therapy for candida esophagitis.

- Acyclovir given either intravenously or orally for 10–14 days treats HSV esophagitis, although some patients may require maintenance therapy.
- Either ganciclovir or foscarnet can be used to treat CMV esophagitis; however, the relapse rate can be as high as 40% in the setting of continued immunosuppression.
- Mycobacterial esophagitis is treated with a multidrug regimen given for up to 9 months.

References

1 Glickman, Michael S, Palmer, Eric G. "Cell-Mediated Defense against Infection." Graman, Paul "Esophagitis." *Principles and Practice of Infectious Diseases*, 6th edn. Edited by Gerald Mandell, John Bennett and Raphael Dolin. Edinburgh: Churchill-Livingstone, 2005.
2 Bonavina L, Incarbone R, Reitano M, Tortorano A, Viviani M, Peracchia A. Candida colonization in patients with esophageal disease: a prospective clinical study. *Dis Esophagus* 2003; **16**: 70–2.
3 Gupta KL, Ghosh AK, Kochhar R, Jha V, Chakrabarti A, Sakhuja V. Esophageal candidiasis after renal transplantation: comparative study in patients on different immunosuppressive protocols. *Am J Gastroenterol* 1994; **89**: 1062–5
4 Moore RD, Chaisson RE. Natural history of opportunistic disease in an HIV-infected urban clinical cohort. *Ann Intern Med* 1996; **124**: 633–42.
5 López-Dupla M, Mora Sanz P, Pintado García V, *et al.* Clinical, endoscopic, immunologic, and therapeutic aspects of oropharyngeal and esophageal candidiasis in HIV-infected patients: a survey of 114 cases. *Am J Gastroenterol* 1992; **87**: 1771–6.
6 Wilcox CM, Schwartz DA. Endoscopic-pathologic correlates of Candida esophagitis in acquired immunodeficiency syndrome. *Dig Dis Sci* 1996; **41**: 1337–45.
7 Wilcox CM, Straub RF, Clark WS. Prospective evaluation of oropharyngeal findings in human immunodeficiency virus-infected patients with esophageal ulceration. *Am J Gastroenterol* 1995; **90**: 1938–41.
8 Wilcox CM, Alexander LN, Clark WS, Thompson SE 3rd. Fluconazole compared with endoscopy for human immunodeficiency virus-infected patients with esophageal symptoms. *Gastroenterology* 1996; **110**: 1803–9.
9 Barbari G, Barbarini G, Calderon W, *et al.* Fluconazole versus itraconazole for Candida esophagitis in acquired immunodeficiency syndrome. *Gastroenterology* 1996; **111**: 1169.
10 Barbaro G, Barbarini G, Calderon W, Grisorio B, Alcini P, Di Lorenzo G. Fluconazole versus itraconazole for candida

esophagitis in acquired immunodeficiency syndrome. *Gastroenterology* 1996; **111**: 1169–77.

11 Villanueva A, Gotuzzo E, Arathoon EG, *et al.* A randomized double-blind study of caspofungin versus fluconazole for the treatment of esophageal candidiasis. *Am J Med* 2002; **113**: 294–9.

12 Itoh T, Takahashi T, Kusaka K, *et al.* Herpes simplex esophagitis from 1307 autopsy cases. *J Gastroenterol Hepatol* 2003; **18**: 1407–11.

13 Connolly GM, Hawkins D, Harcourt-Webster JN, Parsons PA, Husain OA, Gazzard BG. Oesophageal symptoms, their causes, treatment, and prognosis in patients with the acquired immunodeficiency syndrome. *Gut* 1989; **30**: 1033–9.

14 Wilcox CM, Schwartz DA, Clark WS. Esophageal ulceration in human immunodeficiency virus infection. Causes, response to therapy, and long-term outcome. *Ann Intern Med* 1995; **123**: 143–9.

15 Ramanathan J, Rammouni M, Baran J Jr, Khatib R. Herpes simplex virus esophagitis in the immunocompetent host: An overview. *Am J Gastroenterol* 2000; **95**: 2171–6.

16 Baehr PH, McDonald GB. Esophageal infections: risk factors, presentation, diagnosis, and treatment. *Gastroenterology* 1994; **106**: 509–32.

17 Levine MS, Loevner LA, Saul SH, Rubesin SE, Herlinger H, Laufer I. Herpes esophagitis: sensitivity of double-contrast esophagography. *AJR Am J Roentgenol* 1988; **151**: 57–62.

18 Wilcox CM, Rodgers W, Lazenby A. Prospective comparison of brush cytology, viral culture, and histology for the diagnosis of ulcerative esophagitis in AIDS. *Clin Gastroenterol Hepatol* 2004; **2**: 564–7.

19 d'Arminio Monforte A, Mainini F, Testa L, *et al.* Predictors of cytomegalovirus disease, natural history and autopsy findings in a cohort of patients with AIDS. *AIDS* 1997; **11**: 517–24.

20 Wilcox CM, Diehl DL, Cello JP, Margaretten W, Jacobson MA. Cytomegalovirus esophagitis in patients with AIDS. A clinical, endoscopic, and pathologic correlation. *Ann Intern Med* 1990; **113**: 589–93.

21 Wilcox CM, Straub RF, Schwartz DA. Prospective endoscopic characterization of cytomegalovirus esophagitis in AIDS. *Gastrointest Endosc* 1994; **40**: 481–4.

22 Balthazar EJ, Megibow AJ, Hulnick D, Cho KC, Beranbaum E. Cytomegalovirus esophagitis in AIDS: radiographic features in 16 patients. *AJR Am J Roentgenol* 1987; **149**: 919–23.

23 Wilcox CM, Straub RF, Schwartz DA. Prospective evaluation of biopsy number for the diagnosis of viral esophagitis in patients with HIV infection and esophageal ulcer. *Gastrointest Endosc* 1996; **44**: 587–93.

24 Wilcox CM, Straub RF, Schwartz DA. Cytomegalovirus esophagitis in AIDS: A prospective evaluation of clinical response to Ganciclovir therapy, relapse rate, and long-term outcome. *Am J Med* 1995; **98**: 169–76.

25 Eroğlu A, Kürkçüoğlu C, Karaoğlanoğlu N, Yilmaz Ö, Gürsan N. Esophageal tuberculosis abscess: an unusual cause of dysphagia. *Dis Esophagus* 2002; **15**: 93–5.

26 Jain SK, Jain S, Jain M, Yaduvanshi A. Esophageal tuberculosis: is it so rare? Report of 12 cases and review of the literature. *Am J Gastroenterol* 2002; **97**: 287–91.

27 Abid S, Jafri W, Hamid S, *et al.* Endoscopic features of esophageal tuberculosis. *Gastrointest Endosc* 2003; **57**: 759–62.

28 Nagi B, Lal A, Kochhar R, *et al.* Imaging of esophageal tuberculosis: a review of 23 cases. *Acta Radiol* 2003; **44**: 329–33.

29 Walsh TJ, Belitsos NJ, Hamilton SR. Bacterial esophagitis in immunocompromised patients. *Arch Intern Med* 1986; **146**: 1345–8.

30 Abdalla J, Myers J, Moorman J. Actinomycotic infection of the oesophagus. *J Infect* 2005; **51**: 39–43.

31 Bergman S, Geisinger KR. Esophageal aspergillosis in cytologic brushings: report of two cases associated with acute myelogenous leukemia. *Diagn Cytopathol* 2004; **30**: 347–9.

32 Fucci JC, Nightengale ML. Primary esophageal histoplasmosis. *Am J Gastroenterol* 1997; **92**: 530–1.

33 Gill RA, Gebhard RL, Dozeman RL, Sumner HW. Shingles esophagitis: endoscopic diagnosis in two patients. *Gastrointest Endosc* 1984; **30**: 26–7.

34 Kitchen VS, Helbert M, Francis ND, *et al.* Epstein–Barr virus associated oesophageal ulcers in AIDS. *Gut* 1990; **31**: 1223–5.

CHAPTER 37
Strictures, Rings, and Webs

Peter D. Siersema

Department of Gastroenterology and Hepatology, University Medical Center Utrecht, Utrecht, The Netherlands

Summary

Benign esophageal strictures, rings, and webs are a common problem in endoscopic practice. There are various etiologies of benign esophageal strictures with considerable variation in pathologic features. The predominant symptom of all patients is dysphagia. The overall pathologic finding in patients with a benign esophageal stricture, ring, or web is the deposition of fibrous tissue. The initial treatment option for patients with a benign stricture of the esophagus is endoscopic dilation. A subgroup of esophageal strictures, rings, and webs tends to recur and is called refractory, requiring an alternate treatment strategy. This chapter summarizes the etiologies of benign esophageal strictures, rings, and webs, the modalities to diagnose them, and the treatment options that are currently available.

Case

A 55-year-old white man presented with a 10-month history of dysphagia. Over the last 5 years, he had suffered from heartburn and regurgitation, particularly when bending forward and during the night while in bed. These symptoms had quite suddenly resolved and at the same time he noticed dysphagia. His body weight had gradually increased over the past few years. His appetite had not changed. An esophagogastroduodenoscopy was performed which showed a regular, smooth, 1–2-cm-long stricture in the distal esophagus, just above the gastroesophageal junction. The stricture could be passed only with a small-caliber (5.9 mm) endoscope. Biopsies were taken, but only showed a moderate inflammatory reaction and fibrous tissue with no evidence of malignancy. He was diagnosed with a peptic stricture, and the stricture was dilated using various diameter Savary–Gilliard dilators up to 18 mm and he was started on proton pump inhibitors (PPIs). After dilation, the symptoms did not recur and he was able to resume a normal diet.

Definition and Epidemiology

Benign esophageal strictures, rings, and webs are caused by a variety of etiologies with considerable variation in

Practical Gastroenterology and Hepatology: Esophagus and Stomach, 1st edition. Edited by Nicholas J. Talley, Kenneth R. DeVault and David E. Fleischer. © 2010 Blackwell Publishing Ltd.

underlying pathologic mechanisms (Table 37.1) [1] and severity of symptoms (Table 37.2) [2]. In addition, benign esophageal strictures, rings, and webs can be classified according to complexity, which determines the type and number of therapeutic procedures. Strictures that are short, focal, and straight, and allow passage of an endoscope, are considered simple strictures. The main examples of these are peptic strictures, rings, and webs. In general, one to three dilations are needed to relieve dysphagia due to these strictures, with only a quarter requiring additional treatment sessions. There is a subgroup of strictures that is more difficult to treat and tend to recur despite dilation therapy. These strictures are usually longer (>2 cm), angulated, and irregular, and have a severely narrowed diameter. They are defined as an anatomic restriction because of a cicatricial luminal compromise or fibrosis that results in symptoms of dysphagia in the absence of endoscopic evidence of inflammation. This may occur as the result of an inability either to successfully remediate the anatomic problem to a diameter of at least 14 mm over five sessions at 2-week intervals (refractory) or to maintain a satisfactory luminal diameter for 4 weeks once the target diameter of 14 mm has been achieved. These are defined as refractory esophageal strictures [1].

Although dysphagia is a common condition, occurring in 5–8% of the general population over 50 years [3], it is

Table 37.1 Differential diagnosis of esophageal dysphagia [1].

Inflammatory and/or fibrotic strictures
Peptic
Caustic
Pill induced
Radiation induced

Mucosal rings and webs
Schatzki ring
Multiringed esophagus (eosinophilic esophagitis)

Cancer
Primary (squamous, adenocarcinoma)
Secondary (e.g., lung, breast, melanoma)

Intramural lesions
Leiomyoma
Granular cell tumor

Extramural lesions
Aberrant right subclavian artery (dysphagia lusoria)
Mediastinal masses
Lung cancer

Anatomical abnormalities
Hiatus hernia
Esophageal diverticulum

Motility disorders
Achalasia and achalasia-like disorders
Pseudoachalasia
Hypomotility secondary to systemic disease (e.g., scleroderma,
  amyloid, diabetes)

Table 37.2 Dysphagia scoring system to grade severity of dysphagia in patients with benign esophageal strictures, rings, or webs [2].

Score	Definition
0	Able to eat a normal diet
2	Able to swallow semisolid foods
3	Able to swallow liquids only
4	Unable to swallow liquids

difficult to obtain detailed information on incidence and prevalence rates, due to the various etiologies (see Table 37.1) [4]. An estimated 60–70% of benign esophageal strictures are peptic in origin and result from gastroesophageal reflux disease (GERD). The prevalence of strictures among GERD patients undergoing endoscopy is 4–20%, but this may diminish in the future due to the widespread use of PPIs. Another important group of

benign esophageal strictures includes those that are caused by caustic injury [5]. Despite the increasing use of "child-proof" packages and containers for household caustic agents, accidental ingestion by children still occurs with alarming frequency. Among adults, most ingestions of caustic substances are intentional, i.e., for the purpose of suicide. Due to the increasing number of patients undergoing upper digestive tract surgery for a malignancy, anastomotic strictures between the esophagus and the stomach (gastric tube), jejunum, or colon interposition are also increasingly being recognized [6].

Web-like strictures of the esophagus are usually congenital or inflammatory in origin. Symptomatic hypopharyngeal webs with iron-deficiency anemia in middle-aged women constitute the Plummer–Vinson syndrome. The clinical importance of this syndrome is uncertain. Although commonly reported in the past, it is now an uncommon disorder.

Lower esophageal mucosal rings (Schatzki rings) are thin, web-like constrictions located at the squamocolumnar junction or near the border of the lower esophageal sphincter. Schatzki rings are associated with GERD; however, their exact pathogenic mechanism remains uncertain. A relatively new disorder causing rings throughout the esophagus is eosinophilic esophagitis. This inflammatory disorder is increasingly being recognized in the Western world, but it is unknown how often it causes strictures and, as a consequence, dysphagia [7].

Pathophysiology

Benign esophageal strictures result from esophageal injury. The volume, dwell time, concentration, and depth of the injury produced by the underlying causative etiology determine the severity and recurrence risk after treatment of the stricture [8]. The pathologic processes in benign esophageal strictures can be quite diverse. An inflammatory component is found in almost all benign strictures, but not to the same degree or for the same period of time. For example, the initial inflammatory reaction in peptic and caustic strictures can be severe, but this will ultimately resolve with a satisfactory outcome for the stricture as well. On the other hand, transmural (ischemic) insults to the esophagus, such as are seen in postoperative anastomotic and postradiation strictures, may be more difficult and need more time to resolve, and sometimes need prolonged treatment. Any treatment in these situations is a temporizing maneuver, allowing the inflammatory reaction to resolve over time. In particular, if there is ongoing or repeated injury to the esophageal mucosa, the resulting acute inflammation and healing reaction with fibrosis may maintain the stricture.

Clinical Features

Patients with a benign stricture, web, or ring have symptoms in common, but may have some discriminating symptoms depending on the type of injury to the esophageal wall. It is important to obtain a careful history before deciding which investigative algorithm will be used (Table 37.3).

Dysphagia is the primary symptom of any type of esophageal obstruction, although it is often a late symptom. Typically the patient will describe food "stick-

ing" or "holding up," but at times the presenting symptoms may be atypical. Atypical symptoms of dysphagia include meal-related regurgitation (often reported as vomiting), a sense of fullness or filling up retrosternally, or hiccups during meals. Two aims should be met when taking a dysphagia history. The first is to establish whether or not dysphagia is actually present, i.e., to distinguish true dysphagia from globus sensation or a difficulty in swallowing. The second is to determine whether the site of the problem is pharyngeal or esophageal.

If dysphagia is present, it usually starts with difficulty passing larger solid food challenges, typically meat, down the esophagus followed by dysphagia for all solids (see Table 37.2). Solid food obstruction becomes permanent when the esophageal lumen is reduced to approximately 12 mm (which equals 50% of normal). Patients often ignore the early symptoms of dysphagia for some time. They compensate for this by eating softer or minced food, eating slowly, or using variable amounts of fluid to facilitate the passage of food down the esophagus. At a sudden moment, complete obstruction for all food, and a later stage also for fluids, occurs during a meal. This is a challenging problem to endoscopists because it usually occurs during the nighttime, some time after dinner.

Regurgitation during meals, as well as spontaneous regurgitation between meals or at night, is easily separated from vomiting because it is not associated with nausea. Unlike regurgitation that is related to gastroesophageal reflux, the regurgitated fluid and/or food in patients with an esophageal stricture is generally not noxious to taste.

Odynophagia is not always present, but can be present with erosive or ulcerative esophageal disease, or with increased intraesophageal pressure and distension. Examples of the former include benign esophageal strictures with an ongoing inflammatory component, as is seen in GERD, caustic burns, and postradiation esophagitis.

It is important to take a thorough previous medical history, which should take into account the previous application of radiation therapy on the chest (postradiation stricture), the use of medication, e.g., non-steroidal anti-inflammatory drugs (NSAIDs), potassium chloride, alendronate (pill-induced strictures), the accidental or intentional use of caustic fluids (caustic strictures), the performance of a surgical procedure to the esophagus or stomach (anastomotic stricture), a history of heartburn

Table 37.3 Clinical features in patients with benign strictures, rings, or webs.

Symptom	Comment
Dysphagia	Starting with large solids, followed by all solids, then liquids, and finally no food or drinks
Regurgitation	Mostly in advanced cases
Odynophagia	In cases with erosions or ulceration (reflux esophagitis, radiation injury, caustic injury)
Previous medical history	Radiation therapy on chest, esophageal or gastric resection
History of esophageal injury	GERD, caustic, radiation therapy, pills
Other symptoms	Heartburn (GERD), systemic disease (scleroderma)
Sialorrhea	Related to severity of obstruction
Weight loss	Uncommon with benign stricture, rings, or webs (more common with malignancy)
History of smoking and alcohol abuse	Malignant disorder (esophageal cancer, lung cancer)

GERD, gastroesophageal reflux disease.

in GERD, and some other causes (see Tables 37.1 and 37.3).

Diagnosis

The most valuable investigation in patients with esophageal dysphagia is esophagogastroduodenoscopy (EGD). In some cases, a barium swallow or computed tomography (CT) scan of the chest and gastroesophageal junction (GEJ) can be helpful. Endoscopy will, however, frequently obviate the need for a radiographic examination. Finally, esophageal manometry may detect a motility disorder (Table 37.4).

Esophagogastroduodenoscopy

EGD is indicated in virtually all patients with dysphagia. Endoscopy will identify anastomotic strictures, but is also able to detect any coexisting perforation, leak, or fistula. Caustic strictures can be multifocal in the esophagus, with the most proximal location just below the upper esophageal sphincter. Postradiation strictures are mostly localized, and the same is true for pill-induced strictures that are often found in the mid-esophagus. Not surprisingly, peptic strictures and Schatzki rings are always found in the distal esophagus. If no clear

structural abnormality is seen, distal and mid-esophageal biopsies should be considered, to rule out eosinophilic esophagitis, in any case of unexplained dysphagia or food impaction. Infective esophagitis (e.g., that caused by herpes simplex virus, cytomegalovirus, or candida infections) has typical appearances. Strictures should in most cases be biopsied and dilated at the time of endoscopy. The finding of food, fluid, or salivary residue within a dilated esophagus is highly suggestive of dysmotility, particularly achalasia. In these cases, esophageal manometry is the best technique to confirm this diagnosis.

(Barium) Radiography

Radiography with or without the use of contrast medium may have a role in the identification of a (Zenker) diverticulum or a mucosal ring as is seen in eosinophilic esophagitis. This technique is also able to detect a perforation, leak, or fistula, in combination with a stricture. In addition, a CT scan can be used to identify the extent of a malignancy and/or detect a malignancy compressing the esophagus. In some cases, a CT scan will detect a small malignancy close to the GEJ causing so-called pseudoachalasia or explaining dysphagia in combination with hiccups.

It is important to note that normal endoscopy and radiography results do not always rule out a structural esophageal disorder [9]. If a structural disorder is still suspected, it is important to determine whether a barium swallow study included prone views and a marshmallow or pill swallow. Mucosal rings and webs, in particular, are frequently overlooked unless adequate and deliberate distension of the esophagus is achieved by evaluating the esophageal contours in the prone position, preferably while the patient performs the Valsalva maneuver. It can also be considered to repeat endoscopy and perform empirical esophageal dilation. Empirical dilation can have short-term and long-term efficacy, and is safe when endoscopic inspection of the esophagus shows a tiny ring-like stricture or is completely normal. Diagnostic information can also be gained by inspection of the esophagus immediately after removal of the dilator. If one or more mucosal tears are present, this confirms the site and caliber of any constrictions not previously visualized. Furthermore, the absence of post-dilation mucosal trauma correlates reasonably well with a poor clinical response, and indicates that a mucosal web,

Table 37.4 Diagnostic modalities in benign strictures, rings, or webs.

Symptom	Comment
Esophagogastroduodenoscopy	Allows inspection of localization of the stricture In addition, it allows biopsies to be obtained and endoscopic treatment to be performed
Radiography	A barium swallow detects small strictures, rings, or webs and identifies coexisting perforations, leaks, and fistulae A computed tomography scan detects extramural lesions and small tumors around the gastroesophageal junction
Esophageal manometry	Detects motility disorders

ring, or stricture is unlikely to account for the patient's dysphagia.

Differential Diagnosis

The time period for which the dysphagia has been present and whether it is intermittent and/or progressive will help to define the likely cause. Slowly progressive, long-standing dysphagia, particularly against a background of reflux, is suggestive of a peptic stricture. However, the physician should remember that the severity of heartburn correlates poorly with esophageal mucosal damage. Patients who have mucosal changes including strictures and Barrett esophagus could have had minimal or no heartburn in the immediate past. On the other hand, a short history of dysphagia, particularly with rapid progression (weeks or months) and associated weight loss, is highly suggestive of esophageal cancer. Long-standing, intermittent, non-progressive dysphagia purely for solids is indicative of a fixed structural lesion such as a distal esophageal ring or proximal esophageal mucosal web. Finally, it is important to emphasize that the (previous) medical history will also allow a diagnosis to be made (see Table 37.1) [4].

Treatment

The majority of simple strictures can be treated successfully with bougie or balloon dilation. Common etiologies include peptic injury, (Schatzki) rings, or webs. One to three dilations are usually sufficient to relieve symptoms. Complex esophageal strictures are more difficult to treat. The most common causes include caustic ingestion, radiation injury, and postsurgical anastomotic strictures. These strictures often require at least three dilation sessions, and are associated with high recurrence rates. When this is the case, they are considered to be refractory and other treatment modalities will be required (Table 37.5).

It is important to treat esophageal strictures in a stepwise fashion, starting with the least invasive treatment modality (Table 37.6). If this is not sufficient to relieve the dysphagia, the next treatment modality in the algorithm should be applied. In the following, the various treatments for strictures are discussed. At the end, an

Table 37.5 Treatment modalities in benign strictures, rings, or webs.

Dilation therapy:
  bougie
  balloon
  combined antegrade and retrograde dilation (CARD)
Dilation with intralesion steroid injection
Incisional therapy:
  needle knife
  argon plasma coagulation
Stent placement:
  self-expanding metal stent (SEMS)
  self-expanding plastic stent (SEPS)
Self-bougienage

Table 37.6 Treatment algorithm of benign esophageal strictures, rings, and webs.

Step	Action
1	Dilation (Savary–Gilliard or balloon) up to 16–18 mm (up to five sessions)
2	Dilation combined with intralesional four-quadrant triamcinolone acetate injections (max. three sessions) Incisional therapy (max. three sessions) for Schatzki rings and anastomotic strictures
3	Stent placement
4	Self-bougienage Surgery

algorithm for the treatment of refractory strictures is proposed.

Dilation Therapy

Treatment of benign esophageal strictures aims to relieve symptoms of dysphagia, with avoidance of complications and prevention of recurrences. Dilation is the first-line treatment option for benign esophageal strictures [10]. Dilators can be categorized into mechanical (bougie) or balloon-type dilators. Mechanical dilators are further subdivided into bougies that are used with or without a guidewire and/or fluoroscopy. The most commonly used guidewire-assisted bougie is the polyvinyl Savary–Gilliard dilator, which has a tapered tip and is available in multiple sizes. The American dilators are similar products that are impregnated with barium and easier to see fluoroscopically. Balloon dilators can be passed through the scope and are also available with or without a guidewire.

Bougie dilators dilate a stenotic segment by using gradually increasing dilator diameters, resulting not only in a longitudinal, but also in a radial, force on the stricture. Balloon dilation can be performed under direct vision. In contrast to bougies, balloon dilators deliver only a radial force, resulting in a simultaneously applied dilating force across the entire length of the stricture. Despite these mechanistic differences, no clear advantage of either balloon or bougie dilation has been demonstrated in terms of efficacy and safety [11]. An advantage of bougie dilators is that they are more cost-effective because they are reusable, compared with balloon dilators that are intended for single use only.

The most frequently reported complications of esophageal dilation are perforation, hemorrhage, and bacteremia. Perforation rates varying between 0.1% and 0.4% have been reported. In general, it is accepted that the risk of perforation is minimal only when "the rule of three" is applied, meaning that no more than three dilators of progressively increasing diameter should be passed in a single session, corresponding with a total of $3 \times 1 = 3$ mm increase in diameter [12]. Although this "rule" is easily applicable as a clinical guideline, no studies have demonstrated that it indeed improves safety and efficacy. It is commonly advised to limit initial dilation to 39–45 Fr (about 13–15 mm). Nevertheless, there is no evidence that this prevents development of complications. The efficacy and safety of endoscopic dilation without fluoroscopy have been shown. However, it is generally advocated that fluoroscopic guidance be used to enhance safety during dilation of complex strictures.

Combined Antegrade and Retrograde Dilation

Most complex strictures can be endoscopically passed with a guidewire, followed by dilation. Occasionally, it can be difficult to identify the true lumen of a stenotic esophagus, e.g., in postradiation strictures in the cervical esophagus. In these circumstances, the passing of a guidewire for dilation through antegrade endoscopy is unsuccessful. In order to reduce the potential risk of perforation, the combined antegrade and retrograde dilation (CARD) technique can be applied [13]. The principle of the CARD technique is double endoscopic

access to the proximal and distal ends of the stricture, resulting in better control during dilation. This procedure is described in further detail in Chapter 9.

Dilation and Intralesional Steroid Injection Therapy

In the 1960s, the efficacy of intralesional corticosteroid injections into benign esophageal strictures of dogs and children was demonstrated. Over the last decade, this treatment has increasingly been employed in the treatment of refractory benign esophageal strictures. The mechanism of action is suggested to be the local inhibition of the inflammatory response, resulting in a reduction in collagen formation.

It has been demonstrated that there was an increase in intervals between dilations and a reduction in the frequency of dilations when dilation was combined with intralesional injections with triamcinolone acetonide [14]. There is no certainty about the optimal technique of intralesional steroid injection, i.e., what the optimal dose is per session is (varying between 40 and 80 mg), the number of injections per session (four to eight per session), the injection site (upper margin or inside stricture), the interval between treatment sessions, and the maximum number of treatment sessions. Only a few complications (perforation ($n = 2$) and *Candida albicans* infections ($n = 2$)) have been reported.

Incisional Therapy

Strictures at the esophagogastric anastomosis following esophageal resection have been reported in up to 30% of patients. Postoperative complications, such as anastomotic leakage, fistula formation, or ischemia of the proximal gastric tube contribute to anastomotic stricture formation. The success rate of dilation therapy of anastomotic strictures ranges from 70% to 90%, with up to 40% of patients requiring more than three dilation sessions to achieve an adequate result [6]. An alternate treatment option for refractory benign anastomotic strictures is the use of incisional therapy [15], which can be performed with needle knife electrocautery or argon plasma coagulation (APC). The author incises the stricture in four quadrants and, in addition, coagulates the bridging (fibrous) tissue in between the incisions in order to establish a maximum wide luminal diameter (Figure 37.1).

In short anastomotic strictures (<10 mm), a single treatment session is usually effective, whereas longer

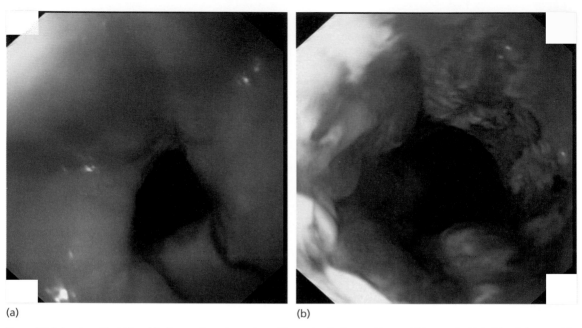

(a)   (b)

Figure 37.1 Anastomotic stricture (a) after esophageal resection with gastric tube interposition, and (b) treated with incisional therapy with needle knife electrocautery.

strictures (≥10 mm) require more electrocautery procedures. Incisional therapy can also be considered in refractory Schatzki rings. Only limited experience but no complications have been reported. More studies are needed to confirm the initial results and define patients most amenable to this treatment.

Stents

Placement of a self-expanding metal stent (SEMS) is frequently used for the palliation of dysphagia from esophageal or gastric cardia cancer. Over the last few years, stents have become increasingly important in various clinical applications such as sealing benign esophageal leaks or perforations and dilating refractory benign esophageal strictures. The introduction of self-expanding plastic stents (SEPSs) has given a further boost to the use of stents for these indications. In benign esophageal strictures, the idea is that dilation for a prolonged period of time will ultimately reduce the risk of recurrent stricture formation [16].

Self-expanding Metal Stents

Until now, more than 150 patients have been reported with a SEMS placed for a benign esophageal stricture [16]. In most, strictures were resistant to (repeat) dilation. Indications for SEMS placement included achalasia, caustic strictures, postradiation strictures, anastomotic strictures, peptic strictures, and some other causes. In initial studies, mainly uncovered SEMSs were used. In the more recent studies, partially or fully covered SEMSs were more common.

A limitation of uncovered and partially covered SEMSs is the occurrence of hyperplastic tissue ingrowth through the uncovered stent meshes. Tissue ingrowth has been considered to be due to a combination of factors, particularly the type of metal used (stainless steel or nitinol), the size and radial force of the stent, and the duration of stenting. The risk of tissue ingrowth increases with stenting time, but it can already be observed as soon as 2–6 weeks after stent placement [17]. This tissue reaction causes the uncovered stent parts to embed in the esophageal wall, which precludes easy removal. An obvious advantage of this anchoring is that migration of uncovered or partially covered SEMSs is rare, although it is more frequent with fully covered SEMSs. Hyperplastic tissue overgrowth at both stent ends can also be observed. Tissue in- or overgrowth is the cause of recurrent dysphagia in 15–20% of patients treated with a SEMS for a benign esophageal stricture, whereas stent migration is seen in 10–15% of patients. SEMSs are relatively safe with major complication, i.e., pain, reflux (esophagitis) seen in 10–20% of patients, and (rarely) perforation [16].

In published series, SEMSs were not removed in all patients. This was likely due to patient-related factors, such as old age and co-morbidity of patients. In addition, it can be imagined that physicians were sometimes reluctant to remove an imbedded SEMS. Limited reports have shown that approximately 40–50% of patients had no clinical evidence of a recurrent stricture after stent removal.

Self-expanding Plastic Stents

SEPSs are the other stent type used for this indication. The Polyflex stent is the only SEPS currently available (Figure 37.2). It is a silicone device with an encapsulated monofilament braid made of polyester. Over the last 5 years, more than 150 patients have been reported with a Polyflex stent for a (refractory) benign esophageal stricture [16]. Indications for stent placement in these series included anastomotic strictures, followed by peptic strictures, caustic strictures, postradiation strictures, and some other causes.

Although initial studies with Polyflex stents showed promising results, more recent studies have shown less favorable results, with high stent migration rates and recurrent strictures after stent removal reported in up to 90% of patients. An advantage of Polyflex stents is that they are easily removable and hyperplastic tissue overgrowth is unusual after Polyflex stent placement for benign esophageal strictures. This is probably due to the non-metal material used, the fully covered design and the relatively low radial force at the stent ends. On the other hand, migration rates are high after Polyflex stent placement, occurring in almost 50% of patients [18,19]. This high migration rate is likely the result of the fully covered stent design, the smooth outer surface of the stent, and the insufficient anchoring support provided by the stricture. Major complications were seen in less than 10% of patients and consisted of perforations, fistulas, bleeding, reflux esophagitis, and pain.

In various studies, Polyflex stents were removed in all patients after stenting times varying between 4 weeks and 18 months. Long-term improvement of dysphagia was seen in only 40% of patients.

Management of Refractory Benign Esophageal Strictures

It is important to treat esophageal strictures in a stepwise fashion, starting with the least invasive treatment modality (see Table 37.6). If this is not sufficient to relieve dysphagia, the next treatment modality in the algorithm should be applied.

Step 1

The first step in managing a benign esophageal stricture is balloon or Savary–Gilliard dilation, preferably to 16–

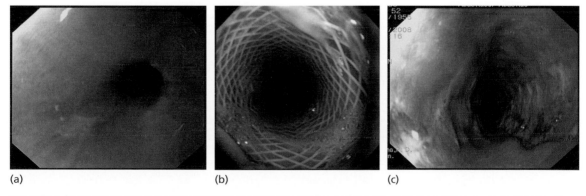

(a) (b) (c)

Figure 37.2 (a) Caustic stricture in the mid-esophagus for which (b) a Polyflex stent was placed. (c) The esophagus was significantly wider after stent removal.

18 mm. It is recommended to perform at least five dilations to the maximum diameter before the decision is taken to switch to an alternate treatment. In the author's institution, dilations are performed once a week or twice weekly in order to reach the maximum diameter in a relatively short time period.

If a stricture is considered to be refractory, the treatment plan should first be discussed with the patient, because in some refractory benign esophageal strictures many endoscopy sessions are indicated (see Figure 37.1). It is important for the patient's cooperation that he or she knows what the treatment options are and what to expect. It can also be imagined that some patients are not willing to undergo a multitude of endoscopy sessions and prefer, already after one or two dilation sessions, to have a stent placed (step 3) or even to opt for a surgical solution (step 4).

Step 2

After maximum dilation, the next step is to combine dilation with intralesional steroid injections. In the author's institution, triamcinolone acetate 20 mg/mL is used for intralesional injection and, in addition, injection of another four aliquots of 0.5 mL at the proximal margin of the stricture. There is, however, no evidence to substantiate this protocol. It is suggested that dilation, combined with intralesional steroid injection, be limited to a maximum of three sessions because, in the author's experience, more treatment sessions are rarely effective.

In refractory Schatski rings and anastomotic strictures, refractory strictures can also be treated with incisional therapy using needle knife electrocautery or APC. Again, it is suggested that a maximum of three treatment sessions be performed mainly due to a lack of further effect with more than three sessions.

Step 3

Stent placement is a treatment option to consider when an adequate luminal diameter has not been established with previous treatment modalities or when the stricture still recurs within a short time interval. The preferred stent in patients with a longer stricture in the mid-esophagus (>2–4 cm), e.g., due to caustic injury or radiation therapy, is a Polyflex stent. In patients with an anastomotic stricture in the proximal esophagus or the distal esophagus, e.g., a peptic stricture, a more flexible, partially covered stent is recommended, because the risk of migration is lower with this stent type (unpublished results).

It is not clear how long a stent should be left in the esophagus. Factors that influence stenting time include the underlying cause, the time since injury to the esophagus, and the length of the stricture. The protocol for stent placement in refractory benign esophageal strictures that is followed in the author's institution is shown in Table 37.7.

When stent placement is not successful and the stricture still persists, consideration can be given to continuing stenting and, depending on the time to the occurrence of hyperplastic tissue in- and overgrowth in a particular patient, replacing the stent at intervals determined by this fibrous tissue growth. As discussed, it is likely that the inflammatory reaction underlying the stricture will finally subside and the luminal diameter achieved at that time will remain.

Step 4

An alternate treatment option is to teach the patient self-bougienage using Maloney dilators. This is not a commonly performed practice, but it is safe and effective when patients have learned this technique. In the author's experience, self-bougienage is most successful when there is a favorable anatomy (e.g., proximal strictures of caustic or anastomotic origin without significant diverticulum formation).

Table 37.7 Guidelines for the use of stents for benign esophageal strictures, rings, and webs.

1 Strictures that are caused by ischemic injury, present within <6–12 months of the injury and/or longer than 5 cm are stented for at least 8–16 weeks
2 In all other cases, stents are inserted for a shorter period, usually 4–8 weeks
3 When symptoms recur after stent removal, a second stent is placed
4 When partially covered SEMSs are used, endoscopy should be performed at 4-week intervals to visualize whether embedding of the uncovered stent part in the esophageal mucosa has occurred; if this is the case, stent removal is performed and another stent is placed, preferably a fully covered stent
5 As fully covered SEMS and Polyflex stents also carry a risk of hyperplastic tissue overgrowth, periodic endoscopy at 6-week intervals is recommended

SEMS, self-expanding metal stent.

There is a subgroup of patients, in whom all efforts to dilate a refractory benign esophageal stricture are unsuccessful. Alternately, there are also patients who are unable to tolerate stent placement, or have just not enough patience to let the stricture resolve. In these patients, a surgical procedure could be considered.

Take-home points

Diagnosis

- Benign esophageal strictures, rings, and webs can be subdivided according to underlying pathologic mechanisms (inflammatory disorder, anatomic disorder, intra- or extramural lesions, or motility disorder).

- Benign esophageal disorders, rings, and webs can also be classified according to treatment response, i.e., simple or complex, with the latter frequently requiring repeat and prolonged treatment.

- Patients with a benign stricture, web, or ring have several symptoms in common (dysphagia, regurgitation, and odynophagia), but may have some discriminating symptoms depending on the type of injury to the esophageal wall.

- The most valuable investigation in patients with esophageal dysphagia is esophagogastroduodenoscopy, followed by radiography (barium swallow or CT of the chest) and esophageal manometry.

Therapy

- Most strictures can be treated with bougie or balloon dilation. Refractory strictures need an alternate treatment, such as intralesional steroid injection, incisional therapy, stent placement, self-bougienage, or surgery.

- It is important to treat esophageal strictures in a stepwise fashion, starting with the least invasive treatment. If this is not sufficient to relieve dysphagia, the next treatment modality in the algorithm should be applied.

- An alternative for repeat dilation in anastomotic strictures is to use incisional therapy with needle knife electrocautery or argon plasma coagulation.

- The idea of dilation for a prolonged period of time, using self-expanding metal stents or self-expanding plastic stents, is that this will reduce the risk of recurrent stricture formation.

- If the various treatment modalities are not effective in relieving dysphagia, a patient can be taught to apply self-bougienage or, ultimately, surgery can be performed.

References

1 Kochman ML, McClave SA, Boyce HW. The refractory and the recurrent esophageal stricture: a definition. *Gastrointest Endosc* 2005; **62**: 474–5.

2 Atkinson M, Ferguson R, Ogylvie AC. Management of malignant dysphagia by intubation at endoscopy. *J R Soc Med* 1979; **27**: 894–7.

3 Lindgren MD, Janzon L. Prevalence of swallowing complaints and clinical findings among 50–70 year old men and women in an urban population. *Dysphagia* 1991; **6**: 187–92.

4 Spechler SJ. AGA technical review on treatment of patients with dysphagia caused by benign disorders of the distal esophagus. *Gastroenterology* 1999; **117**: 233–54.

5 Poley JW, Steyerberg EW, Kuipers EJ, *et al.* Ingestion of acid and alkaline agents: outcome and prognostic value of early upper endoscopy. *Gastrointest Endosc* 2004; **60**: 372–7.

6 Honkoop P, Siersema PD, Tilanus HW, *et al.* Benign anastomotic strictures after transhiatal esophagectomy and cervical esophagogastrostomy: risk factors and management. *J Thorac Cardiovasc Surg* 1996; **111**: 1141–6.

7 Schoepfer AM, Gschossmann J, Scheurer U, *et al.* Esophageal strictures in adult eosinophilic esophagitis: dilation is an effective and safe alternative after failure of topical corticosteroids. *Endoscopy* 2008; **40**: 161–4.

8 Siersema PD, Hirdes MM. What is the optimal duration of stent placement for refractory, benign esophageal strictures? *Nat Clin Pract Gastroenterol Hepatol* 2009; **6**: 146–7.

9 Cook IJ. Diagnostic evaluation of dysphagia. *Nat Clin Pract Gastroenterol Hepatol* 2008; **5**: 393–403.

10 Ferguson DD. Evaluation and management of benign esophageal strictures. *Dis Esophagus* 2005; **18**: 359–64.

11 Saeed ZA, Winchester CB, Ferro PS, *et al.* Prospective randomized comparison of polyvinyl bougies and through-the-scope balloons for dilation of peptic strictures of the esophagus. *Gastrointest Endosc* 1995; **41**: 189–95.

12 Lew RJ, Kochman ML. A review of endoscopic methods of esophageal dilatation. *J Clin Gastroenterol* 2002; **35**: 117–26.

13 Bueno R, Swanson SJ, Jaklitsch MT, *et al.* Combined antegrade and retrograde dilation: a new endoscopic technique in the management of complex esophageal obstruction. *Gastrointest Endosc* 2001; **54**: 368–72.

14 Ramage JI Jr, Rumalla A, Baron TH, *et al.* A prospective, randomized, double-blind, placebo-controlled trial of endoscopic steroid injection therapy for recalcitrant esophageal peptic strictures. *Am J Gastroenterol* 2005; **100**: 2419–25.

15 Hordijk ML, Siersema PD, Tilanus HW, *et al.* Electrocautery therapy for refractory anastomotic strictures of the esophagus. *Gastrointest Endosc* 2006; **63**: 157–63.

16 Siersema PD. Stenting for benign esophageal strictures. *Endoscopy* 2009; **41**: 363–73.

17 Cwikiel W, Willén R, Stridbeck H, *et al.* Self-expanding stent in the treatment of benign esophageal strictures: experimen-

tal study in pigs and presentation of clinical cases. *Radiology* 1993; **187**: 667–71.

18 Holm AN, de la Mora Levy JG, Gostout CJ, *et al.* Self-expanding plastic stents in treatment of benign esophageal conditions. *Gastrointest Endosc* 2008; **67**: 20–5.

19 Dua KS, Vleggaar FP, Santharam R, *et al.* Removable self-expanding plastic esophageal stent as a continuous, non-permanent dilator in treating refractory benign esophageal strictures: a prospective two-center study. *Am J Gastroenterol* 2008; **103**: 2988–94.

CHAPTER 38

Medication-induced Esophageal Disease

Peter Bytzer

Department of Medicine, Køge University Hospital, Køge, Denmark

Summary

Drug-induced esophageal injury should be suspected in any patient with no prior esophageal symptoms who develops retrosternal pain and odynophagia. Esophageal injury is usually caused by direct mucosal contact with tablets or capsules which have disintegrated due to prolonged esophageal passage. More than two-thirds of lesions are located in the mid-esophagus. Tetracycline, bisphosphonates, potassium salts, and NSAIDs are common offenders. Symptoms are usually acute and can often be related to ingestion of an offending drug. Presenting symptoms include chest pain, odynophagia, heartburn, globus, and sometimes dysphagia. Withdrawing the offending agent is key to treatment success. Acid inhibition is only supportive. Patients should be encouraged to take adequate amounts of fluid and to remain upright for 15 to 30 min after drug intake to prevent drug-induced esophageal injury.

Case

An 84-year-old woman with osteoporosis complicated with multiple fractures admitted with a history of vomiting and dysphagia. Approximately 5 months prior to admission she was prescribed alendronate for osteoporosis. Her other medication included furosemide, potassium chloride, low-dose prednisolone, tramadol and vitamin B_{12} injections every 3 months. Endoscopy revealed numerous ulcerations in the lower part of the esophagus. Biopsies showed chronic inflammation and ulceration but no signs of malignancy. She was prescribed esomeprazole 40 mg twice daily and scheduled for a control endoscopy 3 months later. She was readmitted after only 4 weeks because of dehydration due to vomiting and dysphagia. Repeat endoscopy showed progression of the ulcerations, which were now also found in the mid esophagus (Figure 38.1). Alendronate was stopped and she recovered without any further therapy over the next 3 weeks. A control endoscopy at 3 months showed complete healing of the ulcerations.

Practical Gastroenterology and Hepatology: Esophagus and Stomach, 1st edition. Edited by Nicholas J. Talley, Kenneth R. DeVault and David E. Fleischer. © 2010 Blackwell Publishing Ltd.

Definition and Epidemiology

Drug-induced esophageal injury should be suspected in a patient with no prior esophageal symptoms who develops retrosternal pain and odynophagia. The sudden onset of odynophagia in a patient taking potentially offending drugs is suggestive of pill esophagitis. The diagnosis can be confirmed by endoscopy which typically will show multiple, discrete erosions or ulcers in the mid-esophagus. The condition was first recognized in 1970. To date more than 1000 cases involving more than 70 different drugs have been reported in the literature. The true incidence is unknown. Swedish data from the 1970s suggest four cases per 100 000 population per year but this is likely an underestimate as many cases are undetected or not reported [1]. Pill esophagitis may occur at any age but elderly are at increased risk, mainly because of more frequent use of offending medications.

Pathophysiology

Esophageal injury can be caused directly by prolonged

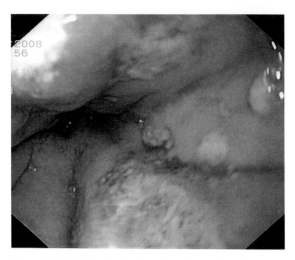

Figure 38.1 Multiple ulcers in the mid-esophagus in a patient taking bisphosphonates.

Table 38.1 Risk factors for drug-induced esophageal injury.

Esophageal strictures
Esophageal motility disorders
Left atrial enlargement
Low volume of liquid taken with medication
Supine position
Hyposalivation
Drug formulation (capsules, slow-release tablets)
Old age

hernia, achalasia, or strictures. A review of 119 cases showed that 70% of lesions were in the mid-esophagus, 21% in the lower third, and 9% in the upper third of the esophagus [4].

Clinical Features

Symptoms are usually acute and can often be related to ingestion of an offending drug. Patients present with chest pain, odynophagia, heartburn, globus, and sometimes dysphagia. Odynophagia can be so severe as to cause dehydration and weight loss. Severe complications are rare and include esophageal perforation, hemorrhage, strictures, and fistulae to the respiratory tract.

Patients with disorders of peristalsis, decreased saliva production, and with any mechanical impediments in the esophagus (stenosis, left atrial enlargement), bedridden patients and patients on polymedication are at particular risk (Table 38.1). However, most patients have no predisposing esophageal disorder or other identifiable risk factors [6].

Types of Drug

More than 70 drugs have been reported to induce esophageal injury [7,8]. Tetracyclines, bisphosphonates, potassium salts, and quinidine are the substances most often reported in the literature (Table 38.2). NSAIDs, including aspirin and COX2-inhibitors, are probably the most common causes of drug-induced esophageal injury. Erosive esophagitis has been demonstrated in 20% or more of patients taking NSAIDs [9]. The mechanism of action is uncertain but may include local chemical effects, systemic effects related to inhibition of platelet aggregation, and exacerbation of pre-existing gastroesophageal reflux disease.

mucosal contact with tablets or capsules. Studies have confirmed poor clearance of tablets from the esophagus in the supine position, especially if taken with inadequate (<100 mL) amounts of liquid [2]. The acidity or alkalinity of a medication is unlikely to be the only factor; other chemical properties may also be important [3]. Factors such as drug dissociation rate, osmolarity, and intrinsic chemical toxicity have also been implicated in the pathogenesis. Sustained-release medications may be more injurious to the esophagus than standard preparations. Some drugs have been formulated to disintegrate rapidly on contact with water and the hygroscopicity of the tablet can cause it to stick to the esophageal mucosa and reach a high ulcerogenic local concentration [4]. For example, deposits of potassium chloride have been demonstrated in biopsies from an esophageal ulcer.

NSAIDs appear to contribute to esophageal pathology by direct cellular toxicity and disruption of the mucosal barrier (local effect) rather than by inhibiting prostaglandin synthesis (systemic effect) [5]. Drugs with anticholinergic properties may facilitate reflux esophagitis by a relaxing effect of the lower esophageal sphincter.

Sites of injury include anatomical sites of narrowing such as the level of the aortic arch in the mid-esophagus whereas more distal lesions may occur in the presence of pre-existing esophageal abnormalities, for example hiatal

Table 38.2 Medications commonly associated with esophageal injury.

Medication	Clinical features
Doxycycline and tetracycline	Young patients Complications rare
NSAIDs including acetylsalicylic acid	Bleeding, strictures, ulcers
Potassium chloride	Progressive dysphagia due to strictures Pain dull or absent
Emepronium bromide	Mostly females
Bisphosphonates (alendronate, pamidronate, etidronate)	Strictures, hemorrhage, perforation
Ferrous sulfate	Progressive dysphagia due to strictures
Quinidine	Profuse esophageal exudates and edema May mimic neoplasia
Chemotherapy (bleomycin, cytarabin, daunorubicin, methotrexate and others)	Often accompanied by oropharyngeal mucositis

Diagnosis

The diagnosis of drug-induced esophageal injury is one of exclusion. Diagnosis may be supported by the temporal relation of drug intake to the onset of symptoms, a history of pill intake with little or no water or pill intake immediately before going to bed, the absence of any other cause, and the resolution of symptoms (and endoscopic findings) after withdrawal of the drug.

In patients who are endoscoped, the site and nature of lesions lend further support to a drug-induced etiology. Typical findings include discrete ulcers from pinpoint to several centimeters in size surrounded by normal mucosa (Figure 38.1). Severe ulcerative esophagitis and thickening of the esophageal wall is sometimes seen. Any area of the esophagus may be injured but lesions are most common in the mid-esophagus. Biopsies show unspecific acute inflammation.

Differential Diagnosis

Medication-induced lesions in the distal esophagus may be confused with reflux esophagitis. The correct diagnosis is usually suggested by the history with sudden onset related to drug ingestion. Opportunistic fungal or viral esophageal infections can also cause ulcers and should be suspected in immunocompromised individuals. Crohn disease can present with aphtous ulcers in the esophagus but these patients usually have other signs of inflammatory bowel disease. In cases of strictures and large ulcers a malignancy should be excluded. Ischemic heart disease must be sought in patients with chest pain without swallowing symptoms.

Therapeutics

Treatment is non-specific and empiric. Most importantly the offending agent should be stopped. Acid inhibition with a proton pump inhibitor or an H_2-blocker is not a substitute for the discontinuation of the suspected drug but should be prescribed in patients where gastroesophageal reflux is believed to exacerbate the injury. Symptomatic treatment may include topical anesthetics, sucralfate, and antacids but the value has not been proven.

Symptoms usually stop within a week with cessation of the offending drug and is accompanied by healing of the lesions, even without specific therapy.

Prognosis and Prevention

Prognosis is usually good if the offending agent is stopped but strictures and even drug-related deaths because of esophageal rupture have been reported [10].

Improper ingestion and inappropriate timing of drug intake, especially of potentially corrosive medications, may result in esophageal injury. To avoid this patients should be encouraged to take adequate amounts of fluid and to remain upright for 15 to 30 min after drug intake [2].

Take-home points

- Acute onset of retrosternal pain, odynophagia, globus, and dysphagia are key symptoms.
- Relationship to recent drug intake is often reported by the patient.

- Tetracycline, bisphosphonates, NSAIDs, potassium chloride, and ferrous sulfate are common offenders.
- Diagnosis is suggested by multiple, small ulcers in the middle part of an otherwise normal esophagus.
- Drug injury is usually observed at anatomical sites of narrowing in the esophagus (middle third).
- Treatment is non-specific: stop the offending agent and give palliative therapy.
- To prevent injury advise patients to take medications with at least 100 mL of liquid in the upright position.

References

1 Carlborg B, Kumlien A, Olsson H. Oesophageal strictures induced by oral drug therapy. *Läkartidningen* 1978; **75**: 4609–11.

2 Hey H, Jørgensen F, Sørensen K, *et al.* Oesophageal transit of six commonly used tablets and capsules. *BMJ* 1982; **285**: 1717–9.

3 Parfitt JR, Driman DK. Pathological effects of drugs on the gastrointestinal tract: a review. *Hum Pathol* 2007; **38**: 527–36.

4 Eng J, Sabanathan S. Drug-induced esophagitis. *Am J Gastroenterol* 1991; **86**: 1127–33.

5 Avidan B, Sonnenberg A, Schnell TG, Sontag SJ. Risk factors for erosive reflux esophagitis: A case-control study. *Am J Gastroenterol* 2001; **96**: 41–6.

6 Kikendall JW, Friedman AC, Oyewole MA, *et al.* Pill-induced esophageal injury. Case reports and review of the medical literature. *Dig Dis Sci* 1983; **28**: 174–82.

7 Jaspersen D. Drug-induced oesophageal disorders. *Drug Safety* 2000; **22**: 237–49.

8 de Groen PC, Lubbe DF, Hirsch LJ, *et al.* Esophagitis associated with the use of alendronate. *N Engl J Med* 1996; **335**: 1016–21.

9 Mantry P, Shah A, Sundaram U. Celecoxib associated esophagitis. Review of gastrointestinal side effects from Cox-2 inhibitors. *J Clin Gastroenterol* 2003; **37**: 61–3.

10 Collins FJ, Matthews HR, Baker SE, Strakova JM. Drug-induced oesophageal injury. *BMJ* 1979; **1**: 1673–6.

CHAPTER 39
Radiation Injury

Matthew D. Callister

Department of Radiation Oncology, Mayo Clinic, Scottsdale, AZ, USA

Summary

Exposure of the esophagus to radiation is common in the treatment of malignancies of the chest and neck. Radiation esophagitis is the most common acute side effect, manifested by odynophagia and weight loss. Radiation esophagitis is usually diagnosed clinically, based on patient symptoms and radiation dose exposure of the esophagus. Treatment includes acid suppression, diet modification, analgesics, empirical treatment for candidiasis, and aggressive nutritional support. Esophageal stricture is the most common late effect of radiation on the esophagus, presenting as progressive dysphagia. Endoscopic dilation is successful therapy in most patients.

Case

A 54-year-old man presents with a T4N2M0 squamous cell carcinoma of the tongue base. He undergoes 7 weeks of external-beam radiotherapy to the oropharynx and neck with concurrent chemotherapy. His tumor responds completely, but 7 months after therapy he develops progressive dysphagia to solids. Barium swallow reveals circumferential narrowing of the proximal esophagus at C6, consistent with a radiation-related stricture. Esophageal dilation resolves his dysphagia. Two months later a second dilation is required for minor recurrence of symptoms.

Definition and Epidemiology

Cases of radiation injury to the esophagus are almost invariably due to therapeutic radiation used in the treatment of malignancy. Thoracic cancers, such as lung, esophageal, and mediastinal tumors, as well as head and neck cancers, are the most common diseases for which radiotherapy may cause esophageal side effects or complications. Modern radiation treatment advances with CT-based planning, improved dose conformality, and daily image guidance often reduce exposure of the esophagus to radiation. Yet, complete exclusion of the esophagus during radiotherapy is often impossible.

The acute effects of radiotherapy on the esophagus occur during radiotherapy or within 3 months of completion. Esophagitis is the predominant acute effect from radiotherapy. Clinically apparent esophagitis is expected in most patients being treated with radiotherapy for thoracic or head and neck malignancies. Severe radiation esophagitis is more prevalent in patients treated for esophageal and lung cancers with significant mediastinal involvement. Concurrent use of chemotherapy with radiation increases the incidence and severity of esophagitis.

The late effects of radiation on the esophagus are observed any time 3 months after treatment completion. Strictures are the most common complication, particularly among head and neck cancer patients. Late ulcerations/perforation and fistula formation are rare and difficult to distinguish from recurrent cancer. Radiation-induced malignancies of the esophagus are rare but have been reported after treatment for breast and head and neck cancers, as well as Hodgkin disease [1]. Dysmotility may also occur and is probably underreported.

Pathophysiology

The acute effect of radiation on the esophagus is due to the relative radiosensitivity of mucosal epithelium. Erythema is initially noted, followed by epithelial

Practical Gastroenterology and Hepatology: Esophagus and Stomach, 1st edition. Edited by Nicholas J. Talley, Kenneth R. DeVault and David E. Fleischer. © 2010 Blackwell Publishing Ltd.

denudation, erosion, and submucosal edema [2]. Epithelium regenerates within weeks of radiotherapy completion. The severity of radiation esophagitis is dependent on multiple treatment factors including daily and cumulative radiation dose, use of concurrent chemotherapy, and volume/length of esophagus exposed [3]. Patient differences in sensitivity to radiotherapy greatly vary.

Late esophageal injury is from subepithelial damage of the lumen wall, causing submucosal and muscle wall fibrosis, lumen narrowing, and mucous gland atrophy [4]. Stricture formation at the tumor site (esophagus cancer) due to replacement by fibrous tissue is not uncommon. Patients with collagen vascular disease (especially systemic lupus and scleroderma), Bloom syndrome, and ataxia–telangiectasia are particularly at risk of late esophageal injury [5].

Clinical Features

Two weeks of external-beam radiotherapy (approximately 20 Gy) is sufficient to induce esophagitis. Initially patients describe tightness or pressure when swallowing which may subsequently progress to burning or sharp pain in the lower neck or substernal thorax, possibly radiating to the back. Symptoms may be indistinguishable from cardiac pain or infectious esophagitis. Pain may be transitory or constant. Dehydration and weight loss will quickly ensue without adequate symptom control. Completion of radiotherapy usually leads to symptom resolution within 1–3 weeks.

Late effects of radiation are characterized by dysphagia rather than pain, consistent with stricture and/or dysmotility. Symptoms generally develop gradually and associated weight loss is common.

Diagnosis

For the vast majority of patients, radiation esophagitis is diagnosed based on symptoms *and* confirmation of radiation exposure of the esophagus. Further work-up is usually not indicated. Indeed, in many cases, radiation esophagitis is expected to develop during the course of therapy.

Although probably safe to perform during radiotherapy, the infrequent indications for esophagogastroduo-

denoscopy (EGD) include worsening obstructive symptoms (exclude tumor progression), unexplained gastrointestinal symptoms (e.g., gastric ulcer), and possible viral esophageal infection in the immunocompromised patient [6]. Endoscopic findings may not correlate with severity of patient symptoms and range from patchy erythema to multiple ulcerative patches and exudates [7]. Esophageal candidiasis is common during radiotherapy but its clinical suspicion alone is not an indication for endoscopy because it can be treated empirically. Biopsy of the acutely irradiated esophagus should be avoided. Radiographic studies are rarely helpful.

Esophageal stricture is the most common late effect of radiotherapy on the esophagus and should be evaluated by EGD and/or radiographic imaging with an esophagogram (Figure 39.1). Early diagnosis and intervention may prevent progression to higher-grade strictures which may be less correctable by dilation. Esophageal dysmotility, evaluated by manometry, should be considered in patients without stricture but for whom radiation-related esophageal dysfunction is suspected [8].

Esophageal ulceration, perforation, and fistula formation are far less common late effects than strictures. As malignant ulceration or fistula may be difficult to distinguish from benign complications, biopsy and thoracic imaging should be strongly considered in such circumstances. Esophageal ulcers secondary to radiotherapy are generally isolated and round, conforming to the long axis of the esophagus [1]. Deep ulceration into esophageal

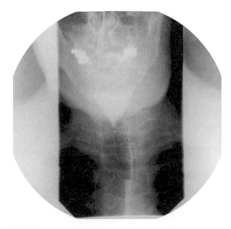

Figure 39.1 Barium esophagogram showing 8 mm severe stricture in proximal esophagus after previous radiotherapy to the neck.

musculature is rare in the absence of exposure to high radiation doses.

Therapeutics

Treatment of radiation esophagitis includes minimizing esophageal irritation, adequate pain control, nutritional support, and empirical treatment for candidiasis (detailed in Table 39.1). Acid suppression with a proton pump inhibitor should be initiated at the start of a course of radiotherapy among patients whose esophagus will be exposed to radiation. Diet modification with soft, bland foods and avoidance of alcohol, tobacco, hot foods, and citrus fruit may benefit the symptomatic patient [3]. Oral sucralfate has been studied extensively as an esophageal mucosal protectant to radiation, but without any observed benefit and poor tolerance in a randomized trial [9]. Percutaneous feeding tube placement is commonly indicated for patients receiving the most aggressive therapies or those who present malnourished before initiation of cancer treatment. Time will relieve radiation esophagitis as the mucosa repopulates. Breaks in radiation treatment schedules may lessen the severity of symptoms and accelerate recovery but may compromise treatment outcomes and are thus avoided. Esophageal irritation for radiation to the chest may also predispose patients to esophageal spasm and treatment with calcium channel antagonists may benefit [10].

Esophageal candidiasis is common during external-beam radiotherapy to the chest or neck, documented in over a quarter of patients [11]. The mucosa is predisposed to infection probably due to interruption of the epithelial barrier [2]. As symptoms may be indistinguishable from and coincident with radiation esophagitis, a low threshold for empirical antifungal therapy should be considered. Lack of visible oral candidiasis on examination should not reduce the suspicion of esophagus infection [6]. In the setting of severe esophagitis in an immunocompromised host, infection with herpes simplex virus or cytomegalovirus should be considered.

Among patients with deeply infiltrative tumors of the proximal tracheobronchial tree and upper/middle esophagus, tumor regression with radiotherapy may predispose the patient to fistula formation as the tumor regresses. Although prognosis of such patients is poor, successful treatment for some has been reported. Patients

Table 39.1 Treatment of radiation esophagitis.

Acid suppression	Full-dose PPI
Diet	Soft, bland diet Avoid alcohol, tobacco, hot foods, cold foods, carbonated beverages
Topical agents	Miracle Mouthwash preparations (diphenhydramine, viscous lidocaine, antacid) Sucralfate suspension*
Analgesics	Oxycodone or hydrocodone in suspension Consider "long-acting" analgesic for severe, persistent pain (transdermal fentanyl patch)
Infection	Empirical treatment of candidiasis (nystatin suspension, fluconazole)
Nutrition/hydration	Push oral hydration, consider IVF Oral nutritional supplements, consider percutaneous gastrostomy tube, TPN (rare)
Esophageal spasm	Consider calcium channel blocker (e.g., nifedipine)
Radiotherapy/chemotherapy	Consider reducing radiation fields, breaking treatment, or holding chemotherapy

*Controversial benefit.
IVF, intravenous feed; PPI, proton pump inhibitor; TPN, total parenteral nutrition.

at greatest risk for the formation of a malignant fistula may be identified by bronchoscopy before initiation of cancer treatment. Placement of an esophageal or tracheobronchial stent should be considered.

Prevention of radiation esophagitis with the radiation cytoprotectant amifostine has been extensively studied with mixed results, but a meta-analysis suggests benefit [12]. Due to concerns about cost, side effects, and tumor protection, its use had not been widely embraced. Indomethacin has also been studied as a protectant against radiation esophagitis [10], but without sufficient evidence to justify its clinical use.

Early detection of esophageal strictures may lead to more successful correction. Benign strictures should be treated with intermittent endoscopic dilation with a success rate of close to 80% [13,14]. Hydrocortisone injection after dilation may also be of benefit [10]. Severe strictures or complete obliteration of the esophagus is rare and would be the exceptional indication for consideration of surgical repair, as would fistula formation [15].

Esophageal ulceration should be managed conservatively with analgesics, acid suppression, and diet modification. In serious cases, consideration could be given to hyperbaric oxygen treatment to promote healing.

Take-home points

Diagnosis

- Radiation esophagitis is a common and often expected side effect of radiotherapy for malignancies within the thorax and neck.

- Radiation esophagitis is clinically diagnosed based on symptoms and confirmation of esophageal radiation exposure.

- Esophageal stricture is the most common late radiation effect, diagnosed by esophagogram and/or barium swallowing study.

Therapy

- Treatment of radiation esophagitis includes acid suppression, analgesics, diet modification, empirical treatment of candidiasis, and nutritional support.

- Esophageal strictures are often successfully treated by esophageal dilatation.

References

1 Fajardo L, Berthrong M, Anderson R. *Radiation Pathology.* New York: Oxford University Press 2001.

2 Chowhan NM. Injurious effects of radiation on the esophagus. *Am J Gastroenterol* 1990; **85**: 115–20.

3 Werner-Wasik M. Treatment-related esophagitis. *Semin Oncol* 2005; **32**(2 Suppl 3): S60–6.

4 Berthrong M, Fajardo LF. Radiation injury in surgical pathology. Part II. Alimentary tract. *Am J Surg Pathol* 1981; **5**: 153–78.

5 Coia LR, Myerson RJ, Tepper JE. Late effects of radiation therapy on the gastrointestinal tract. *Int J Radiat Oncol Biol Phys* 1995; **31**: 1213–36.

6 Perez RA, Early DS. Endoscopy in patients receiving radiation therapy to the thorax. *Dig Dis Sci* 2002; **47**: 79–83.

7 Hirota S, Tsujino K, Hishikawa Y, *et al.* Endoscopic findings of radiation esophagitis in concurrent chemoradiotherapy for intrathoracic malignancies. *Radiother Oncol* 2001; **58**: 273–8.

8 Seeman H, Gates JA, Traube M. Esophageal motor dysfunction years after radiation therapy. *Dig Dis Sci* 1992; **37**: 303–6.

9 McGinnis WL, Loprinzi CL, Buskirk SJ, *et al.* Placebo-controlled trial of sucralfate for inhibiting radiation-induced esophagitis. *J Clin Oncol* 1997; **15**: 1239–43.

10 Zimmermann FB, Geinitz H, Feldmann HJ. Therapy and prophylaxis of acute and late radiation-induced sequelae of the esophagus. *Strahlenther Onkol* 1998; **174**(Suppl 3): 78–81.

11 Soffer EE, Mitros F, Doornbos JF, Friedland J, Launspach J, Summers RW. Morphology and pathology of radiation-induced esophagitis. Double-blind study of naproxen vs placebo for prevention of radiation injury. *Dig Dis Sci* 1994; **39**: 655–60.

12 Sasse AD, Clark LG, Sasse EC, Clark OA. Amifostine reduces side effects and improves complete response rate during radiotherapy: results of a meta-analysis. *Int J Radiat Oncol Biol Phys* 2006; **64**: 784–91.

13 O'Rourke IC, Tiver K, Bull C, Gebski V, Langlands AO. Swallowing performance after radiation therapy for carcinoma of the esophagus. *Cancer* 1988; **61**: 2022–6.

14 Laurell G, Kraepelien T, Mavroidis P, *et al.* Stricture of the proximal esophagus in head and neck carcinoma patients after radiotherapy. *Cancer* 2003; **97**: 1693–700.

15 Moghissi K, Pender D. Management of proximal oesophageal stricture. *Eur J Cardiothorac Surg* 1989; **3**: 93–7; discussion 7–8.

CHAPTER 40
Caustic Esophageal Injury

David A. Katzka

Division of Gastroenterology and Hepatology, Mayo Clinic, Rochester, MN, USA

Summary

Caustic ingestion is one of the most devastating sources of injury to the esophagus. The damage is fast and extensive on contact with the injurious substance. Knowledge of the specific caustic swallowed is important because damage may be minor or catastrophic depending on the type and amount swallowed. Stabilization of the patient is most important initially because esophageal perforation is of greatest concern and will require immediate esophagectomy if suspected and the patient is not moribund. If surgery is not required, then airway assessment and urgent endoscopy are indicated regardless of the degree of oral ulceration, to assess the degree of injury. This will be the most important determinant of prognosis and therapy, with low injury grades requiring observation and higher grades mandating long hospitalizations with total parenteral nutrition and/or jejunostomy tube feeding. There are few evidence-based trials evaluating the routine use of antibiotics and steroids in these patients, so the decision to use them should be case specific and based on clinical judgment. In patients with severe injury, long-term complications, particularly strictures, will need aggressive and often life-long dilations, if not surgical esophageal resection. Although routine screening for esophageal cancer is not wholly endorsed, one must recognize the significantly higher incidence of squamous cell cancer in these patients.

Case

A 25-year-old man is brought to the emergency room with a history of caustic substance ingestion. The man has a long history of depression for which he has been treated with medications in the past. Treatment has included two hospitalizations. Three hours ago he was witnessed by a friend to drink a cup of Drano in an effort to commit suicide, despondent over the fact that his girlfriend broke up with him. On examination, he is in distress, holding his throat and drooling. He has difficulty talking, sounds hoarse, and some mild stridor is present. He is afebrile, his heart rate is 100/min, and his respirations are 20/min. His lips appear erythematous. He can barely open his mouth but his buccal mucosa appears markedly erythematous with blisters. His chest is clear to auscultation. No crepitus is present in the chest or neck. Heart tones are normal. Abdomen is soft, non-tender, and non-distended. Laboratory reveals white blood cell count (WBC) of 11 900 without normal

distribution and Hb 15.5 g. Pulse oxygenation is 94% on room air. Chest radiograph shows clear lung fields without pneumomediastinum or free abdominal air. A request for a gastroenterology consultation is made.

Introduction

Caustic substance ingestion is potentially the most devastating type of injury that the esophagus may sustain. Its damage is rapid, its results potentially catastrophic, and, if the patient lives, the pathologic and symptomatic consequences may last a lifetime. Through careful government regulation, the USA has done much to eliminate potential exposure to caustic substances in our population. Although this has been a great achievement in reducing caustic esophageal injury, paradoxically it leaves us with a problem. Specifically, when a patient with caustic substance ingestion comes under an institution's care the conundrum remains of having to make immedi-

Practical Gastroenterology and Hepatology: Esophagus and Stomach, 1st edition. Edited by Nicholas J. Talley, Kenneth R. DeVault and David E. Fleischer. © 2010 Blackwell Publishing Ltd.

ate and potentially life-threatening decisions with little personal experience behind them. Furthermore, lack of exposure to this condition in the USA results in a minimum of active research in this area, with the vast majority of guidance coming from other countries. In this chapter, a synthesis of what knowledge is available in the evaluation and treatment of patients who have sustained caustic esophageal injury is given to guide care in this potentially devastating condition.

Definitions and Pathophysiology

Caustic esophageal injury is defined as the ingestion, either accidentally or purposefully, of a substance that is capable of extensively damaging the esophageal mucosa. In general, caustic substances are classified into four categories: alkalis, acids, detergents, and bleaches (Table 40.1). Strong alkalis or acids have a higher potential for esophageal injury than detergents or bleach. Ingestion of these substances is somewhat geographically dependent. In less developed countries, strong acids (Table 40.2) tend to be the most common form of caustic substance available because they are inexpensive and used widely as cleaners. In the Western world, alkali ingestion is more common because of the many common household products that contain these substances (Table 40.3). Corrosive

detergents are also readily available in the USA, although, as mentioned, they are not as damaging (Table 40.4).

In general, the degree of esophageal injury depends on the specific caustic agent swallowed, the quantity and concentration of the caustic substance, and the duration of contact time between the esophagus and the ingestant. As a result, the spectrum of injury may range from little to no injury with small amounts of a relatively weak corrosive to complete esophageal necrosis and death with large volumes of highly concentrated caustic agents.

Table 40.3 Common corrosive alkalis.

Examples of products	Major caustic ingredients
Drano (liquid)	NaOH (9.5%)
Drano Professional (liquid)	NaOH (32%)
Drano Crystals	NaOH (54%)
Red Devil Drain Opener	NaOH (96–100%)
Dow Oven Cleaner	NaOH (4%)
Efferdent Extra Strength Tablets	NaOH (0.5–1.0%)
Mr Clean (liquid)	Sodium bicarbonate
Top Job (liquid)	Sodium carbonate/ammonia
Lysol Deodorizing Cleaner	Ammonium chloride (2.7%)
Hair relaxers	Sodium or calcium hydroxide Ammonium hydroxide
Button batteries	Mercuric oxide (30.3%) Manganese oxide (17.6%) Silver oxide (30.3%)

Table 40.1 Types of ingested caustic agents and the injuries produced in the esophagus.

Type of agent	Injury
Alkalis	Liquefaction necrosis
Acid	Coagulation necrosis
Detergents	Mild mucosal injury
Bleaches	Mild mucosal injury

Table 40.4 Common corrosive detergents.

Examples of products	Major caustic ingredients
Oxydol Laundry Detergent	Sodium tripolyphosphate
Electrosol Dishwasher Detergent	Sodium tripolyphosphate
Calgonite Dishwasher Detergent	Sodium phosphates
Cascade Dishwasher Detergent	Phosphates
Comet Cleanser	Trisodium phosphate
Clorox Bleach	Sodium hypochlorite
Peroxide	Hydrogen peroxide
Tilex Instant Mildew Remover	Sodium hypochlorite Sodium hydroxide

Table 40.2 Common corrosive acids.

Examples of products	Major caustic ingredients
Mister Plumber	Sulfuric acid (99.5%)
SnoBol Toilet Bowl Cleaner	Hydrochloric acid (15%)
Saniflush Toilet Bowl Cleaner	Sodium bisulfate (75%)
Vanish Toilet Bowl Cleaner	Sodium bisulfate (75%)

Strong alkalis potentially produce the most devastating injury. In various animal models, including cat, rat, and rabbit, as little as 1 mL of a highly concentrated alkali leads to esophageal necrosis and potentially death [1]. The mechanism of alkali injury is through liquefaction necrosis, which allows easy penetration of the solution into deeper layers of the esophageal wall, leading to coagulation of blood vessels, resultant ischemia, further necrosis, and full-thickness esophageal injury. This rapid transmural injury explains the high incidence of acute perforation acutely, and perforation and stricture formation chronically.

Acid-induced injury is different from alkali-induced injury in many respects, although its ability to destroy the esophagus may be equally potent. The basic form of injury is one of coagulative necrosis rather than liquefaction. This type of injury is theoretically less severe because the coagulum and eschar that form in response to epithelial acid exposure may limit penetration into the deep esophageal layers. Acid also tends to be less viscous than alkali, resulting in faster esophageal transit and therefore less contact time with the esophageal lining. This is a mixed blessing, however, in that more severe gastric injury is facilitated by this. Even so, complete esophageal necrosis, perforation, and death are well recognized with acid-induced injury

Detergents and bleaches cause characteristically milder degrees of injury (see Table 40.4). Although typically alkaline, in general the pH of these solutions is lower than that of strong alkalis and they are composed of substances less toxic than the sodium hydroxide used in corrosive agents. The mechanism of damage is similar, however.

A unique type of caustic injury that must be recognized is that caused by button batteries. There are three mechanisms that occur with button batteries: release of caustic alkali chemicals; electrical injury; and mucosal pressure necrosis most commonly occurring in the area of aortic arch impression on the esophageal wall.

Initial Diagnosis and Assessment

As discussed, the degree of esophageal injury depends on the specific caustic agent swallowed, the quantity and concentration of the caustic agent, and the duration of contact time between the esophagus and the ingestant.

As a result, the initial history from the patient, or the family, if the patient is unable to give a history (such as in a child, in the case of severe oropharyngeal injury that precludes talking, or in catastrophic presentation), should include the type and quantity of corrosive. In general, caustic agents in the form of granules and solids are more likely to cause oropharyngeal and proximal esophageal injury whereas liquids, particularly less viscous ones, are more likely to cause esophageal and gastric injury. Also, in general, ingestion of caustic agents in a suicide attempt is likely to cause more esophageal damage compared with accidental injury, in which a lower volume of corrosive is typically consumed [2] (Figure 40.1). If the substance is unknown to the physician, information about virtually any substance can be obtained through the poison control center.

Initial examination will include vital signs and an assessment of airway function. Patients with severe hypotension, fever not responding to fluids, or respiratory distress will need to be assessed as an emergency with airway stabilization, computed tomography (CT), and surgical consultation for concerns about complete esophageal necrosis. Early clues to perforation may include subcutaneous emphysema and abdominal rigidity. Oropharyngeal and respiratory injury can be initially assessed by the presence of drooling, inability to talk, hoarseness, and stridor. These symptoms may indicate laryngeal edema, injury to the epiglottis, or aspiration of the caustic agent. It is important to note, however, that neither the presence nor the absence of these symptoms reliably predicts the extent of esophageal injury. This holds true specifically for the degree of oropharyngeal involvement where, in fact, some studies suggest that extensive oral injury may predict less severe esophageal injury because of oropharyngeal pooling, expectoration, and subsequently less esophageal exposure [3,4]. Prolonged or concentrated oral exposure may also be protective to the esophagus by reflexively eliciting upper esophageal sphincter hypertonicity as a barrier to esophageal entry by the corrosive substance. Concordantly, a normal oropharyngeal examination by no means predicts limited esophageal injury and several studies have shown that up to a third of patients with severe esophageal injury will have a normal oropharyngeal examination at presentation [5,6]. The bottom line is that further evaluation is needed to assess the degree of esophageal injury, even if the initial oral and systemic evaluation is

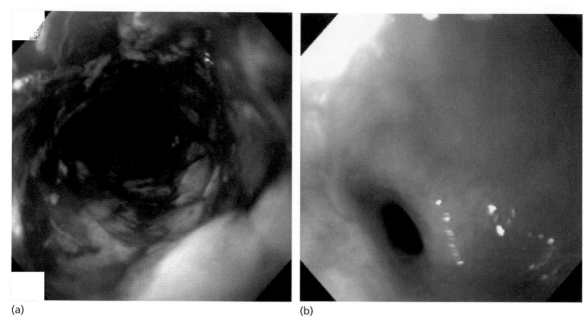

(a)   (b)

Figure 40.1 (a) Endoscopic image of acute caustic esophageal injury approximately 12 h after ingestion of oven cleaner in a failed suicide attempt. There is multifocal ulceration and hemorrhagic exudate. (b) High-grade, fibrotic esophageal stenosis is the sequela of second-degree esophageal injury due to caustic ingestion at subsequent follow-up. The stricture responded poorly to repeated endoscopic dilation therapy. (Courtesy of Dr Gregory G. Ginsberg.)

unimpressive and a highly caustic substance has been ingested.

Airway and Esophageal Visualization

There should be a very low threshold for laryngoscopy requests in patients with caustic substance ingestion. The first reason is that laryngeal injury is common. In one study, of 50 patients 38% had laryngeal injury and 8% required intubation and ventilation for respiratory distress [6]. Other studies have reported similar findings. The second is that absence of oral lesions and symptoms of laryngeal injury, such as stridor or hoarseness, do no preclude laryngeal injury either. As a result, with a history of ingestion of a highly caustic substance, consultation with otorhinolaryngology is essential as a first step in the relatively stable patient. On the other hand, patients with these symptoms should always undergo laryngoscopy as an assessment of airway access because a need for tracheal intubation is not uncommon in these patients.

Once stable, endoscopy should be performed urgently in all patients with corrosive substance ingestion. In the past, authors expressed concern about the safety of endoscopy in the presence of severe esophageal injury but, with the use of newer more flexible endoscopes, this concern has been markedly reduced. Furthermore, older literature has also suggested that the endoscopy should be terminated at the first sight of severe mucosal injury but an extensive literature now documents that, just as there may be poor correlation between oral and esophageal injury, there is also poor correlation between proximal esophageal injury and damage to the more distal esophagus and stomach. As a result, a full endoscopy should be performed if technically possible in all patients with a history of corrosive substance ingestion stable enough to undergo endoscopy.

In addition to guiding initial management, endoscopy is also of great value in staging these patients through the use of various endoscopic esophageal injury scoring systems [6,7]. One such example is given in Table 40.5. These systems are generally similar in classifying endoscopic findings. The strength of these scoring systems is

Table 40.5 Endoscopic grading of caustic esophageal injury.

Grade	Features
0	Normal
I	Edema and erythema of the mucosa
IIa	Friability, blisters, hemorrhage, erosions, severe erythema, white exudates, or superficial ulceration
IIb	IIa plus deep or circumferential ulceration
IIIa	Areas of necrosis, brown–black or grayish discoloration, deep ulceration
IIIb	Extensive necrosis

From Zargar et al. [8].

in their ability to predict the likelihood of long-term esophageal injury and therefore serve as a guide on how aggressively to treat patients at initial presentation. For example, when using the system in Table 40.5, and injury is less than grade IIa, no development of stricture or bleeding occurred in these patients, thus suggesting that initial conservative treatment is adequate. On the other hand, when a grade greater than IIb is present, 93.8% of bleeding and 100% of esophageal strictures are predicted; all patients greater than grade IIIa developed bleeding or stricture. As a result, these data suggest that patients with endoscopic injury greater than grade IIb require total parenteral nutrition and should be considered for therapies such as antibiotics and steroids. Although the grading is by no means perfect, it serves as an excellent starting point for determining initial treatment as well as clinical course over the next few weeks, if not longer.

Case continued

The patient undergoes nasopharyngeal laryngoscopy by an otorhinolargyngologist. Mild laryngeal edema is seen but overall the airway is patent. The patient then undergoes urgent endoscopy which demonstrates grade III injury throughout the esophagus, with sparing of the stomach.

Management of Caustic Esophageal Injury

Management of caustic esophageal injury is generally divided into three stages: initial injury (the first week), the latent phase (1–4 weeks), and the chronic phase (after

Table 40.6 Stages of caustic esophageal injury.

Phase	Duration	Characteristics
Acute	7 days	Acute injury with inflammation and necrosis
Latent	1–4 weeks	Reparative phase, threat of silent perforation
Chronic	> 4 weeks	Fibrosis and stricture formation

4 weeks) (Table 40.6). These phases are defined to some degree by pathologic response. The first phase represents the acute injury, the second stage the start of remodeling and healing, and the third long-term healing with or without fibrotic change.

Initial Management

One of the most difficult decisions to make in the assessment of esophageal caustic injury is the need for emergency esophagectomy (Figure 40.2). This decision is difficult for several reasons. When the patient presents acutely with signs of organ necrosis, perforation, and peritonitis or mediastinitis, or both, the chances of the patient surviving surgery are very small. Furthermore, performance of esophagectomy is difficult electively, but more so in an unstable patient, and is only temporary because anastomoses are not viable in the presence of necrosis and inflammation. As a result, some type of proximal oropharyngeal venting ostomy must be performed, further complicating the procedure and, of course, requiring reoperation at some point to fashion a neo-esophagus. This becomes even more complicated when oropharyngeal reconstruction is required [9]. On the other hand, if a patient has extensive esophageal necrosis with incipient or evident perforation, and esophagectomy and debridement are not performed, death is inevitable. As a result, some investigators have tried to determine criteria for esophagectomy, including high volume of concentrated caustic substance ingested, peritonitis, mediastinitis, acidosis (pH < 7.22), renal failure, hemodynamic instability, and high-grade esophageal injury [10]. The following are the criteria for early surgical management in acute esophageal caustic injury:
- 200 mL highly concentrated acid or alkali ingested
- Rigid abdomen and/or chest wall crepitus
- Cardiovascular shock

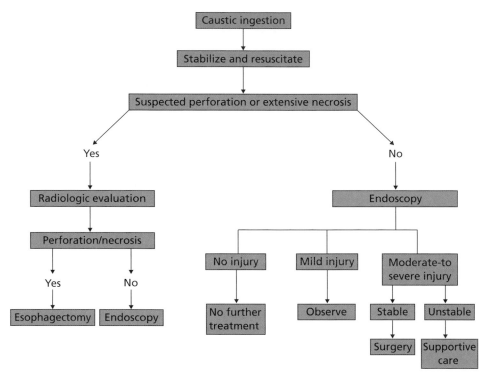

Figure 40.2 Acute management of caustic esophageal injury.

• Sepsis and profound acidosis
• Disseminated intravascular coagulation
• Highest-grade esophageal injury
• Need for hemodialysis.

Even with these criteria, good clinical judgment remains the most important determinant in the success of surgery under these extreme conditions.

If surgery is not indicated, the following non-surgical goals are initially pursued:
• Prevention of perforation
• Prevention of infection
• Prevention of stricture formation
• Maintenance of the esophageal lumen
• Maintenance of nutrition.

In attempting to achieve the first three goals, much attention has been focused on the use of prophylactic antibiotics, acid suppression, and steroids as a part of the initial therapy of severe caustic esophageal injury. This is an area where few data exist and opinion and experience seem to dictate practice. Specifically, very few studies have been performed to accurately define the use of these

agents in caustic injury. Only one controlled trial assessing the efficacy of steroids in children with alkali ingestion was performed almost 20 years ago, with low numbers of patients with severe injury to definitively define a role for or against steroids [11]. There is one meta-analysis of 10 trials suggesting a lack of steroid efficacy in caustic esophageal injury [12], but the trials used for this study were not controlled and had small numbers. There are no controlled trials for the use of antibiotics. As a result of these data, every US review article on caustic esophageal injury in recent times cautions against the use of steroids and antibiotics in this population. This stands in contrast, however, to the fact that investigators of virtually every study performed in a country where corrosive substance ingestion is much more common (e.g., Turkey, Israel, and China) use steroids and antibiotics at the time of initial injury. Furthermore, there is no agreement among physicians who advocate their use of the duration, dose, or type of delivery of steroids (e.g., intravenous, intralesional) or antibiotics. Thus, there are no clear guidelines for their use in this situation. There are no randomized studies using antibiotics or acid suppression in caustic esophageal injury either. At this point, the current author advocates the use of antibiotics initially for patients with evidence of perforation or mediastinitis, high-grade esophageal injury, fever, or leukocytosis. He also uses high-dose proton pump inhibitors to prevent superimposed acid reflux injury to the esophagus, and does not advocate the use of intravenous steroids initially, although he could not argue with those who do advocate their use.

Maintenance of the esophageal lumen is generally advocated in an effort to prevent complete esophageal closure and technically aid a potential need for dilation at a future point. Several ways of achieving this have been proposed. The most commonly used are soft nasogastric tubes and Dobhoff tubes [9,13,14]. The value of these tubes is that they may be inserted early in the course without much difficulty. Some investigators have used strings and, more recently, several uncontrolled studies of small numbers of patients had advocated the use of removable esophageal stents [15,16]. Initial nutrition is usually started with total parenteral nutrition in the first week. If a nasogastric or Dobhoff tube has been inserted, it may be used if the organ at the distal end of the tube and structures beyond (stomach or duodenum, respectively) are healthy and can tolerate feedings.

Case continued

A Dobhoff tube is placed across the esophageal lumen and into the duodenum, and nasojejunal feedings started. As a result of an elevation in WBC to 19 400, with a shift in polymorphonuclear leukocytes and a temperature of 101.5°F, the patient is started on broad-spectrum antibiotics for a week until his WBC becomes normal. He is then observed for another week, with a Gastrografin swallow not demonstrating any leak but showing extensive esophageal wall edema and luminal compromise. A repeat Gastrografin study 1 week later demonstrates some improvement. At 4 weeks, endoscopy is performed which shows a long esophageal stricture measuring 6 mm in diameter without obvious mucosa necrosis or edema. A course of endoscopic dilations is initiated over the next few weeks.

The Latent Phase

In patients with severe injury who survive the acute phase, the latent phase marks the start of healing and formation of granulation tissue. It may appear to be a "quiet" phase but it is often a phase in which silent catastrophes (perforation or infection) occur because the esophageal tissue is at its weakest [15]. As a result, this is a phase where supportive care is emphasized in the hope of sustaining life, and avoiding surgery in an effort to get patients non-surgically to the chronic phase. Endoscopy is contraindicated during this phase because of the high risk of perforation and, if imaging of the esophagus is indicated, contrast esophagography is recommended. For patients with initial high-grade injury, some advocate weekly radiographs to monitor healing and assess for signs of impending perforation such as deep ulceration or gas in the esophageal wall. This is also a phase when longer-term nutritional issues are addressed and, if possible, total parenteral nutrition is converted to enteral feeding, usually through the surgical insertion of a jejunostomy tube if a nasogastric or Dobhoff tube has not been previously inserted. The decision to place a tube rests on the expected necessary time to bypass the esophagus. Patients showing relatively rapid improvement and needing less than 3 weeks before the esophagus may be used can remain on parenteral nutrition. Patients with slower improvement are best converted to enteral tube feedings.

The Chronic Phase

The main goal of the chronic phase is to manage long-term complications of high-grade caustic esophageal injury. For the most part, this means management of esophageal strictures, which will develop in approximately 10% of all patients who sustain caustic ingestion [2]. As discussed previously, grades of IIb or higher predict a high incidence of stricture formation, with grades III or higher almost guaranteeing occurrence of a stricture in some series. The spectrum of stricture formation is wide ranging, from relatively focal esophageal narrowing to complete luminal compromise with only a few millimeters of diameter present. The basic choices of therapy are endoscopic dilation or esophagectomy. Endoscopic dilation can be very effective. In one study of 47 patients with corrosive strictures, satisfactory results were seen in 94% [17]. In this study a median of eight dilations were required for esophageal patency with a high recurrence rate. Thus, although dilation can be effective, the major caveats of dilation are the number required for achieving adequate and sustained results and the attending risk of subsequent perforation. As expected, short concentric strictures have a better chance of responding to therapy when compared with those patients with strictures of a long, eccentric configuration, where the chance of perforation is higher. It is generally for this type of stricture that elective esophagectomy is considered. The proper interval between dilations varies. Recent literature proposes every 3 weeks initially until adequate luminal diameter is achieved, followed by monthly maintenance dilations [18], although others propose initial weekly dilations. One group of authors, interestingly, also suggests that strictures refractory to peroral dilation may be approached retrograde through a gastrostomy insertion [18]. Another study has suggested that intralesional injection of steroids into caustic strictures may reduce the need for a number of dilations [19]. A protocol similar to steroid injection of peptic strictures with triamcinolone may be followed if this method is used. Finally, limited anecdotal literature has suggested the use of an expandable esophageal stent for stricture treatment [20], but more experience is needed. If frequent dilation is required, consideration can be given to having the patient learn to perform self-dilation.

The surgical approach to refractory strictures has many variations. Although most procedures involve replacement of the esophagus with an intestinal interposition or gastric tube formation, the operation depends on several factors. One factor is the location of the proximal and distal margins available for anastomosis, e.g., if only the mid- and distal esophagus are injured the proximal esophagus and stomach may be used on the ends of the interposition. On the other hand, extensive pharyngeal, laryngeal, or gastric caustic injury will mandate different and more difficult surgery, particularly when hypopharyngeal reconstruction is required. Another factor is the segment of intestine used for interposition, e.g., whereas some surgeons use jejunum, others use part of the colon or the proximal stomach. Finally, the comfort of the surgeon with a specific surgical approach will often dictate the surgical therapy. This results from a lack of universal experience, opportunity for study, and hence standardization of the "best" procedure.

Finally, one potential concern in the chronic phase of caustic esophageal injury is the development of esophageal cancer. Retrospectively derived data suggest a thousandfold increase in the risk of squamous cell carcinoma of the esophagus over the general population [21]. Most cancers occur at the tracheal bifurcation, potentially leading to a high rate of reported respiratory tree fistulization. As a result of these issues, some investigators propose endoscopy screening 20 years after injury [22]. Of further note, however, is that some of the literature suggests a longer survival for caustic-induced esophageal cancer due to limitation of spread by the fibrosis [23].

Take-home points

- Devastating caustic esophageal injury may occur with small amounts of a highly toxic substance.

- The degree of injury is determined by the amount, the type, and the contact time of the caustic agent with the esophageal mucosa.

- The initial assessment should be toward stabilization and determination of whether the patient requires, and can survive, esophagectomy if perforation is suspected.

- Assessment and stabilization of the airway are required immediately due to the potential for laryngeal injury.

- If immediate surgery is not required, urgent endoscopy is performed to assess the full extent of injury as neither the presence nor the severity of oropharyngeal injury reliably predicts the extent of more distal esophageal or gastric involvement.

- The degree of endoscopic injury is assessed by a grading scale that may reliably predict prognosis and therapy required.

- Low-grade injury requires observation only, whereas high-grade endoscopic injury requires total parenteral nutrition and/or jejunostomy feedings, and a prolonged hospitalization is to be expected.

- The routine use of antibiotics and steroids has been neither clearly shown nor disproven to be of benefit, but should be administered on a case-by-case basis.

- Long-term complications, particularly strictures, usually require aggressive dilation and, if not, esophagectomy.

- It should be recognized that the incidence of squamous cell carcinoma of the esophagus is significantly increased in these patients, although routine screening has not been advocated.

References

1 Mattos GM, Lopes DD, Mamede RCM, *et al.* Effects of time of contact and concentration of caustic agent on generation of injuries. *Laryngoscope* 2006; **116**: 456–60.

2 Arevalo-Silva C, Eliashar R, Wohlgelernter J, Elidan J, Gross M. Ingestion of caustic substances: a 15-year experience. *Laryngoscope* 2006; **116**: 1422–6.

3 DiConsanzo J, Noirclerc M, Jouglard J, *et al.* New therapeutic approach to corrosive burns of the upper gastrointestinal tract. *Gut* 1980; **21**: 370–5.

4 Symbas PN, Vlasis SE, Hatcher CR Jr. Esophagitis secondary to ingestion of caustic material. *Ann Thorac Surg* 1983; **36**: 73–7.

5 Ramasamy K, Gumaste VV. Corrosive ingestion in adults. *J Clin Gastroenterol* 2003; **37**: 119–24.

6 Dogan Y, Erkan T, Cokugras FC, Kutlu T. Caustic gastro-esophageal lesions in childhood: an analysis of 473 cases. *Clin Pediatr* 2006; **45**: 435–8.

7 Poley JW, Steyerberg EW, Kuipers EJ, *et al.* Ingestion of acid and alkaline agents: outcome and prognostic value of early upper endoscopy. *Gastrointest Endosc* 2004; **60**: 372–7.

8 Zargar SA, Kochhar R, Mehta S, *et al.* The role of fiberoptic endoscopy in the management of corrosive and modified endoscopic classification of burns. *Gastrointest Endosc* 1991; **37**: 165 9.

9 Chirica M, de Chaisemartin C, Goasguen N, *et al.* Colopharyngoplasty for the treatment of severe pharygnoesophageal caustic injuries. An audit of 58 patients. *Ann Surg* 2007; **246**: 721–7.

10 Cheng YJ, Kao EL. Arterial blood gas analysis in acute caustic ingestion injuries. *Surg Today* 2003; **33**: 483–5.

11 Anderson KD, Rouse TM, Randolph JG. A controlled trial of corticosteroids in children with corrosive injury of the csophagus. *N Engl J Med* 1990; **323**: 637–40.

12 Pelclova D, Navratil T. Do corticosteroids prevent esophageal stricture after corrosive ingestion? *Toxicol Rev* 2005; **24**: 125–9.

13 Janousek P, Kabelka Z, Rygl M, *et al.* Corrosive injury of the esophagus in children. *Int Pediatr Otorhinolaryngol* 2006; **70**: 1103–7.

14 Broto J, Asensio M, Vernet JM. Results of a new technique in the treatment of severe esophageal stenosis in children: poliflex stents. *J Pediatr Gastroenterol Nutr* 2003; **37**: 203–6.

15 Wang R-W, Zhou J-H, Fan S-Z, *et al.* Prevention of stricture with intraluminal stenting through laparotomy after corrosive esophageal burns. *Eur J Cardiothorac Surg* 2006; **30**: 207–21.

16 Tuncozgur B, Savas MC, Isik AF, Sarimehmetoglu A, Sanli M, Elbeyli L. Removal of metallic stent by using polyflex sent in esophago-colic anastomotic stricture. *Ann Thorac Surg* 2006; **82**: 1913–14.

17 Broor SL, Bose PP, Lahoti D, *et al.* Long term results of endoscopic dilatation of corrosive esophageal strictures. *Gut* 1993; **34**: 1498–501.

18 Gun F, Abbasoglu L, Celik A, Salman FT. Early and late term management in caustic ingestion in children: a 16 year experience. *Acta Chir Belg* 2007; **107**: 49–52.

19 Kochhar R, Ray JD, Sriram PV, *et al.* Intralesional steroids augment the effects of endoscopic dilation in corrosive esophageal strictures. *Gastrointest Endosc* 1999; **49**: 509–513.

20 Evrard S, Le Moine O, Lazaraki G, Dormann A, El Nadaki I, Deviere J. Self-expanding plastic stents for benign esophageal lesions. *Gastrointest Endosc* 2004; **60**: 894–900.

21 Appelqvist P, Salmo M. Lye carcinoma of the esophagus: a review of 63 cases. *Cancer* 1980; **45**: 2655–8.

22 Isolauri J, Markkula H. Lye ingestion and carcinoma of the esophagus. *Act Chir Scand* 1989; **37**: 233–4.

23 Kochhar R, Sethy PK, Kochhar S, Nagi B, Gupta NM. Corrosive induced carcinoma of the esophagus: report of three patients and review of the literature. *J Gastro Hepatol* 2006; **21**: 777–80.

CHAPTER 41

Surgery for Benign Esophageal Disease

Roger P. Tatum and Carlos A. Pellegrini

Department of Surgery, University of Washington, Seattle, WA, USA

Summary

A wide variety of benign esophageal diseases are amenable to surgical treatment. For gastroesophageal reflux disease, surgery is an effective therapeutic modality but is most commonly reserved for patients who are refractory to medical therapy. In the case of achalasia surgery is the most effective treatment option, and is most often recommended as the first line of treatment. Paraesophageal hernias and esophageal diverticula require surgical management when symptomatic. All of the disorders discussed here may be approached using minimally invasive methods. This chapter will focus on the work-up, surgical techniques, and outcomes for patients with gastroesophageal reflux disease, paraesophageal hiatus hernia, esophageal motility disorders such as achalasia, and esophageal diverticula.

Case

A 50-year-old female who has had acid reflux for 15 years asks if her gastroenterologist will refer her to a surgeon for surgery for her hiatal hernia. Her symptoms are completely controlled on a twice-daily dose of a proton pump inhibitor but she fears her husband will lose his insurance in this difficult economy and she is uncertain if they can continue to pay for medications if he does. In addition to heartburn and regurgitation she sometimes experiences food sticking. She had an endoscopy and a 3-cm hiatal hernia was found with no evidence of esophagitis. She was treated with empiric dilation and that was not of benefit. A 24-h pH-impedance test showed that both acid and non-acid reflux were controlled on the current medications. An esophageal motility study showed a decreased LES pressure and ineffective esophageal motility in the distal esophagus. She is referred to a surgeon with a reputation for expertise with laparoscopic surgery. She asks if the surgery would be good for her? She wants to know how long will the benefit last? She also wants to find out if swallowing will be a problem after surgery since she has some trouble now with food sticking.

Practical Gastroenterology and Hepatology: Esophagus and Stomach, 1st edition. Edited by Nicholas J. Talley, Kenneth R. DeVault and David E. Fleischer. © 2010 Blackwell Publishing Ltd.

Introduction

This chapter focuses on the surgical treatment of common esophageal disorders from a practical perspective. We will discuss in separate sections the operative management of gastroesophageal reflux disease (GERD), paraesophageal hernia, motility disorders such as achalasia, and esophageal diverticula. For each of these diseases we will describe the indications for operation, the work-up, the operation itself, and the outcomes. Today, most surgical procedures for benign diseases of the esophagus are performed using minimally invasive techniques and in keeping with the practicality of the book we will particularly detail those approaches.

Surgery for GERD

Since GERD is such a common disorder, antireflux surgery is the most frequently performed esophageal surgery in the USA. The era of antireflux surgery more or less began in 1956 with the description of the fundoplication by Nissen [1]. Although there are other antireflux procedures, the most effective operation remains the fundoplication. The laparoscopic approach was first described in 1991 by Dallegmagne *et al.* [2], and owing to the great advantages that the minimally invasive approach confers both in terms of visualization of the anatomy and in patient recovery, the number of these procedures performed annually has increased significantly since that time.

The typical patient referred for antireflux surgery is one with severe, daily symptoms of reflux who is already taking acid-suppression therapy, usually with proton pump inhibitors (PPIs). Most frequently heartburn has been relieved to some extent by the medication, but regurgitation continues unabated. Most of these patients have either a long history of reflux or reflux manifested early in life. Surgery is rarely considered to be first-line therapy for reflux, and thus the primary indication is the treatment of severe refractory symptoms and or esophageal damage despite medical therapy. The results of antireflux surgery are best for the relief of "typical" symptoms of GERD, such as heartburn, dysphagia, and regurgitation, and the procedure is somewhat less effective in the control of the "atypical" symptoms, including hoarseness and respiratory symptoms [3]. Therefore, patients with atypical symptoms should be cautioned that the procedure may or may not provide relief of these symptoms. Further, patients with a good response to medical therapy are more likely to have a good result from antireflux surgery. The patient who receives absolutely no relief from PPIs, irrespective of how high the dose, is least likely to benefit from an operation, as reflux may not be the true cause of their symptoms. In these patients, objective demonstration of reflux becomes most important before recommending surgery.

Work-up

Often the first, and certainly the most important, component of the preoperative work-up for an antireflux procedure is esophagogastroduodenoscopy (EGD). This is necessary to first and foremost rule out esophageal cancer, and to assess for the presence of intestinal metaplasia (Barrett esophagus). Additional useful information includes the identification of esophagitis and/or a hiatal hernia. Esophageal manometry is important to rule out a diagnosis of achalasia, which can sometimes mimic GERD with symptoms of dysphagia, regurgitation, and chest pain, and to evaluate esophageal body motility. In most cases, patients with ineffective esophageal motility can be managed in the same manner as those with normal peristalsis (i.e., with a total fundoplication such as the Nissen), but patients with complete aperistalsis, such as many with scleroderma, may do poorly with any antireflux procedure. A pH study is performed both to document the presence of pathologic acid reflux (defined as a pH less than 4.0 in the distal esophagus for 4.2% of a 24-h study period, or a DeMeester score greater than 14.72) and to demonstrate correlation between symptoms experienced by the patient and acid reflux events. A barium esophagram is helpful to define the anatomy preoperatively (particularly the size and type of hiatal hernia), and is of greater benefit to the surgeon than the information provided by endoscopy.

Technique of Laparoscopic Nissen Fundoplication

The patient is placed under general anesthesia, and typically in a low-lithotomy position, well-secured to the operating table. In the most typical operation, five incisions are made on the upper abdomen for placement of the ports, with the laparoscope being used through the incision just above and to the left of the umbilicus. The left lateral segment of the liver is retracted to reveal the gastric cardia and the hiatus, and the esophagogastric junction is then dissected away from the left and right crura of the diaphragm. The short gastric vessels between the gastric fundus and splenic hilum are then divided to mobilize the fundus and be able to create a fundoplication without tension. The esophagus is then freed from its adhesions in the mediastinum until the esophagogastric junction lies at least 3 cm below the level of the hiatus without tension. This is important in preventing the recurrence of the hiatal hernia, which is the most common cause of anatomic failure of this operation. The hiatus is then closed posterior to the esophagus using interrupted sutures to approximate the right and left crus of the diaphragm, taking care not to make this tight around the esophagus. Next, the posterior and superolateral aspect of the fundus is passed behind the esophagogastric junction from left to right. A 50–60 F esophageal dilator is placed by the anesthesiologist. The fundoplication is created by suturing the posterior fundus, now on the right side, to the proximal fundus centered over the esophagogastric junction, with the dilator in place to ensure that the fundoplication is not created too tight.

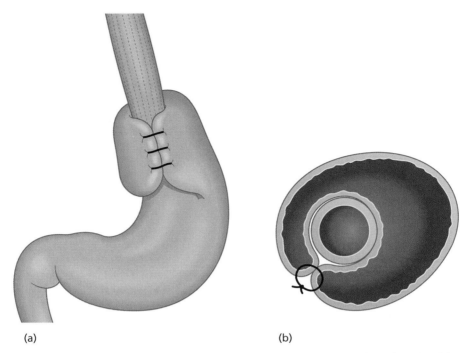

(a)   (b)

Figure 41.1 (a) Completed laparoscopic Nissen fundoplication. (b) Cross-sectional diagram illustrating the configuration of the 360-degree fundoplication around the esophagogastric junction.

The dilator is removed and then the superior aspect of the fundus is sutured to the right and left crus, respectively, to fix the fundoplication in place beneath the diaphragm (Figure 41.1). The ports are then removed and the incisions closed. The patient typically stays overnight in the hospital and is discharged on the first postoperative day. They are instructed to follow a soft diet for approximately 3 weeks after the operation, as some degree of early postoperative dysphagia is inevitable, but resolves over the ensuing 3 weeks to 3 months in the vast majority of cases.

Outcomes

Reports of outcomes after laparoscopic Nissen fundoplication have been quite favorable, with persistent improvement for typical GERD symptoms ranging from 80 to 90% over the long term [4–6]. Atypical symptoms such as cough, hoarseness, and wheezing are improved in approximately 70% of patients with these complaints [7]. In a series of 250 patients, 84% reported satisfactory control of primary reflux symptoms, and 21% were back on medical therapy at 10-year follow-up [5]. Satisfaction

rates were 80% in another series of 239 patients followed for a minimum of 10 years, with 86% of patients stating that they would be willing to undergo the operation again if necessary [6].

Recent trials comparing the efficacy of antireflux surgery to that of long-term proton pump inhibitor therapy have demonstrated the superiority of surgical management. Anvari and colleagues reported significantly improved reflux scores at 1-year follow-up in 52 patients randomized to Nissen fundoplication compared to a group of 52 patients who remained on omeprazole. The medically treated group experienced no overall change in symptom scores, despite escalation of therapy when indicated [8]. The results of another randomized controlled trial reported by Lundell *et al.* revealed significantly higher rates of treatment failure after 7 years in a group of 119 patients treated with omeprazole compared with 99 who underwent antireflux surgery [9].

Ultimately, a combination of thorough patient workup, careful patient selection, and patient preparation are all extremely important in achieving the best outcomes from these procedures.

Paraesophageal Hernia

Paraesophageal hiatus hernias (PEH), in which a portion of the stomach beyond the gastric cardia herniates above the diaphragm, make up approximately 10% of all hiatal hernias. The vast majority of these are mostly likely a progression of the sliding (so-called Type I) hiatus hernia, rather than a separate phenomenon, and are referred to as Type III hernias in which the esophagogastric junction and a portion of the gastric body lie above the diaphragm. True paraesophageal hernias (Type II), in which the fundus herniates through a focal hiatal defect while the esophagogastric junction remains fixed below the hiatus, are quite rare [10]. Symptoms of PEH can include those of reflux as seen with sliding hiatal hernias, as well as anemia (from gastric mucosal erosions known as Cameron lesions), early satiety, and intermittent nausea and vomiting.

Unlike the sliding hernia seen in most patients with GERD, a paraesophageal hernia is an anatomical defect that merits specific consideration as it carries some risk by itself. The stomach flopping above the hiatus can easily become torsed, obstructed, and/or strangulated following the ingestion of food. In fact, the mere discovery of a PEH was considered an indication for surgical repair in the past to prevent these complications. However, a recent meta-analysis of 20 published reports of PEH determined that the annual incidence of complications of PEH requiring emergent surgery was only 1.1%, and that asymptomatic patients were most likely to benefit from watchful waiting [11]. Therefore, we recommend elective PEH repair, which is most commonly performed laparoscopically in a manner similar to an antireflux procedure, and is usually reserved for patients who report one or more of the symptoms (or complications such as anemia) described above.

Work-up

The evaluation of a patient with a paraesophageal hernia is essentially the same as that for a patient with GERD. Frequently, the problem is initially identified as an incidental finding on chest X-ray, in which an air-fluid level is seen above the diaphragm. This will typically lead to the performance of a barium esophagram, which will more precisely define the size and configuration of the hernia (Figure 41.2), and EGD to assess for the presence of esophagitis, Barrett esophagus, and Cameron lesions.

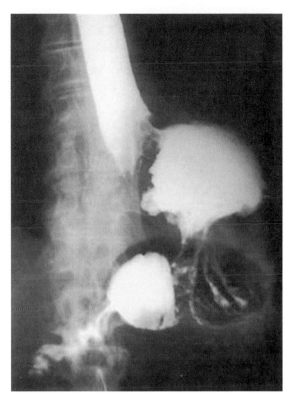

Figure 41.2 Barium esophagram of paraesophageal hernia.

Manometry and pH studies are performed in anticipation of surgical repair.

Surgical Technique

The paraesophageal hernia is approached laparoscopically using the same technique as that for the Nissen fundoplication. The hernia is reduced by pulling the stomach down from the mediastinum, dividing adhesions and the hernia sac in the process. The hiatus is then repaired with sutures as is the case in a sliding hiatus hernia. A fundoplication is typically performed in conjunction with the hernia repair to prevent reflux and also to help maintain the stomach in the subdiaphragmatic position. Notably, the rate of recurrence for PEH after repair can be rather high: 45% when repaired laparoscopically, compared with 15% for those repaired by open surgical techniques, according to one report [12]. Several aspects of the repair are important in reducing the likelihood of recurrence. These include complete excision of the hiatal hernia sac from the mediastinum, full reduction of the esophagogastric junction to a level of at least 3 cm below the hiatus without tension, and adequate crural closure. A fundoplication is typically performed in addition to the hiatal closure.

The existence of the "short esophagus," in which the esophagogastric junction cannot be brought down 3 cm below the diaphragm, is debated. The addition of an esophageal lengthening procedure, whereby a segment of "neoesophagus" is created by separating the gastric cardia from the fundus using a stapling technique, is advocated by some authors who report good results [13–16]. However, these are non-physiologic, can be difficult to perform, and leave acid-secreting mucosa above the hiatus. Alternative strategies to achieve adequate esophageal length in such situations include extensive mediastinal esophageal dissection, which has been demonstrated to yield a median of 3 cm of additional esophageal length below the hiatus [17], and in some cases vagotomy, which can be performed without significant sequelae [18].

Outcomes

As noted above, recurrence of a paraesophageal hernia, with or without symptoms, is high in comparison to sliding hiatus hernias. Therefore, many surgeons currently use a prosthetic mesh to reinforce the suture repair of the hiatus in PEH. In a prospective, randomized multicenter study in which a bioprosthetic mesh was used, hernia recurrence rates were reduced to 9% at 6 month follow-up compared with 24% of patients in whom primary suture repair of the hiatus was performed [19]. Other studies using meshes made of materials such as polypropylene and polytetrafluoroethylene (PTFE) have demonstrated significantly improved recurrence rates as well [20,21]. However, the use of these synthetic materials has been associated with esophageal strictures and erosion into the esophageal or gastric lumen in some cases [22]. Bioprosthetic meshes, which are absorbable and serve as a sort of "scaffold" for fibroblast ingrowth, have not been shown to be associated with these risks [19].

Surgery for Esophageal Motility Disorders

Of the known and classified esophageal motility disorders, achalasia is the one that is most amenable to surgical treatment. Similarly, the results of surgery for hyperten-

sive lower esophageal sphincter are generally favorable [23]. Diffuse esophageal spasm may also respond to surgery, but with less predictable results [24,25]. All three disorders are associated with symptoms of dysphagia and frequently chest pain. Surgical treatment for each of them consists of esophageal myotomy, or division of the muscularis of the LES and distal esophagus.

Work-up

Since each of these problems is most reliably diagnosed by esophageal manometry, this test is essential. Achalasia is identified manometrically by the absence of LES relaxation to swallows together with aperistalsis. Diffuse esophageal spasm is defined as more than 20% of contractions in the esophageal body being simultaneous, and hypertensive LES is a situation in which the LES resting pressure is greater than 45 mmHg, while it relaxes normally to swallows.

EGD is also extremely important to rule out other causes of dysphagia, in particular esophageal cancer. A barium esophagram is also useful to rule out anatomic causes of obstruction. In achalasia, a dilated esophagus is frequently observed together with a tapered narrowing ("bird's beak") distally indicating the non-relaxing LES. The "corkscrew esophagus" pattern (alternating narrow and dilated esophageal segments) is often seen in patients with diffuse esophageal spasm.

Surgical Technique

Invasive procedures to treat benign esophageal disease can be traced back as far as the 1600s, when the English physician Thomas Willis described the use of a whale rib tipped with a sponge for rigid dilation of the lower esophageal sphincter for the treatment of achalasia [26]. The first truly surgical procedure for achalasia was described by Heller in 1913 [27], and the fundamental principles of this operation are still followed today.

For both achalasia and hypertensive lower esophageal sphincter, the most effective procedure is the Heller myotomy. The minimally invasive approach for the treatment of achalasia was introduced in 1992 when a series of 17 patients demonstrated that this approach was possible while hospital stays were reduced substantially [28]. Since then, the minimally invasive approach (primarily via laparoscopy) has largely displaced balloon dilation as the main therapy for achalasia [29].

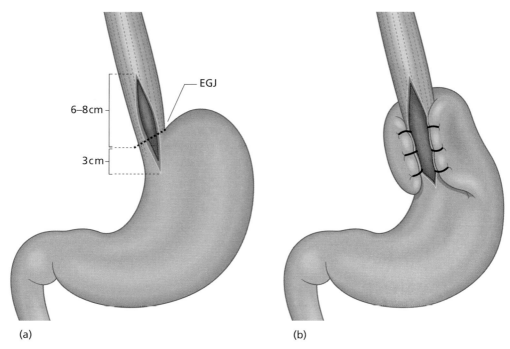

(a)   (b)

Figure 41.3 (a) Length of extended myotomy (shaded area) extending 6–8 cm proximal to the esophagogastric junction (EGJ), and 3 cm distally onto the gastric cardia. (b) Completed laparoscopic extended Heller myotomy and Toupet fundoplication.

The patient is placed under general anesthesia. The positioning and port placements are identical to those for the laparoscopic Nissen fundoplication described above. The gastric fundus is mobilized by dividing the short gastric vessels, and the esophagogastric junction is dissected from the hiatus anteriorly, exposing the distal esophagus. The anterior vagus nerve is identified and carefully preserved, and the epigastric fatpad is dissected away from the gastric cardia. With a lighted dilator placed transorally into the esophagus, the myotomy is begun on the gastric cardia 3 cm distal to the esophagogastric junction, dividing both the outer longitudinal and inner circular muscle layers down to the level of the submucosa. A minimal amount of cautery is used in this dissection to prevent esophageal perforation. The myotomy is continued across the esophagogastric junction and proximally onto the distal esophagus for a distance of 6 to 8 cm. If a perforation does occur, this can be repaired laparoscopically with fine absorbable sutures. Once the myotomy is complete, most surgeons will perform a partial antireflux procedure, such as the Toupet fundoplication wherein the gastric fundus is

passed posterior to the esophagogastric junction and sutured to the right side of the myotomy, while the near aspect of the fundus is sutured to the left edge of the myotomy (Figure 41.3). The ports are removed and the incision is closed. Typically the patient is allowed clear liquids shortly after surgery, and begins a soft diet and is discharged home on the first postoperative day.

Outcomes

With the technique of laparoscopic extended Heller myotomy described above, 95% of patients experienced relief of symptoms without the need for re-intervention at a median follow-up of 63 months. Mean dysphagia scores decreased significantly postoperatively compared to preoperatively, and symptoms of heartburn were minimal [30].

Long Myotomy for Diffuse Esophageal Spasm

A thoracoscopic approach is used in the surgical treatment of diffuse esophageal spasm, in order to permit extension of the myotomy throughout the affected region. First, however, a Heller myotomy must be performed to completely relieve the relative obstruction. The patient is placed in the left lateral decubitus position, and four thoracoscopy ports are placed in the right chest. With the techniques described above, the myotomy is extended proximally to the level of the azygos vein [31]. As noted previously, the results of myotomy for this disorder are somewhat less predictable than those of the Heller myotomy for achalasia.

Surgery for Epiphrenic Diverticulum

Epiphrenic diverticula are diverticula of the pulsion-type which occur in the distal esophagus. They are more common in the elderly population, and are asymptomatic or minimally symptomatic in approximately 60% of patients [32]. When they do cause symptoms, patients most frequently present with dysphagia, regurgitation, and/or weight loss. They are thought to be associated with a motility disorder in the majority of cases, although a variety of motility abnormalities may be observed. In fact, patients presenting with epiphrenic diverticula may exhibit achalasia, diffuse esophageal spasm, hypertensive LES, or ineffective esophageal motility on manometry [32–35]. There is no medical treatment for this problem. Surgery is typically reserved for patients with severe symptoms.

Work-up

The work-up for a patient with a symptomatic epiphrenic diverticulum is similar to that for patients with motility disorders. As the problem has usually been first identified on upper GI radiography, this study has typically been done before the patient is referred to a surgeon. In all cases it is necessary in order to define the size and position of the diverticulum in planning the procedure. As indicated above, manometry helps to identify an associated motility abnormality, and endoscopy is done preoperatively to rule out esophagitis, Barrett esophagus, or esophageal cancer.

Surgical Technique

The fundamental principles of surgery for epiphrenic diverticulum include, for most surgeons, excision of the diverticulum together with a distal esophageal and LES myotomy to relieve the functional obstruction which is thought to lead to the formation of the diverticulum in the first place. Diverticulectomy alone is thought to be more likely to contribute to a risk of esophageal leak as well as recurrence of symptoms [34,35]. As with surgery for motility disorders, an antireflux procedure is frequently added to prevent the occurrence of GERD postoperatively. Left-sided thoracotomy, right-sided thoracoscopy, and laparoscopic approaches are all currently practiced, with the choice of approach being highly dependent on the surgeon and the level of the diverticulum. More distal diverticula are the most amenable to the laparoscopic technique. Advocates of the thoracotomy approach quote lower overall complication rates, particularly of esophageal leak, as well as the ability to readily perform the myotomy up to the level of the aortic arch as advantages of this technique [35]. Thoracoscopic and laparoscopic approaches are typically associated with less postoperative pain and shorter hospital stays as well as potentially better visualization of the anatomy, although notably all authors recommend that these be performed at centers with a high level of experience in minimally invasive esophageal surgery [33,34,36].

For the thoracotomy approach, the patient is placed in the right lateral decubitus position and a left chest incision is performed. The diverticulum is dissected free of mediastinal tissues, and is divided with a surgical stapling device from the esophagus, taking care not to narrow the esophageal lumen. The muscularis is then reapproximated over the staple line with absorbable suture, and an esophageal myotomy is performed on the opposite side of the diverticulectomy starting distal to the esophagogastric junction on the cardia and continuing either up to the level of the diverticulum or past it all the way up to the aortic arch. Subsequently, an antireflux procedure is performed, which is typically a partial fundoplication such as the Belsey Mark IV (240-degree wrap) [35].

The thoracoscopic approach is similar to that sometimes used in the treatment of diffuse esophageal spasm, with the patient in the left lateral decubitus position and three or four thoracoscopic ports through the right chest. The diverticulum is resected using an endoscopic linear cutting stapler, and the myotomy is performed as described above. The muscularis is closed over the staple line with sutures

Laparoscopic approaches all follow the same principles as the procedures above, and are performed using the same positioning and access techniques as in the laparoscopic Heller myotomy. After transhiatal dissection of the distal esophagus and identification and isolation of the epiphrenic diverticulum, an endoscopic linear cutting stapler is used to perform the diverticulectomy, and sutures may be placed to close the muscularis. The myotomy is performed on the opposite side of the esophagus, and a partial fundoplication completes the procedure [36].

Because of the potential for esophageal leak, many surgeons will obtain a water-soluble contrast esophagram one or more days after the procedure to rule out this complication prior to initiating oral feeding. Otherwise, recovery is dependent on the approach, with typically longer hospital stays after thoracotomy compared with minimally invasive techniques.

Outcomes

Results after diverticulectomy and myotomy are favorable, regardless of the operative approach. Varghese *et al.* reported complete resolution of symptoms in 76% of patients in the largest series to date, which included 35 patients operated by left thoracotomy with a mean follow-up of 45 months; 97% reported fair to excellent results. The esophageal leak rate in this series was 6% [35]. Leak rates in other reported series (of both open and minimally invasive techniques) range from zero to 23%, indicating the potential for substantial morbidity from this procedure. Mortality rates as high as 11% have been observed [32–37]. For these reasons, surgical treatment of epiphrenic diverticulum should only be reserved for patients with significant, life-limiting symptoms.

Pharyngoesophageal (Zenker) Diverticulum

The pharyngoesophageal diverticulum, also known as a pharyngeal pouch or more commonly as Zenker diverticulum, is a pulsion phenomenon like the epiphrenic diverticulum. Patients are typically elderly, and when symptomatic they present with dysphagia, regurgitation of undigested food, and/or halitosis [38]. The pouch arises in the cervical esophagus between the thyropharyngeal and cricopharyngeal muscles and is related to poor compliance of the latter [39]. Therefore in order for treatment to be maximally effective, the relative high pressure zone created by the cricopharyngeus must be eliminated. As with the epiphrenic diverticulum, surgery is indicated only for symptomatic patients. Either an open or an endoscopic approach may be employed; both involve division of the cricopharyngeus muscle.

Work-up

Work-up for Zenker diverticulum is similar to that for the other esophageal disorders described previously. EGD and barium esophagography are both important in ruling out any other causes of dysphagia, particularly esophageal cancer, and define the size and position of the pouch. Manometry may demonstrate evidence of upper esophageal sphincter incoordination [38].

Surgical Technique—Open Cricopharyngeal Myotomy With or Without Diverticulectomy

With the patient under general anesthesia and the head turned slightly to the right, a left cervical incision is made along the anterior border of the sternocleidomastoid. After retraction of the thyroid anteromedially and division of the middle thyroid vein and inferior thyroid artery, the pharynx and proximal cervical esophagus are carefully identified posterior to the larynx and trachea and anterior to the spine, taking care not to injure the recurrent laryngeal nerve which runs along the tracheoesophageal groove. The posterior esophagus is bluntly dissected to identify the diverticulum which is then grasped and retracted. Immediately distal to this is the cricopharyngeus muscle. A myotomy is then performed over a right angle clamp inserted between the muscle fibers for a distance of approximately 5 cm distal to the diverticulum. The pouch is then stapled at its neck on the esophagus using a terminal anastomotic surgical stapling device, and is resected [40]. When the diverticulum is 1 cm or less, a myotomy alone is often sufficient, as stapling a pouch this small can lead to narrowing of the esophageal lumen [38]. The wound is then closed without leaving a drain.

Some surgeons will obtain a water-soluble contrast swallow study on the first or second postoperative day to rule out a leak prior to initiating feeding. Patients are typically discharged once they can tolerate a soft diet (2–3 days postoperative).

Surgical Technique—Transoral Endoscopic Stapling

Though endoscopic approaches have been used in one form or another for over 90 years, the endoscopic stapling technique that is in common use currently was first reported by Collard et al. in 1993 [41]. The concept involves the creation of a common lumen between the diverticulum and the esophagus, while simultaneously dividing the cricopharyngeus. With the patient under general anesthesia, a specially designed diverticuloscope with two blades is inserted into the pharynx with one blade being directed down the esophageal lumen and the other into the mouth of the diverticulum. The stapler is then used to divide the common septum between them, firing three rows of staples on either side. Depending on the length of the diverticulum, a second firing of the stapler may be necessary.

This approach has the advantages of shorter operative times, faster recovery, and less morbidity than the open procedure. Notably, however, this technique is not suitable for smaller diverticula (less than 3 cm), because in these cases it will not be possible to perform an adequate myotomy with the stapler [40].

As with the open technique, some surgeons perform a swallow study after the procedure. Patients resume a liquid diet and are discharged on the first postoperative day.

Outcomes

Both the open and endoscopic approaches are associated with good short- and long-term relief of symptoms and a relatively low morbidity. In the largest series comparing both techniques, Bonavina et al. reported that 92% of 181 patients after endoscopic treatment and 94% of 116 patients after open diverticulectomy and myotomy were asymptomatic; in 10-year follow-up of 35 endoscopic and 19 open surgical patients, 82% and 84% remained asymptomatic [40]. Other reports of smaller series have yielded similar results [38,42].

Conclusion

Surgery for benign diseases of the esophagus encompasses a wide variety of disorders and requires knowledge of specialized techniques. Many of the surgical problems described in this chapter involve functional as well as anatomic esophageal abnormalities. While knowledge and treatments of these diseases date back to over 300 years ago, surgical approaches continue to evolve and minimally invasive techniques have recently been developed for each, and are either becoming or already have become the standard of care.

Take-home points

- Surgery for benign esophageal disease has evolved over a long period of time, and currently there are minimally invasive techniques for most of these surgical problems.

- Surgery for GERD is typically reserved for those patients who receive only partial benefit from medical therapy and is most effective in the treatment of typical reflux symptoms such as heartburn, dysphagia, and regurgitation.

- Paraesophageal hiatus hernias can result in reflux symptoms, anemia, or in extreme cases gastric volvulus and/or perforation; they are typically only repaired when symptomatic, and can be approached laparoscopically or thoracoscopically.

- Heller myotomy, most commonly performed laparoscopically, is the most effective treatment for esophageal achalasia and is often recommended as the first line of treatment.

- Treatment of esophageal diverticula, including epiphrenic and pharyngoesophageal (Zenker) diverticula, generally includes division of the distal musculature (LES or cricopharyngeus, respectively) with or without resection of the diverticulum.

References

1 Nissen R. [A simple operation for control of reflux esophagitis.]. *Schweiz Med Wochenschr* 1956; **86** (Suppl. 20): 590–2.

2 Dallemagne B, Weerts JM, Jehaes C, *et al*. Laparoscopic Nissen fundoplication: preliminary report. *Surg Laparosc Endosc* 1991; **1**: 138–43.

3 Oelschlager BK, Quiroga E, Parra JD, *et al*. Long-term outcomes after laparoscopic antireflux surgery. *Am J Gastroenterol* 2008; **103**: 280–7, quiz 8.

4 Morgenthal CB, Shane MD, Stival A, *et al*. The durability of laparoscopic Nissen fundoplication: 11-year outcomes. *J Gastrointest Surg* 2007; **11**: 693–700.

5 Kelly JJ, Watson DI, Chin KF, *et al*. Laparoscopic Nissen fundoplication: clinical outcomes at 10 years. *J Am Coll Surg* 2007; **205**: 570–5.

6 Cowgill SM, Gillman R, Kraemer E, *et al.* Ten-year follow up after laparoscopic Nissen fundoplication for gastroesophageal reflux disease. *Am Surg* 2007; **73**: 748–52, discussion 52–3.

7 Kaufman JA, Houghland JE, Quiroga E, *et al.* Long-term outcomes of laparoscopic antireflux surgery for gastroesophageal reflux disease (GERD)-related airway disorder. *Surg Endosc* 2006; **20**: 1824–30.

8 Anvari M, Allen C, Marshall J, *et al.* A randomized controlled trial of laparoscopic nissen fundoplication versus proton pump inhibitors for treatment of patients with chronic gastroesophageal reflux disease: One-year follow-up. *Surg Innov* 2006; **13**: 238–49.

9 Lundell L, Miettinen P, Myrvold HE, *et al.* Seven-year follow-up of a randomized clinical trial comparing proton-pump inhibition with surgical therapy for reflux oesophagitis. *Br J Surg* 2007; **94**: 198–203.

10 Maziak DE, Todd TRJ, Pearson FG. Massive hiatus hernia: Evaluation and surgical management. *J Thor Cardiovas Surg* 1998; **115**: 53–62.

11 Stylopoulos N, Gazelle GS, Rattner DW. Paraesophageal hernias: operation or observation? *Ann Surg* 2002; **236**: 492–500, discussion 1.

12 Hashemi M, Peters JH, DeMeester TR, *et al.* Laparoscopic repair of large type III hiatal hernia: objective followup reveals high recurrence rate. *J Am Coll Surg* 2000; **190**: 553–60, discussion 60–1.

13 Johnson AB, Oddsdottir M, Hunter JG. Laparoscopic Collis gastroplasty and Nissen fundoplication. A new technique for the management of esophageal foreshortening. *Surg Endosc* 1998; **12**: 1055–60.

14 Luketich JD, Grondin SC, Pearson FG. Minimally invasive approaches to acquired shortening of the esophagus: laparoscopic Collis-Nissen gastroplasty. *Semin Thorac Cardiovasc Surg* 2000; **12**: 173–8.

15 Terry ML, Vernon A, Hunter JG. Stapled-wedge Collis gastroplasty for the shortened esophagus. *Am J Surg* 2004; **188**: 195–9.

16 Youssef YK, Shekar N, Lutfi R, *et al.* Long-term evaluation of patient satisfaction and reflux symptoms after laparoscopic fundoplication with Collis gastroplasty. *Surg Endosc* 2006; **20**: 1702–5.

17 Bochkarev V, Lee YK, Vitamvas M, Oleynikov D. Short esophagus: how much length can we get? *Surg Endosc* 2008; **22**: 2123–7.

18 Oelschlager BK, Yamamoto K, Woltman T, Pellegrini C. Vagotomy during hiatal hernia repair: a benign esophageal lengthening procedure. *J Gastrointest Surg* 2008; **12**: 1155–62.

19 Oelschlager BK, Pellegrini CA, Hunter J, *et al.* Biologic prosthesis reduces recurrence after laparoscopic paraesophageal hernia repair: a multicenter, prospective, randomized trial. *Ann Surg* 2006; **244**: 481–90.

20 Frantzides CT, Madan AK, Carlson MA, Stavropoulos GP. A prospective, randomized trial of laparoscopic polytetrafluoroethylene (PTFE) patch repair vs simple cruroplasty for large hiatal hernia. *Arch Surg* 2002; **137**: 649–52.

21 Granderath FA, Schweiger UM, Kamolz T, *et al.* Laparoscopic Nissen fundoplication with prosthetic hiatal closure reduces postoperative intrathoracic wrap herniation: preliminary results of a prospective randomized functional and clinical study. *Arch Surg* 2005; **140**: 40–8.

22 Tatum RP, Shalhub S, Oelschlager BK, Pellegrini CA. Complications of PTFE mesh at the diaphragmatic hiatus. *J Gastrointest Surg* 2008; **12**: 953–7.

23 Tamhankar AP, Almogy G, Arain MA, *et al.* Surgical management of hypertensive lower esophageal sphincter with dysphagia or chest pain. *J Gastrointest Surg* 2003; **7**: 990–6, discussion 6.

24 Patti MG, Gorodner MV, Galvani C, *et al.* Spectrum of esophageal motility disorders: implications for diagnosis and treatment. *Arch Surg* 2005; **140**: 442–8, discussion 8–9.

25 Tutuian R, Castell DO. Review article: oesophageal spasm—diagnosis and management. *Aliment Pharmacol Ther* 2006; **23**: 1393–402.

26 Willis T. *Pharmaceutice Rationalis Sive Diatribe de Medicamentorum Operationibus in Human Corpore.* London, England: Hagae Comitis, 1674.

27 Heller E. Extramukose kardioplastic beim chronischen kardiospasmus mit dilatation des oesophagus. *Mitt Grenzeb Med Chir* 1913; **27**: 141–9.

28 Pellegrini C, Wetter LA, Patti M, *et al.* Thoracoscopic esophagomyotomy. Initial experience with a new approach for the treatment of achalasia. *Ann Surg* 1992; **216**: 291–6, discussion 6–9.

29 Patti MG, Pellegrini CA, Horgan S, *et al.* Minimally invasive surgery for achalasia: an 8-year experience with 168 patients. *Ann Surg* 1999; **230**: 587–93, discussion 93–4.

30 Wright AS, Williams CW, Pellegrini CA, Oelschlager BK. Long-term outcomes confirm the superior efficacy of extended Heller myotomy with Toupet fundoplication for achalasia. *Surg Endosc* 2007; **21**: 713–8.

31 Patti MG, Pellegrini CA. Endoscopic surgical treatment of primary oesophageal motility disorders. *J R Coll Surg Edinb* 1996; **41**: 137–42.

32 Benacci JC, Deschamps C, Trastek VF, *et al.* Epiphrenic diverticulum: results of surgical treatment. *Ann Thorac Surg* 1993; **55**: 1109–13, discussion 14.

33 Del Genio A, Rossetti G, Maffetton V, *et al.* Laparoscopic approach in the treatment of epiphrenic diverticula: long-term results. *Surg Endosc* 2004; **18**: 741–5.

34 Fernando HC, Luketich JD, Samphire J, *et al.* Minimally invasive operation for esophageal diverticula. *Ann Thorac Surg* 2005; **80**: 2076–80.

35 Varghese TK, Jr., Marshall B, Chang AC, *et al.* Surgical treatment of epiphrenic diverticula: a 30-year experience. *Ann Thorac Surg* 2007; **84**: 1801–9, discussion 9.

36 Rosati R, Fumagalli U, Bona S, *et al.* Diverticulectomy, myotomy, and fundoplication through laparoscopy: a new option to treat epiphrenic esophageal diverticula? *Ann Surg* 1998; **227**: 174–8.

37 Streitz JM, Jr., Glick ME, Ellis FH, Jr. Selective use of myotomy for treatment of epiphrenic diverticula. Manometric and clinical analysis. *Arch Surg* 1992; **127**: 585–7, discussion 7–8.

38 Aly A, Devitt PG, Jamieson GG. Evolution of surgical treatment for pharyngeal pouch. *Br J Surg* 2004; **91**: 657–64.

39 Cook IJ, Blumbergs P, Cash K, *et al.* Structural abnormalities of the cricopharyngeus muscle in patients with pharyngeal (Zenker's) diverticulum. *J Gastroenterol Hepatol* 1992; **7**: 556–62.

40 Bonavina L, Bona D, Abraham M, *et al.* Long-term results of endosurgical and open surgical approach for Zenker diverticulum. *World J Gastroenterol* 2007; **13**: 2586–9.

41 Collard JM, Otte JB, Kestens PJ. Endoscopic stapling technique of esophagodiverticulostomy for Zenker's diverticulum. *Ann Thorac Surg* 1993; **56**: 573–6.

42 Visosky AM, Parke RB, Donovan DT. Endoscopic management of Zenker's diverticulum: factors predictive of success or failure. *Ann Otol Rhinol Laryngol* 2008; **117**: 531–7.

CHAPTER 42

Esophageal Cancer

Michael S. Smith[1] and Charles J. Lightdale[2]

[1] Gastroenterology Section, Department of Medicine, Temple University School of Medicine, Philadelphia, PA, USA

[2] Division of Digestive and Liver Diseases, Columbia University Medical Center, New York, NY, USA

Summary

Esophageal cancer (EC) is a devastating disease because by the time the patient develops symptoms he/she usually has advanced disease and the 5-year survival is only 17%. In the United States, adenocarcinoma is now the predominant histologic type. Worldwide, squamous cell carcinoma is much more common. The two types of EC have different risk factors and pathophysiologies but their clinical symptoms are similar. Most commonly, patients present with dysphagia and weight loss. The key to management of EC is staging, which guides both prognosis and therapy. When possible, resection is the preferred treatment in most cases. Chemoradiation can be used as a primary therapy in inoperable situations or as neoadjuvant therapy. Endoscopic therapy is important for palliative management and its role as curative therapy has grown as screening for both adenocarcinoma (primarily in patients with Barrett esophagus) and for precursors of squamous cell cancer has led to the diagnosis at earlier stages and the potential for better outcomes.

Case

A 57-year-old man comes to your office for evaluation. He notes difficulty swallowing steak over the past 6 months, which had improved by cutting smaller pieces. Recently, however, the sensation has returned, and other foods are "getting stuck" as well. There is a long history of heartburn and intermittent reflux of acid. He does not weigh himself, but notes having to pull his belt tighter to hold up his pants. On examination, he is obese and smells of cigarette smoke. He comes with images from a recent barium esophagram which shows an irregularity in the distal esophageal lumen. Esophagogastroduodenoscopy (EGD) identifies a long segment Barrett esophagus with an exophytic mass arising from within intestinal metaplasia. Biopsies confirm adenocarcinoma, and endoscopic ultrasound is performed, showing a T3 lesion with a suspicious periesophageal lymph node. The patient is referred to an oncologist. A computed tomography/positron emission tomography (CT/PET) scan is obtained that shows no evidence of distant metastases. He begins neoadjuvant chemoradiation with plans for surgical resection.

Practical Gastroenterology and Hepatology: Esophagus and Stomach, 1st edition. Edited by Nicholas J. Talley, Kenneth R. DeVault and David E. Fleischer. © 2010 Blackwell Publishing Ltd.

Epidemiology

Esophageal cancer (EC) is a highly lethal malignancy with a rapidly growing incidence. Approximately 16 470 patients are diagnosed with esophageal cancer each year in the United States, with 14 280 deaths expected annually from the disease [1]. Despite widespread improvements in diagnosis, staging, and treatment, data from the Surveillance, Epidemiology, and End Results (SEER) Program of the National Cancer Institute demonstrate continued poor patient outcomes. While the 5-year survival rate from 1975 to 1977 was 6%, it climbed to only 17% from 1996 to 2002.

Two main histologic subtypes dominate the diagnosis of EC. Worldwide, squamous cell carcinoma (SCC) remains the most common cancer, with the highest incidence rates in Asia (southern Russia, China, and Singapore), northern Iran and Turkey, and Africa. In the United States, a nearly sixfold rise in the incidence of adenocarcinoma (AC) since 1975 has made it the most common EC subtype. Other tumors are uncommon, accounting for only a few percent of cases. They include extrapulmonary small cell cancer, metastatic disease, and, very rarely, other primary tumors including granular cell tumors, choriocarcinoma, sarcoma, melanoma, and lymphoma. Given the predominance of SCC and AC, this chapter will focus on these two malignancies.

Risk Factors for Squamous Cell Cancer

While EC often is considered a single disease when discussing treatment and prognosis, in fact the SCC and AC subtypes are somewhat divergent with respect to their risk factors (Table 42.1). Overall, SCC appears more associated with men (particularly outside of endemic regions) and occurs most frequently in the sixth decade. One recent study estimated that, within the Unites States, a history of tobacco use (especially cigarettes), alcohol consumption, and a diet poor in fruits and vegetables accounted for nearly 90% of ECC cases [2]. Other dietary factors include the chewing of Betel nuts, a popular habit

Table 42.1 Major risk factors for development of squamous cell carcinoma and adenocarcinoma.

Risk factor	Squamous cell carcinoma	Adenocarcinoma
Male sex	√	√
Caucasian race		√
Increased age	?	√
Obesity		√
Tobacco use	√	√
Alcohol consumption	√	
Diet poor in fruits/ vegetables	√	√
Vitamin deficiencies	√	?
Ingestion of N-nitroso compounds	√	√
History of prior esophageal disease	√	
Barrett esophagus/GERD		√
Conditions with increased esophageal acid exposure (ZES, impaired LES function)		√

GERD, gastroesophageal reflux disease; LES, lower esophageal sphincter; ZES, Zollinger–Ellison syndrome.

in some regions of Asia, as well as low levels of selenium, zinc, and vitamins A and C. Foods that contain carcinogenic N-nitroso compounds, such as pickled vegetables, also appear to increase the risk of developing SCC, as does consumption of maté, a beverage popular in parts of South America made from a maté herb. Exposure to polycyclic aromatic hydrocarbons from various environmental sources has been postulated to be a potential etiologic factor in all areas of the world.

Additional factors also appear to increase the risk of developing SCC. These include a history of prior esophageal disease, such as achalasia or caustic (lye) ingestion, exposure to ionizing radiation, and the presence of human papilloma virus. Patients with Plummer–Vinson syndrome and tylosis, a disease involving hyperkeratosis of the palms and soles of the hands and feet, also are at an increased risk of developing SCC. While patients with a history of prior SCC of the head, neck, or airway also appear to have a higher risk of developing esophageal SCC, this may be due to overlapping risk factors and not a direct link between the two malignancies.

Risk Factors for Adenocarcinoma

While SCC and AC share a few common risk factors, including smoking, a fruit and vegetable-poor diet and intake of N-nitroso compounds, the main drivers associated with AC are very different. The majority of AC arises from Barrett esophagus, a condition where chronic gastroesophageal reflux leads to replacement of the normal squamous mucosal lining of the esophagus with columnar mucosa, including specialized intestinal metaplasia. The presence of gastroesophageal reflux disease (GERD), thought to be the force behind the development of Barrett metaplasia, also has been linked to AC, with the severity and duration of acid exposure correlating with the risk of malignancy. Obesity, which has been linked to GERD, also increases the risk of development of AC, with higher body mass index (BMI) leading to greater risk of cancer, probably mostly related to accumulation of excess intra-abdominal or visceral fat [3]. There is no relationship, however, between obesity and SCC. Increased esophageal acid exposure, from hypersecretory states such as Zollinger–Ellison syndrome or conditions that impair lower esophageal sphincter (LES) function such as scleroderma, presence of a hiatal hernia, prior myotomy or dilation, and use of certain medications that relax the LES, also have been implicated.

Unlike SCC, there appears to be an ethnic disparity in patients who develop AC. Caucasians are far more likely to develop AC, at double the rates of Hispanic patients and four times that of Asians and Blacks, according to a study performed in the United States [4]. Men also appear far more likely to develop this malignancy, and, as with SCC, the risk of developing AC appears to increase with age.

There are some factors that appear to be protective against AC. A Swedish study discovered a moderate decrease in risk of developing AC in the setting of high fiber intake, thought to neutralize conversion of salivary nitrites into nitrosamines [5]. Other nutritional studies have suggested that vitamins A, B_6, C, and E, as well as folate, are also protective. While still under investigation, some studies suggest a chemopreventive role for use of non-steroidal anti-inflammatory medications (NSAIDs) such as aspirin, which inhibit cyclo-oxyenase-2. In contrast to SCC, alcohol use does not predispose to AC, and drinking wine may even decrease the risk of developing malignancy [6]. However, this is not firmly established and decreased risk could be related to other factors in moderate wine drinkers.

Pathophysiology

Squamous Cell Cancer

Most squamous cell malignancies arise in the middle third of the esophagus. Tumors arise from denuded epithelium, plaques, or small polypoid excrescences [7]. On a molecular level, cell proliferation increases, most frequently from mutations in the cyclin D1 gene leading to poor regulation of the G1 phase of the cell cycle. These tumors are often initially flat in appearance, and characteristically invade the submucosa at a relatively early stage. This facilitates local lymph node invasion due to the presence of lymphatics in the lamina propria and not deep to the muscularis mucosa, as seen in other gastrointestinal organs. Metastasis also can occur into adjacent structures, such as the trachea and aorta, and to regional lymph nodes in the periesophageal, periaortic, and, sometimes, celiac stations. About a third of patients demonstrate distant metastasis, with liver, bone (including marrow), and lung being the most frequently involved organs. Spread to the peritoneum and distant lymph nodes is less common, and brain metastasis is very rare.

Adenocarcinoma

As previously stated, AC appears to arise from Barrett mucosa, and therefore is most often found in the distal third of the esophagus. The predominant molecular defect appears to be hypermethylation of the *p16* promoter region, leading again to increased cell cycling along with aneuploidy. The lesion can be flat, nodular, or ulcerated in early stages, whether or not it is associated with intestinal metaplasia. Like SCC, early spread is seen due to the relatively shallow lymphatics, though involvement of more caudal regional lymph nodes (celiac and gastrohepatic) are seen due to the predominance of more distal lesions in the esophageal lumen. Similar distant metastatic patterns are seen.

Clinical Features

Unfortunately, many esophageal cancers do not generate symptoms until they reach an advanced stage. The most common initial presentation is one of progressive dysphagia, particularly to solid foods, and is often accompanied by weight loss due to decreased oral intake from dysphagia and dietary changes, or tumor-associated anorexia. Retrosternal discomfort or burning can occur, but is non-specific and often ignored by patients or treated with empiric acid control medication. Once the tumor has advanced, additional symptoms can be observed, including regurgitation of saliva or undigested food, hoarseness due to involvement of the recurrent laryngeal nerve, and back pain due to mediastinal invasion by the tumor. Occasionally, aspiration pneumonia is seen, particularly in the setting of a tracheoesophageal fistula. Iron-deficiency anemia from chronic blood loss associated with the tumor is common, but hematemesis and melena are far less frequently identified in these patients. The exception to this is when an aortoesophageal fistula has formed, at which point a life-threatening bleed may occur.

Diagnosis and Staging

Making a diagnosis of esophageal cancer sometimes begins with radiographic imaging of the esophagus, most frequently a barium esophagram. However, to make the actual diagnosis, tissue is required, almost always using

EGD. Lesions can take several forms, including flat plaques, ulcerations or ulcerated masses, and stricturing lesions (Figure 42.1). In the case of flat lesions suspicious for SCC, application of Lugol iodide solution for chromoendoscopy can identify neoplastic tissue, which does not stain due to the absence of glycogen molecules found in normal squamous mucosa. Similarly for AC arising from Barrett esophagus, use of advanced imaging techniques such as narrow-band imaging and confocal microscopy can identify abnormal vascular and cellular patterns suspicious for advanced neoplasia and malignancy. Once the suspected lesion is identified, targeted endoscopic biopsies should be performed. To improve diagnostic accuracy, the endoscopist should consider increasing the number of biopsies obtained and adding brush cytology specimens [8].

Staging of esophageal cancer is performed soon after the tissue diagnosis is made. Similar to other tumors, a widely accepted staging system has been developed by the American Joint Commission on Cancer [9] (Table 42.2). A variety of studies are used to assess both the primary tumor and look for metastatic spread. The first technique employed is frequently computed tomography (CT) scan of the chest and abdomen. CT has the benefit of being a minimally invasive test, and is particularly helpful in both identifying distant metastatic disease, as well as excluding a T4 lesion by looking for preservation of the anatomic fat plane between the esophagus and adjacent structures. However, CT is far less successful in determining the depth of tumor invasion (T stage) and has a relatively low sensitivity for detecting locoregional disease and small metastases. Thus, additional testing is performed on those with CT scans that do not show metastases.

Endoscopic ultrasound (EUS) is used to fill in the staging gaps left by CT. This technique utilizes a high frequency transducer embedded within the tip of the endoscope and, when introduced into the esophagus, can approximate the appropriate anatomic structures to provide the most accurate T and N staging (Video 16). These data can be crucial in identifying and selecting the optimal therapeutic approach. For example, tumors staged as a T1, which do not involve the muscularis propria, may be amenable to endoscopic mucosal resection in place of surgical intervention if no evidence of lymphatic spread is present. In one meta-analysis, the accuracy of EUS for determining T stage was 89% [10].

In some cases, however, EUS T staging is more difficult due to a long tumor, location at the gastroesophageal (GE) junction, or when a stenotic tumor prevents safe advancement of standard equipment to the proper location for imaging. Dilation of the tumor to allow complete EUS evaluation is discouraged owing to the risk of perforation. To traverse these narrowed lumens, a catheter-based miniature EUS probe inserted through the endoscopic biopsy channel may be used, but its resolution is inferior to that of the endoscope-mounted probe, particularly when evaluating lymph nodes. Another option is to use a 7 mm diameter wire-guided echoendoscope which does not contain fiberoptics, but this equipment is not widely available.

EUS also offers the added benefit of fine needle aspiration (FNA) where, in many cases, tissue sampling of suspicious lymph nodes can be performed (Video 17). Possible exceptions occur when these nodes lie directly behind the tumor mass, or if the patient must remain on constant anticoagulation. When certain endosonographic criteria are met (diameter greater than 10 mm, round or oval shape, well-defined endoscopic borders), the endoscopist may choose not to sample and instead empirically treat these findings as positive for regional nodal spread.

Given the length of the esophagus, regional lymph nodes for EC vary based on the anatomic location of the primary lesion. Regional lymph nodes for tumors in the thoracic or middle third of the esophagus include both upper and lower periesophageal as well as subcarinal stations. For EC near the GE junction, the lower periesophageal station is included, as well as the diaphragmatic, pericardial, left gastric, and celiac stations. For the rare tumors found in the cervical esophagus, the regional nodal stations differ significantly and include scalene, internal jugular, cervical (upper and lower), upper periesophageal, and supraclavicular nodes. A thorough examination of all stations is performed, however, as positive findings outside the appropriate region are considered distant metastatic disease.

Those patients whose CT and EUS findings suggest they remain candidates for resection generally proceed to a scan integrating CT with positron emission tomography (PET), which uses ^{18}F-fluorodeoxyglucose to identify areas of hypermetabolic activity suspicious for tumor. The role of this combined technique is not fully explored in clinical studies, but is generally accepted as the optimal

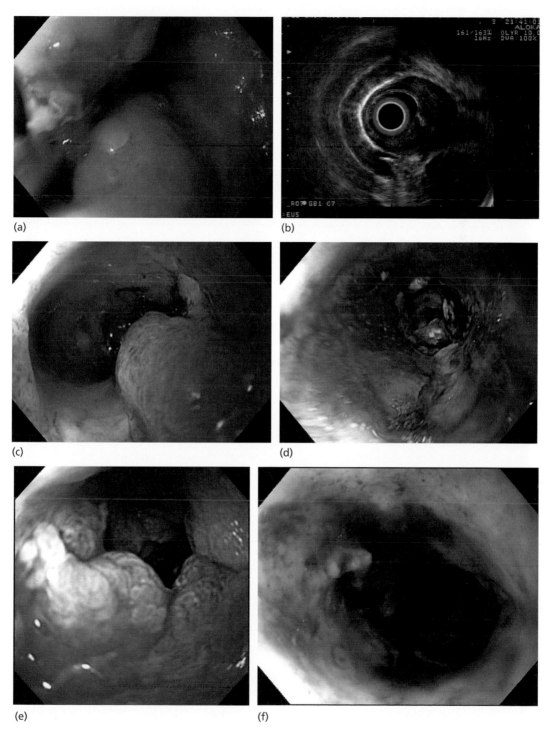

(a)

(b)

(c)

(d)

(e)

(f)

Figure 42.1 Endoscopic diagnosis, staging and treatment of esophageal cancer. Squamous cell carcinoma of the esophagus (a) found to be a T3 lesion on endoscopic ultrasound (b). Adenocarcinoma of the esophagus before (c, e) and after (d, f) palliative ablation using an Nd:YAG laser.

Table 42.2 TNM staging for esophageal cancer.

Primary tumor (T)		Regional lymph nodes (N)		Distant metastasis (M)	
Tx	Cannot be assessed	Nx	Cannot be assessed	Mx	Cannot be assessed
T0	No evidence of primary tumor			M0	No distant metastasis
Tis	Intramucosal carcinoma (*carcinoma in situ*)			M1*	Distant metastasis
T1a	Invades only to mucosa or lamina propria	N0	No nodes involved	**M1 classification:*	
T1b	Invades submucosa			Upper thoracic tumors:	
T2	Invades muscularis propria			M1a: cervical nodes involved	
				M1b: other distant metastasis	
T3	Invades adventitia	N1	Regional node metastasis	Midthoracic tumors:	
				All lesions are M1b	
T4	Invades adjacent structures			Lower thoracic tumors:	
				M1a: celiac nodes involved	
				M1b: other distant metastasis	

imaging for distant metastasis at this point in the staging process.

Two additional procedures should be considered prior to surgical resection in some patients. For locally advanced tumors located at or above the level of the carina, guidelines published by the National Comprehensive Cancer Network recommend performing bronchoscopy to rule out airway invasion [11]. For tumors of the GE junction, there is some support for use of diagnostic laparoscopy, particularly when there is suspicion of intraperitoneal metastasis, but its use remains controversial.

Therapeutics

Endoscopic Approaches

Curative endoscopic-based intervention is reserved for those patients who are found to have tumor that does not involve the submucosa (Table 42.3). Because of the low risk of lymph node metastases, high-grade dysplasia (Tis, carcinoma *in situ*) and intramucosal carcinoma (T1a) can be treated with a variety of techniques, with some variation depending on tumor subtype. Lesions found to be high-grade dysplasia or intramucosal adenocarcinoma can be treated with the same techniques available for eradication of Barrett esophagus. These include endoscopic mucosal resection (EMR), radiofrequency ablation (for flat lesions only), and cryoablation (see Chapter 33). Photodynamic therapy, which uses light to activate

a photosensitizing agent predisposed to collecting within neoplastic cells, can be used, but recently has fallen out of favor due to a relatively high risk of complication and poor tolerance compared to alternative approaches. EMR, which creates a pseudopolyp containing the lesion using a saline injection and/or endoscope-mounted cap with band placement, can be considered for lesions that extend into the submucosa (T1) (Video 18). Utilization of this technique provides the added benefit of obtaining a deeper tissue sample which can confirm or adjust EUS-based staging based on the pathology result. Lesions that invade submucosa likely are not candidates for EMR-based monotherapy given the higher likelihood of lymphatic spread. Highly-skilled endoscopists, mainly in Japan, have utilized endoscopic submucosal dissection (ESD) with needle-knife type devices for *en bloc* resection of early esophageal cancer for accurate pathological staging and definitive therapy with excellent results. This procedure, however, is more expensive and time consuming with higher complication rates than with EMR technique.

Surgical Approaches

Esophagectomy has been the core treatment for esophageal cancer for many years. Primary resection is indicated for the treatment of stage I and II lesions (approximately one in three patients). There are two common approaches to the resection. The first is a transhiatal esophagectomy (THE), which utilizes an upper midline laparotomy and left neck incision with gastric interposition and creation

Table 42.3 Preferred initial treatment for esophageal cancer according to TNM classification.

Stage grouping by TNM classification				Preferred initial therapy
Stage 0	Tis	N0	M0	Endoscopic removal
Stage 1	T1	N0	M0	Endoscopic removal vs. esophagectomy ± chemoradiotherapy, based on depth of invasion into submucosa
Stage IIa	T2	N0	M0	Esophagectomy vs. chemoradiotherapy, consider both
	T3	N0	M0	
Stage IIb	T1	N1	M0	Neoadjuvant chemoradiotherapy followed by esophagectomy if indicated after restaging
	T2	N1	M0	
Stage III	T3	N1	M0	
	T4	Any N	M0	
Stage IV	Any T	Any N	M1	Chemotherapy with palliative measures as required
IVa	Any T	Any N	M1a	
IVb	Any T	Any N	M1b	

of a cervical anastomosis. A thoracotomy is not required for this procedure, which decreases the risk of complications, but this also prevents a full exploration and resection of thoracic lymph nodes, and does not allow for visualization of the mid-thoracic dissection during the operation. An alternative approach is the Ivor–Lewis transthoracic esophagectomy, which utilizes a right thoracotomy as well as a laparotomy. During this procedure, a full lymphadenectomy is performed and there is direct visualization of the thoracic esophagus during dissection; however, the proximal resection margin is limited, and there is a greater risk of complications, including bile reflux (due to a lower anastomosis) and pulmonary compromise. Modified and even combined versions of these two techniques are performed by some surgeons, depending on the specifics of individual tumors. Variations include extended lymphadenectomy, common in Japan, and interposition of a section of jejunum or colon as a conduit to replace the esophagus instead of a gastric pull-up. Data has shown similar rates of complications and success for both procedures [12,13]. Five-year survival rates are in the range of 20%.

Where the esophagectomy is performed plays an important role in perioperative mortality rates, according to several studies. One study showed that high-volume centers have a significantly lower risk of mortality compared to hospitals which rarely perform the procedure [14]. The adjusted odds ratio for centers performing 20 or more procedures per year was 0.36 (95% CI 0.26–0.50) when compared to hospitals performing less than two esophagectomies yearly. Regardless of where and how the esophagectomy was performed, there is a significant risk of postoperative complications, including anastomotic leakage, the need for reoperation, and tumor recurrence.

Surgical management of EC (nearly always SCC) located within the cervical esophagus, which extends from the cricopharyngeus to the thoracic inlet, is different than that of mid- and distal esophageal tumors. These lesions are treated similarly to SCC of the head and neck, with extensive resections involving the pharynx, larynx, thyroid, and esophagus, along with radical neck dissection and lymphadenectomy. Reconstruction of the gastrointestinal tract can be accomplished using a gastric pull-up with pharyngeal anastomosis, a jejunal interposition or myocutaneous flap (either deltopectoral or pectoralis major).

Curative Radiation and Chemotherapy

Alternatives to surgical monotherapy must be considered, given that the majority of patients are not candidates for resection at presentation, and additional patients are found to have locoregional or distant metastasis during surgery. Both radiotherapy and chemotherapy have been considered, alone or in combination, for use as both definitive and adjuvant agents, though there is little support for radiation monotherapy in either role.

Chemotherapy regimens generally consist of cisplatin and 5-fluorouracil, and sometimes newer agents such as irinotecan or a taxane. While chemotherapy alone has been considered for definitive treatment, combination chemoradiotherapy (CRT), thought to benefit from the radiosensitizing properties of some chemotherapeutic agents, is favored. CRT became the preferred option based on the results of a key trial performed by the Radiation Therapy Oncology Group [15,16]. This study compared the response to radiation alone and CRT in patients with locoregional thoracic esophageal cancer (90% SCC). Interim analysis demonstrated a significant 2-year survival advantage for patients receiving CRT (38 vs. 10%), and subsequent data showed a 5-year survival of 26%, comparable to that of esophagectomy. These results have led to definitive CRT becoming the preferred option in patients who are not surgical candidates, either due to an inoperable lesion or expected poor tolerance of surgery.

CRT also has become the standard of care in a neoadjuvant setting for those patients with locoregional spread found on initial evaluation. These patients are treated and then re-staged prior to any surgical intervention. It is believed that CRT can improve both macro- and micrometastatic disease, resulting in a higher percentage of patients achieving a pathologic complete response (pCR) when the esophagectomy specimen is examined. Multiple studies have shown that patients with persistent disease have poorer outcomes than those who achieve pCR. Use of preoperative CRT in patients with limited tumor burden, however, is more controversial.

Palliation

When treatment without curative intent is planned there are multiple modalities that can be employed (Table 42.4). Systemic chemotherapy can be considered for stage IV disease to decrease overall tumor burden and possibly extend life expectancy; radiotherapy is not administered as it would be ineffective in treating distant metastases outside the targeted anatomic area. Other options generally focus on treating the primary symptom of dysphagia or other sequelae of advanced disease.

Esophagectomy and esophageal bypass are two surgical options for palliation, neither of which is performed frequently due to the high rates of perioperative morbidity and mortality. Radiation therapy has been shown to improve swallowing function in patients. However, the

Table 42.4 Options for palliation of inoperable esophageal cancer.

Location of treatment	Treatment type
Extracorporeal/systemic	Systemic chemotherapy
	External beam radiotherapy
Luminal-based treatments	Stenting (metal or plastic)
	Dilation
	Laser therapy
	Argon plasma coagulation
	Cryoablation
	Photodynamic therapy
	Brachytherapy
	Intratumoral alcohol injection
	Intratumoral chemotherapy injection
	Esophagectomy
	Esophageal bypass surgery

need for multiple sessions makes it less desirable for those with a relatively short expected lifespan, and the short duration of benefits from treatment decreases its benefit in those with longer predicted survival. Concomitant brachytherapy, where a radioactive source is placed intraluminally to provide additional treatment, improves outcomes versus external radiation alone, but increases the risk of fistula formation in patients with local recurrence or prior CRT and should not be used with salvage chemotherapy.

Much of the focus on palliative intervention has shifted to endoscopic-based treatments. Temporary relief of dysphagia can be accomplished by dilation up to 17 mm using a variety of techniques, though repeat sessions are frequently needed and there is an inherent risk of perforation [17]. More permanent symptomatic relief is obtained by using one of several ablative devices. These include laser palliation (infrequently performed now, but in the recent past neodymium-yttrium-aluminum-garnet or Nd:YAG lasers were mostly used), argon plasma coagulation, photodynamic therapy, and cryoablation. Chemical ablations with absolute alcohol injection and intratumoral chemotherapy injection also have been described.

Self-expanding endoluminal stents have become the mainstay of palliative interventions for advanced EC. Currently available devices, which have a pre-deployment diameter of under 10 mm, are far superior to their predecessors in that they are self-expanding and do not require significant dilation prior to placement. They can be placed with or without fluoroscopic guidance. Stents come in a variety of metal alloys or are made from plastic, and are available in multiple lengths. This allows the endoscopist to select a stent approximately 4 cm longer than the lesion and ensure that the entire stenotic segment is opened. Coating the stents with a semipermeable membrane to create a "covered" stent has decreased the amount of tumor or regenerative hyperplastic or fibrotic ingrowth seen with bare stents; however, it also has increased the likelihood of stent migration out of the optimal position. While stents with greater diameters can be used to maximize the likelihood of maintaining patency, these stents carry a greater risk of complications including fistulization and hemorrhage. As an alternative, reintervention with placement of a second stent is common when dysphagia recurs.

While stenting is the preferred method for treatment of fistulae and a favored approach for symptomatic relief in the presence of a malignant stricture, endoscopists must consider several factors when deciding whether and how to utilize this technique. Tumor location is critical. Placement of proximal esophageal stents is technically challenging, and while symptoms improve, efficacy is less than what is seen when treating more distal lesions [18]. Stents deployed across lesions near the GE junction maintain a patent channel for acid reflux which can adversely affect quality of life. Thus, high-dose proton pump inhibitor therapy is recommended post-procedure. Stents in this location also cannot have significant segments within the stomach, and may create ulceration through trauma of the opposing gastric wall. In cases of suspected tracheal compression by the tumor, tracheal stenting must be considered to maintain airway patency. A trial of balloon dilation prior to esophageal stenting can lead to prophylactic tracheal stent placement to prevent respiratory compromise.

Take-home points

Epidemiology:
- Adenocarcinoma is now the most common esophageal cancer in the United States, due to a rapid and continuing rise in incidence for the past several decades, associated with increased rates of GERD and obesity.
- Squamous cell carcinoma remains the most common subtype worldwide, and in the United States is linked closely to tobacco and alcohol use.

Diagnosis:
- Patients often present with dysphagia to solid foods and weight loss.
- Endoscopic biopsy to obtain a tissue diagnosis is required.
- A combination of CT, EUS, PET/CT, and in some cases bronchoscopy, is used to stage patients, particularly those who are potential surgical candidates.

Therapy:
- Endoscopic-based therapy is reserved for T0 or T1 lesions.
- Surgical intervention, using either a transhiatal or transthoracic approach, historically has been the mainstay of curative treatment for stage I and II lesions.
- Chemoradiotherapy has become the standard of care for definitive treatment in non-surgical candidates, and is given as neoadjuvant treatment prior to surgery in patients with only locoregional spread.
- Palliative options, both externally and endoluminally applied, are available for treatment of the sequelae of advanced disease, particularly dysphagia and tracheoesophageal fistula.

References

1 Jemal A, Siegel R, Ward E, et al. Cancer statistics, 2008. CA Cancer J Clin 2008; **58**: 71–96.

2 Engel LS, Chow WH, Vaughan TL, et al. Population attributable risks of esophageal and gastric cancers. J Natl Cancer Inst 2003; **95**: 1404–13.

3 Hampel H, Abraham NS, El-Serag HB. Meta-analysis: obesity and the risk for gastroesophageal reflux disease and its complications. Ann Intern Med 2005; **143**: 199–211.

4 Kubo A, Corley DA. Marked multi-ethnic variation of esophageal and gastric cardia carcinomas within the United States. Am J Gastroenterol 2004; **99**: 582–8.

5 Terry P, Lagergren J, Ye W, et al. Inverse association between intake of cereal fiber and the risk of gastric cardia cancer. Gastroenterology 2001; **120**: 387–91.

6 Gammon MD, Schoenberg JB, Ahsan H, et al. Tobacco, alcohol, and socioeconomic status and adenocarcinomas of the esophagus and gastric cardia. J Natl Cancer Inst 1997; **89**: 1247–84.

7 Holscher AH, Bollschweiler E, Schneider PM, et al. Prognosis of early esophageal cancer: comparison between adeno- and squamous cell carcinoma. Cancer 1995; **76**: 178–86.

8 Graham DY, Schwartz JT, Cain GD, et al. Prospective evaluation of biopsy number in the diagnosis of esophageal and gastric carcinoma. Gastroenterology 1982; **82**: 228–31.

9　Greene FL, ed. *AJCC Cancer Staging Manual*, 6th edn. New York: Springer-Verlag, Inc., 2002.

10　Rosch T. Endosonographic staging of esophageal cancer: a review of literature results. *Gastrointest Endosc Clin N Am* 1995; **5**: 537–47.

11　National Comprehensive Cancer Network. *NCCN Clinical Practice Guidelines in Oncology™: Esophageal Cancer*, V.1, 2009, Accessed via http://www.nccn.org/professionals/physician_gls/f_guidelines.asp.

12　Orringer MB, Marshall B, Chang AC, *et al.* Two thousand transhiatal esophagectomies: changing trends, lessons learned. *Ann Surg* 2007; **246**: 363–72.

13　Griffin SM, Shaw IH, Dresner SM. Early complications after Ivor Lewis subtotal esophagectomy with two-field lymphadenectomy: risk factors and management. *J Am Coll Surg* 2002; **194**: 285–97.

14　Birkmeyer JD, Siewers AE, Finlayson EV, *et al.* Hospital volume and surgical mortality in the United States. *N Engl J Med* 2002; **346**: 1128–37.

15　Herskovic A, Martz K, al-Sarraf M, *et al.* Combined chemotherapy and radiotherapy compared with radiotherapy alone in patients with cancer of the esophagus. *N Engl J Med* 1992; **326**: 1593–8.

16　Cooper JS, Guo MD, Herskovic A, *et al.* Chemoradiotherapy of locally advanced esophageal cancer: long-term follow-up of a prospective randomized trial (RTOG 85-01). *JAMA* 1999; **281**: 1623–7.

17　Boyce HW Jr. Palliation of dysphagia of esophageal cancer by endoscopic lumen restoration techniques. *Cancer Control* 1999; **6**: 73.

18　Bethge N, Sommer A, Vakil N. A prospective trial of self-expanding metal stents in the palliation of malignant esophageal strictures near the upper esophageal sphincter. *Gastrointest Endosc* 1997; **45**: 300–3.

PART 6

Diseases of the Stomach

CHAPTER 43
Peptic Ulcer Disease

Vincent W.S. Wong and Francis K.L. Chan

Department of Medicine and Therapeutics, The Chinese University of Hong Kong, Shatin, NT, Hong Kong SAR, China

Summary

Unlike many chronic medical conditions, peptic ulcer disease is a potentially curable or avoidable condition because *Helicobacter pylori* infection and the use of non-steroidal anti-inflammatory drugs (NSAIDs) account for the vast majority of cases. The key to successful management rests on choosing appropriate *H. pylori* diagnostic tests according to specific clinical settings (e.g., avoid using urease tests in the presence of proton-pump inhibitor therapy), obtaining a careful drug history to identify NSAID exposure (e.g., over-the-counter NSAIDs), and assessing both gastrointestinal and cardiovascular risks of individual patients before prescribing NSAIDs. With declining prevalence of *H. pylori* infection, ulcers not associated with *H. pylori* or NSAID use are increasingly recognized. In patients presenting with peptic ulcer bleeding, endoscopic therapy is highly effective in achieving hemostasis. However, early rebleeding is common and causes significant morbidity and mortality. The use of a proton-pump inhibitor before and after endoscopic diagnosis of peptic ulcer bleeding has significantly improved clinical outcome but fails to reduce mortality.

Case

An 85-year-old female presented with weakness and an occasional episode of dizziness. She had noticed no other symptoms, but did report that her stools were darker than the past. Her medical history was significant for osteoarthritis and a possible TIA several years in the past. Medications included propranolol, daily 81-mg aspirin and 2–3 200-mg ibuprofen most days. On physical examination, she was pale and her pulse was 120 BPM. She had mild epigastric tenderness and her rectal exam showed dark, but not black stool that was heme positive on testing. Initial laboratory testing was significant for an Hgb of 7.8 with microcytic indices. A colonoscopy one year ago had been normal.

She was started on omeprazole 20 mg daily, was told to stop ibuprofen, and was transfused with two units of packed RBCs. The next day she was feeling much better and underwent an EGD. This demonstrated a normal esophagus and a 2.5-cm bland-appearing ulcer in the antrum. The duodenum was normal. Biopsy from the ulcer was benign, but showed moderate numbers of *Helicobacter pylori*

organisms. Her omeprazole was increased to twice daily, and she was given 10 days of amoxicillin and clarithromycin. At the conclusion of the 10 days, her omeprazole was decreased to once daily. A follow-up endoscopy 6 weeks later showed the ulcer to be healed and biopsies did not show *Helicobacter*. At one year she remained on daily omeprazole and had returned to the occasional use of ibuprofen without additional episodes of bleeding.

Background and Epidemiology

Peptic ulcer disease and its complications are leading causes of morbidity and mortality worldwide. It is the most common cause of acute upper gastrointestinal bleeding. The incidence of acute upper gastrointestinal bleeding ranges from 36 to 172 per 100 000 population. Despite major improvements in clinical care, the mortality rate after an episode of acute upper gastrointestinal bleeding remains high at 5 to 14% [1]. In contrast, due to advances in endoscopic treatment, operations for peptic ulcer complications have fallen by 80% in the last three decades.

Practical Gastroenterology and Hepatology: Esophagus and Stomach, 1st edition. Edited by Nicholas J. Talley, Kenneth R. DeVault and David E. Fleischer. © 2010 Blackwell Publishing Ltd.

Etiologies

The most common causes of peptic ulcer disease are *Helicobacter pylori* and the use of non-steroidal anti-inflammatory drugs, including low-dose aspirin. As the prevalence of *H. pylori* infection is declining, ulcers associated with the use of NSAIDs and low-dose aspirin have become increasingly important in the elderly. Interestingly, the incidence of ulcers not associated with *H. pylori* or NSAID use is also rising [2].

Helicobacter pylori

The discovery of *H. pylori* by Marshall and Warren revolutionized our understanding of upper gastrointestinal disorders. *H. pylori* infection is associated with gastritis, peptic ulcers, mucosa-associated lymphoid tissue lymphomas, and gastric cancer. The infection affects up to half of the world's population, and is more common in developing countries. The mode of transmission is believed to be fecal–oral or oral–oral and is usually acquired during childhood. *H. pylori* is present in saliva and on eating utensils, and the transmission is increased in population where mothers chew their infants' food and people share eating utensils [3].

One characteristic feature of *H. pylori* is its ability to produce the enzyme urease. The enzyme functions best at pH 7.2 and pH 3. By generating ammonia to buffer hydrogen ions, urease is essential for the colonization and survival of the bacteria. When *H. pylori* migrates to the gastric mucosa, bacterial products are translocated to the host epithelial cells, resulting in gastritis and tissue injury.

Aspirin and Non-steroidal Anti-inflammatory Drugs

Non-steroidal anti-inflammatory drugs (NSAIDs), including low-dose aspirin, are the most commonly used drugs worldwide. It has been estimated that about 70% of people aged 65 years or older use NSAIDs at least once a week. Around 40 to 50% of bleeding peptic ulcers are etiologically linked to aspirin or NSAIDs. The proportion is expected to rise in aging populations.

Topical injury was once thought to be an important mechanism of NSAID-induced gastric ulceration. Now there is good evidence that NSAIDs damage the stomach by suppressing gastric prostaglandin synthesis. The discovery of two isoforms of cyclo-oxygenase (COX-1 and COX-2) has led to the development of COX-2-selective NSAIDs as gastric-sparing anti-inflammatory analgesics. Current evidence indicates that COX-2-selective NSAIDs induce fewer ulcers than non-selective NSAIDs. In animal experiments, neutrophil adherence to the gastric microcirculation plays a critical role in initiating NSAID injury. Emerging evidence also indicates that the protective functions of prostaglandins in the stomach can be carried out by other gaseous mediators such as nitric oxide and hydrogen sulfide [4].

A history of peptic ulcer bleeding is the most important factor predicting recurrent ulcer complications associated with aspirin and NSAID use. Other risk factors include old age (>75), co-morbid illnesses, coexisting *H. pylori* infection, and concomitant use of aspirin, corticosteroids, or anticoagulants. Although corticosteroids and anticoagulants are not ulcerogenic themselves, they markedly increase the risk of gastrointestinal bleeding if used together with aspirin or NSAIDs [5].

Non-NSAID Non-*H. pylori* Idiopathic Ulcers

As the prevalence of *H. pylori* infection is declining, the proportion of ulcers not associated with *H. pylori* or NSAID use is increasing. Previously, it was thought that the relative proportion of idiopathic ulcers increased only as a consequence of the declining prevalence of *H. pylori*-related ulcers. Current evidence, however, indicates that there is a genuine rise in the absolute incidence of non-NSAID, non-*H. pylori* idiopathic ulcers [2]. The pathogenesis of idiopathic ulcer remains uncertain and but several studies suggested that this condition probably accounts for up to 20% of all peptic ulcer disease [2,6]. Compared to patients with *H. pylori*-related bleeding ulcers, those with non-NSAID, non-*H. pylori* idiopathic bleeding ulcers are older, suffer from more severe illnesses, and have a higher risk of recurrent ulcer bleeding [2].

Before making a diagnosis of idiopathic ulcers, however, one should scrutinize the patient's drug history carefully to exclude any surreptitious use of NSAIDs. In addition, recent use of acid suppressants or antibiotics and blood in the stomach are important causes of false-negative tests for *H. pylori*. A recent study showed that some patients with idiopathic ulcers actually had *H. pylori* detected in duodenal metaplasia [7]. Repeating diagnostic tests for *H. pylori*, including duodenal biopsy, is advisable. Finally, uncommon but well-recognized conditions such as Crohn disease, cytomegalovirus disease, and Zollinger–Ellison syndrome should also be considered.

Clinical Features

Patients with peptic ulcers often complain of dyspepsia. However, dyspepsia is a poor predictor of peptic ulcers because this non-specific symptom is common in other upper gastrointestinal conditions. On the other hand, up to 80% of patients receiving NSAIDs develop ulcer complications without any warning symptoms. Among patients with a history of ulcer who receive a COX-2 inhibitor or combination of a proton-pump inhibitor and a non-selective NSAID, it has been shown that those who develop breakthrough dyspepsia have a significantly higher likelihood of developing recurrent ulcers than their asymptomatic counterparts [8]. In patients presenting with upper gastrointestinal bleeding, fresh blood hematemesis, hypotension, anemia, and co-morbid illnesses are predictors of poor clinical outcome such as death. The presence of chronic liver stigmata, however, may indicate variceal bleeding. Chronic pyloric and duodenal ulcers may result in gastric outlet obstruction. Patients present with epigastric distension and repeated vomiting. On physical examination, epigastric distension and succussion splash may be found. Perforated peptic ulcer is a surgical emergency. Abdominal tenderness, rebound tenderness, guarding, and sluggish bowel sounds may be found. It is important to note that some perforated peptic ulcers may seal off spontaneously, and peritonism may not be apparent. If this possibility is not considered and endoscopy is arranged, unsealing of the perforation may occur.

Diagnosis

Peptic ulcer can be diagnosed by barium meal or esophagogastroduodenoscopy (EGD). All patients with peptic ulcer should be tested for *H. pylori* infection regardless of any history of NSAID use. It is important to biopsy gastric ulcers to exclude dysplasia or carcinoma, and follow-up endoscopy is necessary to confirm ulcer healing. In addition, physicians should obtain a detail

drug history to identify any recent use of prescription or over-the-counter NSAIDs. The diagnosis of *H. pylori* infection is described in Chapter 44. A note of caution is that both the rapid urease test and histology have low sensitivity during acute bleeding and in the presence of acid-suppressive therapy [9]. Thus, patients with bleeding peptic ulcers should be tested for *H. pylori* after the acute bleeding episode has subsided and at least one week after stopping acid-suppressive therapy. Alternatively, a serology test can be performed at the time of acute bleeding.

In patients with gastric outlet obstruction, a plain radiograph may show dilated gastric shadow with displaced transverse colon and small bowel loops. The stomach should be decompressed with a sump drain or nasogastric tube before endoscopy to reduce the risk of aspiration.

In patients suspected to have perforated peptic ulcer, a plain chest radiograph may show free gas under the diaphragm. If the plain film is non-diagnostic, a contrast computer tomography scan may show free peritoneal gas, fluid in the peritoneum, or inflammatory changes at the site of perforation.

Therapeutics

H. pylori Ulcers

There is good evidence from meta-analysis of randomized trials that eradication of *H. pylori* alone is sufficient to heal symptomatic and bleeding peptic ulcers such that additional acid-suppressive therapy is not required [10]. Therefore, the treatment of *H. pylori*-related peptic ulcer is to ensure successful eradication of the bacterium. This goal can be achieved in 80 to 90% of cases with 7- to 14-days of proton pump inhibitor (PPI)-based triple therapies.

In patients with duodenal ulcer, confirmation of *H. pylori* eradication by non-invasive methods (e.g., ^{13}C-urea breath test or *H. pylori* stool antigen test) is a validated surrogate marker for healing of duodenal ulcer. Eradication of *H. pylori* also effectively heals gastric ulcers. For patients with large (>1.5 cm) gastric ulcers, however, adding a PPI to *H. pylori* eradication therapy is recommended to promote ulcer healing. Unlike duodenal ulcers, gastric ulcer healing needs to be confirmed endoscopically because delayed healing is not uncommon in patients with large gastric ulcers and biopsy is mandatory to exclude malignancy.

In patients with *H. pylori*-related bleeding peptic ulcers, an additional course of PPI therapy is advisable to prevent early rebleeding although there are data showing that eradication of *H. pylori* alone is sufficient to heal bleeding peptic ulcers [11]. After ulcer healing and successful eradication of *H. pylori*, maintenance acid-suppressive therapy is not required because recurrent ulcer or ulcer bleeding is very uncommon [12] (refer to Chapter 44 for treatment of *H. pylori* infection).

NSAID Ulcers

Treatment of Active Ulcers

Patients should stop taking NSAIDs in the presence of active ulcers. If continuous NSAID therapy is required, standard doses of histamine-2 receptor antagonists (H₂RAs) effectively heal duodenal ulcers but not gastric ulcers. Current evidence indicates that PPI is superior to standard-dose H₂RA therapy and full-dose misoprostol in healing ulcers [13]. Since *H. pylori*-related ulcers cannot be differentiated from NSAID-induced ulcers and *H. pylori* infection is a risk factor for peptic ulcers associated with NSAID use, all patients should be tested for *H. pylori* and, if present, the infection should be eradicated. Data derived from *post hoc* subgroup analysis suggested that eradication of *H. pylori* might impair ulcer healing. This finding, however, was not confirmed by a prospective randomized trial [14].

Prevention of Ulcers

Aspirin- and NSAID-induced ulcer is an avoidable, iatrogenic condition. Before prescribing these drugs, physicians should review whether the benefits will outweigh their risks. Simple analgesics (e.g., acetaminophen) should be the first-line therapy for pain relief in degenerative arthritis. When NSAIDs are deemed necessary, one should use the least ulcerogenic NSAID at the lowest effective dose and for the shortest duration. Test-and-treat *H. pylori* infection before prescribing NSAIDs has been shown to reduce the risk of peptic ulcers [15]. All patients with a history of peptic ulcer should be tested for *H. pylori* infection.

Patients who require NSAIDs can be stratified according to their levels of gastrointestinal risk, namely, low risk (absence of risk factors), moderate risk (presence of one or two risk factors), and high risk (history of ulcer com-

plications, multiple risk factors, or concomitant use of corticosteroids or anticoagulant therapy). Low-risk patients should receive the least ulcerogenic NSAIDs (e.g. ibuprofen) at their lowest effective doses. Moderate-risk patients should receive prophylaxis with a PPI or misoprostol. There is evidence from randomized trials that a COX-2-selective NSAID alone is comparable to a nonselective NSAID plus a PPI in terms of the risk of ulcer bleeding [16]. High-risk patients should avoid taking NSAIDs if possible because neither a COX-2 inhibitor alone nor a non-selective NSAID plus a PPI can eliminate the ulcer risk [8]. Short-term corticosteroid therapy can be considered for acute, self-limiting arthritis (e.g., gout). If long-term NSAID therapy is required, the combination of a COX-2 selective NSAID and a PPI or misoprostol provides the best protection [17,18].

NSAID Users with High Cardiovascular Risk

Patients with a history of coronary artery disease or multiple cardiovascular risk factors should receive low-dose aspirin. Current evidence suggests that COX-2 selective NSAIDs and some non-selective NSAIDs such as diclofenac and ibuprofen increase the risk of myocardial infarction. In addition, concomitant use of ibuprofen and low-dose aspirin should be avoided because ibuprofen has been shown to attenuate the cardioprotective effect of aspirin. Meta-analyses of randomized trials [19] and observational studies [20] indicated that full-dose naproxen (500 mg twice daily) does not increase the risk of myocardial infarction and is the preferred NSAID in patients with increased cardiovascular risk. However, naproxen is very ulcerogenic and concomitant use of low-dose aspirin will markedly increase the risk of ulcer complications such that prophylaxis with a PPI or misoprostol is recommended (Table 43.1).

Antiplatelet Therapy in Patients with High Ulcer Risk

For many years, the American Heart Association and the American College of Cardiology have strongly recommended the use of clopidogrel in patients with major gastrointestinal intolerance to aspirin. This recommendation, however, was largely based on *post hoc* secondary analysis of safety data of clinical trials that were not designed to evaluate the gastrointestinal safety of clopidogrel [21]. In a double-blind, randomized comparison of clopidogrel with aspirin plus a PPI in patients with prior peptic ulcer bleeding, the recurrent ulcer bleeding

Table 43.1 Recommendations for the use of NSAIDs according to gastrointestinal and cardiovascular risk.

Cardiovascular risk	Gastrointestinal risk*		
	Low	Moderate	High
Low CV risk	NSAID	NSAID + PPI/misoprostol or COX-2 inhibitor	COX-2 inhibitor + PPI
High CV risk†	Naproxen + PPI/misoprostol	Naproxen + PPI/misoprostol	Avoid NSAIDs or COX-2 inhibitors

*Gastrointestinal risk is defined as low (no risk factors), moderate (presence one or two risk factors), or high (multiple risk factors, or previous ulcer complications, or concomitant use of corticosteroids or anticoagulants). All patients with a history of ulcers who require NSAIDs should be tested for *H. pylori* and, if the infection is present, eradication therapy should be given.
†High cardiovascular risk (CV) risk is defined as the requirement for low-dose aspirin for prevention of myocardial infarction.
NSAID, non-steroidal anti-inflammatory drug; PPI, proton pump inhibitor; COX, cyclo-oxygenase.

rate in 1 year was significantly lower in the aspirin plus a PPI group (0.7%) than in the clopidogrel group (8.6%) [22]. In an updated expert consensus report, aspirin plus a PPI is recommended in patients requiring antiplatelet therapy with high gastrointestinal risk [23]. However, recent observational data suggest that PPI cotherapy may increase the risk of recurrent myocardial infarction in patients receiving clopidogrel [24,25].

Non-NSAID Non-*H. pylori* Idiopathic Ulcers

The optimal management of patients with non-NSAID non-*H. pylori* ulcers remain uncertain since the pathogenesis and natural history of this condition is poorly understood. One should caution not to over-diagnose this condition due to false-negative *H. pylori* test or failure of obtaining a detail drug history. There is evidence that the risk of recurrent ulcer bleeding is high among patients with a history of non-NSAID non-*H. pylori* ulcer bleeding [2]. Long-term prophylaxis with a PPI is therefore advisable.

Peptic Ulcer Bleeding

Peptic ulcer bleeding is a serious complication of peptic ulcers. Advances in endoscopic and pharmacological treatment have improved the outcomes of peptic ulcer bleeding. Surgical treatment for peptic ulcer bleeding is rarely performed nowadays. Despite interobserver variability, the Forrest classification is still commonly used to predict the risk of recurrent bleeding based on the presence of stigmata of recent hemorrhage (Table 43.2). A number of risk-stratification schemes are also available to aid clinicians determine the prognosis and the risk of

Table 43.2 Forrest classification of peptic ulcers.

Forrest class	Description	Risk of rebleeding if untreated (%)
IA	Arterial spurting	100
IB	Arterial oozing	55
IIA	Non-bleeding visible vessel	43
IIB	Adherent blood clot	22
IIC	Pigmented spot	10
III	Clean base	5

rebleeding, such as the Rockall score and the Glasgow–Blatchford bleeding score (GBS). Recently, a prospective cohort study compared the GBS score with the Rockall score in patients admitting to general hospitals with upper gastrointestinal bleeding [26]. It was found that the GBS score was superior to the Rockall score for prediction of need for intervention or death. In addition, patients who were classified as low risk (GBS score of 0) were managed safely as outpatients without adverse events [26].

Endoscopic Hemostasis

Endoscopic hemostasis can be achieved by injection therapy, thermal devices, and mechanical devices. Diluted epinephrine (1:10000) injection around bleeding ulcers is commonly performed because of its efficacy and simplicity of use. Thermal device such as a heater probe is another commonly used method for hemostasis. It works by compressing the walls of the bleeding vessel together and sealing it off by thermal energy—a condition called coaptive coagulation. The success of heater probe treatment requires the application of firm pressure over the bleeding point. This can be technically demanding in difficult locations such as the posterior duodenal wall. Hemoclip is a mechanical device that controls bleeding by obliterating the feeding vessel. The deployment can be difficult if the ulcer base is fibrotic or if the location of ulcer only allows tangential application.

A meta-analysis of randomized trials indicates that dual endoscopic therapy (epinephrine injection plus a thermal or mechanical device) reduces early rebleeding and the need for surgical intervention compared to epinephrine injection alone. In contrast, dual endoscopic therapy has not been shown to be superior to monotherapy using a thermal or mechanical device. Although epinephrine injection alone is inferior to other mono- or dual-therapies, none of the endoscopic hemostatic strategies can improve survival when compared to epinephrine injection alone [27].

Acid-suppressive Therapy

Platelets function optimally at neutral pH. This explains why acute upper gastrointestinal bleeding can be torrential and lethal. Potent suppression of gastric acid leads to clot stabilization and is expected to reduce the risk of bleeding. Systematic review of randomized trials has shown that both oral and intravenous PPI initiated after endoscopic diagnosis of peptic ulcer bleeding reduces the risk of rebleeding and surgical requirement but fails to reduce mortality [28]. The optimal dose and route of administration of adjuvant PPI therapy remains controversial. To date, the use of intravenous high-dose PPI (e.g., 80 mg of omeprazole bolus injection followed by 8 mg/h infusion for 72 h) after endoscopic hemostatic therapy is the most studied and best proven strategy.

Should PPI therapy be initiated before endoscopy in patients presenting with hematemesis or melena? In a double-blind randomized trial of high-dose PPI infusion before endoscopy the next morning, patients receiving pre-emptive PPI required significantly less endoscopic treatment than in the placebo group [29]. A systematic review found that both oral and intravenous PPI given before endoscopy reduce the need for endoscopic therapy when compared to placebo or H$_2$RAs [30]. It follows that pre-emptive PPI is particularly useful in hospitals where 24-h emergency endoscopy is not readily available. However, clinicians should not have the misconception that pre-emptive PPI can substitute timely endoscopic

treatment because the former does not reduce rebleeding, surgical requirement, and mortality [30].

Rebleeding

Close monitoring is required after endoscopic therapy for peptic ulcer bleeding. Repeating endoscopy and surgery are both effective in controlling recurrent ulcer bleeding. The mortality does not differ using either approach [31]. Endoscopy results in less complications, but is more likely to fail if the patient develops hypotension during rebleeding or the ulcer is more than 2 cm in size. Scheduled second-look endoscopy after initial hemostasis may reduce the risk of rebleeding, but has no effect on the duration of hospitalization or mortality [32]. Emerging evidence suggests that angiographic embolization is also effective in managing refractory bleeding [33]. Figure 43.1 shows an algorithm for the management of peptic ulcer bleeding.

Take-home points

- *Helicobacter pylori* infection and the use of non-steroidal anti-inflammatory drugs (NSAIDs), including low-dose aspirin, are the two most common causes of peptic ulcer disease.

- Eradication of *H. pylori* infection alone heals peptic ulcer and prevents ulcer relapse.

- NSAID-induced ulcer complications are potentially avoidable. Risk factors include history of ulcer, old age, the use of high-dose or multiple NSAIDs, concomitant use of aspirin, anticoagulants, or corticosteroids, and *H. pylori* infection.

- Combination of a non-selective NSAID and a gastroprotective agent (proton-pump inhibitor or misoprostol) or substitution for a cyclo-oxygenase (COX)-2 selective NSAID reduces the risk of ulcer complications.

- COX-2 selective and some non-selective NSAIDs increase the risk of myocardial infarction.

- Physicians should assess patients' gastrointestinal (GI) and cardiovascular (CV) risk before prescribing NSAIDs. Patients with low CV risk can be managed according to the number and type of GI risk factors. Naproxen is preferred in patients with high cardiovascular risk.

- Patients with high GI risk who require aspirin should receive PPI prophylaxis.

- Clopidogrel is not an alternative to aspirin in patients with high GI risk.

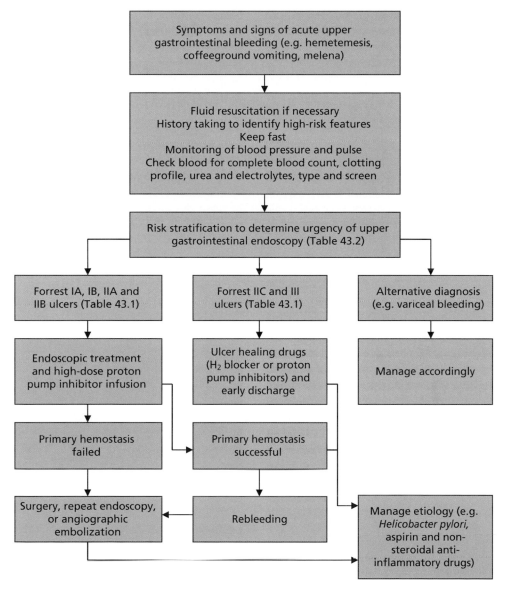

Figure 43.1 Management of peptic ulcer bleeding.

- Endoscopic therapy using epinephrine injection plus a thermal or mechanical device is superior to epinephrine injection alone reduces early rebleeding and surgical requirement.
- Infusion of high-dose proton pump inhibitor after endoscopy for bleeding peptic ulcers reduces early rebleeding, transfusion, requirement of surgery, and the duration of hospital stay but has no effect on mortality.

References

1 Rockall TA, Logan RF, Devlin HB, *et al.* Incidence of and mortality from acute upper gastrointestinal haemorrhage in the United Kingdom. Steering committee and members of the National Audit of Acute Upper Gastrointestinal Haemorrhage. *BMJ* 1995; **311**: 222–6.

2 Hung LC, Ching JY, Sung JJ, *et al.* Long-term outcome of

Helicobacter pylori-negative idiopathic bleeding ulcers: a prospective cohort study. *Gastroenterology* 2005; **128**: 1845–50.

3 Covacci A, Telford JL, Del Giudice G, *et al. Helicobacter pylori* virulence and genetic geography. *Science* 1998; **284**: 1328–33.

4 Wallace JL. Prostaglandins, NSAIDs, and gastric mucosal protection: why doesn't the stomach digest itself? *Physiol Rev* 2008; **88**: 1547–65.

5 Chan FK. Primer: managing NSAID-induced ulcer complications—balancing gastrointestinal and cardiovascular risks. *Nat Clin Pract Gastroenterol Hepatol* 2006; **3**: 563–73.

6 Laine L, Hopkins RJ, Girardi LS. Has the impact of *Helicobacter pylori* therapy on ulcer recurrence in the United States been overstated? A meta-analysis of rigorously designed trials. *Am J Gastroenterol* 1998; **93**: 1409–15.

7 Pietroiusti A, Forlini A, Magrini A, *et al.* Isolated *H. pylori* duodenal colonization and idiopathic duodenal ulcers. *Am J Gastroenterol* 2008; **103**: 55–61.

8 Chan FK, Hung LC, Suen BY, *et al.* Celecoxib versus diclofenac plus omeprazole in high-risk arthritis patients: results of a randomized double-blind trial. *Gastroenterology* 2004; **127**: 1038–43.

9 Gisbert JP, Abraira V. Accuracy of *Helicobacter pylori* diagnostic tests in patients with bleeding peptic ulcer: a systematic review and meta-analysis. *Am J Gastroenterol* 2006; **101**: 848–63.

10 Ford AC, Delaney BC, Forman D, Moayyedi P. Eradication therapy in *Helicobacter pylori* positive peptic ulcer disease: Systematic review and economic analysis. *Am J Gastroenterol* 2004; **99**: 1833–55.

11 Sung JJ, Leung WK, Suen R, *et al.* One-week antibiotics versus maintenance acid suppression therapy for Helicobacter pylori-associated peptic ulcer bleeding. *Dig Dis Sci* 1997; **42**: 2524–8.

12 Gisbert JP, Calvet X, Feu F, *et al.* Eradication of *Helicobacter pylori* for the prevention of peptic ulcer rebleeding. *Helicobacter* 2007; **12**: 279–86.

13 Hawkey CJ, Karrasch JA, Szezepanski L, *et al.* Omeprazole compared with misoprostol for ulcers associated with nonsteroidal antiinflammatory drugs: Omeprazole versus Misoprostol for NSAID-induced Ulcer Management (OMNIUM) Study Group. *N Engl J Med* 1998; **338**: 727–34.

14 Chan FK, Sung JJ, Suen R, *et al.* Does eradication of *Helicobacter pylori* impair healing of nonsteroidal anti-inflammatory drug associated bleeding peptic ulcers? A prospective randomized study. *Aliment Pharmacol Ther* 1998; **12**: 1201–5.

15 Chan FK, To KF, Wu JC, *et al.* Eradication of *Helicobacter pylori* and risk of peptic ulcers in patients starting long-term treatment with non-steroidal anti-inflammatory drugs: a randomised trial. *Lancet* 2002; **359**: 9–13.

16 Chan FK, Hung LC, Suen BY, *et al.* Celecoxib versus diclofenac and omeprazole in reducing the risk of recurrent ulcer bleeding in patients with arthritis. *N Engl J Med* 2002; **347**: 2104–10.

17 Chan FK, Wong VW, Suen BY, *et al.* Combination of cyclo-oxygenase-2 inhibitor and a proton-pump inhibitor for prevention of recurrent ulcer bleeding in patients at very high risk: a double-blind, randomised trial. *Lancet* 2007; **369**: 1621–6.

18 Targownik LE, Metge CJ, Leung S, Chateau DG. The relative efficacies of gastroprotective strategies in chronic users of nonsteroidal anti-inflammatory drugs. *Gastroenterology* 2008; **134**: 937–44.

19 Kearney PM, Baigent C, Godwin J, *et al.* Do selective cyclo-oxygenase-2 inhibitors and nonselective non-steroidal anti-inflammatory drugs increase the risk of atherothrombosis? Meta-analysis of randomised trials. *BMJ* 2006; **332**: 1302–8.

20 McGettigan P, Henry D. Cardiovascular risk and inhibition of cyclooxygenase: a systematic review of the observational studies of selective and nonselective inhibitors of cyclooxygenase 2. *JAMA* 2006; **296**: 1633–44.

21 Braunwald E, Antman EM, Beasley JW, *et al.* ACC/AHA guideline update for the management of patients with unstable angina and non-ST-segment elevation myocardial infarction–2002: summary article: a report of the American College of Cardiology/American Heart Association Task Force on Practice Guidelines (Committee on the Management of Patients with Unstable Angina). *Circulation* 2002; **106**: 1893–900.

22 Chan FK, Ching JY, Hung LC, *et al.* Clopidogrel versus aspirin and esomeprazole to prevent recurrent ulcer bleeding. *N Engl J Med* 2005; **352**: 238–44.

23 Bhatt DL, Scheiman J, Abraham NS, *et al*; American College of Cardiology Foundation Task Force on Clinical Expert Consensus Documents. ACCF/ACG/AHA 2008 expert consensus document on reducing the gastrointestinal risks of antiplatelet therapy and NSAID use: a report of the American College of Cardiology Foundation Task Force on Clinical Expert Consensus Documents. *Circulation* 2008; **118**: 1894–909.

24 Juurlink DN, Gomes T, Ko DT, *et al.* A population-based study of the drug interaction between proton-pump inhibitors and clopidogrel. *CMAJ* 2009; **180**: 713–8.

25 Ho PM, Maddox TM, Wang L, *et al.* Risk of adverse outcomes associated with concomitant use of clopidogrel and proton-pump inhibitors following acute coronary syndrome. *JAMA* 2009; **301**: 937–44.

26 Stanley AJ, Ashley D, Dalton HR, *et al.* Outpatient manage-

ment of patients with low-risk upper-gastrointestinal haemorrhage: multicentre validation and prospective evaluation. *Lancet* 2009; **373**: 42–7.

27 Marmo R, Rotondano G, Piscopo R, *et al.* Dual therapy versus monotherapy in the endoscopic treatment of high-risk bleeding ulcers: a meta-analysis of controlled trials. *Am J Gastroenterol* 2007; **102**: 279–89.

28 Leontiadis GI, Sreedharan A, Dorward S, *et al.* Systematic reviews of the clinical effectiveness and cost-effectiveness of proton pump inhibitors in acute upper gastrointestinal bleeding. *Health Technol Assess* 2007; **11**: 1–164.

29 Lau JY, Leung WK, Wu JC, *et al.* Omeprazole before endoscopy in patients with gastrointestinal bleeding. *N Engl J Med* 2007; **356**: 1631–40.

30 Dorward S, Sreedharan A, Leontiadis GI, *et al.* Proton pump inhibitor treatment initiated prior to endoscopic diagnosis in upper gastrointestinal bleeding. *Cochrane Database Syst Rev* 2006; **4**: CD005415.

31 Lau JY, Sung JJ, Lam YH, *et al.* Endoscopic retreatment compared with surgery in patients with recurrent bleeding after initial endoscopic control of bleeding ulcers. *N Engl J Med* 1999; **340**: 751–6.

32 Marmo R, Rotondano G, Bianco MA, *et al.* Outcome of endoscopic treatment for peptic ulcer bleeding: Is a second look necessary? A meta-analysis. *Gastrointest Endosc* 2003; **57**: 62–7.

33 Cheung FK, Lau JY. Management of massive peptic ulcer bleeding. *Gastrointest Clin North Am* 2009; **38**: 231–43.

CHAPTER 44
Helicobacter pylori

Barry J. Marshall, Helen M. Windsor, and Kazufumi Kimura

School of Biomedical, Biomolecular and Chemical Sciences, University of Western Australia, Perth, WA, Australia

Summary

Helicobacter pylori infection of the stomach is the most important cause of peptic ulcer disease. Half the world's population is infected by *H. pylori* including about 25% of those in developed countries and the majority in developing countries. It is probably transmitted by via dirty water and saliva, acquired in early childhood and is permanent unless specifically treated. Decades after the acute *H. pylori* infection, 20% develop peptic ulcer disease. The remainder are asymptomatic but carry a 1–5% risk of stomach cancer in later life.

Diagnosis is via serology, urea breath test, and fecal antigen test; or urease test, histology, and culture of gastric biopsies. Therapy cures 85% using an acid pump blocker concurrently with two antibiotics for 7–10 days. Cure of peptic ulcer, remission of lymphoma, and decreased cancer risk follow the bacteriologic cure. Reinfection is uncommon.

Case

A 38-year-old female patient presents with upper abdominal discomfort. This symptom has been present for the past 2 years. It is made worse with meals, particularly large and fatty meals. She has no real heartburn, dysphagia, or other esophageal symptoms. There is some nausea, no vomiting, and she has gained 5 kg over the past year. Her bowel movements are normal. There are no fever, chills, or other associated symptoms. Her internist ordered an upper abdominal ultrasound and upper GI X-ray, both of which were normal. On further questioning, she is somewhat concerned since her father (in her home country of Paraguay) died of gastric cancer and she has heard that those problems tend to run in families. Her physical exam and general screening laboratories were both normal.

Bacteriology

Helicobacter pylori is a Gram-negative, spiral-shaped organism measuring approximately 0.5 μm in diameter and 3 to 5 μm in length. It has two to six polar sheathed

Practical Gastroenterology and Hepatology: Esophagus and Stomach, 1st edition. Edited by Nicholas J. Talley, Kenneth R. DeVault and David E. Fleischer. © 2010 Blackwell Publishing Ltd.

flagella which allow the bacterium to move in the viscous environment of the gastric mucus.

Prior to the first isolation and characterization of this organism in 1982 [1], it was assumed that the human stomach was sterile because bacteria are usually killed by acid at pH below 3.0. A new genus, *Helicobacter*, was created and since then at least 30 new species have been added, mainly isolated from the stomach and gastrointestinal tracts of mammals.

The genome of *H. pylori* was sequenced in 1997 [2]. It has a single circular chromosome of 1.7 Mb with 1500 genes of which only 1000 are present in all strains. The small size of the *H. pylori* genome confirmed that it has fewer regulatory genes than other bacteria, supporting the hypothesis that *H. pylori* lives only in the human stomach as it does not possess enzymatic pathways to survive in other environments.

H. pylori is nutritionally fastidious and can be cultivated in the laboratory from gastric biopsies on agar plates which contain blood or serum, under microaerobic conditions or in the presence of air enriched with 10% CO_2. Optimum growth is obtained at 37°C after 4–5 days for primary culture or 2 days for subsequent subculture. The growth of small translucent, water droplet-like colonies which are urease, catalase, and oxidase positive and which show the characteristic spiral morphology is usually adequate for the identification of *H. pylori*. Large amounts of urease are produced, which is used to break down urea to ammonia and bicarbonate allowing the organism to survive in acid. Diagnosis by culture is usually reserved for cases where bacterial susceptibility data is required or for research studies.

Epidemiology and Transmission

H. pylori infects more than half the people on earth, especially those in developing countries where the majority of population may be infected. In Western countries and in countries emerging from a developing to a Western economy, the prevalence of *H. pylori* in the community is decreasing due to improved standards of hygiene, smaller families, and awareness of the infection. In the United States for example, *Helicobacter* infected about 60% of the population in 1965 but currently infects only about 30% of the population, immigrants being infected proportional to the prevalence rate in their home country [3,4].

The transmission of *H. pylori* is not totally understood because it can rarely be cultured from environmental samples. It has occasionally been cultured from feces, saliva and dental plaque but, for the most part, lives only in the stomach. Thus saliva transfer is thought to be a likely means of transmission, particularly between mother and child. In support of this, *H. pylori* does seem to run in families and children are more likely to have exactly the same strain as their mother. The major mode of transmission of *H. pylori* in developing countries is probably via contaminated water [5].

Emphasizing the possible transmission of *H. pylori* via feces or gastric secretions are papers showing that medical staff, nursing staff, and, especially, gastroenterologists are likely to be infected by *H. pylori*. Similarly, persons who experienced a vomiting illness were likely to spread the infection within their family [6].

In Table 44.1 the approximate percentages of *H. pylori* infection in the general population are shown throughout the world. These change over time and in Figure 44.1 the example of *H. pylori* age-related prevalence is shown in a developing country (e.g., The Gambia in Africa) versus a developed country (e.g., Japan).

Reinfection after treatment is uncommon in Western countries (1–2%) but common in countries with a high prevalence. Our poor understanding of the transmission of *H. pylori* is reflected in data such as those from Malaysia, an emerging economy, where the reinfection rate is only about 2%, even though the prevalence is high and varies greatly between different racial groups [7].

Pathogenesis and Disease Associations

Upon entering the stomach *H. pylori* colonizes the mucus layer above the secreting gastric epithelial cells. Adherent

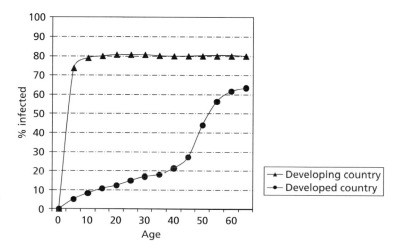

Figure 44.1 Epidemiology of *H. pylori*. In a developed country such as Japan elderly people have a high prevalence of infection, reflecting the conditions during their childhood, whereas those born after 1970 have a much lower prevalence. The continuing spread of *H. pylori* can usually be inferred by looking at the prevalence rate in young children. In developing countries, most children are infected by the age of 10 years. As soon as transmission is controlled, young children will be found not to be infected.

Table 44.1 Prevalence of *H. pylori* in different countries.

Country	Prevalence (%)	Date	Age range	Sample size	Diagnostic test	Reference
Australia	15.1	2002	1–59	2413	Serology	[20]
Bangladesh	60	2009	0–2	238	Stool antigen	[21]
Canada	23	2007	50–80	1306	Serology	[22]
China	62.5	1993	all	830	Serology	[23]
	49.3	2003	3–92	1471		
Czech Republic	41.6	2008	5–100	2509	UBT	[24]
Germany	49	2007	50–74	9444	Serology	[25]
Estonia	69	2007	25–50	240	Serology	[26]
Iceland	36	2007	25–50	447		
Sweden	11	2007	25–50	359		
India	80	2007	30–79	500	Biopsy	[5]
Japan	3.7	2007	2	108	Stool antigen	[27]
Japan	70	2008	40–60	5209	Serology	[28]
Netherlands	1.2	2007	2–4	1258	Serology	[29]
Russia	44	1995	2–19	307	Serology	[30]
	13	2005	2–19	370		
South America (rural)	91	2002	<14	201	Serology	[31]
Taiwan	11.2	2007	9–15	1950	Serology	[32]
	45.1	2007	> 25	253		

H. pylori organisms can inject toxin, called cag A, into the epithelial cells which release interleukin 8 thus attracting polymorphonuclear leukocytes and components of the innate immune system. This acute inflammatory reaction produces interleukin 1B, which serves to inhibit acid secretion. Thus, in the first few days of the acute infection, acid secretion falls to near zero and the syndrome of "acute gastritis with hypochlorhydria" develops, probably as a mild illness which is largely unnoticed in young children. This status of low acidity may continue for months, years, or possibly even a lifetime in some people. Subsequently, acute inflammation settles and chronic inflammation sets in. IgM, then IgG and IgA antibodies develop as *H. pylori* colonization reaches a stable form. In this mid stage, lasting most of the lifetime of the person, acid secretion returns but there may be no symptoms.

In some people, gastritis impairs normal secretion of somatostatin thereby permitting increased secretion of gastrin [8]. People with duodenal ulcer thus tend to have a raised fasting basal acid secretion. After decades of infection, the chronic inflammation can lead to intestinal metaplasia in the gastric mucosa with atrophy of the acid-secreting tissue and the return of a low-acid state.

When *Helicobacter* is eradicated, the inflammation largely resolves and a mild infiltrate of lymphocytes and plasma cells remain. Intestinal metaplasia does not resolve and the presence of associated atrophy marks a continuing cancer risk even after the eradication of *H. pylori*. This cancer risk probably declines over 5 years.

Duodenal and Gastric Ulcers

In duodenal ulcer, the *H. pylori* infection causes chronic gastritis of the antrum but acid secretion is normal or high because the upper 75% of the stomach is mostly spared. Duodenal ulcers are associated with infected islands of gastric metaplasia (a normal anatomical variant) in the duodenal bulb. Duodenal ulcers and gastric ulcers form a continuum through the pylorus. Duodenal ulcers are not associated with gastric cancer whereas gastric ulcers do carry a risk of malignancy and therefore should be biopsied. In duodenal ulcer the gastric mucosa returns to near normality after the *Helicobacter* has been eradicated. After *H. pylori* eradication, 80–90% of patients may experience a total ulcer cure. Gastric ulcers are more likely to be associated with non-steroidal anti-inflammatory drugs (NSAIDs) than duodenal ulcers. In Western countries, the *H. pylori* contribution to peptic ulcer has decreased because of widespread treatment and lower prevalence. As a result, NSAIDs now account for about 50% of "peptic ulcers."

Gastric MALT Lymphoma

Lymphoma of the mucosa-associated lymphoid tissue (MALT) is the most common lymphoma of the gastrointestinal tract. This indolent B-cell gastric tumor is strongly associated with *H. pylori*; 75% of people undergo clinical remission of the disease when *H. pylori* is eradicated [9]. Those with undifferentiated MALT lymphoma of the stomach or associated MALT lymphoma outside the stomach are not cured, although occasional exceptions occur so the bacterium should always be eliminated. Histological studies of patients in clinical remission still reveal a clonal population of lymphocytes in the gastric epithelium. Thus, follow-up to prove continuing absence of *H. pylori* (with a combination of tests such a urea breath test plus serology) is essential for their long-term care.

Gastric cancer is associated with chronic gastritis. In Japan, where gastric cancer was, until recently, the most common malignancy, almost everyone with gastric cancer has evidence of current or past *H. pylori* infection, evidenced by specific antibodies, atrophy of the gastric acid secreting glands, and intestinal metaplasia. The chronic inflammation may attract circulating bone marrow stem cells which then colonize the damaged gastric glands and are susceptible to malignant change leading to adenocarcinoma [10]. Some countries with a high prevalence of *H. pylori* do not have a correspondingly high incidence of gastric cancer (e.g., Thailand, the Middle East) [11]. Bacterial factors (cagA toxin activity) but also dietary (high salt diet) and cultural factors may also affect cancer risk.

Persons with intestinal metaplasia and widespread gastric atrophy carry a cancer risk which continues after eradication of *H. pylori* but possibly reduces in time [12]. In persons who do not have these changes in the gastric mucosa, eradication of *H. pylori* negates the risk of gastric cancer.

Other Conditions Associated with *H. pylori*

Numerous other conditions have been associated with *H. pylori* infections. Many of these are rare and anecdotal but still warrant brief mention.

The syndrome of non-ulcer dyspepsia refers to the presence of epigastric discomfort, hyperacidity, belching, bloated feelings, distension, etc., which occurs in the absence of peptic ulcer disease. In prospective double-blind studies where *H. pylori* has been eradicated, complete symptomatic cures have been noted in about 15% of persons and a similar percentage have been markedly improved [13].

Iron deficiency associated with *H. pylori* infection is presumably from slight chronic gastric mucosal iron loss. In prospective studies in Japan, iron levels increased after eradication of *H. pylori*. The effect of treatment is small but in a population with low iron intake, some persons probably do develop iron deficiency anemia related to *H. pylori*. Therefore, in all persons with iron deficiency anemia, who do not have a serious source identified, eradication of *H. pylori* is justified.

Atherosclerotic cardiovascular disease has been reported to be more common in persons with *H. pylori* infection. In Italy, persons who had suffered recent myocardial infarction were more likely to be infected with *H. pylori* and were also more likely to have the antibody towards *H. pylori* cytotoxin (cagA) in their serum. In case-controlled studies this association was not noticed. So far, there is no good evidence that antibiotic treatment for *H. pylori* protects against cardiovascular disease. Interestingly however, persons with elevated C-reactive protein are more likely to suffer from cardiovascular disease and it is known *Helicobacter* infection does cause elevation of C-reactive protein [14].

Idiopathic thrombocytopenic purpura (ITP) has been reported to be associated with *H. pylori*. Since other treatments for ITP are hazardous, a course of antibiotics to eradicate *H. pylori* is an excellent first choice with a cure rate of 30–59% in some studies. Therefore, always test and treat *H. pylori* in patients with ITP [15].

Some of the other recorded associations with *H. pylori* are listed in Table 44.2. These are collections of anecdotal cases not validated by prospective trials. It is possible that

Table 44.2 Non-gastric conditions associated with *H. pylori*.

Studies/reports	Diseases	
Substantial evidence from several studies	Iron deficiency	Proven association; possible clinical relevance when nutrition poor [33]
	Idiopathic thrombocytopenic purpura (ITP)	Several reports but prospective data are weak [33]
	Atherosclerotic heart disease	Correlation between *H. pylori* infection and atherosclerosis and cerebral infarction reported [33]
	Chronic urticaria	Systematic review concluded that bacterial eradication correlated with remission [34]
Several anecdotal reports and small clinical series	Hepatic encephalopathy (HE) in cirrhotic patients	HE was more frequently observed in patients with *H. pylori* infection than those without [35]
	Bronchiectasis	High incidence of *H. pylori* seropositivity was reported in the patients [36]
	Alzheimer disease	Correlation was reported [33]
	Guillain–Barré syndrome	High *H. pylori* prevalence was reported among the patients [33]
Isolated anecdotal reports	Ocular rosacea	Improvement after eradication was reported [37]
	Blepharitis	High *H. pylori* prevalence was reported among the patients [38]
	Type B insulin resistant diabetes mellitus	A case report [39]
	Acute anterior uveitis and spondyloarthropathies	Relationship with these diseases was reported [40]

uncommon disease associations vary by strain of *H. pylori* and by country.

Diagnosis

Accurate diagnosis of *H. pylori* is essential for good treatment compliance from the patient and enthusiastic participation by the physician. Diagnostic tests can be characterized as non-invasive versus invasive and also as tests for active disease versus past disease. Serology for specific IgG antibodies against *H. pylori* is highly sensitive so that *H. pylori* infection can be virtually excluded if the test is negative. The IgG level may stay in the positive range for years after eradication of *H. pylori*.

The urea breath test (UBT) is based on the ability of *H. pylori* to secrete a large amount of urease enzyme, which splits urea into CO_2 and ammonia. Therefore by giving the patient a small dose of urea labeled with ^{13}C or ^{14}C, the patient with *H. pylori* will breathe out the labeled CO_2. Breath tests are highly specific and can be used for initial diagnosis of *H. pylori* in a similar role to serology. However, they are essential for non-invasive follow-up testing of *H. pylori* since they test for the actual live *H. pylori* organisms in the gastric mucosa. Since antibiotic treatment only cures 85% of people, 15% of persons will have a positive UBT when re-tested 4 weeks after antibiotic treatment. During breath testing it is important that the patient not be taking any medications that inhibit *H. pylori*. Acid pump blockers should be ceased for 7 days before performing the UBT. An alternative test for active disease is the *Helicobacter* fecal antigen test. Organisms shed from the stomach are passed into the intestine and appear in the feces. This test is particularly useful in pediatric patients who may not be able to perform a breath test [16].

At endoscopy, accurate diagnosis of *H. pylori* is made by studying biopsy samples of the gastric mucosa (Figure 44.2). These tests may be negative when the patient is taking an inhibitory compound in the days before endoscopy. In persons with active *H. pylori* disease at least two biopsies should be taken from opposite sides of the gastric antrum for histology and examined with hematoxylin and eosin stain and either a Giemsa, toluidine blue, or silver stain for *H. pylori* organisms. Immunohistochemical stains can be used to prove the organisms are *H. pylori*. *H. pylori* are usually less abundant in the corpus but corpus biopsies are useful to see the extent of the gastritis and the state of the parietal cells.

A useful addition to diagnosis is the rapid urease test. An antral biopsy is taken from the prepyloric lesser curve and placed into a medium that contains urea. In the

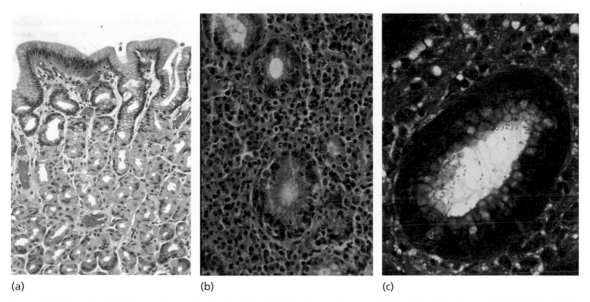

(a)   (b)   (c)

Figure 44.2 Example of histology sections stained with different stains: (a) normal mucosa (II&E ×100), (b) active gastritis (H&E stain ×250); (c) numerous bacilli (toluidine blue stain ×500).

presence of *H. pylori* the urea is split into CO_2 and ammonia which raises the pH whereby an indicator dye gives a color change in about 10 min. This allows the gastroenterologist to make a diagnosis in the endoscopy room.

Gastric biopsies may also be cultured in order to determine the antibiotic sensitivities of the organism. This information is worthwhile in patients who have failed previous therapies. *H. pylori* are almost universally sensitive to penicillin and tetracycline and most strains are initially sensitive to clarithromycin and metronidazole but after being exposed to these latter two drugs the organism usually becomes resistant. Antibiotic resistance develops in *H. pylori* because of its high spontaneous mutation rate.

Treatment

There are three groups of medication that are used in a successful *H. pylori* eradication therapy. These are:
1 Drugs that can be used repeatedly as *H. pylori* remains susceptible
2 Drugs that can only be used once as *H. pylori* becomes resistant

3 Drugs that decrease acid secretion and assist antibiotic action.

The drugs that can be used over and over again are amoxicillin, tetracycline, and bismuth ("Pepto-Bismol"— bismuth subsalicylate in USA or bismuth subcitrate, elsewhere). These are usually given in a 7 to 14-day course, which leads to widespread suppression of the organism but given alone they only rarely cure the infection. Therefore, a second antibiotic drug is given concurrently. In this group are metronidazole, clarithromycin, the quinolones, and the rifamycins such as rifabutin. These drugs must always be given with a suppressive agent from the first group. If treatment needs to be repeated, a different drug from this group should be used.

Finally, in order for antibiotics to work effectively in the gastric mucosa, acid secretion must be completely eliminated. This is done with high-dose proton pump inhibitors (PPI).

The most widely used therapy in the United States is a 10-day course of a PPI twice daily, amoxicillin 1 g twice daily and clarithromycin 500 mg twice daily. In Australia and Europe this "triple therapy" treatment is only given for 7 days.

Quadruple therapy comprises bismuth, a PPI, metronidazole, and tetracycline for 14 days and is equivalent to triple therapy. A capsule containing bismuth subcitrate (140 mg), metronidazole (125 mg), and tetracycline (125 mg) is available and FDA approved. The dosing is three capsules four times daily plus a PPI twice daily.

Recently the concept of "sequential therapy" has been promoted because it gives an improved cure rate with decreased side effects. Typical therapy consists of a total 10-day treatment of high-dose PPI with amoxicillin added in the first 5 days then changing this to both clarithromycin and metronidazole for the second 5 days. A cure rate of 89% is expected with this therapy [17]. Simplified treatment packs of sequential therapy are presently unavailable so they are less convenient to prescribe.

In practice, patients are given the standard 7-day treatment with PPI, amoxicillin, and clarithromycin. If UBT results show that the treatment has failed, the patient undergoes a second treatment with a higher dose of PPI, a higher dose of amoxicillin, plus a quinolone and rifabutin. The authors use PPI and amoxicillin for the full 10 days and give the added quinolone (ciprofloxacin) plus rifabutin in the last 5 days of the course. For patients who are allergic to penicillin, replace amoxicillin with bismuth. If this treatment fails, furazolidone can be added but it is less well tolerated. Once a patient fails two attempts at eradication they should be referred to a physician experienced in this type of management.

Controversies in Management

Who to Diagnose and Who to Treat

Anyone with persistent epigastric discomfort, pain, acidic symptoms, or suspicion of upper GI disease might reasonably be tested for *H. pylori* and treated if the organism is present. In persons who come from a country where gastric cancer is common, then endoscopic diagnosis is preferred as a way of excluding malignancy and diagnosing *H. pylori* at the same time (e.g., Hong Kong). In Western countries where gastric cancer is relatively uncommon, below the age of 50, persons with simple dyspepsia without alarm symptoms (e.g., weight loss, GI bleeding, etc.) may reasonably be subjected to "test and treat" strategies whereby the primary-care physician performs a convenient diagnostic test for *H. pylori*, prescribes treatment to eradicate it if the test is positive, then follows the patient up 1 month later with a test of active disease, for example UBT, to confirm eradication. If treatment fails the primary-care physician may choose to treat the patient on a second occasion. If symptoms persist then the patient should be referred to a gastroenterologist for endoscopy.

Well-known indications for *H. pylori* eradication are any history of peptic ulcer, gastric cancer in the patient's family, gastric lymphoma, presence of *H. pylori* associated disease in other family members, and, less definitely, presence of any of the "disease associations." It is not cost effective to screen and treat *H. pylori* in asymptomatic people except in populations at risk of gastric cancer, such as Japanese Americans [18]. One strategy is to perform a serologic test for *H. pylori* at age 50 and give positive patients antibiotic therapy to eradicate *H. pylori*.

Children and *H. pylori*

Children infected with *H. pylori* are generally asymptomatic. However, the presence of chronic GI symptoms should be investigated with a non-invasive test (serology, UBT, or fecal antigen test) to exclude presence of the organism. If *H. pylori* is present then the organism should be treated and eradication should be confirmed with a UBT or a fecal antigen test. Double-blind data proving the value of this strategy are sparse.

Cancer Prevention

First-degree relatives of persons with gastric adenocarcinoma have an increased risk of cancer caused by their *H. pylori* infection [19]. Therefore, even asymptomatic family members of gastric cancer patients should be screened, and treated for *H. pylori* if it is present. Prospective treatment studies have shown some protection from gastric cancer, that is new cancer cases are less in persons from whom *H. pylori* has been eradicated. However, some cancers still occur in the stomach after *H. pylori* was cured. The presence of atrophic gastritis and intestinal metaplasia served to prolong the risk of gastric adenocarcinoma for several years after *H. pylori* eradication.

After eradication of *H. pylori*, hypochlorhydric patients with widespread asymptomatic gastritis might increase their acid secretion, thereby unmasking an incompetent lower esophageal sphincter. On a population basis, it is inevitable that gastroesophageal reflux disease (GERD) and adenocarcinoma of the esophagus could increase if the whole asymptomatic population was treated for *H. pylori*. On the other hand the risk of a continuing low-acid state due to atrophic gastritis is known to confer at least a sixfold increased rate of gastric adenocarcinoma in individuals with persistent *H. pylori*. The practical response to this controversy is to test and treat any patients who have *H. pylori* but be on the look out for new GERD symptoms. These can be readily treated with PPIs. The physician should appropriately discuss the pros and cons of *H. pylori* therapy with the patient. Most patients are concerned about the small cancer risk of *H. pylori*, the potential for transmitting the organism to other members of the family, and the possibility that eradication of chronic inflammation of the gastric mucosa might lead to symptom relief.

Case continued

Given the presentation of ulcer-negative dyspepsia in an emigrant from a country with a high prevalence of *H. pylori*, a test and treat strategy could be considered, although the number needed to treat to achieve a cure of these symptoms may be quite high (since significant ulcer disease was excluded with the barium test). On the other hand, given this patient's family history and concerns, an esophagogastroduodenoscopy (EGD) could be justified. She underwent an EGD that demonstrated diffuse erythema of the stomach. Biopsy confirmed *H. pylori* infection, but there were no areas of histological concern. Eradication therapy produced a partial improvement in her upper gastrointestinal symptoms and follow-up breath testing confirmed eradication.

Take-home points

- *Helicobacter pylori* is a bacterial pathogen causing gastritis, peptic ulcers, and gastric cancer (both adenocarcinoma and MALT lymphoma).
- The route of transmission poorly understood.
- Disease outcome is dependent upon bacterial and host factors.
- Diagnosis may be made by endoscopic biopsy, breath testing, stool tests, and serology.
- Eradication is by antibiotic therapy.

References

1 Marshall BJ, Royce H, Annear DI, *et al*. Original isolation of *Campylobacter pyloridis* from human gastric mucosa. *Microbios Lett* 1984; **25**: 83–8.

2 Tomb JF, White O, Kerlavage AR, *et al*. The complete genome sequence of the gastric pathogen *Helicobacter pylori*. *Nature* 1997; **388**: 539–47.

3 Parsonnet J, Friedman GD, Vandersteen DP, *et al*. *Helicobacter pylori* infection and the risk of gastric carcinoma. *N Engl J Med* 1991; **325**: 1127–31.

4 Perez-Perez GI, Olivares AZ, Foo FY, *et al*. Seroprevalence of *Helicobacter pylori* in New York City populations originating in East Asia. *J Urban Health* 2005; **82**: 510–6.

5 Ahmed KS, Khan AA, Ahmed I, *et al*. Impact of household hygiene and water source on the prevalence and transmission of *Helicobacter pylori*: a South Indian perspective. *Singapore Med J* 2007; **48**: 543–9.

6 Perry S, de la Luz Sanchez M, Yang S, *et al*. Gastroenteritis and transmission of *Helicobacter pylori* infection in households. *Emerg Infect Dis* 2006; **12**: 1701–8.

7 Goh KL, Parasakthi N. The racial cohort phenomenon: seroepidemiology of *Helicobacter pylori* infection in a multiracial South-East Asian country. *Eur J Gastroenterol Hepatol* 2001; **13**: 177–83.

8 El-Omar EM, Oien K, El-Nujumi A, *et al*. *Helicobacter pylori* infection and chronic gastric acid hyposecretion. *Gastroenterology* 1997; **113**: 15–24.

9 Bayerdorffer E, Neubauer A, Rudolph B, *et al*. Regression of primary gastric lymphoma of mucosa-associated lymphoid tissue type after cure of *Helicobacter pylori* infection. MALT Lymphoma Study Group. *Lancet* 1995; **345**: 1591–4.

10 Houghton J, Wang TC. *Helicobacter pylori* and gastric cancer: a new paradigm for inflammation-associated epithelial cancers. *Gastroenterology* 2005; **128**: 1567–78.

11 Yamaoka Y, Kato M, Asaka M. Geographic differences in gastric cancer incidence can be explained by differences between *Helicobacter pylori* strains. *Intern Med* 2008; **47**: 1077–83.

12 Asaka M, Sugiyama T, Nobuta A, *et al*. Atrophic gastritis and intestinal metaplasia in Japan: results of a large multicenter study. *Helicobacter* 2001; **6**: 294–9.

13 Moayyedi P, Soo S, Deeks J, *et al*. Eradication of *Helicobacter pylori* for non-ulcer dyspepsia. *Cochrane Database Syst Rev* 2006; **2**: CD002096.

14 Stettin D, Waldmann A, Strohle A, Hahn A. Association between *Helicobacter pylori*-infection, C-reactive protein and status of B vitamins. *Adv Med Sci* 2008; **53**: 205–13.

15 Stasi R, Sarpatwari A, Segal JB, *et al*. Effects of eradication of *Helicobacter pylori* infection in patients with immune thrombocytopenic purpura: a systematic review. *Blood* 2009; **113**: 1231–40.

16 Gisbert JP, de la Morena F, Abraira V. Accuracy of monoclonal stool antigen test for the diagnosis of *H. pylori* infection: a systematic review and meta-analysis. *Am J Gastroenterol* 2006; **101**: 1921–30.

17 Vaira D, Zullo A, Vakil N, *et al*. Sequential therapy versus standard triple-drug therapy for *Helicobacter pylori* eradication: a randomized trial. *Ann Intern Med* 2007; **146**: 556–63.

18 Talley NJ, Fock KM, Moayyedi P. Gastric Cancer Consensus conference recommends *Helicobacter pylori* screening and treatment in asymptomatic persons from high-risk populations to prevent gastric cancer. *Am J Gastroenterol* 2008; **103**: 510–4.

19 Motta CR, Cunha MP, Queiroz DM, *et al*. Gastric precancerous lesions and *Helicobacter pylori* infection in relatives of gastric cancer patients from Northeastern Brazil. *Digestion* 2008; **78**: 3–8.

20 Gibney KB, Mihrshahi S, Torresi J, *et al*. The profile of health problems in African immigrants attending an infectious disease unit in Melbourne, Australia. *Am J Trop Med Hyg* 2009; **80**: 805–11.

21 Bhuiyan TR, Qadri F, Saha A, Svennerholm AM. Infection by *Helicobacter pylori* in Bangladeshi children from birth to two years: relation to blood group, nutritional status, and seasonality. *Pediatr Infect Dis J* 2009; **28**: 79–85.

22 Naja F, Kreiger N, Sullivan T. *Helicobacter pylori* infection in Ontario: prevalence and risk factors. *Can J Gastroenterol* 2007; **21**: 501–6.

23 Chen J, Bu XL, Wang QY, *et al*. Decreasing seroprevalence of *Helicobacter pylori* infection during 1993–2003 in Guangzhou, southern China. *Helicobacter* 2007; **12**: 164–9.

24 Bures J, Kopacova M, Koupil I, *et al*. Epidemiology of *Helicobacter pylori* infection in the Czech Republic. *Helicobacter* 2006; **11**: 56–65.

25 Weck MN, Stegmaier C, Rothenbacher D, Brenner H. Epidemiology of chronic atrophic gastritis: population-based study among 9444 older adults from Germany. *Aliment Pharmacol Ther* 2007; **26**: 879–87.

26 Thjodleifsson B, Asbjornsdottir H, Sigurjonsdottir RB, *et al*. Seroprevalence of *Helicobacter pylori* and cagA antibodies in Iceland, Estonia and Sweden. *Scand J Infect Dis* 2007; **39**: 683–9.

27 Okuda M, Miyashiro E, Booka M, *et al*. *Helicobacter pylori* colonization in the first 3 years of life in Japanese children. *Helicobacter* 2007; **12**: 324–7.

28 Yanaoka K, Oka M, Yoshimura N, *et al*. Risk of gastric cancer in asymptomatic, middle-aged Japanese subjects based on serum pepsinogen and *Helicobacter pylori* antibody levels. *Int J Cancer* 2008; **123**: 917–26.

29 Mourad-Baars PE, Verspaget HW, Mertens BJ, Mearin ML. Low prevalence of *Helicobacter pylori* infection in young children in the Netherlands. *Eur J Gastroenterol Hepatol* 2007; **19**: 213–6.

30 Tkachenko MA, Zhannat NZ, Erman LV, *et al*. Dramatic changes in the prevalence of *Helicobacter pylori* infection during childhood: a 10-year follow-up study in Russia. *J Pediatr Gastroenterol Nutr* 2007; **45**: 428–32.

31 Robinson LG, Black FL, Lee FK, *et al*. *Helicobacter pylori* prevalence among indigenous peoples of South America. *J Infect Dis* 2002; **186**: 1131–7.

32 Lin DB, Lin JB, Chen CY. Seroprevalence of *Helicobacter pylori* infection among schoolchildren and teachers in Taiwan. *Helicobacter* 2007; **12**: 258–64.

33 Suzuki H, Marshall BJ, Hibi T. Overview: *Helicobacter pylori* and extragastric disease. *Int J Hematol* 2006; **84**: 291–300.

34 Federman DG, Kirsner RS, Moriarty JP, Concato J. The effect of antibiotic therapy for patients infected with *Helicobacter pylori* who have chronic urticaria. *J Am Acad Dermatol* 2003; **49**: 861–4.

35 Chen SJ, Wang LJ, Zhu Q, *et al*. Effect of *H. pylori* infection and its eradication on hyperammo-nemia and hepatic encephalopathy in cirrhotic patients. *World J Gastroenterol* 2008; **14**: 1914–8.

36 Tsang KW, Lam SK, Lam WK, *et al*. High seroprevalence of *Helicobacter pylori* in active bronchiectasis. *Am J Respir Crit Care Med* 1998; **158**: 1047–51.

37 Dakovic Z, Vesic S, Vukovic J, *et al*. Ocular rosacea and treatment of symptomatic *Helicobacter pylori* infection: a case series. *Acta Dermatovenerol Alp Panonica Adriat* 2007; **16**: 83–6.

38 Sacca SC, Pascotto A, Venturino GM, *et al*. Prevalence and treatment of *Helicobacter pylori* in patients with blepharitis. *Invest Ophthalmol Vis Sci* 2006; **47**: 501–8.

39 Imai J, Yamada T, Saito T, *et al*. Eradication of insulin resistance. *Lancet* 2009; **374**: 264.

40 Otasevic L, Zlatanovic G, Stanojevic-Paovic A, *et al*. *Helicobacter pylori*: an underestimated factor in acute anterior uveitis and spondyloarthropathies? *Ophthalmologica* 2007; **221**: 6–13.

CHAPTER 45

Gastritis

Massimo Rugge[1,2] *and David Y. Graham*[2]

[1] Department of Diagnostic Medical Sciences and Special Therapies, Pathology Unit, University of Padova, Italy

[2] Michael E. DeBakey Veterans Affairs Medical Center and Baylor College of Medicine, Houston, TX, USA

Summary

Gastritis is defined as inflammation of stomach mucosa and its classification is based on etiology. Diagnostic tools includes clinical evaluation, serology (pepsinogens, and antibodies against infectious agents and/or autoantigens), endoscopy (standardized biopsy protocols should be applied), and histology. Histology distinguishes non-atrophic versus atrophic gastritis (atrophy = loss of appropriate glands). Atrophy and (even more) non-invasive neoplasia are precancerous lesions. The histology report should be clinically informative: a recently suggested histology reporting format (OLGA staging system) relates the gastric disease to its cancer risk. According to their etiology, the main forms of gastritis are infectious (*H. pylori*), chemical, and autoimmune.

Definitions

Gastritis is defined as inflammation of the stomach [1–5]. Gastritis is a widely misused term as it is often used to denote endoscopic finding such as redness or symptoms such as those experienced after eating spicy foods. Clinically, gastric abnormalities associated with clinical or endoscopic findings are divided into inflammatory conditions and non-inflammatory or focally inflammatory conditions called gastropathies [6]. While this distinction is theoretically appropriate, histologically they almost always reveal an inflammatory component such as associated with NSAID-induced erosions [7].

Assessment

The approach to gastritis is both clinical and histological. Clinical features assist in interpretation of both the endoscopic and histological findings. For example, interpretation of endoscopic findings of multiple, small, antral erosions would be advanced by knowing that the patient

Practical Gastroenterology and Hepatology: Esophagus and Stomach, 1st edition. Edited by Nicholas J. Talley, Kenneth R. DeVault and David E. Fleischer. © 2010 Blackwell Publishing Ltd.

took aspirin the morning of the procedure. Similarly, the finding of antral and corpus atrophy in a patient with vitamin B_{12} deficiency (pernicious anemia) would point toward the process being the end result of a chronic *Helicobacter pylori* infection rather than an autoimmune phenomena.

A diagnosis of gastritis implies that one has histologically examined the gastric mucosa. Most often the tissue specimens are obtained at endoscopy. Standardized biopsy protocols should be used and many different biopsy sampling protocols have been proposed [4,8]. The most recent is the Sydney System or its modifications in which mucosa from the oxyntic, antral, and incisura angularis areas are sampled (Figure 45.1) as well as additional specimens from any focal lesions seen [9]. Generally, all antral specimens including the incisura biopsy can be placed in one bottle and the corpus biopsies in a separate one. If more extensive sampling of the corpus is done (e.g., two lesser curve and two greater curve specimens) three bottles should be used to separate the lesser and greater curve corpus specimens. This is based on the notion that atrophy extends proximally more quickly along the lesser curve than the greater curve.

Biopsy samples should be handled as little as possible and after fixation should be embedded on edge. The basic stain is H&E. When *H. pylori* is suspected, a special stain such as a modified Giemsa, a triple stain such as the

Genta or El-Zimaity, or immunohistochemical staining should be used [10,11].

The histology report should be clinically informative and the terminology suggested by the Sydney System or, more recently, by an international group of gastroenterologists and pathologists and called the OLGA staging system [12]. The OLGA system categorizes gastritis in five stages according to the progressively increasing extension of atrophy (histologically assessed in both antral and oxyntic compartments: OLGA-staging system Stages I to IV) (Table 45.1). OLGA staging is particularly useful in regions where gastric cancer is still prevalent as it provides information about the cancer risk and also includes assessment of the etiology of gastritis (*H. pylori*, autoimmune, etc.).

Non-invasive tests can also provide information regarding important information that can complement or supplant histologic mapping studies; for example, pepsinogens levels: pepsinogen I (PgI) is present in fundic chief cells whereas PgII is present in the antrum and corpus [13,14].

Gastrin 17 levels provide evidence regarding acid secretion (high gastrin 17 = low acid secretion; low gastrin 17 = typically, high acid secretion). Antiparietal cells antibodies assist in diagnosis of autoimmune gastritis.

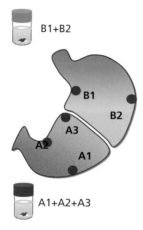

Figure 45.1 Biopsy protocol sampling in the routine assessment of gastritis. Biopsy samples from antral (A1, A2), oxyntic (B1, B2), and incisura angularis (A3) mucosa should be obtained; antral specimens (including incisura angularis) can be placed in one vial and the corpus biopsies in a separate one.

Basic Morphology

Inflammatory Infiltrate: Mononuclear Cells

The inflammatory infiltrate mainly consists of lymphocytes, plasmocytes, histiocytes, and granulocytes within the lamina propria and may also infiltrate single glands units. Lymphocytes may be dispersed or organized in follicular (or nodular) structures.

The term "lymphocytic gastritis" is applied to those conditions in which single lymphocytes are detected within the columnar epithelia of the majority of the glandular structures and suggests, but is not diagnostic of, an

Table 45.1 OLGA system for gastritis staging [9]. The gastritis stage results from the combination of the atrophy scores detected at the antral mucosa and at the corpus mucosa.

Atrophy score		Corpus			
		No atrophy (score 0)	Mild atrophy (score 1)	Moderate atrophy (score 2)	Severe atrophy (score 3)
Antrum	No atrophy (score 0) (including incisura angularis)	Stage 0	Stage I	Stage II	Stage II
	Mild atrophy (score 1) (including incisura angularis)	Stage I	Stage I	Stage II	Stage III
	Moderate atrophy (score 2) (including incisura angularis)	Stage II	Stage II	Stage III	Stage IV
	Severe atrophy (score 3) (including incisura angularis)	Stage III	Stage III	Stage IV	Stage IV

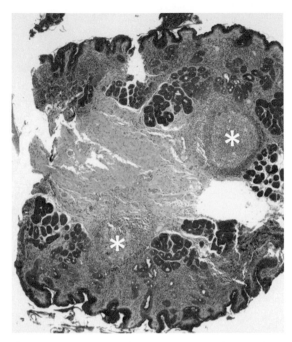

Figure 45.2 Gastric biopsy obtained from the antral mucosa (PAS stain). Lamina propria is expanded by inflammatory infiltrate, both diffuse and nodular; two lymphoid follicles are marked *. The population of original antral glands seems partially lost; high-grade inflammatory infiltrate displaces the antral glands (are they lost?); the histological diagnosis of "gastritis indefinite for atrophy" is appropriate.

immunomediated pathogenesis [15]. A more severe (nodular) lymphocyte intraglandular infiltrate may destroy the continuity of the glandular epithelia: such a "lymphoepithelial lesion" is considered almost pathognomonic of primary gastric (almost always, *H. pylori*-associated) lymphomas.

The presence of the inflammatory infiltrate, particularly in *H. pylori* gastritis, may make it difficult or impossible to determine whether glandular units are absent (atrophy) or pushed apart (pseudoatrophy). In such cases, it is best to use a temporary diagnosis such as "indefinite for atrophy" and defer final judgment until after *H. pylori* eradication when the inflammation has resolved (Figure 45.2). This "indefinite" category is borrowed from the classification of intraepithelial neoplasia (dysplasia) in the gastrointestinal tract and is not intended to represent a biological entity (see atrophy definition, below) [16].

Inflammatory Infiltrate: Polymorphs (Neutrophils and Eosinophils)

When neutrophils are detected within the lamina propria and/or into the glandular lumen the patient has an "active gastritis". The presence of a predominant eosinophil population is assessed as eosinophilic gastritis.

Fibrosis of the Lamina Propria and Smooth Muscle Hyperplasia

Irrespective of its etiology, the expansion of the collagen tissue of the lamina propria (fibrosis) couples with loss of glandular units and the lesion is assessed as mucosa atrophy. Fibrosis of the lamina propria may be also focal (i.e., scar of peptic ulcer).

Hyperplasia of the muscularis mucosae may result from long-term PPI therapy; smooth muscle fascicles may push apart the glandular coils, realizing a pseudoatrophic pattern.

Hyperplasia of Glandular Elements

All inflammatory conditions of the gastric mucosa are associated with some degree of regenerative epithelial modifications and this is typically seen adjacent to peptic ulcers and erosions (regenerative hyperplasia). Expansion of the proliferative compartment of the gastric glands (neck region) results in foveolar hyperplasia. Chemical (biliary reflux into the stomach or NSAID use) or infectious stimuli increasing the cellular turnover result in hyperplastic foveolae. Atypical regeneration of the glandular neck and/or expansion of the glandular proliferative compartment may cause difficulty in differentiating regenerative from dysplastic lesions (see lesions indefinite for non-invasive neoplasia).

Changes occurring in the oxyntic epithelia as result of proton pump inhibitors in response to the inhibition of the acid secretion are sometimes considered a hyperplastic change but may simply represent a remodeling of the epithelia structure due to cytoskeletal rearrangements.

Glandular Atrophy

Atrophy is defined as the "loss of appropriate gastric glands". Different phenotypes of atrophic transformation may be present (Table 45.2) including: (i) vanishing or evident shrinkage of glandular units replaced by fibrosis ("scarring") of the lamina propria (such a situation results in a reduced glandular mass, but does not imply any modification of the original (mucosecreting or oxyntic) cell phenotype); and (ii) metaplastic replacement of the native glands by glands featuring a new cellular commitment (= intestinal and/or pseudopyloric metaplasia). The number of glands is not necessarily lower, but the metaplastic replacement of the original glandular units decreases the population of the native glands (which are "appropriate" for the compartment considered). A formal classification of atrophic changes has been proposed (Table 45.2; Figure 45.3).

Table 45.2 Atrophy in gastric mucosa.

Atrophy	Histological type	Location and key lesions		Grading
		Antrum	Corpus	
0 Absent (= score 0)				
1 Indefinite (no score is applicable)				
2 Present	2.1 Non-metaplastic	Glands: shrinking/vanishing Lamina propria: fibrosis	Glands: shrinking/vanishing Lamina propria: fibrosis	2.1.1 Mild = G1 (1–30%) 2.1.2 Moderate = G2 (31–60%) 2.1.3 Severe = G3 (>60%)
	2.2 Metaplastic	Intestinal metaplasia	Intestinal metaplasia Pseudopyloric metaplasia	2.2.1 Mild = G1 (1–30%) 2.2.2 Moderate = G2 (31–60%) 2.2.3 Severe = G3 (>60%)

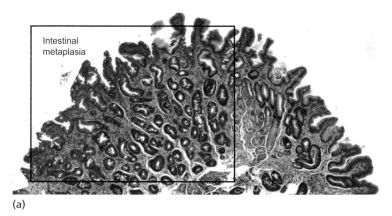

(a)

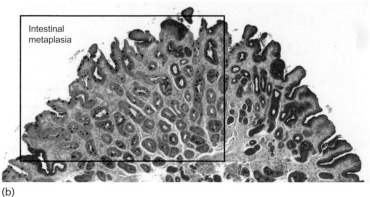

(b)

Figure 45.3 Gastric biopsy obtained from the antral mucosa; (a) H&E, (b) PAS stain. The native population of the antral glands (dark red with PAS; right side of the biopsy sample, outside the square) is replaced by metaplastic glands (area in the square). With PAS stain, metaplastic intestinalized glands (inside the square) show a purple (PAS +ve) "globular" secretion (= goblet cells).

Metaplasia Phenotypes

By definition, metaplasia is a transformation of the native commitment of a cell. Within the stomach, the metaplastic transformation always implies loss of appropriate (native) glands (i.e., atrophy). Two main histotypes of gastric glands metaplasia are described. Pseudopyloric metaplasia of native corpus epithelia is characterized by antral-appearing mucosa obtained from what was anatomically corpus mucosa. It is particularly important for the endoscopist to identify the location of the biopsy specimens otherwise the pathologist will likely miss the fact that the antral-appearing mucosa is a metaplastic epithelia. The original commitment of a pseudopyloric-metaplastic epithelium can be revealed by positive immunostain for pepsinogen I which is only found in the corpus (oxyntic) mucosa.

The most frequent variant of metaplasia is of the intestinal type. Intestinal metaplasia may arise in native mucosecreting (antral) epithelia or in previously antralized oxyntic glands (pseudopyloric metaplasia). Different subtypes of intestinal metaplasia have been proposed based on whether the metaplastic epithelium phenotype resembles large bowel epithelia (colonic type intestinal metaplasia) or small intestinal mucosa [17,18].

Endocrine Cells Hyperplasia

Most frequently, endocrine cell hyperplasia is secondary to gastric achlorhydria, usually associated with corpus atrophy. In such a condition the hyperplasia of the endocrine enterochromaffin-like (ECL) cells may be micronodular or diffuse. Less frequently, (neuro)endocrine (nodular) tumors (well-differentiated endocrine tumors; i.e., Type I carcinoids) may develop. Such tumors almost never metastasize and, when indicated, they should be simply resected. They often regress following removal of the source of gastrin (i.e., antral resection).

Non-invasive Neoplasia (Synonym: Intraepithelial Neoplasia; Formerly Defined as Dysplasia)

In longstanding (atrophic) gastritis, mainly due to *H. pylori* infection, the glands may undergo neoplastic transformation confined within the basal membrane, formerly defined as gastric dysplasia. Because molecular studies have detected a number of the genotypic alterations common to both to gastric dysplasia and gastric cancer, both are recognized as neoplastic. Dysplasia has therefore been redefined as an intraepithelial or non-invasive neoplasia (i.e., confined by the dysplastic glands' basal membrane) [19,20]. The continuity/integrity of the dysplastic glands' basal membrane separates the dysplastic epithelia from the stroma (i.e., lamina propria) excluding the potential for invasion required for any metastatic implant. It was previously thought that cancer often arose from intestinal metaplastic cells, but more recent studies have challenged that hypothesis and currently the cell of origin is considered unknown.

Classification

Current classifications are based on etiology. Table 45.3 summarizes the etiological classification of gastritis.

Main Forms of Gastritis

Helicobacter pylori Gastritis

H. pylori gastritis is by far the most frequent and important form of gastritis. In never-treated, infected patients, *H. pylori* is usually easy detectable within the mucous gel layer covering gastric mucosa. It is more abundant in the antrum and cardia than in oxyntic mucosa and, while it can be detected with the H&E stain, randomized controlled trials have shown that accuracy is best with special stains. In cases with extensive gastric intestinalization and in patients treated with proton pomp inhibitors, *H. pylori* detection may be difficult and may be difficult to diagnose even with special stains. In our experience, less-experienced pathologists often over diagnose the infection based on the presence of a few silver-stained particles in otherwise non-inflamed tissue.

The presence of the infection is suggested by both mononuclear and neutrophil (i.e., "active") inflammation (neutrophils may fill the foveolar lumen producing pit microabscesses). Lymphoid follicles are also frequently detected. After successful eradication therapy, neutrophils quickly disappear whereas the mononuclear component remains detectable for many weeks to months. However, the persistence of neutrophils and/or mononuclear infiltrate should suggest the possibility of therapeutic failure even if organisms are not seen. This is especially a problem when PPI therapy is continued.

Table 45.3 Etiological classification of gastritis.

Etiological category	Agents	Specific etiology	Clinical presentation	Notes
Transmissible agents	Virus	Cytomegalovirus	acute	Non-atrophic †
		Herpes virus	acute	Non-atrophic †
	Bacteria	*Helicobacter pylori*	acute or chronic	Non-atrophic and atrophic, Type B
		Mycobacterium tuberculosis	? acute	Non-atrophic *
		Mycobacterium avium complex	? acute	Non-atrophic *
		Mycobacterium diphtheriae	acute	Non-atrophic *
		Actinomyces	acute	Non-atrophic *
		Spirochaeta	acute	Non-atrophic *
	Fungi	*Candida*	acute	Non-atrophic †
		Histoplasma	acute	Non-atrophic *
		Phycomycosis	acute	Non-atrophic *
	Parasites	*Cryptosporidium*	acute	Non-atrophic *
		Strongyloides	acute	Non-atrophic *
		Anisakis	acute	Non-atrophic *
		Ascaris lumbricoides	acute	Non-atrophic *
Chemical agents (most frequently gastropathies)	Environment (dietary and drug-related)	Dietary factors	chronic	Non-atrophic and atrophic ‡
		Drugs: NSAIDs, ticlopidine	acute	Non-atrophic; Type C ‡
		Alcohol	acute	Non-atrophic; Type C †
		Cocaine	acute	Non-atrophic; Type C*
		Bile (reflux)	acute or chronic chronic chronic	Non-atrophic; Type C ‡
Physical agents	Radiations		acute or chronic	Non-atrophic and atrophic *
Immunomediated	Different pathogenesis	Autoimmune	chronic	Atrophic (corpus); Type A. †
		Drugs (ticlopidine)	acute	
		? Gluten	chronic	Lymphocytic gastritis †
		Food sensitivity	acute or chronic	Eosinophilic gastritis †
		H. pylori (autoimmune) component)	chronic	Non-atrophic and atrophic
		Graft-versus-host disease	acute or chronic	Non-atrophic and atrophic *
		Idiopathic	acute or chronic	
Idiopathic		Crohn disease	? chronic	Non-atrophic/focal atrophy †
		Sarcoidosis	? chronic	Non-atrophic or focal atrophy*
		Wegener granulomatosis	? chronic	Non-atrophic or focal atrophy*
		Collagenous gastritis	acute	Non-atrophic*

*Very rare.
†Infrequent.
‡Common.

H. pylori infection is the major cause of gastric atrophy. Atrophic changes (metaplastic and non-metaplastic) detected in a biopsy sample obtained from both angularis incisura and antral mucosa should be primarily considered as part of an *H. pylori* gastritis. In long-standing infection (i.e., elderly subjects) or in young infected patients with concomitant risk factors, atrophic changes also occur in oxyntic mucosa typically as pseudopyloric metaplasia often coexisting with multifocal (antral and corpus) intestinal metaplasia. Such patients are at increased risk of gastric cancer [21].

H. pylori gastritis is also strongly suggested endoscopically by the presence of follicular gastritis which represents the endoscopic visualization of the multiple lymphoid follicles in the antrum. Experienced endoscopists are often able to correctly assess atrophy/intestinal metaplasia, which should feature an irregular surface often with patchy pink and pale areas (Figure 45.4).

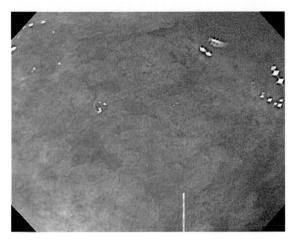

Figure 45.4 Extensive intestinal metaplasia seen endoscopically. The pattern of irregular pink patches within a white, often velvety, background is typical of intestinal metaplasia. When extensive, both the white and pink mucosa typically show intestinal metaplasia histologically.

Chemical Gastritis/Gastropathies

The exposure of gastric mucosa to bile reflux (due to both partial gastrectomy or dysmotility syndrome) or to aspirin or other non-steroidal anti-inflammatory agents (NSAIDs), or to other chemical injuries (possibly alcohol, etc.) may result a wide spectrum of mucosal changes [22]. The histological lesions range from minimal to severe (also hemorrhagic) mucosal damage. Based on their trivial inflammatory trait, these conditions have been defined as chemical gastropathies. The pathogenesis of such abnormalities is not completely understood and it differs slightly according to the different etiologies.

Postgastrectomy gastric reflux of bile salts and pancreaticoduodenal secretions alters the mucus barrier and allows increased back-diffusion of hydrogen ions. The exposure of gastric mucosa to this noxious chemical environment accelerates the turnover of the gastric epithelium; the overproliferation of the epithelial compartment may result in polypoid lesions. Concomitant histamine-mediated vascular response and release of other proinflammatory cytokines produce vascular ectasia, edema, muscularis mucosa hyperplasia, and variable mucosal fibrosis. It is not clear whether there is any relation between the histological findings and symptoms. Most chemical gastropathies are asymptomatic and non-atrophic. In intact stomachs, the reflux of duodenal content may also result in similar abnormalities.

In 10–50% of long-term NSAIDs users, endoscopy and/or histology document variable gastric mucosa alterations. NSAIDs reduce the synthesis of prostaglandins, which results into inefficient protection of the superficial epithelial layer (decreased secretions of both mucus and bicarbonate). The variable unbalance of the cytoprotection and the characteristics of chemical agent are thought to be the main determinants of the severity of the mucosal damage. Mucosa lesions range from minimal alterations (only detectable at histology: low-grade interfoveolar edema, foveolar hyperplasia, and vascular ectasia) to multiple erosions/ulcers, with bleeding. Concomitant *H. pylori* infection is a risk factor for more severe gastric lesions; the concomitant infection is likely responsible for an inflammatory component which is usually undetectable in "pure" chemical forms.

Autoimmune Gastritis

Autoimmune gastritis is a corpus-restricted inflammation due to a selective autoimmune damage of parietal cells (antiparietal cell and anti-intrinsic factor antibodies). The clinical manifestations of the full-blown disease include hypoachlorhydria, hypergastrinemia, low pepsinogen I/pepsinogen II ratio (which parallels the loss of oxyntic gland population), and vitamin B_{12}-deficient macrocytic anemia. The disease may coexist with immunomediated diseases (Hashimoto thyroditis, insulin-dependent diabetes, vitiligo).

In the early stage, oxyntic mucosa shows rich, full-thickness lymphocyte infiltrate (non-atrophic stage). In advanced cases, the corpus-restricted gastritis is characteristically atrophic. The native oxyntic glands are replaced by metaplastic glandular units (pseudopyloric metaplasia comes first; gland intestinalization represents a more advanced stage). The native nature of the oxyntic glands can be disclosed by demonstrating the residue attitude of pyloric-type glands to the pepsinogen I secretion (see above). Hypochlorhydria triggers gastrin hypersecretion (hyperplasia of gastrin secreting cells in antral mucosa), which stimulates the ECL cells of the oxyntic compartment. Such a situation may result in ECL cell hyperplasia (linear and micronodular). Micronodular ECL cell hyperplasia may evolve into well-differentiated endocrine tumors (type I carcinoid) [23,24]. It is important to note that such a type of tumor is only locally invasive. While extensive gastric metaplastic atrophy is the major risk factor for adenocarcinoma it not clear that autoimmune gastritis without concomitant *H. pylori* infection carries a significant cancer risk. The same clinical syndrome of pernicious anemia can also occur in patient with *H. pylori* infection and is characterized by both antral and corpus atrophy rather than only corpus atrophy.

Take-home points

- Gastritis is defined as inflammation of the gastric mucosa.
- Worldwide, *Helicobacter pylori* infection is the most prevalent etiology.
- Atrophic pangastritis is the major risk factor for gastric cancer.
- Reporting gastritis in terms of staging (OLGA staging system: Stages 0–IV) provides an estimate of gastritis-associated cancer risk.
- Non-invasive testing may complement or supplant more expensive invasive procedures; the most informative tests are: the urea breath test and the stool antigen test for *H. pylori* infection; serum levels of pepsinogen I and II for atrophy; serum gastrin 17 and antiparietal cells antibody levels for autoimmune gastritis.
- Chemical gastritis is mostly non-atrophic (low cancer risk).
- Autoimmune atrophic gastritis is associated with an increased risk of neuroendocrine well-differentiated tumors (Type I) and possibly also of gastric adenocarcinoma.

References

1 Owen DA. Gastritis and carditis. *Mod Pathol* 2003; **16**: 325–41.

2 Correa P. Chronic gastritis: a clinico-pathological classification. *Am J Gastroenterol* 1988; **83**: 504–9.

3 Price AB. The Sydney System: histological division. *J Gastroenterol Hepatol* 1991; **6**: 209–22.

4 Dixon MF, Genta RM, Yardley JH, *et al*. Classification and grading of gastritis. The updated Sydney System. International Workshop on the Histopathology of Gastritis, Houston 1994. *Am J Surg Pathol* 1996; **20**: 1161–81.

5 Whitehead R. The classification of chronic gastritis: current status. *J Clin Gastroenterol* 1995; **21** (Suppl. 1): S131–4.

6 Srivastava A, Lauwers GY. Pathology of non-infective gastritis. *Histopathology* 2007; **50**: 15–29.

7 Sepulveda AR, Patil M. Practical approach to the pathologic diagnosis of gastritis. *Arch Pathol Lab Med* 2008; **132**: 1586–93.

8 Sipponen P, Stolte M. Clinical impact of routine biopsies of the gastric antrum and body. *Endoscopy* 1997; **29**: 671–8.

9 Rugge M, Correa P, Di Mario F, *et al*. OLGA staging for gastritis: a tutorial. *Dig Liver Dis* 2008; **40**: 650–8.

10 Genta RM, Robason GO, Graham DY. Simultaneous visualization of Helicobacter pylori and gastric morphology: a new stain. *Hum Pathol* 1994; **25**: 221–6.

11 el-Zimaity HM, Wu J, Graham DY. Modified Genta triple stain for identifying Helicobacter pylori. *J Clin Pathol* 1999; **52**: 693–4.

12 Rugge M, Genta RM. Staging gastritis: an international proposal. *Gastroenterology* 2005; **129**: 1807–8.

13 Pasechnikov VD, Chukov SZ, Kotelevets SM, *et al*. Invasive and non-invasive diagnosis of Helicobacter pylori-associated atrophic gastritis: a comparative study. *Scand J Gastroenterol* 2005; **40**: 297–301.

14 Sipponen P, Graham DY. Importance of atrophic gastritis in diagnostics and prevention of gastric cancer: application of plasma biomarkers. *Scand J Gastroenterol* 2007; **42**: 2–10.

15 Haot J, Hamichi L, Wallez L, *et al*. Lymphocytic gastritis: a newly described entity: a retrospective endoscopic and histological study. *Gut* 1988; **29**: 1258–64.

16 Rugge M, Correa P, Dixon MF, *et al*. Gastric mucosal atrophy: interobserver consistency using new criteria for classification and grading. *Aliment Pharmacol Ther* 2002; **16**: 1249–59.

17 Filipe MI. Mucins in the human gastrointestinal epithelium: a review. *Invest Cell Pathol* 1979; **2**: 195–216.

18 Filipe MI, Munoz N, Matko I, *et al*. Intestinal metaplasia types and the risk of gastric cancer: a cohort study in Slovenia. *Int J Cancer* 1994; **57**: 324–9.

19 Rugge M, Correa P, Dixon MF, *et al*. Gastric dysplasia: the Padova international classification. *Am J Surg Pathol* 2000; **24**: 167–76.

20 Rugge M, Cassaro M, Di Mario F, *et al*. The long term outcome of gastric non-invasive neoplasia. *Gut* 2003; **52**: 1111–16.

21 Uemura N, Okamoto S, Yamamoto S, *et al*. *Helicobacter pylori* infection and the development of gastric cancer. *N Engl J Med* 2001; **345**: 784–9.

22 De Nardi FG, Riddell RH. Reactive (Chemical) gastropathy and gastritis. In: Graham DY, Genta RM, Dixon MF, ed. *Gastritis*. Philadelphia: Lippincott Williams & Wilkins; 1999: 125–46.

23 Rindi G, Kloppel G, Alhman H, *et al*. TNM staging of foregut (neuro)endocrine tumors: a consensus proposal including a grading system. *Virchows Arch* 2006; **449**: 395–401.

24 Rindi G, Kloppel G. Endocrine tumors of the gut and pancreas tumor biology and classification. *Neuroendocrinology* 2004; **80** (Suppl. 1): 12–15.

Gastroparesis

Henry P. Parkman

GI Motility Laboratory, Temple University School of Medicine, Philadelphia, PA, USA

Summary

Gastroparesis is a disorder characterized by symptoms of, and evidence for, gastric retention in the absence of mechanical obstruction. Evaluation consists of demonstrating delayed gastric emptying in a patient with appropriate symptoms, with the absence of mechanical obstruction or mucosal disorders such as an ulcer. Treatment for gastroparesis primarily involves use of several treatment options, including dietary management, antiemetic agents, and prokinetic agents. Treatment of patients with medically refractory gastroparesis may include domperidone, symptom modulators, gastric electric stimulator, or a jejunostomy feeding tube.

Case

A 19-year-old female presents with nausea and vomiting. Approximately 1 year ago, she became ill while on a cruise ship in the Caribbean. Several other passengers also became ill, but no clear etiology was ever determined. Her acute illness resolved, but she remained nauseated. Three months ago she began to experience episodic vomiting. Initially this occurred on a weekly basis, but has progressed to several episodes of vomiting each day. She usually is well in the morning, but as she begins to eat, she gets more and more nausea and usually begins to vomit in the early afternoon. She feels distended and uncomfortable all the time, has limited her diet to mostly liquids and has lost weight from 70 to 55 kg. She is fatigued, but otherwise has no other symptoms and has no significant past medical, social or family history.

Upper endoscopy demonstrated a moderate amount of retained gastric content despite a 12-hour fast. The underlying mucosa to the third portion of the duodenum was normal. A small bowel x-ray was also negative with a normal appearing terminal ileum. Nuclear medicine gastric emptying testing demonstrated delayed gastric emptying at 2 hours (65% retention; normal <60%) and 4 hours (25%

retention; normal <10%). A trial of metoclopramide was not tolerated due to severe worsening in her fatigue. Erythromycin actually increased her nausea. Her father was able to obtain domperidone from Canada and on a dose of 20 mg four times daily she is now able to tolerate a low-residue diet and has stabilized her weight loss.

Introduction

Gastroparesis is a disorder characterized by symptoms of, and evidence for, gastric retention in the absence of mechanical obstruction. Gastroparesis can occur in many clinical settings with varied symptoms and severity of symptoms. The most frequently reported symptoms include nausea, vomiting, early satiety, and postprandial fullness. Abdominal pain, weight loss, malnutrition, and dehydration may be prominent in severe cases. In diabetics, gastroparesis may adversely affect glycemic control. Diagnostic evaluation in patients with symptoms suggestive of gastroparesis generally consists of esophagogastroduodenoscopy (EGD) and a gastric emptying test. Management of this condition can be particularly challenging. This chapter will cover the evaluation and management of patients with gastroparesis.

Practical Gastroenterology and Hepatology: Esophagus and Stomach, 1st edition. Edited by Nicholas J. Talley, Kenneth R. DeVault and David E. Fleischer. © 2010 Blackwell Publishing Ltd.

Etiology of Gastroparesis

Gastroparesis can occur in many settings with varied symptoms and severity of symptoms [1]. Gastroparesis was initially described as an infrequent complication of long-standing diabetes, especially in association with other complications of diabetes such as neuropathy. The true prevalence of gastroparesis is not known, however it has been estimated that up to 4% of the population experiences symptomatic manifestations of this condition [2]. Diabetic, postsurgical, and idiopathic etiologies comprise the majority of cases. Diabetes mellitus is the most common systemic disease associated with gastroparesis. A similar number of patients present with gastroparesis of an idiopathic nature. Postsurgical gastroparesis, often with vagotomy or damage to the vagus nerve, represents the third most common etiology of gastroparesis. Delayed gastric emptying can also be seen in patients with gastroesophageal reflux disease where reflux symptoms may predominate. In a series of 146 patients with gastroparesis [3], the three major categories of gastroparesis were idiopathic (36%), diabetic (29%), and postsurgical (13%). Whatever the cause, gastroparesis more commonly affects female patients and has significant impact on quality of life.

Diabetic Gastroparesis

Gastroparesis is a well-recognized complication of diabetes mellitus. Classically, gastroparesis occurs in patients with long-standing type 1 diabetes mellitus who have other associated complications of diabetes, such as retinopathy, nephropathy, and peripheral neuropathy. Many affected patients may have other signs of autonomic dysfunction, including postural hypotension. Gastroparesis may also occur in patients with type 2 diabetes. The prevalence of gastroparesis in patients with either type 1 or type 2 diabetes has been reported from academic centers to range from 25 to 50%, although the magnitude of gastric delay is modest in many cases. Patients who have had diabetes for a relatively short time may have accelerated emptying from impairment of fundic relaxation caused by vagal dysfunction.

In diabetic patients, delayed gastric emptying contributes to erratic glycemic control because of unpredictable delivery of food into the duodenum. Delayed gastric emptying of nutrients in conjunction with insulin administration may produce hypoglycemia. Conversely, acceleration of the emptying of nutrients with prokinetic agents has been reported to cause early postprandial hyperglycemia. Difficulty in the control of blood glucose levels may be an early indication that a diabetic patient is developing gastric motor dysfunction.

Hyperglycemia itself can reversibly interfere with gastric motility in several ways: decreasing antral contractility; causing decreases in phase III of the migrating motor complex; increasing pyloric contractions; causing disturbances in gastric myoelectric activity; delaying gastric emptying; and modulating fundic relaxation.

Postsurgical Gastroparesis

Gastroparesis may occur as a complication of a number of abdominal surgical procedures. In the past, most cases resulted from vagotomy performed in combination with gastric drainage to correct medically refractory or complicated peptic ulcer disease. Since the advent of laparoscopic techniques for the treatment of gastroesophageal reflux disease (GERD), gastroparesis has become a recognized complication of fundoplication (possibly from vagal injury during the surgery).

Approximately 5% of patients undergoing vagotomy with antrectomy and gastrojejunostomy (Billroth I procedure) develop severe postsurgical gastroparesis. In these patients, the antrum is not present to triturate solids, and the proximal stomach is unable to generate sufficient pressure to empty solid food residue. The combination of vagotomy, distal gastric resection, and Roux-en-Y gastrojejunostomy predisposes to severe gastric stasis resulting from slow emptying from the gastric remnant and delayed small bowel transit in the denervated Roux efferent limb. The Roux-en-Y stasis syndrome—characterized by postprandial abdominal pain, bloating, nausea, and vomiting—is particularly difficult to manage.

Idiopathic Gastroparesis

Idiopathic gastroparesis refers to a symptomatic patient from delayed gastric empting with no detectable primary underlying abnormality for the delayed gastric emptying. This may represent the most common form of gastroparesis [3]. Most patients with idiopathic gastroparesis are women, typically young or middle aged. Symptoms of idiopathic gastroparesis overlap with those of functional dyspepsia and in some patients it may be difficult to provide a definitive distinction between the two. Abdominal pain/discomfort typically is the predominant symptom in functional dyspepsia, whereas nausea, vomiting, early satiety, and bloating predominate in idiopathic gastroparesis.

A subset of patients with idiopathic gastroparesis report sudden onset of symptoms after a viral prodrome, suggesting a potential viral etiology for their symptoms [1,3]. Previously healthy subjects develop the sudden onset of nausea, vomiting, diarrhea, fever, and cramps suggestive of a systemic viral infection. However, instead of experiencing resolution of symptoms, these individuals note persistent nausea, vomiting, and early satiety. Viruses that have been implicated in these cases include cytomegalovirus, Epstein–Barr virus, and varicella zoster. These patients may have slow resolution of their symptoms over several years.

Some patients have cyclic, or episodic nature of vomiting episodes suggesting cyclic vomiting syndrome (CVS). Over time, some of these patients develop more frequent symptom episodes, that is coalescent CVS. In some patients, differentiating gastroparesis from cyclic vomiting syndrome in an adult can be challenging.

Clinical Presentation of Gastroparesis

Symptoms of gastroparesis are variable and include early satiety, nausea, vomiting, bloating, and upper abdominal discomfort. In one series of 146 patients with gastroparesis, nausea was present in 92%, vomiting in 84%, abdominal bloating in 75%, and early satiety in 60% [3]. Complications of gastroparesis include esophagitis, Mallory–Weiss tear, and vegetable-laden bezoars.

Symptoms of gastroparesis may simulate symptoms related to other structural disorders of the stomach and proximal GI tract such as peptic ulcer disease, partial gastric or small bowel obstruction, gastric cancer, and pancreaticobiliary disorders. There also is an overlap between the symptoms of gastroparesis and functional dyspepsia. Indeed, idiopathic gastroparesis can be considered one of the causes of functional dyspepsia.

Although it has been a common assumption that the gastrointestinal symptoms can be attributed to delay in gastric emptying, most investigations have observed only weak correlations between symptom severity and the degree of gastric stasis. In recent studies, early satiety, postprandial fullness, and vomiting have been reported associated with delayed emptying in patients with functional dyspepsia [4]. In patients with diabetes, abdominal fullness and bloating were found to be associated with delayed gastric emptying. In individuals with symptoms of gastroparesis who have normal rates of gastric emptying, other motor, myoelectric, or sensory abnormalities may be responsible for the symptoms.

Abdominal discomfort or pain is present in 46–89% of patients with gastroparesis but is usually not the predominant symptom, in contrast to its prominence in functional dyspepsia. Nevertheless, treatment of abdominal pain in gastroparesis can be challenging. Patients with functional dyspepsia exhibit increased sensitivity to gastric distension suggestive of afferent neural dysfunction as a contributing factor for the symptoms. Similarly, in diabetic patients with dyspeptic symptoms, gastric distension elicits exaggerated nausea, bloating, and abdominal discomfort, suggesting that sensory nerve dysfunction may participate in symptom genesis in some patients with gastroparesis.

A symptom questionnaire, the Gastroparesis Cardinal Symptom Index (GCSI), has been developed and validated in university-based clinical practices for quantifying symptoms in gastroparesis [5]. The GCSI is based on three subscales (postprandial fullness/early satiety, nausea/vomiting, and bloating) and represents a subset of the longer Patient Assessment of Upper Gastrointestinal Disorders-Symptoms (PAGI-SYM) [6].

Evaluation of Patients with Suspected Gastroparesis

A careful history and careful physical examination is an important part of patient evaluation. Symptom onset and progression of the disease with understanding the periods of exacerbations are particularly important. History should include reviewing the patient's medications to help identify and eliminate drugs that can aggravate symptoms. Physical examination may reveal signs of dehydration or malnutrition. The presence of a succussion splash, detected by auscultation over the epigastrium while moving the patient side to side or rapidly palpating the epigastrium, indicates excessive fluid in the stomach from gastroparesis or mechanical gastric outlet obstruction.

Laboratory studies should be performed to identify electrolyte abnormalities such as hypokalemia and metabolic alkalosis, renal insufficiency, anemia, pancreatitis, or thyroid dysfunction. In females with the recent onset of symptoms, a pregnancy test should be obtained. An abdominal obstruction series can be performed to evaluate for mechanical gastric outlet or small bowel obstruction. Most patients will need an EGD or a radiographic upper gastrointestinal series to exclude mechanical obstruction or ulcer disease. The presence of retained food in the stomach after overnight fasting without evidence of mechanical obstruction is suggestive of gastroparesis. Bezoars may be found in severe cases.

The diagnosis of gastroparesis is made when a delay in gastric emptying is present and laboratory studies rule out metabolic causes of symptoms and endoscopic and/or radiographic testing exclude luminal blockage. The classic test for measurement of gastric emptying is scintigraphy. Two new methods are available to measure gastric emptying. First, a pH and pressure recording capsule (SmartPill, Inc., Buffalo, NY), can assess gastric emptying by the acidic gastric residence time of the capsule. Secondly, a ^{13}C-ocanoate breath test (OBT) can be used for measuring gastric emptying, and has been shown to correlate significantly with gastric emptying for solids by scintigraphy. These tests are discussed in depth below.

Gastric Emptying Scintigraphy

Gastric emptying scintigraphy of a solid-phase meal is considered the standard for diagnosis of gastroparesis as it quantifies the emptying of a physiologic caloric meal. Measurement of gastric emptying of solids is more sensitive for detection of gastroparesis as liquid emptying may remain normal even in the presence of advanced disease.

For solid-phase testing, most centers use a ^{99m}Tc sulfur colloid–labeled egg sandwich as the test meal with standard imaging at 0, 1, 2, and 4 h. The radiolabel should be cooked into the meal to ensure radioisotope binding to the solid phase. Scintigraphic assessment of emptying should be extended to at least 2 h after meal ingestion. Even with extension of the scintigraphic study to this length, there may be significant day-to-day variability (up to 20%) in rates of gastric emptying. For shorter durations, the test is less reliable due to larger variations

of normal gastric emptying. Extending scintigraphy to 4 h improves the accuracy in determining the presence of delayed gastric emptying. A 4-h gastric emptying scintigraphy test using radiolabeled EggBeaters meal with jam, toast, and water is advocated by the Society of Nuclear Medicine and the American Neurogastroenterology and Motility Society [7,8].

Emptying of solids typically exhibits a lag phase followed by a prolonged linear emptying phase. A variety of parameters can be calculated from the emptying profile of a radiolabeled meal such as half emptying time and duration of the lag phase. The simplest approach for interpreting a gastric emptying study is to report the percent retention at defined times after meal ingestion usually 2 and 4 h, with normal being less than 60% remaining in the stomach at 2 h and less than 10% remaining at 4 h [7].

Patients should discontinue medications that may affect gastric emptying. For most medications, this will be 48–72 h. Opiate analgesics and anticholinergic agents delay gastric emptying. Prokinetic agents that accelerate emptying may give a falsely normal gastric emptying result. Serotonin receptor antagonists such as ondansetron, which have little effect on gastric emptying, may be given for severe symptoms before performance of gastric scintigraphy. Hyperglycemia (glucose level >270 mg/dL) delays gastric emptying in diabetic patients. It is not unreasonable to defer gastric emptying testing until relative euglycemia is achieved to obtain a reliable determination of emptying parameters in the absence of acute metabolic derangement.

Dual labeling of solids with ^{99m}technetium and liquids with ^{111}indium allows for assessment of gastric emptying of solids and liquids which may be useful for patients after gastric surgery to assess their differential handling by the postsurgical stomach. This will help determine if symptoms result from delayed solid emptying or rapid liquid emptying. Continued imaging of ^{111}indium may be used to assess small bowel transit.

Gastric emptying measures the net output of solids or liquids from the stomach but fails to define the pathophysiologic mechanisms that may contribute to impair gastric emptying. Advances in scintigraphy provide information on fundic and antral abnormalities. Regional gastric emptying can assess intragastric meal distribution and transit from the proximal to distal portions of the stomach. Proximal retention has been described in

GERD, distal retention in functional dyspepsia, and global retention in gastroparesis.

pH and Pressure-Sensing Capsule (SmartPill)

The SmartPill is an ingestible capsule that measures pH, pressure, and temperature using miniaturized wireless sensor technology. The SmartPill capsule is swallowed by the patient and information is recorded as it travels through the gastrointestinal tract. Gastric emptying is determined from the time the SmartPill is swallowed until there is a rapid increase in the pH recorded by the SmartPill, indicating emptying from the acidic stomach to the alkaline duodenum. In addition, the SmartPill capsule characterizes pressure patterns and provides motility indices for the stomach, small intestine, and colon. The gastric residence time of the SmartPill had a high correlation (85%) with the T-90% of gastric emptying scintigraphy, suggesting that the gastric residence time of the SmartPill represents a time near the end of the emptying of a solid meal [9]. A 5-h cut-off value of the SmartPill gastric residence time was best to identify subjects with delayed or normal gastric emptying based on scintigraphy on the day of the test, with sensitivity of 83% and specificity of 83%. The SmartPill GI Monitoring System was recently approved by the United States Food and Drug Administration (FDA) for the assessment of gastric pH, gastric emptying, and total GI transit time.

Breath Testing for Gastric Emptying

Breath tests using the non-radioactive isotope ^{13}C bound to a digestible substance have been validated for measuring gastric emptying [10]. Most commonly, ^{13}C-labeled octanoate, a medium-chain triglyceride, is bound into a solid meal such as a muffin. Other studies have bound ^{13}C to acetate or to proteinaceous algae (*Spirulina*). After ingestion and stomach emptying, ^{13}C-octanoate is absorbed in the small intestine and metabolized to $^{13}CO_2$, which is then expelled from the lungs during respiration. The rate-limiting step is the rate of solid gastric emptying. Thus, octanoate breath testing provides a measure of solid-phase emptying. The octanoate breath test provides reproducible results that correlate with findings on gastric emptying scintigraphy. ^{13}C breath tests do not use ionizing radiation and can be used to test patients in the community or even at the bedside, where gamma camera facilities are not readily available. Breath samples can be

preserved and shipped to a laboratory for analysis. Most octanoate breath testing is performed for clinical research and pharmaceutical studies. The penetrance of this diagnostic modality into clinical practice has been limited.

Treatment of Gastroparesis

The general principles for treating symptomatic gastroparesis are: (i) to correct and prevent fluid, electrolyte, and nutritional deficiencies; (ii) to control symptoms; and (iii) to identify and rectify the underlying cause of gastroparesis, if possible [1,11].

Management of this condition can be particularly challenging. Care of patients generally relies on dietary modification, medications that stimulate gastric motor activity (Table 46.1), and antiemetic drug therapy (Table 46.2) [11,12]. Although in most cases rigorous investigations have not assessed therapeutic responses as a function of symptom severity, a number of basic recommendations can be made (Table 46.3) [11]. For mild symptoms, dietary modifications should be tried. When possible, patients should avoid the use of medications that delay gastric emptying. If needed, low doses of antiemetic or prokinetic medications can be taken on an as-needed basis. Diabetic patients should strive for optimal glycemic control to minimize effects of hyperglycemia on gastric function. For individuals with compensated gastroparesis, treatment recommendations

Table 46.1 Prokinetic medication classes for treatment of gastroparesis.

Class of agent	Presently available	Available under special circumstances
Dopamine D_2 receptor antagonists	Metoclopramide	Domperidone
Motilin receptor agonists	Erythromycin Clarithromycin Azithromycin	
5-HT$_4$ receptor agonists		Cisapride Tegaserod
Muscarinic receptor agonists	Bethanechol	
Acetylcholinesterase inhibitors	Physostigmine Neostigmine	

Table 46.2 Antiemetic therapy for gastroparesis.

Prokinetic agents with antiemetic properties	Metoclopramide (Reglan)
(antagonize dopamine receptors)	Domperidone (Motilium)
Phenothiazine derivatives	Prochlorperazine (Compazine)
(antagonize dopamine receptors in area postrema)	Trimethobenzamide (Tigan)
Antihistamines	Diphenhydramine (Benadryl)
(H_1 receptor antagonists)	Promethazine (Phenergan) Meclizine (Antivert)
Anticholinergic agents	Scopolamine
Antiserotoninergic	Ondansetron (Zofran)
(5-HT_3 receptor antagonists)	Granisetron (Kytril) Dolasetron (Anzemet) Palonosetron (Aloxi)
Substance P/neurokinin-1 receptor antagonists	Aprepitant (Emend)

commonly involve a combination of antiemetic and prokinetic medications given at regularly scheduled intervals to relieve more chronic symptoms of nausea, vomiting, fullness, and bloating. Unfortunately, these agents frequently have no effect on the pain and discomfort which may be associated with gastroparesis. In these patients, measures need to be directed at pain control but these should be measures that do not exacerbate other symptoms of gastroparesis. For patients with severe gastroparesis, care may include enteral nutritional support through a jejunostomy tube and/or other surgical intervention such as gastric electric stimulation.

Dietary Treatment

Increasing the liquid nutrient component of the ingested meal should be emphasized because liquid emptying often is preserved. Fats and fiber tend to decrease gastric emptying; thus, their intake should be minimized. Indigestible fiber and roughage may predispose to bezoar formation. Foods that cannot be reliably chewed into smaller constituency should be avoided. Multiple fre-

Table 46.3 American Neurogastroenterology and Motility Society consensus recommendations for the treatment of gastroparesis. A stepped care approach in a top-down vertical manner is recommended, which is dependent on the severity of gastroparesis. Treatments from different categories (columns) are often used in combination.

Psychological measures	Glycemic control	Nutritional care	Prokinetic medications	Antiemetic therapies	Pain control
Empathy and education	Twice-daily long-acting insulin plus periprandial short-acting insulin	Small, frequent meals, low in fat and fiber	Metoclopramide or erythromycin PRN	Phenothiazine or dopamine receptor antagonist PRN	Acetaminophen or non-steroidal agents
Patient support groups	Insulin pump	Primarily liquid diet Liquid nutrient supplements	Metoclopramide or erythromycin scheduled dosing	Muscarinic receptor antagonist or 5-HT_3 antagonist	Tramadol or propoxyphene
Behavioral or relaxation therapy	Pancreas transplant	Enteral feedings	Domperidone	Tricyclic agents	Tricyclic agents
Hypnosis		Central or peripheral parenteral nutrition short term	Pyloric botulinum toxin	Tetrahydrocannabinol, lorazepam, or alternative therapies Gastric electrical stimulation	Newer antidepressants TCAs, SNRIs Fentanyl patch or methadone Referral for pain specialist Nerve block

Adapted from Abell TL, Bernstein RK, Cutts T, Farrugia G, Forster J, Hasler WL, McCallum RW, Olden KW, Parkman HP, Parrish CR, Pasricha PJ, Prather CM, Soffer EE, Twillman R, Vinik AI. Treatment of gastroparesis: a multidisciplinary review. *Neurogastroenterology and Motility* 2006; **18**: 263–83.
PRN, as needed; TCA, tricyclic antidepressant; SNRI, serotonin–norepinephrine reuptake inhibitor.

quent, but small, meals are often recommended to limit the calorie intake with each meal but to achieve adequate total calories during the day.

Metabolic Control

Diabetic patients with gastroparesis frequently exhibit labile blood glucose concentrations with prolonged periods of significant hyperglycemia. Hyperglycemia itself can delay gastric emptying. Hyperglycemia can also counteract the accelerating effects of prokinetic agents on gastric emptying. Improvement of glucose control increases antral contractility, corrects gastric dysrhythmias, and accelerates emptying. To date, there have been no long-term studies confirming the beneficial effects of maintenance of near euglycemia on gastroparetic symptoms. Nevertheless, the consistent findings of physiologic studies in healthy volunteers and diabetic patients provide a compelling argument to strive for near-normal blood glucose levels in affected diabetic patients [13].

Prokinetic Agents

Current prokinetic agents for treatment include the oral agents metoclopramide (Reglan) and erythromycin (Table 46.1).

Metoclopramide

Metoclopramide (Reglan), a substituted benzamide structurally related to procainamide, exhibits both prokinetic and antiemetic actions. The drug serves as a dopamine receptor antagonist both in the CNS and in the stomach. The prokinetic properties of metoclopramide are limited to the proximal gut. Metoclopramide, with its antinausea and prokinetic actions, is widely used for the treatment of gastroparesis. Metoclopramide provides symptomatic relief and accelerates gastric emptying of solids and liquids in patients with idiopathic, diabetic, and postvagotomy gastroparesis. Metoclopramide is effective for the short-term treatment of gastroparesis for up to several weeks; however, symptomatic improvement does not necessarily accompany improvement in gastric emptying. The long-term utility of metoclopramide has not been proven. Metoclopramide is approved for the treatment of diabetic gastroparesis and for the prevention of postoperative and chemotherapy-induced nausea and vomiting. The usual dosage is 10 mg four times a day. In some patients, rather than using the pill form, liquid metoclopramide is used which might be better tolerated

by patients. Metoclopramide is also available for parenteral use (intravenous or intramuscular). Unfortunately, side effects are relatively common with metoclopramide; it can cause both acute and chronic CNS side effects in some patients. Acute side effects include dystonic reactions resulting from an idiosyncratic reaction. Longer treatment can produce depression or anxiety. Rare cases of tardive dyskinesia have been reported with long-term treatment and the FDA has issued a "black box" warning, which has markedly decreased the use of this agent. If used, the health-care provider should discuss and document these potential risks. These side effects should be discussed with the patient prior to treatment and documented in the patient's medical record.

Erythromycin

The macrolide antibiotic erythromycin exerts prokinetic effects via action on gastroduodenal receptors for motilin, an endogenous peptide responsible for initiation of the phase III migrating motor complex in the upper gut. Clinically, erythromycin has been shown to stimulate gastric emptying in diabetic gastroparesis, idiopathic gastroparesis, and postvagotomy gastroparesis. Erythromycin may be most potent when used intravenously. Limited data exist concerning the clinical efficacy of erythromycin in reducing symptoms of gastroparesis. In studies on oral erythromycin with symptom assessment as a clinical end point, improvement was noted in 43% of patients [11].

Oral administration of erythromycin should be initiated at low doses (e.g., 125 mg three or four times daily). Liquid suspension erythromycin may be preferred because it is rapidly and more reliably absorbed. Intravenous erythromycin (100 mg every 8 h) is used for inpatients hospitalized for severe refractory gastroparesis. Side effects of erythromycin at higher doses include nausea, vomiting, and abdominal pain. Because these symptoms may mimic those of gastroparesis, erythromycin may have a narrow therapeutic window in some patients. Erythromycin may be associated with higher mortality from cardiac disease, especially when combined with agents that inhibit cytochrome P-450, such as calcium channel blockers.

Domperidone

The effects of domperidone on the upper gut are similar to those of metoclopramide, including stimulation of antral contractions and promotion of antroduodenal coordination. Domperidone does not readily cross the blood–brain barrier; therefore, it is much less likely to cause extrapyramidal side effects than metoclopramide. In addition to prokinetic actions in the stomach, domperidone exhibits antiemetic properties via action on the area postrema, a brainstem region with a porous blood–brain barrier. Side effects of domperidone include galactorrhea and amenorrhea.

The FDA has developed a program for physicians who would like to prescribe domperidone for their patients with severe upper GI motility disorders that are refractory to standard therapy even though it is not approved in the USA. Use of this investigational new drug (IND) mechanism for use of domperidone also requires Institutional Review Board (IRB) approval as well as the patient paying for the medication.

Antiemetic Medications

Antiemetic agents are given acutely for symptomatic nausea and vomiting (Table 46.2). The principal classes of drugs that have been used for symptomatic treatment of nausea and vomiting are phenothiazines, antihistamines, anticholinergics, dopamine receptor antagonists, and, more recently, serotonin receptor antagonists. The antiemetic action of phenothiazine compounds appear to be mediated primarily through a central antidopaminergic mechanism in the area postrema of the brain. Commonly used agents include prochlorperazine (Compazine), trimethobenzamide (Tigan), and promethazine (Phenergan).

Serotonin (5-HT-3) receptor antagonists, such as ondansetron (Zofran) and granisetron (Kytril), have been shown to be helpful in treating or preventing chemotherapy-induced nausea and vomiting. The primary site of action of these compounds is probably the chemoreceptor trigger zone, since there is a high density of 5-HT-3 receptors in the area postrema. Ondansetron is now frequently used for nausea and vomiting of a variety of other etiologies. They are best given on an as-needed basis due to their expense.

Psychotropic Medications as Symptom Modulators

Tricyclic antidepressants may have significant benefits in suppressing symptoms in some patients with nausea and vomiting as well as patients with abdominal pain [14]. Doses of tricyclic antidepressants used are lower than those used to treat depression. A reasonable starting dose for a tricyclic drug is 10–25 mg at bedtime. If benefit is not observed in several weeks, doses are increased by 10- to 25-mg increments up to 50–100 mg. Side effects are common with use of tricyclic antidepressants and can interfere with management and lead to a change in medication in 25% of patients. The secondary amines, nortriptyline and desipramine, may have fewer side effects. There are limited data on the use of selective serotonin reuptake inhibitors in gastroparesis or functional dyspepsia.

Pyloric Botulinum Toxin Injection

Gastric emptying is a highly regulated process reflecting the integration of the propulsive forces of proximal fundic tone and distal antral contractions with the functional resistance provided by the pylorus. Manometric studies of patients with diabetic gastroparesis show prolonged periods of increased pyloric tone and phasic contractions, a phenomenon termed pylorospasm. Botulinum toxin is a potent inhibitor of neuromuscular transmission and has been used to treat spastic somatic muscle disorders as well as achalasia. Several open-label studies have tested the effects of pyloric injection of botulinum toxin in small numbers of patients with diabetic and idiopathic gastroparesis and have observed mild improvements in gastric emptying and modest reductions in symptoms for several months. Two double-blind, placebo-controlled studies have been reported that show an improvement in gastric emptying, but no improvement in symptoms compared to placebo [15,16]. Thus, botulinum toxin injection into the pylorus is not a long-term treatment option for gastroparesis.

Gastric Electric Stimulation

Gastric electric stimulation is an emerging treatment for refractory gastroparesis. Currently, it involves an implantable neurostimulator that delivers a high-frequency (12 cpm), low-energy signal with short pulses. With this device, stimulating wires are sutured into the gastric muscle along the greater curvature during laparoscopy or laparotomy. These leads are attached to the electric stimulator, which is positioned in a subcutaneous abdominal pouch. Based on the initial studies that have shown symptom benefit especially in patients with diabetic gastroparesis [17], the gastric electric neurostimulator was granted humanitarian approval from the FDA for the treatment of chronic, refractory nausea and vomiting secondary to idiopathic or diabetic gastroparesis. The main complication of the implantable neurostimulator has been infection, which has necessitated device removal in approximately 5–10% of cases. More recently, a small minority of patients can, at times, have a shocking sensation. Symptoms of nausea and vomiting can improve with stimulation; however abdominal pain often does not. In general, diabetic patients with primary symptoms of nausea and/or vomiting, who are not taking narcotic pain medications and do not have an adequate response to antiemetic and prokinetic medications, appears to be the profile of patients that appear to have a favorable response to gastric electric stimulation [18]. Further investigation is needed to confirm the effectiveness of gastric stimulation in a long-term blinded fashion, which patients are likely to respond, the optimal electrode position, and the optimal stimulation parameters, none of which have been rigorously evaluated to date. Future improvements may include devices that sequentially stimulate the stomach in a peristaltic sequence to promote gastric emptying.

Take-home points

- Diagnosis of a patient with gastroparesis consists of appropriate symptoms, negative endoscopy, and delayed gastric emptying.

- Dietary management, and prokinetic and antiemetic agents are beneficial to treat patients with gastroparesis. Side effects of medications need to be discussed with the patient prior to their use.

- Treatment of refractory gastroparesis involves several options including domperidone, symptom modulators, jejunostomy feeding tubes, and gastric electric stimulation.

- Botulinum toxin injection into the pylorus is not a long-term treatment option for gastroparesis. Although anecdotally it may provide short-term improvement in some patients, recent placebo-controlled studies have not demonstrated a significant clinical improvement of symptoms.

- Gastric electric stimulation is used for refractory gastroparesis. Generally, diabetic patients with refractory symptoms of nausea and vomiting respond best to this treatment.

References

1 Parkman HP, Hasler WL, Fisher RS. American Gastroenterological Association technical review on the diagnosis and treatment of gastroparesis. *Gastroenterology* 2004; **127**: 1592–622.

2 Wang YR, Fisher RS, Parkman HP. Trends of gastroparesis-related hospitalizations in the United States, 1995–2004. *Am J Gastroenterol* 2008; **103**: 313–22.

3 Soykan I, Sivri B, Sarosiek I, *et al.* Demography, clinical characteristics, psychological profiles, treatment and long-term follow-up of patients with gastroparesis. *Dig Dis Sci* 1998; **43**: 2398–404.

4 Stanghellini V, Tosetti C, Paternic A, *et al.* Risk indicators of delayed gastric emptying of solids in patients with functional dyspepsia. *Gastroenterology* 1996; **110**: 1036–42.

5 Revicki DA, Rentz AM, Dubois D, *et al.* Development and validation of a patient-assessed gastroparesis symptom severity measure: the Gastroparesis Cardinal Symptom Index. *Aliment Pharmacol Ther* 2003; **18**: 141–50.

6 Rentz AM, Kahrilas P, Stanghellini V, *et al.* Development and psychometric evaluation of the patient assessment of upper gastrointestinal symptom severity index (PAGI-SYM) in patients with upper gastrointestinal disorders. *Qual Life Res* 2004; **13**: 1737–49.

7 Tougas G, Eaker EY, Abell TL, *et al.* Assessment of gastric emptying using a low fat meal: establishment of international control values. *Am J Gastroenterol* 2000; **95**: 1456–62.

8 Abell TL, Camilleri M, Donohoe K, *et al.* Consensus recommendations for gastric emptying scintigraphy. A joint report of the Society of Nuclear Medicine and the American Neurogastroenterology and Motility Society. *Am J Gastroenterol* 2008; **103**: 753–63.

9 Kuo B, McCallum RW, Koch K, *et al.* Comparison of gastric emptying of a non-digestible capsule to a radiolabeled meal in healthy and gastroparetic subjects. *Aliment Pharmacol Ther* 2008; **27**: 186–96.

10 Bromer MQ, Kantor SN, Wagner DA, *et al.* Simultaneous measurement of gastric emptying with a simple muffin meal using 13C-octanocate breath test and scintigraphy in normal subjects and patients with in dyspeptic symptoms. *Dig Dis Sci* 2002; **47**: 1657–63.

11 Abell TL, Bernstein RK, Cutts T, *et al.* Treatment of Gastroparesis: a multidisciplinary review. *Neurogastroenterol Motil* 2006; **18**: 263–83.

12 Quigley EMM, Hasler W, Parkman HP. AGA technical review on nausea and vomiting. *Gastroenterology* 2001; **120**: 263–86.

13 Camilleri M. Clinical practice—diabetic gastroparesis. *N Engl J Med* 2007; **356**: 820–9.

14 Prakash C, Lustman PJ, Freedland KE, Clouse RE. Tricyclic antidepressants for functional nausea and vomiting: clinical outcome in 37 patients. *Dig Dis Sci* 1998; **43**: 1951–6.

15 Friedenberg FK, Palit A, Parkman HP, *et al.* Botulinum toxin A for the treatment of delayed gastric emptying. *Am J Gastroenterol* 2008; **103**: 416–23.

16 Arts J, Holvoet L, Caenepeel P, *et al.* Clinical trial: a randomized-controlled crossover study of intrapyloric injection of botulinum toxin in gastroparesis. *Aliment Pharmacol Ther* 2007; **26**: 1251–8.

17 Abell T, McCallum R, Hocking M, *et al.* Gastric electrical stimulation for medically refractory gastroparesis. *Gastroenterology* 2003; **125**: 421–8.

18 Maranki JL, Lytes V, Meilahn JE, *et al.* Predictive factors for clinical improvement with Enterra gastric electric stimulation treatment for refractory gastroparesis. *Dig Dis Sci* 2008; **53**: 2072–8.

CHAPTER 47

Non-variceal Upper Gastrointestinal Bleeding

Thomas J. Savides

Division of Gastroenterology, University of California, San Diego, CA, USA

Summary

The most common cause of severe upper gastrointestinal (UGI) bleeding is peptic ulcer disease (gastric and duodenal ulcer), followed by a variety of other etiologies including varices, esophagitis, Mallory–Weiss tear, Cameron erosions, and tumors. A careful history will narrow the differential diagnosis. Medical resuscitation with fluids and transfusions is the most important first step. Urgent endoscopy will diagnose the lesion, and allow endoscopic treatment of lesions at highest risk for rebleeding. Pharmacologic therapy is playing an increasingly important role in the management of peptic ulcer and variceal bleeding. Interventional radiology and surgery are reserved only for rare cases not controlled medically and endoscopically. Improvement in patient outcomes will occur with increased knowledge of risk factors for UGI bleeding, and successful management of acute UGI bleeding with medical and endoscopic therapy.

Case

A 70-year-old man presents with melena and syncope. His past medical history is notable for coronary artery disease and atrial fibrillation. He takes a baby aspirin and warfarin on a daily basis, and 3 weeks ago started ibuprofen for neck pain. On exam he has orthostatic hypotension. His stool is black and guaiac positive. Blood tests reveal hematocrit 25%, mean cell volume (MCV) 82 fL, and international normalized ratio (INR) 3.1. He is admitted and transfused red blood cells and fresh frozen plasma. He is started on intravenous proton pump inhibitor (PPI) medication. Esophagogastrodudenoscopy (EGD) reveals a 15-mm duodenal ulcer with a visible vessel, which is endoscopically treated with epinephrine injection and a hemoclip. Gastric biopsies reveal no *Helicobacter pylori* infection. He is observed for the next 72 h while being switched to an oral PPI and advancing diet. He is discharged home and advised to take long-term PPI medication.

Introduction

Upper gastrointestinal (UGI) bleeding is a common problem in the USA, with an estimated annual hospital-

Practical Gastroenterology and Hepatology: Esophagus and Stomach, 1st edition. Edited by Nicholas J. Talley, Kenneth R. DeVault and David E. Fleischer. © 2010 Blackwell Publishing Ltd.

ization rate of 160 admissions per 100 000 population, with peptic ulcers being the most common lesion [1]. Despite advances in medical therapy, intensive unit care (ICU) care, and endoscopy, the mortality rate remains unchanged over the past 30 years at 5–10%, most likely due to increasing numbers of elderly patients who die from comorbidities related to bleeding. This chapter focuses on severe acute bleeding from the esophagus, stomach, and duodenum that requires hospitalization.

Initial Assessment and Management of UGI Bleeding

There are several important definitions of GI bleeding that are important in the initial assessment of a patient with UGI bleeding (Figure 47.1). Hematemesis includes vomiting large amounts of red blood, which suggests active bleeding, or dark material ("coffee-ground emesis"), which suggests older non-active bleeding. (These specific types of upper gastrointestinal bleeding are discussed further in Chapter 30.) Melena is defined as black tarry stool, which suggests passage of old blood, usually from an UGI source, but possibly from the small bowel or proximal

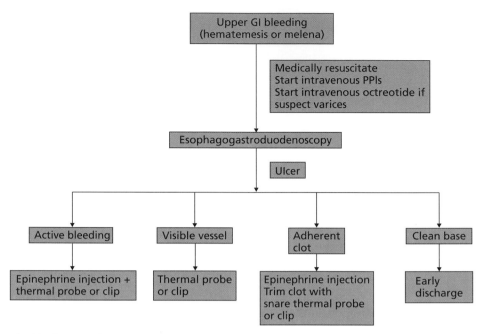

Figure 47.1 Algorithm for approach to upper gastrointestinal (GI) bleeding. PPIs, proton pump inhibitors.

colon. Hematochezia is bright red blood per rectum, and will represent a UGI source only if the patient is also hypotensive due to massive ongoing bleeding.

Initial patient assessment should focus on the history, with attention to a history of gastroesophageal reflux disease (GERD), peptic ulcers, abdominal pain, weight loss, aspirin/non-steroidal antiinflammatory drugs (NSAIDs), alcohol abuse, cirrhosis, and abdominal aortic aneurysm. Physical examination focuses on the presence of orthostatic hypotension, which suggests significant volume depletion, as well as signs of chronic liver disease such as spider angiomas, palmar erythema, gynecomastia, ascites, and splenomegaly. Blood tests should include standard hematology, chemistry, liver, coagulation studies, and crossmatch for blood transfusion.

Nasogastric (NG) tube placement to aspirate and characterize gastric contents can be useful to determine if large amounts of red blood, coffee-grounds, or nonbloody fluid are present. Patients who have witnessed emesis do not need an NG tube for diagnostic purposes, but may need one to clear gastric contents before endoscopy and to minimize aspiration risk.

Initial medical resuscitation is usually performed in the emergency room. Intravenous saline is given to try to keep the systolic blood pressure >100 mmHg and the pulse lower than 100 beats/min. Patients are transfused with packed red blood cells, platelets, and fresh frozen plasma as necessary to ideally keep the hematocrit >24%, platelet count >50 000/mm^3, and prothrombin time <15 s. Patients with ongoing active bleeding (i.e., red blood in NG tube or hypotension) warrant ICU admission and urgent endoscopy, whereas patients with moderate bleeding (melena and resolved hypotension) are admitted to a medical ward or intermediate care unit and undergo semiurgent endoscopy.

Endotracheal intubation should be considered in patients with active, ongoing hematemesis and/or altered mental status in order to prevent aspiration pneumonia. Patients older than 60 years, with chest pain or a history of cardiac problems, should also be evaluated for myocardial infarction with electrocardiograms and serial troponin measurements.

Patients with severe UGI bleeding are usually started on intravenous proton pump inhibitor (PPI) medications before endoscopy. Several studies and meta-analyses have shown that intravenous (IV) PPIs before endoscopy accelerate the resolution of endoscopic stigmata of bleeding ulcers and reduce the need for endoscopic therapy, but do not result in improved clinical outcomes such as decreased transfusions, rebleeding, surgery, or death rates [2,3]. Patients with a strong suspicion for variceal bleeding should also be started on empirical intravenous octreotide because this can reduce rebleeding to rates similar to after endoscopic sclerotherapy [4].

Clinical scoring systems have been developed to try to determine which UGI bleed patients are at highest risk for rebleeding or death. The most commonly used is the Rockall scoring system, which includes clinical as well as endoscopic data [5]. Although important for research studies, the utility of scoring systems is limited in routine clinical practice.

Endoscopy in UGI Bleeding

A large-channel therapeutic upper endoscope should be used to allow for rapid removal of bleed from the stomach and to utilize larger endoscopic hemostasis accessories. Well-trained assistants who are familiar with endoscopic hemostasis devices are critical to successful endoscopic hemostasis. At times it may be worth delaying a procedure in order to utilize assistants who are competent at using accessories in emergency situations. A number of different endoscopic hemostasis devices have been developed over the past 20 years, as described below.

Thermal Contact Probes
These are the mainstay of endoscopic hemostasis. The most commonly used probes are bipolar probes with heat created by current flowing between two intertwined electrodes on the probe tip. These probes can be pressed against the bleeding lesion to physically tamponade the bleeding site, followed by application of the tip of the probe to thermally seal the underlying vessel (coaptive coagulation). Thermal contact probes can seal arteries up to 2 mm. The risks of thermal probes include perforation and inducing more bleeding.

Injection Therapy
This is performed using an endoscopic sclerotherapy needle to inject diluted epinephrine 1:10000 into the submucosa around the bleeding site. The advantages of this are that it is widely available and relatively inexpensive, and can be used in the setting of coagulopathy. In addition, it can be used with less risk of perforation or subsequent thermal burn damage. Injection can also be performed with a sclerosant, such as ethanolamine.

Endoscopic Clips
These are similar to surgical clips in that they apply mechanical pressure to a bleeding site. However, they differ from surgical clips in that they currently do not have as much compressive force and do not have complete apposition of the prongs. Clips have an advantage of not causing thermal injury, but the disadvantage is that they can be challenging to deploy depending on scope position and lesion location.

Band Ligation
This involves aspiration of mucosa/submucosa into the tip of a plastic cap attached to the end of the scope, followed by pulling a tripwire, which rolls a rubber band off the cylinder and over the mucosa/submucosa in the cylinder. The rubber band ligates the lesion, and eventually the banded lesion sloughs off.

Peptic Ulcer Bleeding

Peptic ulcers are the most common source of UGI bleeding. Most ulcers are caused by decreased mucosal defenses due to aspirin/NSAIDs and/or *H. pylori* infection. Resected bleeding ulcers reveal underlying exposed arteries (mean diameter 0.7 mm) or a small clot overlying the bleeding site in the vessel [6].

Poor prognostic factors for bleeding peptic ulcers include the following: age >60 years, comorbid medical illness, orthostatic hypotension, coagulopathy, bleeding onset in the hospital, multiple blood transfusions, red blood in the NG tube, posterior duodenal bulb ulcer, and most importantly endoscopic findings of arterial bleeding or visible vessels.

Endoscopic stigmata of bleeding peptic ulcers provide excellent predictability of the likelihood of rebleeding (Figures 47.2, 47.3, 47.4, and 47.5). Table 47.1 shows that the ulcers at highest risk for rebleeding have active arterial bleeding, a non-bleeding visible vessel, and an adherent clot [7]. The risk of rebleeding is greatest in the first 72 h after presentation.

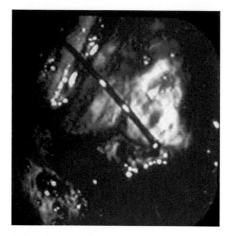

Figure 47.2 Active arterial bleeding peptic ulcer.

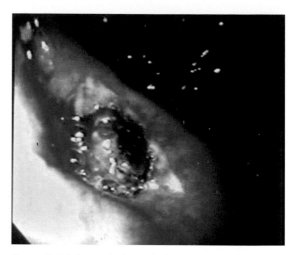

Figure 47.4 Adherent clot in peptic ulcer.

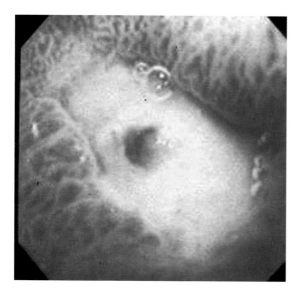

Figure 47.3 Non-bleeding visible vessel in peptic ulcer.

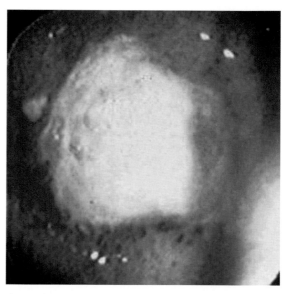

Figure 47.5 Clean-based peptic ulcer.

Active Bleeding and NON-bleeding Visible Vessels

Many well-conducted, randomized controlled trials, meta-analyses, and consensus conferences have confirmed that endoscopic hemostasis with either epinephrine injection or coaptive probe therapy significantly decreases the rate of ulcer rebleeding, the need for urgent surgery, and the mortality in patients with high-risk stigmata such as active bleeding and non-bleeding visible vessels (see Figures 47.2 and 47.3) [8,9]. The rebleeding rates of peptic ulcers with various endoscopic stigmata are shown in Table 47.2. Most of these studies were performed before the widespread use of PPIs, and predominantly used injection therapy, bipolar-probe coagulation therapy, or a combination of injection and probe therapy. In general, for the highest-risk lesions of active bleeding or non-bleeding visible vessels, endoscopic hemostasis alone will decrease the rebleed rate to approximately

Table 47.1 Suspected source of upper gastrointestinal bleeding based on patient history.

Patient history and symptoms	Suspected source of bleeding
Recurrent nose bleeds Prior head and neck malignancy	Nasopharynx
Hemoptysis	Lungs
Heavy alcohol use Gastroesophageal reflux disease Heartburn	Esophagitis
Dysphagia Weight loss	Esophageal cancer
Vomiting Heavy alcohol use	Mallory–Weiss tear
Liver disease Heavy alcohol use	Esophageal or gastric varices/portal hypertensive gastropathy
History of peptic ulcer disease Frequent aspirin or non-steroidal antiinflammatory drug use Epigastric discomfort	Peptic ulcer
Recurrent severe acute unexplained bleeds	Dieulafoy lesion Aortoenteric fistula—primary
Early satiety Weight loss	Gastric cancer
Vomiting Weight loss	Duodenal cancer Gastric outlet obstruction
Prior abdominal aortic aneurysm surgical repair with synthetic graft	Aortoenteric fistula—secondary
Recent ERCP with sphincterotomy	Ampulla of Vater
Recent liver biopsy or cholangiogram	Bile duct system
Pancreatitis, pseudocyst, pancreatogram	Pancreatic duct system

ERCP, endoscopic retrograde cholangiopancreatography.

20–25%. The adjunctive use of PPIs decreases this rate even further, as discussed later.

The most commonly used treatment in the world is injection therapy, because it is widely available, easy to perform, safe, and inexpensive. Therapy with epinephrine alone seems more effective in high doses (13–20 mL) compared with low doses (5–10 mL) [10]. Injection of epinephrine will result in an increase in circulating plasma epinephrine, but rarely causes any clinically significant cardiovascular events. Although epinephrine injection alone is effective compared with placebo, numerous studies and meta-analyses have shown that the addition of a thermal or mechanical modality will further significantly decrease rebleeding, surgery, and

mortality rates [11]. Several studies suggest that the only benefit of adding epinephrine injection to thermal probe therapy occurs in patients with active bleeding, and that there is no benefit in non-bleeding visible vessels [12].

Mechanical endoscopic clips have not been studied as well as injection and thermal probe techniques, but seem to be more effective than epinephrine injection alone, and probably as effective as thermal probe therapy alone. Clips have the advantage of being possible to use in patients with severe coagulopathy with the risk of inducing bleeding. However, the disadvantage of clips is that they can be difficult to deploy, depending on the scope position needed to reach an ulcer.

Table 47.2 Peptic ulcer rebleeding rates.

Endoscopic appearance	Rebleed rate (%)		
	Without endoscopic treatment	After endoscopic treatment alone	After endoscopic treatment + intravenous proton pump inhibitor
Active arterial bleeding	90	25	<10
Visible vessel	50	25	<10
Adherent clot	25	<5	<5
Clean-based ulcer	<5	<5	<5

Adherent Clots

Adherent clots (see Figure 47.4) are blood clots resistant to several minutes of vigorous water irrigation. The rebleeding rate with medical therapy using H_2-receptor antagonists alone is approximately 30% [13]. Randomized controlled studies have shown that endoscopic treatment of adherent clots can decrease the rebleeding rate to <5% [13,14].

Clean-based Ulcers

Patients with clean-based ulcers at endoscopy (see Figure 47.5) have a rebleed rate of <5%. Laine showed that there was no difference between immediate refeeding of these patients versus waiting several days to start eating [15]. Longstreth has shown that selected low-risk compliant patients with mild UGI bleeds and clean-based ulcers can be discharged home safely with significant cost savings [16].

Proton Pump Inhibitors and Peptic Ulcer Bleeding

Gastric pH >6.8 is needed for optimal coagulation and clot formation. Intravenous H_2-receptor antagonists can raise the intragastric pH acutely, but tolerance rapidly develops. PPIs can consistently keep gastric pH >4–6 over a prolonged period. Several studies have found that PPIs initiated after endoscopic diagnosis of peptic ulcer bleeding significantly reduce rebleeding and surgery rates compared with placebo or H_2-receptor blockers [17]. The initiation of PPIs before endoscopy significantly decreases the proportion of patients with stigmata of a recent bleed (i.e., visible vessels) and a need for endoscopic hemostasis, but does not reduce mortality, rebleeding, or surgery risks compared with H_2-receptor blockers or placebo [2,3]. The effects of PPIs are more pronounced in Asian compared with non-Asian populations.

H. pylori Testing

Falsely negative histology for *H pylori*, as well as falsely negative rapid urease, urea breath test, and stool antigen testing, may occur in the setting of acute ulcer bleeding. If infection is not detected, it is important to repeat the evaluation at a later date to confirm the initial result.

Rebleeding after Peptic Ulcer Hemostasis

After successful endoscopic hemostasis and with the use of PPIs, the risk of rebleeding is <10% [18]. In the event of rebleeding, a second endoscopy should be performed rather than surgery, because the outcomes are generally similar with fewer complications. Patients who fail a second attempt at endoscopic hemostasis should undergo either angiography with embolization or surgery.

Variceal Bleeding

Esophageal variceal bleeding is the second most common cause of severe UGI bleeding after peptic ulcers. Variceal bleeding is a manifestation of cirrhosis due to endstage liver disease, with an estimated 1-year survival rate of 50%, and most deaths within the first 2 weeks of the bleed [19]. Patients can bleed from esophageal or gastric varices. Medical management of patients with variceal bleeding includes intravenous octreotide, which causes selective splanchnic vasoconstriction. A meta-analysis suggested that octreotide is as good as endoscopic sclerotherapy for controlling variceal bleeding with fewer adverse events [20]. Patients with variceal bleeding should receive antibiotics, because up to 20% have bacterial infections at admission and antibiotics decrease bacterial infections and mortality [21].

Endoscopic hemostasis was initially performed most commonly with injection of sclerosants (i.e., ethanolamine), but this has mostly been replaced using rubber band ligation of varices, which has a similar acute hemostasis rate of 85% and a rebleed rate of 30%, but fewer local complications such as esophageal strictures [22]. Gastric varices are much more difficult to treat, and the most successful endoscopic therapy is injection of cyanoacrylate glue, but this is not available in the USA as a result of risks of embolization as well as scope damage.

Portosystemic shunts, in which portal pressure is reduced by bypassing the cirrhotic liver with a shunt between the portal and the hepatic veins, are very effective in stopping bleeding and reducing rebleeding. Initially this was done surgically, but this has mostly been replaced by interventional radiologically placed transjugular intrahepatic portosystemic shunts (TIPSs), in which a percutaneously placed, self-expanding, metal stent is placed between the hepatic and portal veins. A TIPS is more effective than endoscopic therapy for preventing variceal bleeding, but it has a slightly higher rate of hepatic encephalopathy and requires periodic checks or revisions to maintain stent patency.

Esophagitis

Patients with severe erosive esophagitis can present with UGI bleeding. Risk factors include alcohol abuse, cirrhosis, and anticoagulant use. This is treated with PPIs. Endoscopy is needed for diagnosis, but is rarely needed for therapy. However, all patients with severe erosive esophagitis should undergo repeat EGD 12 weeks after 12 weeks of daily PPI therapy in order to make sure that there has been complete healing and there is no underlying Barrett esophagus or malignancy.

Stress Ulcers

Stress ulcers occur in the UGI tract of severely ill patients, most likely due to a combination of decreased mucosal protection and mucosal ischemia. They usually occur in the stomach or duodenum. Bleeding due to ICU stress ulcers occurs in 1.5% of ICU patients. Patients with the risk factors of coagulopathy or on mechanical intubation for >48 h have a risk of clinically significant bleeding of 3.7% compared with 0.1% without these risk factors [23]. Intravenous H_2-receptor blockers have been shown to decrease the risk of bleeding in these high-risk ICU patients compared with placebo. PPIs are as good as or better than intravenous H_2-receptor blockers at preventing stress ulcers in ICU patients. A potential risk of prophylactic acid suppression in ICU patients is that decreased gastric pH may allow bacteria to grow in the stomach, which can then be aspirated and cause ventilator-associated pneumonia.

Generally, patients with bleeding stress ulcers should be supported medically, and these ulcers will heal as the patient's overall medical status improves. These lesions tend to have high rebleeding rates, and do not seem to respond as well to endoscopic therapy as peptic ulcers that start to bleed before hospitalization; they are better treated with clips rather than thermal probes which can cause perforation of the non-fibrotic ulcer base [24].

Dieulafoy Lesion

A Dieulafoy lesion (Figure 47.6) is a large (1–3 mm), aberrant, submucosal artery that protrudes through the mucosa but is not associated with ulceration. It can occur anywhere in the GI tract, although usually within the proximal stomach. The etiology is unknown, but may be congenital. Dieulafoy lesions can be difficult to identify due to intermittent bleeding. They are usually found

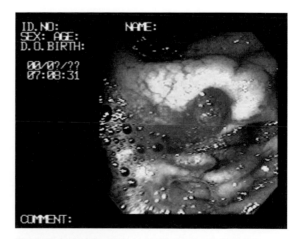

Figure 47.6 Dieulafoy lesion in proximal stomach. Note the bleeding site without adjacent ulceration or mass.

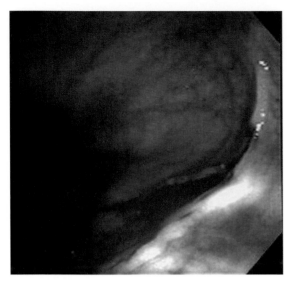

Figure 47.7 Mallory–Weiss tear at gastroesophageal junction.

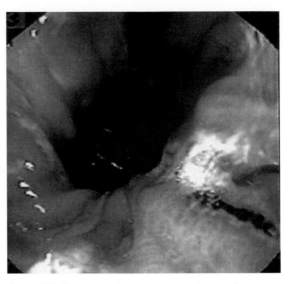

Figure 47.8 Cameron erosions due to mucosal trauma from a hiatus hernia pinch.

when actively bleeding, or in the setting of blood in the stomach and a protruding vessel. They can be successfully treated endoscopically with injection, thermal probes, clips, or band ligation. Although endoscopic hemostasis is usually successful and has low reported rebleeding risks, it is prudent to mark the area around a Dieulafoy lesion with a permanent endoscopic tattoo in case rebleeding occurs in the future that requires endoscopy or surgery.

Mallory–Weiss Tear

Mallory–Weiss tears (Figure 47.7) are mucosal lacerations that occur at the gastroesophageal junction and generally extend distally into a hiatus hernia. Patients generally present with hematemesis or coffee-ground emesis. Typically there is a history of antecedent non-bloody vomiting or heavy alcohol use. Endoscopy can be used to treat the actively bleeding tears with epinephrine injection, thermal probe, or clips. Most tears are mild, and will heal without treatment in less than 48 h. Patients do not need long-term PPI treatment. Those patients who present with Mallory–Weiss tear and are also found to have esophageal varices should have therapy directed toward the varices with band ligation or sclerotherapy.

Cameron Erosions

Cameron erosions (Figure 47.8) are scattered linear erosions or ulcers located circumferentially in the proximal stomach at a hiatus hernia pinch. They are caused by mechanical mucosal trauma from the hiatus hernia compression. Although they can present as acute overt bleeding, they are more commonly a source of obscure bleeding with iron deficiency anemia. Treatment is usually satisfactory with daily oral PPIs, but may need surgical correction of the hernia.

UGI Malignancy

Malignancy accounts for 1% of severe UGI bleeds, from an esophageal, gastric, or duodenal cancer. Endoscopic hemostasis can be used to temporarily control bleeding, but long-term management requires medical or surgical oncologic treatment of the tumor. Angiography should be considered for patients with acute ongoing UGI tumor bleeding that cannot be controlled endoscopically.

Gastric Antral Vascular Ectasia

Gastric antral vascular ectasia (GAVE; also known of "watermelon stomach") is characterized by rows of ectatic mucosal blood vessels that radiate from the pylorus proximally into the antrum. The etiology is unknown, but may represent mucosal trauma associated with antral contraction waves. It has been associated with older age, cirrhosis, chronic renal insufficiency, and systemic sclerosis. Endoscopic thermal therapy can generally control the bleeding, although several sessions may be required. Rarely surgical antrectomy may be warranted to control bleeding.

Portal Hypertensive Gastropathy

Portal hypertensive gastropathy is characterized by a mosaic or snake-skin appearance of the proximal gastric body mucosa, due to high-pressure gastropathy caused by portal hypertension. Patients usually present with chronic blood loss, but can have acute bleeding. Treatment is toward reducing portal pressure, either medically with β-blockers or with TIPS. Generally, there is no endoscopic role for treatment.

Hemobilia

Bleeding from the bile duct that exits the ampulla into the duodenum is usually iatrogenic, such as after a percutaneous liver biopsy or recent biliary endoscopic retrograde cholangiopancreatography (ERCP), but can also occur from hepatocellular carcinoma, cholangiocarcinoma, or biliary parasites. Patients often present with the combination of GI bleeding and increasing liver tests. Bleeding is usually self-limited, but if ongoing will generally be managed with angiographic embolization.

Hemosuccus Pancreaticus

Hemosuccus pancreaticus is bleeding from the pancreatic duct out of the ampulla and into the duodenum. This is best visualized with a side-viewing duodenoscope. It can occur in the setting of acute pancreatitis, chronic pancreatitis, pancreatic pseudocyst, pancreatic cancer, recent ERCP with pancreatic duct manipulation, or splenic artery aneurysm rupture in the pancreatic duct. Computed tomography (CT) can demonstrate pancre-

atic pathology if previously unsuspected. Management of ongoing bleeding is done with angiographic embolization or surgery.

Postsphincterotomy Bleeding

Post-ERCP sphincterotomy bleeding occurs in approximately 2% of patients [25]. Risk factors include coagulopathy, anticoagulation, portal hypertension, renal failure, intraprocedure bleeding, and type and length of sphincterotomy. Successful hemostasis of postsphincterotomy bleeding is usually achieved with endoscopic methods, such as injection of epinephrine, hemoclips, or bipolar probe coagulation. Rarely angiographic embolization is needed.

Aortoenteric Fistula

Aortoenteric fistulas can be primary (new) or secondary (related to implanted graft). A primary aortoenteric fistula is a communication between the native abdominal aorta (usually an atherosclerotic abdominal aortic aneurysm) and the third portion of the duodenum [26]. Often there will be a self-limited "herald bleed" hours to months before a more exsanguinating bleed. Occasionally the diagnosis can be suspected by palpating a pulsatile abdominal mass. The endoscopic diagnosis can be difficult if not actively bleeding and if not suspected. An abdominal CT scan showing an aneurysm suggests the diagnosis [27].

Secondary aortoenteric fistulas usually occur between the small intestine and an infected abdominal aortic aneurysm graft or stent. The fistula usually occurs between the third part of the duodenum and the proximal aspect of the graft, but may occur elsewhere in the GI tract as well. Fistulas usually form between 3 and 5 years after graft placement, although they have been reported sooner or later than that. Patients also often develop a subsequent "herald bleed" which is usually mild and self-limited, but can be intermittent [28]. A secondary fistula can also occur between the third part of the duodenum and an endovascular stent, in which the fistula can occur as a result of pressure from the graft against the duodenum, infection of the stent, or possibly expansion of the native aneurysm [29].

Patients with an acute UGI bleed and a history of an aortic aneurysm repair should have an urgent CT scan, EGD to evaluate the third part of the duodenum for any compression or blood, as well as to rule out any other bleeding sources, and a vascular surgery consultation. CT may show inflammation around the graft. Surgical treatment is required, during which the infected graft is removed. There is no role for therapeutic endoscopy in management of bleeding from aortoenteric fistulas.

Angiomas

Angiomas are occasional causes of UGI bleeding, but usually occur as part of GAVE syndrome, or are found in either the mid-distal small intestine or the right colon. If found in the UGI tract, they can generally be treated with multipolar-probe endoscopic hemostasis.

Take-home points

- The etiology of UGI bleeding can be suspected by taking a good history.
- Peptic ulcers are the most common cause of severe UGI bleeding.
- Endoscopic appearance of bleeding ulcers helps to predict the rebleeding rate.
- Endoscopic hemostasis can reduce the rebleed rate from peptic ulcers.
- PPIs reduce rebleeding rates after endoscopic hemostasis.

References

1 Lewis JD, Bilker WB, Brensinger C, Farrar JT, Strom BL. Hospitalization and mortality rates from peptic ulcer disease and GI bleeding in the 1990s: relationship to sales of non-steroidal anti-inflammatory drugs and acid suppression medications. *Am J Gastroenterol* 2002; **97**: 2540–9.

2 Dorward S, Sreedharan A, Leontiadis GI, Howden CW, Moayyedi P, Forman D. Proton pump inhibitor treatment initiated prior to endoscopic diagnosis in upper gastrointestinal bleeding. *Cochrane Database Syst Rev* 2006; (4): CD005415.

3 Lau JY, Leung WK, Wu JC, *et al.* Omeprazole before endoscopy in patients with gastrointestinal bleeding. *N Engl J Med* 2007; **356**: 1631–40.

4 Yan BM, Lee SS. Emergency management of bleeding esophageal varices: drugs, bands or sleep? *Can J Gastroenterol* 2006; **20**: 165–70.

5 Rockall TA, Logan RF, Devlin HB, Northfield TC. Risk assessment after acute upper gastrointestinal haemorrhage. *Gut* 1996; **38**: 316–21.

6 Swain CP, Storey DW, Bown SG, *et al.* Nature of the bleeding vessel in recurrently bleeding gastric ulcers. *Gastroenterology* 1986; **90**: 595–608.

7 Gralnek IM, Barkun AN, Bardou M. Management of acute bleeding from a peptic ulcer. *N Engl J Med* 2008; **359**: 928–37.

8 Barkun A, Bardou M, Marshall JK. Consensus recommendations for managing patients with nonvariceal upper gastrointestinal bleeding. *Ann Intern Med* 2003; **139**: 843–57.

9 Adler DG, Leighton JA, Davila RE, *et al.* ASGE guideline: The role of endoscopy in acute non-variceal upper-GI hemorrhage. *Gastrointest Endosc* 2004; **60**: 497–504.

10 Lin HJ, Hsieh YH, Tseng GY, Perng CL, Chang FY, Lee SD. A prospective, randomized trial of large- versus small-volume endoscopic injection of epinephrine for peptic ulcer bleeding. *Gastrointest Endosc* 2002; **55**: 615–19.

11 Vergara M, Calvet X, Gisbert JP. Epinephrine injection versus epinephrine injection and a second endoscopic method in high risk bleeding ulcers. *Cochrane Database Syst Rev* 2007; (2): CD005584.

12 Chung SS, Lau JY, Sung JJ, *et al.* Randomised comparison between adrenaline injection alone and adrenaline injection plus heat probe treatment for actively bleeding ulcers. *BMJ* 1997; **314**: 1307–11.

13 Jensen DM, Kovacs TO, Jutabha R, *et al.* Randomized trial of medical or endoscopic therapy to prevent recurrent ulcer hemorrhage in patients with adherent clots. *Gastroenterology* 2002; **123**: 407–13.

14 Bleau BL, Gostout CJ, Sherman KE, *et al.* Recurrent bleeding from peptic ulcer associated with adherent clot: a randomized study comparing endoscopic treatment with medical therapy. *Gastrointest Endosc* 2002; **56**: 1–6.

15 Laine L, Cohen H, Brodhead J, Cantor D, Garcia F, Mosquera M. Prospective evaluation of immediate versus delayed refeeding and prognostic value of endoscopy in patients with upper gastrointestinal hemorrhage. *Gastroenterology* 1992; **102**: 314–16.

16 Longstreth GF, Feitelberg SP. Successful outpatient management of acute upper gastrointestinal hemorrhage: use of practice guidelines in a large patient series. *Gastrointest Endosc* 1998; **47**: 219–22.

17 Leontiadis GI, Sharma VK, Howden CW. Proton pump inhibitor treatment for acute peptic ulcer bleeding. *Cochrane Database Syst Rev* 2006; (1): CD002094.

18 Lau JY, Sung JJ, Lee KK, *et al*. Effect of intravenous omeprazole on recurrent bleeding after endoscopic treatment of bleeding peptic ulcers. *N Engl J Med* 2000; **343**: 310–16.

19 Graham DY, Smith JL. The course of patients after variceal hemorrhage. *Gastroenterology* 1981; **80**: 800–9.

20 D'Amico G, Pietrosi G, Tarantino I, Pagliaro L. Emergency sclerotherapy versus vasoactive drugs for variceal bleeding in cirrhosis: a Cochrane meta-analysis. *Gastroenterology* 2003; **124**: 1277–91.

21 Soares-Weiser K, Brezis M, Tur-Kaspa R, Paul M, Yahav J, Leibovici L. Antibiotic prophylaxis of bacterial infections in cirrhotic inpatients: a meta-analysis of randomized controlled trials. *Scand J Gastroenterol* 2003; **38**: 193–200.

22 Laine L, el Newihi HM, Migikovsky B, Sloane R, Garcia F. Endoscopic ligation compared with sclerotherapy for the treatment of bleeding esophageal varices. *Ann Intern Med* 1993; **119**: 1–7.

23 Cook DJ, Fuller HD, Guyatt GH, *et al*. Risk factors for gastrointestinal bleeding in critically ill patients. Canadian Critical Care Trials Group. *N Engl J Med* 1994; **330**: 377–81.

24 Jensen DM, Machicado GA, Kovacs TOG, *et al*. Current treatment and outcome of patients with bleeding "stress ulcers" (abstract). *Gastroenterology* 1988; **94**: A208.

25 Freeman ML, Nelson DB, Sherman S, *et al*. Complications of endoscopic biliary sphincterotomy. *N Engl J Med* 1996; **335**: 909–18.

26 Ihama Y, Miyazaki T, Fuke C, *et al*. An autopsy case of a primary aortoenteric fistula: A pitfall of the endoscopic diagnosis. *World J Gastroenterol* 2008; **14**: 4701–4.

27 Hagspiel KD, Turba UC, Bozlar U, *et al*. Diagnosis of aortoenteric fistulas with CT angiography. *J Vasc Interv Radiol* 2007; **18**: 497–504.

28 Odemis B, Basar O, Ertugrul I, *et al*. Detection of an aortoenteric fistula in a patient with intermittent bleeding. *Nat Clin Pract Gastroenterol Hepatol* 2008; **5**: 226–30.

29 Bergqvist D, Bjorck M, Nyman R. Secondary aortoenteric fistula after endovascular aortic interventions: a systematic literature review. *J Vasc Interv Radiol* 2008; **19**(2 Pt 1): 163–5.

CHAPTER 48

Gastric Adenocarcinomas

Kazuki Sumiyama[1] and Hisao Tajiri[2]

[1] Department of Endoscopy, The Jikei University School of Medicine, Minato-ku, Tokyo, Japan
[2] Division of Gastroenterology and Hepatology, Department of Internal Medicine, The Jikei University School of Medicine, Minato-ku, Tokyo, Japan

Summary

Gastric cancer is the second most common cause of cancer mortality worldwide after lung cancer, and 90% of cases are histologically confirmed as adenocarcinoma. Surgery is the sole standard treatment option for the therapeutic management for gastric cancer. Overall survival remains dismal but has steadily improved as a result of innovation in various therapeutic options, such as chemotherapy and endoscopic intervention.

Case

A 58-year-old man complained of newly developed non-specific dyspepsia. Blood tests revealed mild iron-deficiency anemia. Prompt endoscopy detected a tumor with ulceration in the lower body of the stomach. Biopsies from the tumor at the initial endoscopic study revealed intestinal-type adenocarcinoma. Multidetector row computed tomography (MDCT) showed a thickened gastric wall, regional lymph node swelling, and no distant metastasis. Endoscopic ultrasonography (EUS) confirmed the absence of serosal invasion of the tumor. Distal subtotal gastrectomy with a more extensive lymphadenectomy (D2) was performed with curative intent. The disease was staged as stage II (T2N1M0) from the results of the surgery. Although radical surgical excision of the tumor was successful, chemoradiation therapy was performed to minimize the chance of recurrence.

Definition and Epidemiology

Gastric cancer is the fourth most common cancer and in 2002 was the second most common cause of cancer mortality after lung cancer worldwide [1]: 90% of gastric cancers are histologically confirmed as adenocarcinoma. Fortunately, the incidence of gastric adenocarcinoma

Practical Gastroenterology and Hepatology: Esophagus and Stomach, 1st edition. Edited by Nicholas J. Talley, Kenneth R. DeVault and David E. Fleischer. © 2010 Blackwell Publishing Ltd.

has diminished markedly in the USA and other economically developed countries. From the 1930s gastric cancer was ranked first in men and third in women as the leading cause of cancer-related death, even in the USA. Although gastric cancer has recently fallen to seventh as the cause of cancer-related death in the USA, approximately 21 260 cases were newly diagnosed with gastric cancer and 13 940 patients died of this disease in 2007 [2].

From a global viewpoint, there are significant geographic variations in the incidence of gastric adenocarcinoma [3]. Two-thirds of gastric adenocarcinomas occur in economically less developed countries. Also, gastric adenocarcinoma remains one of the most frequent gastrointestinal cancers in eastern Asian. Japan has the highest global gastric cancer incidence rate—the incidence being about eightfold higher than in the USA. Even within individual countries, a similar diversity in the incidence rates of gastric cancer can be observed. Ethnic populations in the USA have a higher risk of gastric cancer than non-Hispanic white Americans, e.g., African Americans and Asian Americans/Pacific Islanders have a mortality rate from gastric cancer that is approximately twice that for non-Hispanic white Americans. This racial variation may be partially explained by differences in the socioeconomic background of the groups. Several studies have demonstrated a link between the incidence of gastric cancer and socioeconomic status—a higher incidence rate was associated with lower socioeconomic levels. In addition, the high gastric adenocarcinoma incidence trend in Asian populations appears to reflect the same causative factors associated with historically high incidence rates, including a high infection rate with *Helicobacter pylori* in Asia. The incidence of gastric adenocarcinoma in migrant populations from regions associated with a high incidence has slowly declined in subsequent generations to approximate the incidence associated with the host country [4].

Despite the marked reduction in the total gastric cancer incidence, the incidence of adenocarcinoma of the proximal stomach and the esophagogastric junction has been rising in the last three decades. Both cancer types share etiologic backgrounds including gastroesophageal reflux disease (GERD), Barrett esophagus, and obesity, which have been generically problematic in economically developed countries [5].

The risk of gastric cancer is 1.8–2.0 times higher in men than in women. The median age of diagnosis for gastric cancers in the USA from 2000 to 2004 was 71 years (Surveillance Epidemiology and End Results Program (SEER) of the National Cancer Institute).

Pathophysiology

Gastric adenocarcinoma can be subdivided into two pathologic subtypes: intestinal and diffuse. There are distinct differences in etiology and prognosis between the two subtypes among patients from different backgrounds [6]. The intestinal-type cancer has intestinal gland-like tubular structures and develops with a multistep cancerization process similar to the adenoma–carcinoma sequence in colon cancer (Figure 48.1). This type of gastric adenocarcinoma is the predominant pathologic type in high incidence countries and is more common in men than women. Also, the incidence of intestinal-type gastric cancer progressively increases with age at a higher rate than the diffuse-type cancer. By comparison, the diffuse-type cancer is more poorly differentiated with a lack of gland structures, is more common in women than men, frequently develops in younger patients, and is associated with a worse prognosis.

Gastric cancers can also be divided into early and advanced stages. Early stage cancer is defined as a lesion without muscular layer involvement, regardless of lymph node metastasis.

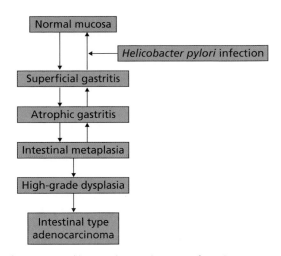

Figure 48.1 Multistep carcinogenesis process of gastric adenocarcinoma. The bidirectional arrows refer to processes that are potentially reversible.

Environmental Risk Factors

Helicobacter pylori

In 1994, the International Agency for Research on Cancer (IARC) classified *H. pylori* as a group I (definite) carcinogenic agent for gastric cancer, based on evidence from a series of large-scale epidemiologic studies. The prevalence of *H. pylori* infection is now about 30% in the USA [7] and economically developing countries, and can rise to up to 80% in children and more than 90% for adults [8]. Pathogenesis of *H. pylori* infection on gastric cancer development can vary according to anatomic location. A meta-analysis of 12 prospective cohort studies demonstrated that *H. pylori* infection is a risk factor only for non-proximal cancer, not for proximal cancer (odds ratio (OR) 2.97, 95% confidence interval (CI) 2.34–3.77) [9]. There was no such significant difference in prevalence of *H. pylori* infection between histologic subtypes or between the intestinal- and diffuse-type gastric cancers. In the intestinal-type cancer, there is a theoretical explanation of the cancer pathway. Correa and colleagues suggest a model in which a cumulative process of precancerous change leads to the development of intestinal-type gastric cancer (see Figure 48.1). This cancer pathway is initiated by superficial gastritis triggered by chronic *H. pylori* infection. Although it is difficult to verify this model in humans, the process has been reproduced in animal experiments using rodent models [10–12].

It is recognized that *H. pylori*-induced atrophic gastritis with suppressed acid secretion reduces the risk of GERD. As expected, an inverse relationship has been reported between *H. pylori* infection and the development of proximal gastric and esophageal adenocarcinomas. However, controversy still exists about the preventive effect of *H. pylori* infection against esophagitis and its carcinogenic sequelae. Several studies reported that eradication of *H. pylori* did not increase the risk of esophagitis, proximal gastric, or esophageal adenocarcinoma [4].

Dietary Factors

Various dietary factors have been postulated as risk factors for gastric cancer development. As previously described, the incidence of gastric cancer has declined in economically developed countries. This downward trend in the rate of gastric cancer may be due in part to the widespread use of refrigeration of food, and the concomitant increase in the intake of fresh fruit and vegetables as an alternative to reliance on food preserved by pickling and salting [13–15].

Vitamin C may be one of the most important protective nutrients associated with the influence of diet on gastric cancer risk. A case–control study demonstrated that a higher intake of vitamin C significantly reduced the risk of gastric cancer development [16]. However, a large meta-analysis, which included 20 randomized trials, 8 of which focused on vitamin C, concluded that there is no convincing evidence of a protective effect for antioxidant supplements, including vitamin C, against the development of gastric cancer or other gastrointestinal cancers [17]. Moreover, this study cautioned that antioxidant supplement intake may increase overall mortality.

Salt and *N*-nitroso compounds, frequently used as a food preservative, have consistently been implicated as carcinogenic agents in gastric cancer development. Case–control studies demonstrated that a high-salt diet was associated with an increased risk of gastric cancer [13,17,18]. Although *N*-nitroso compounds caused gastric cancer in animal models [19], results of clinical studies remain conflicting [20–22].

Genetic Predisposition

Similar to other malignancies, heredity plays an important role in the development of gastric cancer. Approximately 10–15% of gastric cancers arise in individuals with a family history [23]. Individuals with a first-degree relative with a history of gastric cancer have a two- to threefold increased risk [24,25]. Hereditary diffuse gastric cancer (HDGC) syndrome is inherited in an autosomal dominant pattern. Many patients with HDGC are diagnosed before age 35 years (the average age at diagnosis is 38 years of age). The histologic types of HDGC are diffuse type and/or signet ring cell, and they commonly appear as linitis plastica. An increased risk of gastric cancer is also identified in the other dominantly inherited cancer predisposition syndromes such as familial adenomatous polyposis, Lynch syndrome, and Peutz–Jeghers syndrome.

Smoking

Smoking has been consistently demonstrated as an independent risk factor for gastric cancer. There is a significant dose-dependent relationship between cigarette smoking and gastric cancer risk [26–28].

Clinical Features

The vast majority of gastric adenocarcinomas without significant muscular layer invasion are asymptomatic. Weight loss and abdominal pain are the most common symptoms of more advanced gastric cancer. Dysphagia, melena, anemia, anorexia, and other non-specific dyspeptic symptoms are also frequently observed [29]. In most cases, these symptoms indicate advanced disease and are therefore not helpful in the detection of curable disease or improvement of survival [30]. The appearance of symptoms may vary according to the anatomic location of the tumor. Tumors involving the cardiac antrum tend to cause dysphagia whereas those affecting the pylorus may cause gastric outlet obstruction [31].

Gastric cancers can metastasize hematogenously to the liver, lung, and other solid organs. Some common distant metastatic sites for gastric cancer include the Sister Mary Joseph nodule (umbilicus), Krukenberg tumor (ovary), Virchow node (left supraclavicular lymph node), and Blumer shelf (pouch of Douglas). The existence of these distant metastatic lesions leads to difficulty in curative surgical excision of gastric cancer.

Diagnosis

A final diagnosis of gastric adenocarcinoma should be made by histologic confirmation with endoscopic or surgical tissue sampling. The American Gastroenterological Association (AGA) recommended prompt endoscopic examination for individuals with new onset of dyspepsia after the age of 55 years, and in patients before the age of 55 with "alarm symptoms" that include unintended weight loss, gastrointestinal bleeding, progressive dysphagia, odynophagia, unexplained iron-deficiency anemia, persistent vomiting, palpable mass or lymphadenopathy, and jaundice. A younger age cutoff of 45 or 50 years may be recommended for Asian, Hispanic, or African American individuals [32].

Differential Diagnosis

In the USA, 80% of patients diagnosed with gastric cancer have advanced disease. More than half of advanced gastric cancers are associated with ulceration and may mimic benign peptic ulcers at initial endoscopy (Figure 48.2). The macroscopic appearance of ulcerated gastric cancers has some discriminatory characteristics to distinguish this cancer from benign peptic ulcers, including being relatively larger, poorly marginated tumors with irregular, heaped-up, overhanging edges, with the level of the ulcer floor protruding into the gastric lumen and surrounded by irregularly converging folds with a nodular surface (Figure 48.2a). Multiple biopsies should be taken from the ulcer margin to optimize tissue acquisition, because the center of the ulcer is usually covered with necrotic tissue and a tumor can be covered by normal mucosa. Biopsies should also be taken from ulcer scars because some malignant gastric ulcers can heal

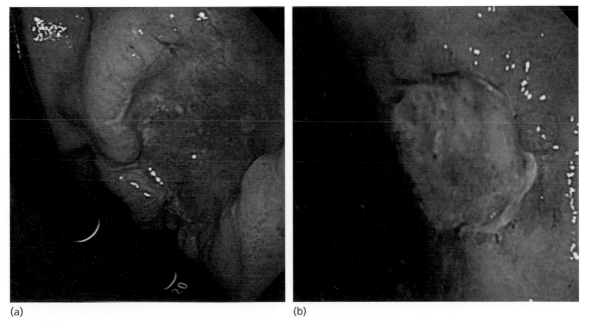

(a)   (b)

Figure 48.2 Endoscopic appearance of an advanced gastric adenocarcinoma with (a) ulceration and (b) a benign peptic ulcer. (a) A large, poorly marginated, malignant ulcer surrounded by irregular heaped-up overhanging edges—the level of the ulcer floor protruding into the gastric lumen. (b) A round benign ulcer marginated with clear and sharp edges—the ulcer floor distinctly depressed from the level of the surrounding normal mucosa.

partially. A single biopsy sample provides a sensitivity of 70% in detecting gastric cancer, whereas eight biopsies improve the sensitivity up to more than 99% [33].

Linitis plastica is a diffusely infiltrating gastric cancer that does not form a discrete luminal mass. In linitis plastica cases, the appearance of the stomach is similar to a "leather bottle." The gastric wall is markedly thickened and less elastic due to cancer cell infiltration of all layers of the gastric wall. Endoscopic studies show that the stomach does not fully distend in linitis plastic cases, despite air insufflation.

Staging

Accurate staging is essential to determine the appropriate therapeutic strategy and to predict the prognosis. The American Joint Committee on Cancer (AJCC) has designated gastric cancer staging using the TNM (tumor, node, metastasis) classification (Table 48.1). For T staging, EUS is useful to evaluate invasion depth within the gastric wall, including serosal involvement. Recent

Table 48.1 TNM classification for gastric cancer designated by the American Joint Committee on Cancer.

Stage	T	N	M
0	Tis	N0	M0
IA	T1	N0	M0
IB	T1	N1	M0
	T2a/b	N0	M0
II	T1	N2	M0
	T2a/b	N1	M0
	T3	N0	M0
IIIA	T2a/b	N2	M0
	T3	N1	M0
	T4	N0	M0
IIIB	T3	N2	M0
VI	T4	N1–3	M0
	T1–3	N3	M0
	Any T	Any N	M1

T, depth of tumor invasion, N, lymph node involvement, M, distant metastasis—yes or no.
Reproduced from the American Joint Committee on Cancer with permission, Chicago, IL. The original source for this material is the American Joint Committee on Cancer [34].

advances in MDCT and magnetic resonance imaging (MRI) have achieved T-staging quality comparable to EUS by using contrast agents. Furthermore, MDCT and MRI allow M and N staging from the same image [35] (see Video 19). Laparoscopy with peritoneal lavage for cytology may be recommended for the preoperative detection of peritoneal metastasis, especially in T3–4 cancers.

For early stage cancers, morphologic staging in addition to TNM staging may help to predict the prognosis of the disease and the curability of the treatment before endoscopic treatment (Figure 48.3) [36]. A flow chart for managing patients with gastric cancer according to stage of disease is shown in Figure 48.4.

Screening

In Japan, mass screening with a standardized double-contrast barium technique has been practiced since the 1960s and many private practices provide ready access to endoscopy for screening. This nationwide screening program in Japan affords great benefit in survival from gastric cancer, which is solely and exclusively high (52%) compared with other regions (21% in the USA and 27% in western Europe) [2]. In Western countries, diagnostic endoscopy is mostly performed for patients with symptoms indicating gastric cancer. The prevalence of early stage cancer is less than 20% of diagnosed cases, which is significantly lower than approximately 50% in Japan [37]. However, there is no solid evidence to recommend routine screening endoscopy for asymptomatic patients in Western countries with lower prevalence of gastric cancer.

An Asian Pacific Gastric Cancer Consensus group has recommended population-based screening and treatment of *H. pylori* for very high-risk populations but this remains to be implemented [38].

Therapeutics

Surgery

Radical surgical excision remains the standard treatment for gastric cancer without distant metastasis and is a major predictive factor for survival. There are three surgical treatment options for gastric cancer:

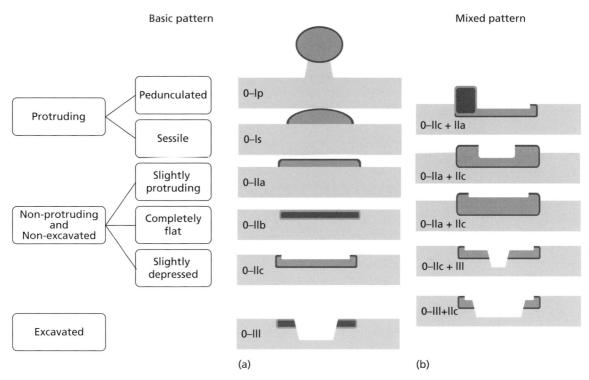

Figure 48.3 Macroscopic classification of early stage gastric cancer. (a) Basic pattern: appearance of the early gastric cancer subdivided into protruding (0–I), non-protruding and non-excavated (0–II), or excavated lesions (0–III). (b) The non-protruding and non-excavated lesions can be subclassified into three groups: protruding (0–IIa), flat (0–IIb), and depressed (0–IIc). (From Endoscopic Classification Review Group [36].)

1 Distal subtotal gastrectomy for cancers localized in the middle and lower third of the stomach

2 Proximal subtotal gastrectomy or total gastrectomy with esophagectomy for cancers involving the cardia.

3 Total gastrectomy for cancers involving the upper third of the stomach without a margin by a distance of >6 cm to the cardia.

Regional lymphadenectomy is routinely performed as a standard procedure in addition to these gastrectomies. However, the extent to which lymphadenectomy provides a cure remains controversial. Surgical resection as a palliative option should be confined to patients with continued bleeding or obstruction.

Chemotherapy

Adjuvant chemotherapy is frequently used as a perisurgical treatment to reduce the chance of tumor recurrence after surgery, whereas neoadjuvant chemotherapy is used as a means to preoperatively limit tumor spread before

surgery to reduce the surgical burden. Chemotherapy may also be given to prolong survival and palliate symptoms without surgery. Perioperative chemotherapy or chemoradiation therapy is recommended as a standard treatment option to improve outcome for patients with resectable gastric cancer based on the evidence from large randomized phase III studies [5]. 5-Fluorouracil (5FU) is the main chemotherapy agent, although a series of chemotherapy agents is available in clinical practice. However, no single-agent regimen is successful in achieving a remarkable survival benefit for patients with inoperable cancer. Various combination therapies have therefore been investigated. The epirubicin, cisplatin, and 5-FU (ECF) regimen has been widely accepted as the reference standard. The National Cancer Institution lists the following as standard options: the single-agent use of 5-FU or cisplatin; cisplatin and 5-FU (CF); etoposide, leucovorin, and 5-FU (ELF); and 5-FU, doxorubicin, and methotrexate (FAMTX). Clinical evaluations for other

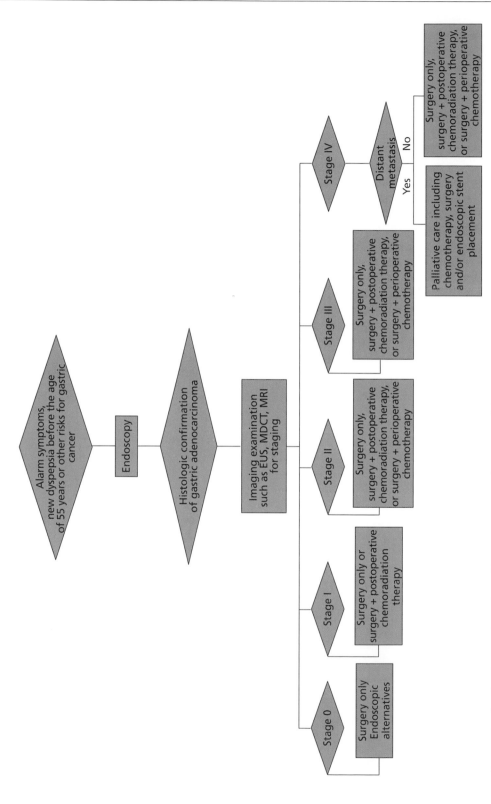

Figure 48.4 A flow chart for managing patients with gastric cancer according to stage of disease. EUS, endoscopic ultrasonography; MDCT, multidetector row computed tomography; MRI, magnetic resonance imaging.

options such as leucovorin, 5-FU, and oxaliplatin (FOLFOX), folic acid, 5-FU, and irinotecan (FOLFIRI), and irinotecan and cisplatin are currently ongoing. In Japan, oral fluoropyrimidine (S-1) is accepted as a first-line drug for gastric cancer chemotherapy. Phase II studies of S-1 have demonstrated responses of 44–45% in patients with advanced gastric cancer and a randomized phase III study verified a significant advantage of S-1 in combination with cisplatin compared with S-1 alone [39]. Furthermore, a randomized study in Japan revealed a distinct benefit of adjuvant chemotherapy with S-1 alone for patients with stage II, IIIA, and IIIB gastric cancer, even after surgery with D2 or more extensive lymph-node dissection with no residual tumor [40].

Endoscopic Treatment

Endoscopic mucosal resection (EMR) offers minimally invasive endoscopic treatment for superficial mucosal cancers. It has been demonstrated that small, differentiated, mucosal cancers can be curatively treated by endoscopic local excision with equivalent long-term outcome relative to surgery [41]. The cap-assisted technique is the most widely used because of technical simplicity, although there is increasing use of the band-ligation, mucosal resection technique, particularly in Western countries. This cap technique is initiated by injecting a small amount of saline into the submucosal tissue plane to isolate the diseased mucosa from the deeper muscular layer, to minimize the risk of perforation. The lesion is then suctioned into the cap attachment fitted on to the tip of the endoscope. The mucosal tissue excision is achieved within the cap using a prelooped snare inside the cap. The current indication of EMR is limited by the size of the lesions (<2 cm in diameter), because the piecemeal resection is necessitated to remove larger lesions due to the limited size of the cap and the snare, which may give rise to incomplete tumor removal [42]. The endoscopic submucosal dissection (ESD) technique was developed in Japan to enable endoscopic excision of the larger lesions en bloc (see Video 20). In ESD, the lesion is securely marginated from the surrounding normal mucosa and then completely excised from the muscularis propria, with repetitive electrosurgical dissections using a specialized needle knife. Although the en-bloc resection rate has been dramatically improved, more than 90% and larger lesions >10 cm in diameter can be removed en bloc. The procedure is difficult and time-consuming, and

is associated with a higher complication rate, including critical complications such as perforation and severe post-therapeutic bleeding.

It is important to confirm *H. pylori* has been eradicated, and if not to treat this infection. Japanese studies have shown that *H. pylori* eradication significantly reduces the subsequent risk of gastric cancer after treatment of early gastric cancer [43].

In order to resolve gastric outlet obstruction, endoscopic placement of a self-expanding metallic stent may be performed for palliative care, which may improve not only quality of life, but also survival of end-stage patients with advanced gastric cancer.

Prognosis

The overall 5-year survival rates of gastric cancer in the USA have shown slight but steady improvement (1975–7: 16%, 1984–6: 18%, 1996–2002: 24%) [2]. The fact that approximately 80% of patients die within 5 years of diagnosis suggests that a cure for stomach cancer remains elusive. The presence of one of the "alarm symptoms" is associated with poor prognosis (26%), which is equivalent to the overall survival rate in the USA because gastric cancer evaluation is usually performed for patients with these symptoms. An increase in the number of symptoms, especially weight loss, dysphagia, and palpable abdominal mass, implies a poorer prognosis [44]. The establishment of a practical endoscopy-based screening system for appropriately assessed high-risk populations is desirable for improvements in overall survival from gastric cancer.

Take-home points

Diagnosis

- A final diagnosis of gastric cancer needs to be confirmed histologically with endoscopic or surgical tissue sampling.

- Prompt endoscopy is recommended for the detection of gastric cancer in individuals with " alarm symptoms," including weight loss, gastrointestinal bleeding, dysphagia, anemia, vomiting, palpable abdominal mass, and the development of new dyspepsia after the age of 55 years.

- The incidence of gastric cancer in men relative to women is approximately double. Ethnic populations and individuals with a family history of gastric cancer are also associated with a higher risk.

> **Therapy**
> - Surgery remains the standard treatment to cure patients with advanced gastric cancer.
> - Perisurgical chemotherapy may increase the opportunity for survival.
> - Endoscopic treatment has been steadily evolving as a less invasive alternative to surgery for mucosal cancers with curative intent and as a palliative option for end-stage patients.

References

1 Parkin DM, Bray F, Ferlay J, Pisani P. Global cancer statistics, 2002. *CA Cancer J Clin* 2005; **55**: 74–108.

2 Jemal A, Siegel R, Ward E, Murray T, Xu J, Thun MJ. Cancer statistics, 2007. *CA Cancer J Clin* 2007; **57**: 43–66.

3 Crew KD, Neugut AI. Epidemiology of gastric cancer. *World J Gastroenterol* 2006; **12**: 354–362.

4 Lochhead P, El-Omar EM. Gastric cancer. *Br Med Bull* 2008; **85**: 87–100.

5 Van Cutsem E, Van de Velde C, Roth A, *et al*. Expert opinion on management of gastric and gastro-oesophageal junction adenocarcinoma on behalf of the European Organisation for Research and Treatment of Cancer (EORTC)—gastrointestinal cancer group. *Eur J Cancer* 2008; **44**: 182–94.

6 Wachtel MS, Zhang Y, Chiriva-Internati M, Frezza EE. Different regression equations relate age to the incidence of Lauren types 1 and 2 stomach cancer in the SEER database: these equations are unaffected by sex or race. *BMC Cancer* 2006; **6**: 65.

7 Graham DY, Malaty HM, Evans DG, Evans DJ Jr, Klein PD, Adam E. Epidemiology of *Helicobacter pylori* in an asymptomatic population in the United States. Effect of age, race, and socioeconomic status. *Gastroenterology* 1991; **100**: 1495–501.

8 Das JC, Paul N. Epidemiology and pathophysiology of *Helicobacter pylori* infection in children. *Indian J Pediatr* 2007; **74**: 287–90.

9 Helicobacter and Cancer Collaborative Group. Gastric cancer and *Helicobacter pylori*: a combined analysis of 12 case control studies nested within prospective cohorts. *Gut* 2001; **49**: 347–53.

10 Crowe SE. Helicobacter infection, chronic inflammation, and the development of malignancy. *Curr Opin Gastroenterol* 2005; **21**: 32–8.

11 Hatakeyama M, Brzozowski T. Pathogenesis of *Helicobacter pylori* infection. *Helicobacter* 2006; **11**(Suppl 1): 14–20.

12 Pritchard DM, Przemeck SM. Review article: How useful are the rodent animal models of gastric adenocarcinoma? *Aliment Pharmacol Ther* 2004; **19**: 841–59.

13 Ramon JM, Serra L, Cerdo C, Oromi J. Dietary factors and gastric cancer risk. A case-control study in Spain. *Cancer* 1993; **71**: 1731–5.

14 Hansson LR, Engstrand L, Nyren O, Lindgren A. Prevalence of *Helicobacter pylori* infection in subtypes of gastric cancer. *Gastroenterology* 1995; **109**: 885–8.

15 Correa P, Haenszel W, Cuello C, *et al*. Gastric precancerous process in a high risk population: cohort follow-up. *Cancer Res* 1990; **50**: 4737–40.

16 Neugut AI, Hayek M, Howe G. Epidemiology of gastric cancer. *Semin Oncol* 1996; **23**: 281–91.

17 Bjelakovic G, Nikolova D, Simonetti RG, Gluud C. Antioxidant supplements for preventing gastrointestinal cancers. *Cochrane Database Syst Rev* 2008; (3): CD004183.

18 Hansson LE, Nyren O, Bergstrom R, *et al*. Diet and risk of gastric cancer. A population-based case-control study in Sweden. *Int J Cancer* 1993; **55**: 181–9.

19 Sugimura T, Fujimura S, Baba T. Tumor production in the glandular stomach and alimentary tract of the rat by *N*-methyl-*N*′-nitro-*N*-nitrosoguanidine. *Cancer Res* 1970; **30**: 455–65.

20 van Loon AJ, Botterweck AA, Goldbohm RA, Brants HA, van Klaveren JD, van den Brandt PA. Intake of nitrate and nitrite and the risk of gastric cancer: a prospective cohort study. *Br J Cancer* 1998; **78**: 129–35.

21 Shikata K, Kiyohara Y, Kubo M, *et al*. A prospective study of dietary salt intake and gastric cancer incidence in a defined Japanese population: the Hisayama study. *Int J Cancer* 2006; **119**: 196–201.

22 Tokui N, Yoshimura T, Fujino Y, *et al*. Dietary habits and stomach cancer risk in the JACC Study. *J Epidemiol* 2005; **15**(Suppl 2): S98–108.

23 Zanghieri G, Di Gregorio C, Sacchetti C, *et al*. Familial occurrence of gastric cancer in the 2-year experience of a population-based registry. *Cancer* 1990; **66**: 2047–51.

24 La Vecchia C, Negri E, Franceschi S, Gentile A. Family history and the risk of stomach and colorectal cancer. *Cancer* 1992; **70**: 50–5.

25 Ottini L, Palli D, Falchetti M, *et al*. Microsatellite instability in gastric cancer is associated with tumor location and family history in a high-risk population from Tuscany. *Cancer Res* 1997; **57**: 4523–9.

26 Gonzalez CA, Pera G, Agudo A, *et al*. Smoking and the risk of gastric cancer in the European Prospective Investigation Into Cancer and Nutrition (EPIC). *Int J Cancer* 2003; **107**: 629–34.

27 Koizumi Y, Tsubono Y, Nakaya N, *et al*. Cigarette smoking and the risk of gastric cancer: a pooled analysis of two prospective studies in Japan. *Int J Cancer* 2004; **112**: 1049–55.

28 Nishino Y, Inoue M, Tsuji I, *et al*. Tobacco smoking and gastric cancer risk: an evaluation based on a systematic

review of epidemiologic evidence among the Japanese population. *Jpn J Clin Oncol* 2006; **36**: 800–7.

29 Voutilainen M, Mantynen T, Kunnamo I, Juhola M, Mecklin JP, Farkkila M. Impact of clinical symptoms and referral volume on endoscopy for detecting peptic ulcer and gastric neoplasms. *Scand J Gastroenterol* 2003; **38**: 109–13.

30 Axon A. Symptoms and diagnosis of gastric cancer at early curable stage. *Best Pract Res Clin Gastroenterol* 2006; **20**: 697–708.

31 Tucker HJ, Snape WJ Jr, Cohen S. Achalasia secondary to carcinoma: manometric and clinical features. *Ann Intern Med* 1978; **89**: 315–18.

32 Talley NJ, Vakil NB, Moayyedi P. American gastroenterological association technical review on the evaluation of dyspepsia. *Gastroenterology* 2005; **129**: 1756–80.

33 Sancho-Poch FJ, Balanzo J, Ocana J, *et al.* An evaluation of gastric biopsy in the diagnosis of gastric cancer. *Gastrointest Endosc* 1978; **24**: 281–2.

34 American Joint Committee on Cancer. *AJCC Cancer Staging Manual*, 6th edn. New York: Springer Science + Business Media LLC; 2002.

35 Kwee RM, Kwee TC. Imaging in local staging of gastric cancer: a systematic review. *J Clin Oncol* 2007; **25**: 2107–116.

36 Endoscopic Classification Review Group. Update on the Paris classification of superficial neoplastic lesions in the digestive tract. *Endoscopy* 2005; **37**: 570–8.

37 Yamazaki H, Oshima A, Murakami R, Endoh S, Ubukata T. A long-term follow-up study of patients with gastric cancer detected by mass screening. *Cancer* 1989; **63**: 613–17.

38 Fock KM, Katelaris P, Sugano K, *et al.* Second Asia-Pacific consensus guidelines for *Helicobacter pylori* infections. *J Gastroenterol Hepatol* 2009; **24**: 1578–600.

39 Koizumi W, Narahara H, Hara T, *et al.* S-1 plus cisplatin versus S-1 alone for first-line treatment of advanced gastric cancer (SPIRITS trial): a phase III trial. *Lancet Oncol* 2008; **9**: 215–21.

40 Sakuramoto S, Sasako M, Yamaguchi T, *et al.* Adjuvant chemotherapy for gastric cancer with S-1, an oral fluoropyrimidine. *N Engl J Med* 2007; **357**: 1810–20.

41 Shim CS. Endoscopic mucosal resection: an overview of the value of different techniques. *Endoscopy* 2001; **33**: 271–5.

42 Sumiyama K, Gostout CJ. Novel techniques and instrumentation for EMR, ESD, and full-thickness endoscopic luminal resection. *Gastrointest Endosc Clin North Am* 2007; **17**: 471–85, v–vi.

43 Uemura N, Muraki T, Okamoto S. Effect of *Helicobacter pylori* eradication on subsequent development of cancer after endoscopic resection of early gastric cancer. *Cancer Epidemiol Biomarkers Prev* 1997; **6**: 639–42.

44 Maconi G, Manes G, Porro GB. Role of symptoms in diagnosis and outcome of gastric cancer. *World J Gastroenterol* 2008; **14**: 1149–55.

CHAPTER 49

Other Gastric Tumors (Benign and Malignant)

Yasser M. Bhat[1] and Michael L. Kochman[2]

[1] Division of Digestive Diseases, David Geffen School of Medicine at UCLA, Los Angeles, CA, USA
[2] Division of Gastroenterology, University of Pennsylvania Health System, Philadelphia, PA, USA

Summary

Gastric tumors, other than adenocarcinoma, are frequently encountered during clinical gastrointestinal practice. A variety of epithelial and subepithelial lesions may arise within the stomach. These are usually found incidentally during endoscopy or a radiographic study. These lesions include both benign and malignant etiologies. Endoscopy alone is often insufficient in defining the full extent of the process and endoscopic ultrasound (EUS) has become a major breakthrough in the evaluation of these diseases. For the purposes of this chapter, these lesions have been grouped into mucosal and submucosal lesions. The common ones are discussed.

Case

A 54-year-old male who has symptoms of reflux undergoes an endoscopy because of concern about Barrett esophagus. His medications include a proton pump inhibitor and two additional antibiotics because the blood work showed that he "tested positive for *H. pylori*." He has a hiatal hernia but no evidence of esophagitis or Barrett esophagus. An "incidental" 2-cm polypoid lesion is seen in the body of the stomach. Biopsies of the lesion show "normal mucosa" and biopsies from both the body and antrum reveal atrophic gastritis with *H. pylori*. The patient has a family history of stomach cancer and the question of a MALT lymphoma was raised because of the *H. pylori*. Therefore an EUS is scheduled. The lesion is determined to be submucosal and endoscopic mucosal resection is performed. The pathology reveals that the lesion is a carcinoid, thought to be related to high gastrin levels from the atrophic gastritis. It was determined the entire lesion was removed by EMR. Testing for MEN1 syndrome was negative.

Practical Gastroenterology and Hepatology: Esophagus and Stomach, 1st edition. Edited by Nicholas J. Talley, Kenneth R. DeVault and David E. Fleischer. © 2010 Blackwell Publishing Ltd.

Mucosal Tumors (Table 49.1)

Gastric Polyps

Gastric polyps are abnormal epithelial growths of the normally uniform and smooth lining of the gastric mucosa. The polyps may be hyperplastic, adenomatous, fundic gland, or hamartomatous on pathologic examination. They may be sessile or pedunculated and single or multiple. Endoscopic and clinical features may be predictive in distinguishing the type of polyp but tissue sampling or resection is often required for accurate diagnosis.

Hyperplastic polyps are the most common polypoid lesions, accounting for 70–90% of gastric polyps (Figure 49.1). They consist of hyperplastic gastric glands with edematous stroma, often with cystic dilation, without any change in the microcellular configuration. The risk of malignant transformation is considered low (0.5–4%). Adenomatous polyps are true neoplastic lesions with dysplastic epithelium and nuclear atypia. The malignant potential is increased (up to 75% in some series) and increases significantly in polyps greater than 2 cm in diameter, although adenomatous polyps with carcinoma less than 2 cm have been reported. Fundic gland polyps

Table 49.1 List of common etiologies that present as gastric tumors and thickened gastric folds.

Mucosal tumors	Submucosal tumors
Gastric polyps	Leiomyomas and leiomyosarcoma
Lymphoma	Lipoma and liposarcoma
MALToma	GIST
Menetrier disease	Gastric carcinoid
Zollinger-Ellison Syndrome	Granular cell tumor
Kaposi sarcoma	Pancreatic rest
Gastritis cystica profunda	Duplication cyst

MALToma, mucosa-associated lymphoid tissue lymphoma; GIST, gastrointestinal stromal tumor.

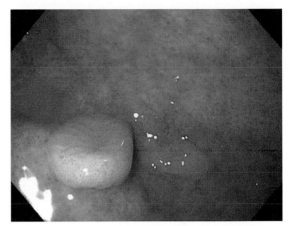

Figure 49.2 Endoscopic image demonstrating a fundic gland polyp. Notice the smooth borders and uniform "pits" on the surface.

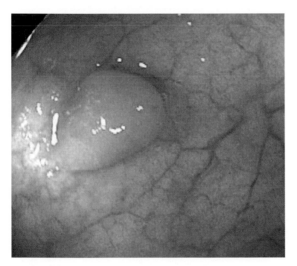

Figure 49.1 Endoscopic image of a typical hyperplastic polyp.

are composed of hypertrophic fundic gland mucosa and are generally benign (Figure 49.2). However, rare cases of malignant transformation in large fundic gland polyps in the setting of familial adenomatous polyposis (FAP) have been reported. Hamartomatous polyps consist of branching smooth muscle bands surrounded by glandular epithelium. They have no malignant potential [1,2]. Gastric polyps may be associated with syndromes including FAP, Peutz–Jeghers syndrome (PJS), and familial juvenile polyposis.

Endoscopic appearance and biopsy samples are sometimes insufficient to reliably diagnose polyp histology. For complete diagnosis excision should be considered. Smaller polyps (<5 mm) may be removed with multiple biopsy forceps while larger ones (>5 mm) may be resected with snare polypectomy. If multiple polyps are present,

the larger lesions (>1 cm) should be resected to confirm histology and absence of dysplasia before setting forth treatment or surveillance strategies. Endoscopic ultrasound (EUS) is a helpful adjunctive tool to delineate the layer of origin before resection. Surgical resection should be considered in those polyps thought to be too large to excise endoscopically [3].

Adenomatous and hyperplastic polyps are associated with chronic gastritis and may be late manifestations of type A chronic gastritis (pernicious anemia) or *Helicobacter pylori* infection. In addition to resection of the polyps, biopsy sampling of the surrounding stomach should be performed to examine for chronic gastritis and intestinal metaplasia. Careful examination should be performed of the remaining gastric mucosa and any surface abnormalities should be biopsied. Eradication of *H. pylori* infection should be undertaken, although it is unclear if this affects polyp recurrence or development of metaplasia as the infection was likely long standing. If intestinal metaplasia is diagnosed, endoscopic surveillance should be considered dependent upon the clinical situation. Finally, an increased prevalence of gastric polyps (hyperplastic, adenomatous and fundic gland) has been reported in patients with FAP and attenuated FAP.

Gastric Lymphoma and MALToma

Lymphomas of the stomach account for up to 5% of gastric malignancies and may be divided into primary gastric lymphomas or those with disseminated nodal disease and secondary gastric involvement [4]. More than 95% of gastric lymphomas are of the non-Hodgkin type. Clinical presentation is similar to adenocarcinoma and the disease can be indolent in the early stage. Abdominal pain, weight loss, nausea, anorexia, and gastrointestinal hemorrhage are the most common symptoms and signs. On endoscopy it can appear as a discrete polypoid lesion, ulcerated mass, or thickened gastric folds due to submucosal infiltration. Endoscopic forceps biopsies are not always diagnostic and snare biopsies or needle aspirates may be required. EUS is helpful in identifying submucosal involvement and identifying perigastric lymph nodes. If the diagnosis remains elusive, surgical full-thickness biopsies may be considered [5,6].

Mucosa-associated lymphoid tissue (MALT) lymphoma is classified as an extranodal marginal zone lymphoma. Numerous lymphoid follicles, plasma cell infiltrates and dense B-cell lymphocytic infiltrates are seen on histology. Clinical presentation may be with bleeding from an ulcerated mass (Figure 49.3) or thickened gastric folds seen on endoscopy or cross-sectional imaging. Diagnosis is usually made on endoscopy with "jumbo" forceps biopsies. The majority of MALTomas are low grade and run an indolent course and are associated with *H. pylori* infection. Gastric biopsies should also be performed to examine for atrophic gastritis, chronic active gastritis, and intestinal metaplasia. EUS is extremely useful in assessing the depth of invasion. Low-grade MALTomas may demonstrate focal thickening of the mucosal and submucosal layers while transmural thickening and perigastric lymphadenopathy indicates high-grade disease (Figure 49.4). Treatment options include *H. pylori* eradication, radiation, and chemotherapy. For low-grade disease limited to the submucosa, eradication of *H. pylori* may regress the tumor in 60–75% of patients. EUS is helpful in objective assessment of response to therapy post-treatment.

Menetrier Disease

Menetrier disease is a condition characterized by marked foveolar hyperplasia with cystic dilation resulting in giant gastric rugal folds with antral sparing. The submucosa may be penetrated, though this is rare. The pathogenesis is unclear and may involve transforming growth factor alpha (TGF-α). The symptoms may include abdominal pain, weight loss, gastrointestinal hemorrhage, and

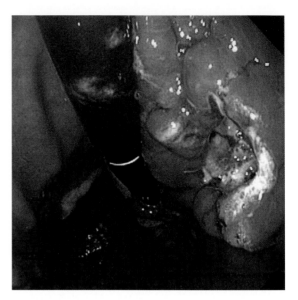

Figure 49.3 Endoscopic image of a ulcerated mass along the lesser curvature of the stomach. This patient presented with melena. Biopsies confirmed a diagnosis of a MALT lymphoma.

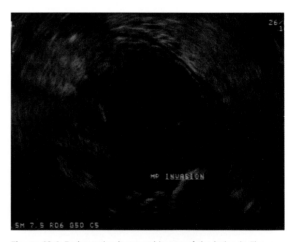

Figure 49.4 Endoscopic ultrasound image of the lesion in Figure 49.3. Note the extension of the mass through the muscularis propria.

protein leakage leading to hypoalbuminemia. EUS may demonstrate thickening of the deep mucosal layer and "jumbo" forceps biopsies or snare resection may be needed to confirm the diagnosis. Various treatment options (antacids, H_2 receptor blockers, proton pump inhibitors, steroids, and prostaglandins) have been tried with limited effect. Subtotal gastrectomy may be considered in refractory cases. The natural history is unclear and some reports have demonstrated the evolution from Menetrier disease to gastric atrophy over a 4 to 8-year time span, with return of the serum albumin concentration to normal. The risk of gastric cancer is also not well characterized but is estimated at 2–15% [7].

In pediatric patients, the disease presents more acutely with abrupt-onset vomiting, abdominal pain, anorexia, and hypoproteinemia. Ascites and pedal edema may then occur with laboratory values demonstrating hypoalbu minemia, a normocytic anemia, and peripheral eosinophilia. In children, an additional histologic feature includes intranuclear inclusion bodies consistent with cytomegalovirus (CMV). Pediatric patients generally respond well to supportive treatment with complete clinical resolution.

Zollinger–Ellison (ZE) Syndrome

ZE syndrome is a condition characterized by hyperplastic gastropathy of the body and fundus of the stomach leading to hypersecretion of gastric acid due to a gastrinoma. Thickened proximal gastric folds are formed due to parietal cell hyperplasia. Most patients develop duodenal or jejunal ulcers and diarrhea may be present; diarrhea and esophagitis and esophageal strictures may also be found at presentation [8]. Up to a third of patients have metastatic disease at presentation (liver, axial skeleton) and it may be part of a MEN1 syndrome (multiple endocrine neoplasia). Localization of the tumor is essential for curative resection and is generally achieved with a combination of somatostatin receptor scintigraphic scanning, EUS examination of the pancreas, and intraoperative exploration. In patients with metastatic or MEN1 disease, medical therapy with proton pump inhibitors is instituted.

Submucosal Tumors (Table 49.1)

Leiomyoma

Leiomyoma are one of the commonest gastric submucosal tumors. EUS is highly accurate in defining the wall layer of origin and also to differentiate from extraluminal compression or isolated gastric vascular structures like varices. Leiomyomas are seen as hypoechoic lesions arising from the muscularis propria and may grow either with an intraluminal or extraluminal pattern. They can range in size from less than 0.5 cm to as large as 30 cm and are most often associated with the esophagus. Microscopically, leiomyomas are formed of fascicles of benign-appearing spindle cells without nuclear atypia. Lesions less than 3 cm in size have a low risk for malignancy and can be observed with serial endosonography.

Gastrointestinal Stromal Tumor (GIST)

Gastrointestinal stromal tumors (GISTs) are mesenchymal tumors thought to be arising from the interstitial cells of Cajal (gastrointestinal pacemaker cells). In the past, they were thought to be of smooth muscle origin but better understanding of the tumor biology has led to reclassification of many formerly diagnosed leiomyomas, leiomyosarcomas, schwannomas, or leiomyoblastomas as GISTs. Most (70%) GI tract GISTs occur in the stomach in older patients (age 50–60) with a wide variety of sizes from few millimeters to 30 cm.

Endoscopic appearance is of a smooth submucosal mass (Figure 49.5; see Video 21). EUS findings include a hypoechoic, typically homogenous lesion with well-defined borders arising from the muscularis propria or muscularis mucosa (Figures 49.6 and 49.7; see Video 22). Larger lesions may show features of liquefactive necrosis, cystic, and hyaline degeneration. The malignant potential is difficult to predict without histologic evaluation; smaller lesions are typically benign in biologic behavior. EUS features (heterogeneous lesions >4 cm

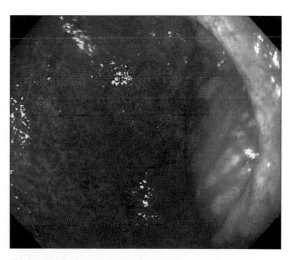

Figure 49.5 Endoscopic image demonstrating a submucosal mass in the antrum with smooth superficial mucosa.

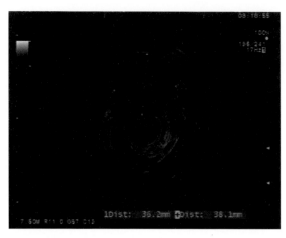

Figure 49.6 Endoscopic ultrasound image of the lesion in Figure 49.5. A hypoechoic mass measuring 36 mm × 38 mm arising from the muscularis propria is seen.

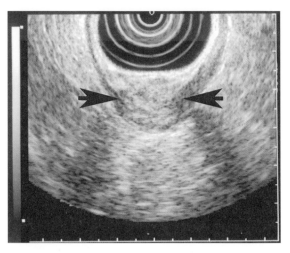

Figure 49.8 Endoscopic ultrasound image of gastric lipoma demonstrating that it is relatively hyperechoic and within the submucosa.

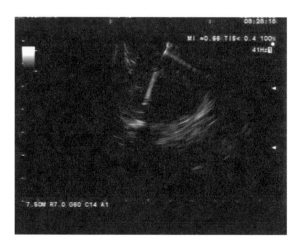

Figure 49.7 Endoscopic ultrasound guided fine needle aspiration (FNA) of the lesion described in Figure 49.6.

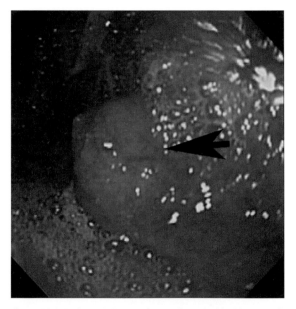

Figure 49.9 Endoscopic image of a gastric carcinoid with mucosal extension.

with irregular extraluminal borders and cystic spaces) may be suggestive of malignancy [9].

GISTs are distinguishable by their molecular features. C-kit (a stem cell receptor called CD117) or PDGFRA (platelet derived growth factor-α receptor) expression is characteristic. Other markers found in GISTs include CD34, smooth muscle actin, and s100 protein. Surgery is clearly indicated for lesions greater than 3 cm in size or other malignant features. Unresectable lesions should be treated with the tyrosine kinase inhibitor imatinib mesylate (STI571; Gleevec, Novartis, USA).

Lipoma

Lipomas are benign tumors composed of matures lipocytes. They are typically found incidentally on endoscopy and colonoscopy. Rarely they may be symptomatic, presenting with bleeding, abdominal pain, or obstruction. Endoscopy will demonstrate an isolated solitary

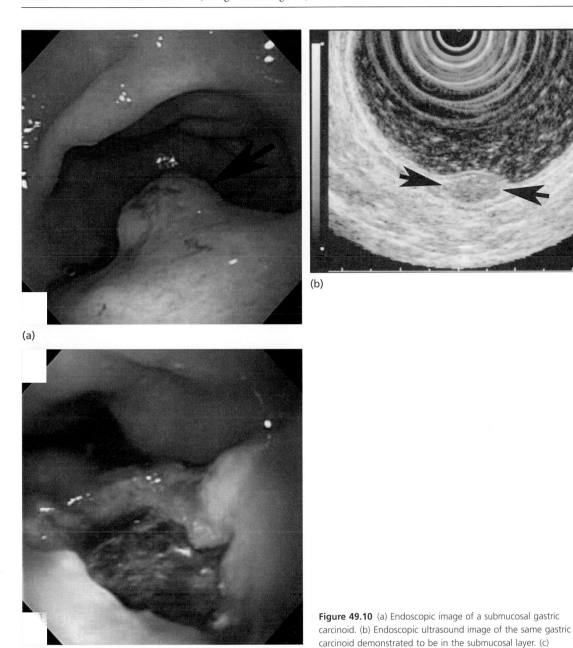

(a)

(b)

(c)

Figure 49.10 (a) Endoscopic image of a submucosal gastric carcinoid. (b) Endoscopic ultrasound image of the same gastric carcinoid demonstrated to be in the submucosal layer. (c) Endoscopic image demonstrating clean endoscopic resection.

bulge with normal overlying mucosa, a yellowish hue, and a smooth regular appearance. A "pillow" sign may be elicited when an indentation in created with palpation by an endoscopic device. EUS will demonstrate a hyperechoic lesion arising from the submucosa. Diagnosis is reliably made based on the typical endoscopic and EUS appearances (Figure 49.8). Expectant management is adequate without need for endoscopic surveillance. Excision should be performed if symptomatic or if unable to distinguish from a liposarcoma.

Gastric Carcinoids

Gastric carcinoids represent 2–3% of all gastrointestinal carcinoids but only 0.3% of all gastric tumors. They are usually located in the body or fundus of the stomach and are generally submucosal and may appear polypoid (Figure 49.9). They arise from gastrointestinal neuroendocrine cells and some are thought to develop as a result of high circulating gastrin which is stimulating to the enterochromaffin cells of the proximal stomach. Therefore, pernicious anemia and chronic atrophic gastritis are risk factors for the typically benign macro- and microcarcinoids but no such lesions have been observed in humans as a result of hypergastrinemia from prolonged proton pump inhibitor use. While circulating vasoactive peptides may be identified, these are frequently incidental as true carcinoid syndrome does not develop without liver involvement. Endoscopy often demonstrates a submucosal mass with a central dimple and EUS is very helpful in defining wall layer involvement. Carcinoids due to pernicious anemia and atrophic gastritis or MEN1 tend to have a benign course and for lesions less than 2 cm and without involvement of the muscularis propria, endoscopic resection may be best (Figure 49.10a–c). Larger lesions would require surgical excision. Antrectomy to reduce G-cell burden may be effective in reducing smaller carcinoid tumors in this setting. Sporadic carcinoid which are autonomous and present in the setting of gastric acid secretion and normal serum gastrin should be treated as malignant and surgically excised as they have a higher rate of regional lymph node involvement [10].

Granular Cell Tumor (GCT)

GCTs are rare submucosal tumors of Schwann cell origin. Immunostaining is positive for s100 protein. They are generally benign but malignant transformation for tumors greater than 4 cm in size has been described. Smaller lesions may be able to be resected or ablated endoscopically, though larger lesions may need surgical resection

Pancreatic Rest

This lesion is often referred to as aberrant pancreas or ectopic pancreas. They are rare submucosal lesions consisting of cystically dilated exocrine pancreatic glandular tissue. They are most commonly observed in the distal stomach or duodenum and endoscopy shows a submucosal nodule with a central dimpling (Figure 49.11). EUS findings are an echovariable hypoechoic, heterogeneous

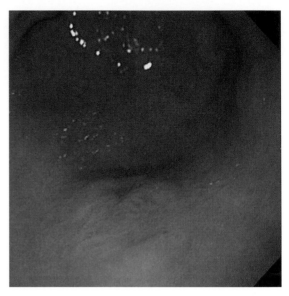

Figure 49.11 Endoscopic image showing a submucosal nodule with central dimpling. Biopsies confirmed the diagnosis of a pancreatic rest.

lesion with indistinct borders arising from the submucosa or muscularis propria. Diagnosis is made by forceps biopsy or snare excision. Management is expectant unless symptomatic or suspicion exists for malignancy.

Take-home points

- Most gastric mucosal and submucosal tumors are asymptomatic and found incidentally. Endoscopy alone is often insufficient for diagnosis. EUS is useful and should be performed for complete evaluation in selected patients.

- Gastric polyps are of many types with varied malignant potential. In general, resection is recommended to establish diagnosis and for therapy.

- Most gastric lymphomas are of the non-Hodgkin type and should be treated as such.

- For low-grade MALTomas, eradication of associated *H. pylori* infection may be sufficient but chemotherapy or radiation is required for high-grade tumors.

- Apparent submucosal tumors may be intramural or due to extramural causes.

- Leiomyomas and lipomas represent the most frequently encountered intramural submucosal tumors and are generally benign when they are small in size.

- In general, submucosal tumors less than 3 cm can be managed expectantly while larger ones should be evaluated for resection.

References

1 Deppish LM, Rona VT. Gastric epithelial polyps: A ten year study. *J Clin Gastroenterol* 1989; **11**: 110–15.

2 Cristallini E, Ascani S, Bolis G. Association between histologic type of polyp and carcinoma of the stomach. *Gastrointest Endosc* 1992; **38**: 481–4.

3 Hirota WK, Zuckerman MJ, Adler DG, *et al.* ASGE guideline: the role of endoscopy in the surveillance of premalignant conditions of the upper GI tract. *Gastrointest Endosc* 2006; **63**: 570–80.

4 Wotherspoon A. Gastric lymphoma of mucosa-associated lymphoid tissue and *Helicobacter pylori. Annu Rev Med* 1998; **49**: 289–99.

5 Kolve M, Fischbach W, Wilhelm M. Primary gastric non-Hodgkin's lymphoma: Requirements for diagnosis and staging. *Recent Results Cancer Res* 2000; **156**: 63–68.

6 Amer MH, el-Akkad S. Gastrointestinal lymphoma in adults: clinical features and management of three hundred cases. *Gastroenterology* 1994; **106**: 846–58.

7 Scharschmidt B. The natural history of hypertrophic gastropathy (Menetrier's diseases). *Am J Med* 1997; **63**: 644–52.

8 Roy PK, Venzon DJ, Shojamanesh H, Abou-Saif A, Peghini P, Doppman JL. Zollinger-Ellison syndrome. Clinical presentation in 261 patients. *Medicine (Baltimore)* 2000; **79**: 379–411.

9 Chak A, Canto MI, Rosch T, *et al.* Endosonographic differentiation of benign and malignant stromal cells. *Gastrointest Endosc* 1997; **45**: 468–73.

10 Gilligan C, Lawton G, Tang L, *et al.* Gastric carcinoid tumors: The biology and therapy of an enigmatic and controversial lesion. *Am J Gastroenterol* 1995; **90**: 338–52.

CHAPTER 50

Eosinophilic Gastroenteritis

Joseph Y. Chang[1] and Nicholas J. Talley[2]

[1] Division of Gastroenterology and Hepatology, Mayo Clinic, Rochester, MN, USA
[2] Faculty of Health, University of Newcastle, NSW, Australia

Summary

Eosinophilic gastroenteritis (EG) is a rare and heterogeneous disorder characterized by gastrointestinal (GI) symptoms and eosinophilic infiltration of the GI tract. Symptoms are dependent upon site of the GI tract involved and depth of involvement. The diagnostic criteria include: (i) the presence of GI symptoms, (ii) histopathology demonstrating predominant eosinophilic infiltration, (iii) the absence of other conditions that cause eosinophilia, and (iv) no eosinophilic involvement of organs outside the GI tract.

Diagnosis requires a clinical history, physical exam, and documentation of any history of atopic disorders, allergies, and drug allergies. Laboratory evaluation includes a complete blood count with differential to evaluate for peripheral eosinophilia. Endoscopic evaluation with random biopsies remains the cornerstone for diagnosis. Histopathologic diagnosis typically requires an infiltration level of 20 or more eosinophils per high power field. Management strategies are based upon severity of symptoms and include antidiarrheals, dietary adjustments, and steroid therapy.

Case

A 41-year-old male presents with a 3-month history of recurring abdominal pain with nausea and vomiting. Complete blood count is notable for peripheral eosinophilia at 5% of total leukocytes. Serologic and stool studies are negative for parasitic infection. Contrast-enhanced computed tomographic views of the abdomen demonstrates thickening of the antrum and second part of the duodenum. The patient undergoes esophagogastroduodenoscopy which reveals stenosis from the antrum through the pylorus, and extending to the second portion of the duodenum. Antral and duodenal biopsies are obtained with histopathology demonstrating marked eosinophilic infiltration of the lamina propria. He is started on steroid therapy with prednisone and has rapid clinical improvement with resolution of his previous symptoms.

symptoms and eosinophilic infiltration of the GI tract. Originally described by Kaijser in 1937 [1], EG has a myriad of clinical manifestations; symptoms are dependent upon both site of the GI tract involved, as well as depth of involvement of the gut wall.

EG has been found to affect all age groups from infants to adults, usually presents in the third decade of life, and has been reported to have a slight male predominance [2,3,6].

Patients may present with a wide spectrum of symptoms ranging from abdominal pain to ascites [2]. Concurrent extraintestinal manifestations have also been reported including eosinophilic splenitis, hepatitis, and cystitis [7,8].

Definition and Epidemiology

Eosinophilic gastroenteritis (EG) is a rare and heterogeneous disorder characterized by gastrointestinal (GI)

Pathophysiology

Accumulation of eosinophils in the gastrointestinal tract is a common finding in many GI disorders such as inflammatory bowel disease and gastroesophageal reflux [9–13]. However, EG is a primary eosinophilic GI disorder with histopathology demonstrating abundant accumulation of eosinophils. Although the exact etio-

Practical Gastroenterology and Hepatology: Esophagus and Stomach, 1st edition. Edited by Nicholas J. Talley, Kenneth R. DeVault and David E. Fleischer. © 2010 Blackwell Publishing Ltd.

pathogenesis for this disorder is unclear, it is believed that the eosinophilic infiltration of the GI tract secondary to food allergy, drugs or toxins, or possibly unrecognized infection results in an adverse immunologic response. Th-2 cytokines and the eotaxin subfamily of chemokines are implicated as eosinophil-specific mediators in regulating this accumulation [14–16]. Furthermore, there is growing evidence of the specific interaction between eotaxin and expression of the CCR3 receptor, a 7-transmembrane-spanning G protein-coupled receptor expressed on eosinophils, in modulating eosinophil infiltration [14]. This has resulted in the consideration of eotaxin- or CC3-specific blocking agents as possible therapeutic interventions.

Following eosinophil localization in the GI tract, it is thought that cellular degranulation with release of cytotoxic proteins results in tissue destruction. Major basic protein (MBP) and eosinophil cationic protein are believed to play key roles, and have been found at immunohistochemically elevated levels in small bowel tissue of patients with EG [14].

There appears to be evidence of the association between eosinophilic gastrointestinal disorders and allergy as many patients have coexisting atopic disorders such as asthma, seasonal rhinitis, eczema, and food allergies [6,14].

Clinical Features

The Klein classification system for EG is the most widely accepted and is based upon depth of tissue infiltration [17]. Patients are divided into those with disease of the mucosa, muscle layer, or serosa, and each group appears to have differing clinical symptoms. Predominant disease of the mucosa appears to be the most commonly reported subclass in clinical studies (25–100%) [3].

Mucosal involvement usually presents with nonspecific symptoms of abdominal pain, nausea, vomiting, diarrhea, anemia, and even malabsorption or protein losing enteropathy with small bowel involvement. Given these non specific symptoms, patients may be inadvertently diagnosed with functional bowel disorder or inflammatory bowel disease [3].

Eosinophilic infiltration of the muscular layer accounts for 13–70% of EG cases and often presents with symptoms of gastric outlet or small intestinal obstruction [2,3].

Finally, involvement of the serosal layer is most uncommon and typically presents as ascites [2,3]. When compared to other types, serosal disease may have significantly higher levels of circulating eosinophils and may have a better treatment response to steroids [3].

Children with EG may present with growth failure, delayed puberty, amenorrhea, and more often have a history of allergy [18,19].

Diagnosis

A careful clinical history and physical exam is paramount in the initial evaluation of a patient (Table 50.1). A history of atopic disorders or allergies, and any pets, should be documented. Consider drug allergies when taking the history (e.g., recent use of azathioprine, co-trimoxazole).

Laboratory evaluations may include a complete blood count, and peripheral eosinophilia may alert the clinician but is absent in at least 20% of cases. In cases of elevated circulating eosinophils, other GI disorders associated with eosinophilia need to be excluded including parasitic infections, malignancies, vasculitis such as Churg–Strauss syndrome, and inflammatory bowel disease. Consider hypereosinophilic syndrome if the absolute eosinophil count is over 1500 cells/μL; a cardiac echo and other investigations are then needed to exclude suspected systemic disease.

Stool studies should be obtained to exclude parasites. In difficult cases, a duodenal aspirate for parasites can be

Table 50.1 Generally accepted diagnostic criteria for eosinophilic gastroenteritis.

1 Presence of gastrointestinal symptoms
2 Biopsies with histopathology demonstrating predominant eosinophilic infiltration
3 Absence of parasitic or extraintestinal diseases that may cause eosinophilia
4 No eosinophilic involvement of the heart or other organs outside the GI tract [2,3]
5 Peripheral eosinophilia may be commonly found, but it is not required for diagnosis as it is not a universal finding [2,4,5]

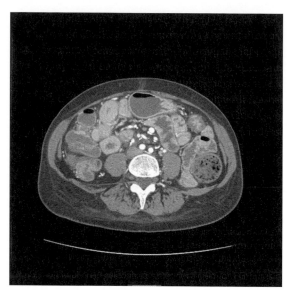

Figure 50.1 Computed tomographic enterography demonstrating thickened jejunal folds from eosinophilic gastroenteritis.

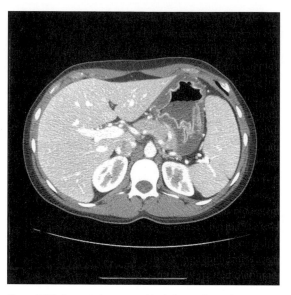

Figure 50.2 Computed tomographic abdomen illustrating gastric wall edema and hyperenhancement of the gastric mucosa from eosinophilic gastritis.

helpful. Dog hookworm infestation classically causes ileocolonic disease; stool studies usually are negative but patients will typically respond to empiric mebendazole (100 mg twice daily for 3 days).

No pathognomonic features are found in radiographic studies. Findings of irregular and thickened intestinal walls have been reported [20]. Plain abdominal radiographs or CT scanning may demonstrate findings of bowel obstruction as seen in EG with disease of the muscular layer (Figures 50.1 and 50.2). Abdominal ultrasound may also demonstrate ascites in serosal disease. Novel radiographic techniques previously used for inflammatory bowel disease have been applied to EG including bowel scintigraphy using radiolabeled granulocytes with technetium-99 with hexamethyl-propylenamine oxime (Tc-99 HMPAO) labeled WBC SPECT, which can be used to assess extent of disease and response to therapy [21].

Endoscopic evaluation with biopsies remains the cornerstone for diagnosis. Thickened gastric or small intestinal folds with or without nodules may be present; the differential diagnosis of enlarged small bowel folds includes Whipple disease, amyloid, lymphoma, paraproteinemia, and intestinal lymphangiectasia. Random biopsies should be taken from both normal and abnormal appearing mucosa in the stomach and small intestine

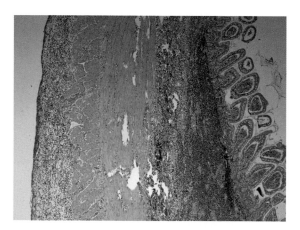

Figure 50.3 Small bowel biopsy from the jejunum that demonstrates dense eosinophilic infiltration involving the submucosa as well as serosa. Note the dense "sheet-like" configuration of the eosinophils within the submucosa. (Courtesy of Dr Thomas C. Smyrk, Mayo Clinic College of Medicine.)

as eosinophilic infiltration may exist despite bland endoscopic appearance [22,23] (Figures 50.3 and 50.4.)

If endoscopic biopsies are negative but there remains a high level of clinical suspicion, then full-thickness laparoscopic biopsies can be considered. Biopsies should be sent for histopathology to evaluate for degree of eosino-

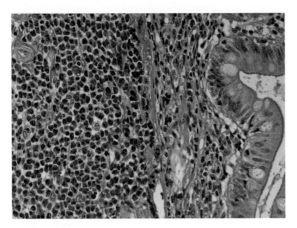

Figure 50.4 Taken from the same jejunal biopsy as Figure 50.3, this higher magnification view of the subserosa demonstrates the significant submucosal accumulation of eosinophils. (Courtesy of Dr Thomas C. Smyrk, Mayo Clinic College of Medicine.)

philic infiltration. Although no generally accepted histopathologic criteria for EG exists, many studies have used 20 or more eosinophils per HPF (high-power-field) as meeting diagnostic requirement [2,23,24]. Ascites with suspected serosal EG should be evaluated with abdominal paracentesis and ascitic fluid should be evaluated for a high eosinophil count.

Therapeutics

Therapeutic strategies for EG are largely based upon anecdotal experience. There have not been any prospective, randomized, controlled trials for potential therapies.

Common management strategies for EG revolve around the severity of symptoms and diseases. For patients with mild symptoms, symptomatic management can be first attempted (e.g., as needed loperamide for diarrhea), dietary adjustments, and close observation can be tried as some cases of EG spontaneously resolve without therapy [23]. Elimination diets may be an option but there is insufficient evidence in adults.

The mainstay of therapy for patients with significant symptoms, such as obstruction or malabsorption, continues to be steroids. Although differing regimens have been reported, many recommend a prednisone taper therapy, with initial 8-week course of therapy with

1–2 mg/kg, to be followed with a 6–8-week taper; 90% respond [3]. Repeated courses may be required as recurrence has been reported either during the taper (15%) or following the tapering process (one-third to one-half). For refractory cases where the patient cannot be tapered off oral prednisone, transition to budesonide has been reported as a possible alternative [25]. Other successful approaches reported in the literature include sodium cromoglycate and montelukast [26–29].

Take-home points

Diagnosis:
- Clinical manifestations of eosinophilic gastroenteritis (EG) are dependent upon the site of disease involvement, as well as depth of tissue involvement of the gut wall.
- Peripheral eosinophilia raises suspicion for EG but is not required for diagnosis.
- Gastric and/or duodenal biopsies with more than 20 eosinophils per high-power field is commonly accepted as confirming the diagnosis of EG, in the absence of parasitic infection.

Therapy:
- Mild disease may be monitored or symptomatically managed with dietary exclusions, as some cases resolve spontaneously.
- Steroids remain the cornerstone of therapy with often dramatic clinical response.
- Relapse after steroid induced remission occurs in up to 50%.

References

1 Kaijser R. Zur Kenntnis der allegischen Affektioner desima Verdauungskanal von Standpunkt desima Chirurgen aus. *Arch Klin Chir* 1937; **188**: 36–64.

2 Talley NJ, Shorter RG, Phillips SF, Zinsmeister AR. Eosinophilic gastroenteritis: a clinicopatholical study of patients with disease of the mucosa, muscle layer, and subserosal tissues. *Gut* 1990; **31**: 54–8.

3 Khan S. Eosinophilic gastroenteritis. *Best Pract Res Clin Gastroenterol* 2005; **19**: 177–98.

4 Chen MJ, Chu CH, Lin SC, *et al*. Eosinophilic gastroenteritis: Clinical experience with 15 patients. *World J Gastroenterol* 2003; **9**: 2813–16.

5 Johnstone J, Morson B. Eosinophilic gastroenteritis. *Histopathology* 1978; **2**: 335–48.

6 Kelly KJ. Eosinophilic gastroenteritis. *J Pediatr Gastroenterol Nutr* 2000; **30**: S28–S35.

7 Robert F, Mura E, Durant JR. Mucosal eosinophilic gastroenteritis with systemic involvement. *Am J Med* 1977; **62**: 39–43.

8 Gregg JA, Utz DC. Eosinophilic cystitis associated with eosinophilic gastroenteritis. *Mayo Clin Proc* 1974; **49**: 185–7.

9 Walsh RE, Gaginella TS. The eosinophil in inflammatory bowel disease. *Scand J Gastroenterol* 1991; **26**: 1217–24.

10 Sarin SK, Malhotra V, Sen Gupta S, *et al.* Significance of eosinophil and mast cell counts in rectal mucosa in ulcerative colitis: a prospective controlled study. *Dig Dis Sci* 1978; **32**: 363–7.

11 Winter HS, Madara JL, Stafford JL, *et al.* Intraepithelial eosinophils: a new diagnostic criterion for reflux esophagitis. *Gastroenterology* 1982; **83**: 818–23.

12 Brown LF, Goldman H, Antonioli DA. Intraepithelial eosinophils in endoscopic biopsies of adults with reflux esophagitis. *Am J Surg Pathol* 1984; **8**: 899–905.

13 Rothenberg ME, Mishra A, Brandt EB, *et al.* Gastrointestinal eosinophils. *Immunol Rev* 2001; **179**: 139–55.

14 Rothenberg ME. Eosinophilic gastrointestinal disorders (EGID). *J Allergy Clin Immunol* 2004; **113**: 11–28.

15 Jose PJ, Griffiths-Johnson DA, Collins PD, *et al.* Eotaxin: a potent eosinophil chemoattractant cytokine detected in a guinea pig model of allergic airways inflammation. *J Exp Mode* 1994; **179**: 881–7.

16 Matthews AN, Fried DS, Zimmerman N, *et al.* Eotaxin is required for the baseline level of tissue eosinophils. *Proc Natl Acad Sci USA* 1998; **95**: 6273–8.

17 Klein NC, Hargrove RL, Sleisenger MH, *et al.* Eosinophilic gastroenteritis. *Medicine* (Baltimore) 1970; **49**: 299–319.

18 Goldman H, Proujansky R. Allergic proctitis and gastroenteritis in children: clinical and mucosal biopsy features in 53 cases. *Am J Surg Pathol* 1986; **10**: 75–86.

19 Moon A, Kleinman RE. Allergic gastroenteropathy in children. *Ann Allergy* 1995; **74**: 5–12.

20 Teele, RL, Katz AJ, Goldman H, *et al.* Radiographic features of eosinophilic gastroenteritis (allergic gastroenteropathy) of childhood. *Am J Roentgenol* 1979; **132**: 575–80.

21 Lee KJ, Hahm KB, Kim YS, *et al.* The usefulness of Tc-99m HMPAO labeled WBC SPECT in eosinophilic gastroenteritis. *Clin Nucl Med* 1997; **22**: 536–41.

22 Straumann A, Spichtin HP, Bucher KA, *et al.* Eosinophilic esophagitis: red on microscopy, white on endoscopy. *Digestion* 2004; **70**: 109–16.

23 Lee M, Hodges WG, Huggins TL, *et al.* Eosinophilic gastroenteritis. *South Med J* 1996; **89**: 189–94.

24 Lee CM, Changchien CS, Chen PC, *et al.* Eosinophilic gastroenteritis: 10 years experience. *Am J Gastroenterol* 1993; **88**: 70–4.

25 Tan AC, Kruimel JW, Naber TH. Eosinophilic gastroenteritis treated with non-enteric coated budesonide tablets. *Eur J Gastroenterol Hepatol* 2001; **13**: 425–7.

26 Van Dellen RG, Lewis JC. Oral administration of cromolyn in a patient with protein-losing enteropathy, food allergy, and eosinophilic gastroenteritis. *Mayo Clin Proc* 1994; **69**: 441–4.

27 Perez-Millan A, Martin-Lorente JL, Lopez-Morante A, *et al.* Subserosal eosinophilic gastroenteritis treated efficaciously with sodium cromoglycate. *Dig Dis Sci* 1997; **42**: 342–4.

28 Neustrom MR, Friesen C. Treatment of eosinophilic gastroenteritis with montelukast. *J Allergy Clin Immunol* 1999; **104**: 506.

29 Schwartz DA, Pardi DS, Murray JA. Use of montelukast as steroid sparing agent for recurrent eosinophilic gastroenteritis. *Dig Dis Sci* 2001; **46**: 1787–90.

CHAPTER 51
Hernias and Volvulus

Rebecca R. Cannom[1], Rodney J. Mason[2], and Tom R. DeMeester[3]

[1]Division of Thoracic Foregut Surgery, Department of Surgery, Keck School of Medicine, University of Southern California, Los Angeles, CA, USA

[2]Division of General and Laparoscopic Surgery, University of Southern California, Los Angeles, CA, USA

[3]Department of Surgery, Keck School of Medicine, University of Southern California, Los Angeles, CA, USA

Summary

Diaphragmatic hernias include acquired hiatal hernias and those of traumatic and congenital origin. Type I (sliding) hiatal hernias are frequently associated with gastroesophageal reflux disease (GERD). Type II hiatal hernias, known as paraesophageal hernias, can cause acute gastric volvulus, which is a surgical emergency. Gastric volvulus typically presents with Borchardt triad: epigastric pain, retching without emesis, and difficulty or inability to pass a nasogastric tube (NGT). A computed tomography (CT) scan is typically the first diagnostic study performed when these patients present to the emergency room (ER) or their primary care physician. A contrast video esophagram followed by an esophagogastroduodenoscopy (FGD) confirms the diagnosis. Prompt surgical repair is indicated.

Case

A 52-year-old female presents to the ER with a 1-week history of new-onset chest pain with dysphagia. The patient had a 4-year history of reflux symptoms including heartburn and regurgitation. Her new complaints were felt to be cardiac in etiology. Cardiac work-up was normal and the patient was discharged home.

Definition and Epidemiology

A hernia is a protrusion of the abdominal cavity beyond its fascial or muscular walls through fascial or muscular openings or defects. Diaphragmatic hernias include acquired hernias through the esophageal hiatus and hernias through traumatic or congenital defects in the diaphragm.

Hiatal hernias result from an enlargement of the esophageal hiatus and are the most common type of diaphragmatic hernia. Hiatal hernias frequently allow for transdiaphragmatic migration of intra-abdominal contents [1]. They are classified based on the location of

Practical Gastroenterology and Hepatology: Esophagus and Stomach, 1st edition. Edited by Nicholas J. Talley, Kenneth R. DeVault and David E. Fleischer. © 2010 Blackwell Publishing Ltd.

the gastroesophageal junction (GEJ) and the hernia sac contents. Ninety percent of diaphragmatic hernias are Type I hiatal hernias or sliding hiatal hernias. The gastroesophageal junction is intrathoracic with the hernia sac containing gastric cardia and fundus. Type II hiatal hernias or paraesophageal hernias constitute 3–5% of acquired diaphragmatic hernias. The gastroesophageal junction is intra-abdominal and the hernia sac contains gastric fundus and body. Type III hiatal hernias are a combination of Types I and II; the gastroesophageal junction is located in the chest, but remains in its normal location in relation to the fundus of the stomach. Type IV hiatal hernias contain another intra-abdominal organ in the hernia sac, in addition to the stomach.

Sliding hiatal hernias are the most frequent abnormality detected on barium studies. Their incidence is unknown and in most situations they are asymptomatic and detected unsuspectedly. Those who estimate their incidence state that 70% of patients over age 70 have a hiatal hernia. Paraesophageal hernias, in contrast to sliding hiatal hernias, are quite rare with an incidence of less than 1% [2]. Hiatal hernias are twice as likely to occur in women, and the incidence in women increases with advancing age [2].

A paraesophageal hernia, or type II hernia, can lead to gastric volvulus. Volvulus is a more than 180-degree rotation of a hollow organ about its mesentery, with possible sequelae of luminal obstruction, impaired venous return, and tissue ischemia [1]. More common types of volvulus are cecal and sigmoid volvulus [1]. Gastric volvulus has a peak incidence in the fifth decade of life, with men and women affected equally [3].

Traumatic hernias are much less common than nontraumatic hernias. Blunt abdominal trauma results in a traumatic rupture of the diaphragm 5% of time. Penetrating trauma to the anterior chest, inferior to the nipple line, has a 42% incidence of diaphragmatic injury and hernia [4].

The most common congenital diaphragmatic hernia is the Bochdalek hernia. This is a posterolateral diaphragmatic hernia and occurs in approximately 1/3000 live births. Morgagni hernias are rare, accounting for only 3% of surgically treated diaphragmatic hernias [5]. They are parasternal and typically the result of postnatal trauma. Eventration of the diaphragm is an attenuation of one leaf of the diaphragm resulting in a unilateral elevation of the diaphragm and the organ underneath [5]. When the left diaphragm is involved it can lead to a gastric volvulus underneath the high riding diaphragm. Eventrations of the diaphragm commonly are confused with a hiatal hernia.

Pathophysiology

Hiatal hernias are caused by an enlargement of the esophageal hiatus due to developmental defects, increased intra-abdominal pressure, and depletion of elastic fibers in the phrenoesophageal membrane with aging [6,7]. The acquired hiatal enlargement allows the gastroesophageal junction to herniate into the chest (Type I) or for the gastric fundus to migrate alongside the gastroesophageal junction and into the chest (Type II) [2].

Paraesophageal hernias are the most common cause of gastric volvulus in both adults and children [1]. Less frequent causes include diaphragmatic defects secondary to eventration or trauma, abdominal adhesions, or a Bochdalek hernia, commonly seen in children [8]. Secondary gastric volvulus occurs when the stomach ascends into the chest and the greater curvature rotates anteriorly with respect to the fixed duodenum and gastroesophageal junction.

There are two ways the stomach can rotate. Organo-axial rotation, which accompanies two-thirds of gastric volvulus, occurs when the stomach ascends into the chest and the greater curvature rotates horizontally on its longitudinal axis between the pylorus and the gastroesophageal junction [1,9]. In one-third of patients, the stomach rotates vertically on a line parallel to the gastrohepatic ligament, known as mesenteroaxial rotation [1] (Figure 51.1).

Primary gastric volvulus is associated with eventration of the left diaphragm and results from laxity of the stomach's ligamentous attachments (gastrohepatic, gastrocolic, gastrosplenic, and gastrophrenic) allowing the stomach to abnormally rotate within the abdomen [3].

Clinical Features

Most hiatal hernias are asymptomatic, consequently type I and III hiatal hernias are found incidentally when an upper gastrointestinal (UGI) barium study or an EGD is performed for other reasons [6]. When symptoms occur the patient usually complains of heartburn and regurgitation [6]. In contrast, Type II hiatal hernias are usually symptomatic, but can be diagnosed incidentally when the chest X-ray reveals an air–fluid level in the mediastinum or the left chest [2] (Figure 51.2). Unlike Type I or III hiatal hernias, patients with Type II hiatal hernias tend not to present with reflux symptoms [7]. Rather, they complain of non-specific complaints such as epigastric pain, dysphagia, postprandial fullness, chest pain, shortness of breath, or palpitations. They can even present with arrhythmias and cardiac tamponade secondary to mediastinal compression [1,2]. Consequently, the diagnosis of a paraesophageal hernia can be illusive.

When paraesophageal hernias are complicated with acute gastric volvulus, obstruction, strangulation, and/or perforation can occur [2]. This surgical emergency presents with Borchardt triad of epigastric pain, retching without emesis, and difficulty or inability to pass a nasogastric tube (NGT). Borchardt triad occurs in 70% of all patients with a paraesophageal hernia and nearly 100% of those with an associated organoaxial volvulus [3]. Patients with acute gastric volvulus may present with minimal abdominal complaints as the incarcerated or strangulated stomach is intrathoracic [8]. In mesenteroaxial volvulus, the obstruction is usually partial and the

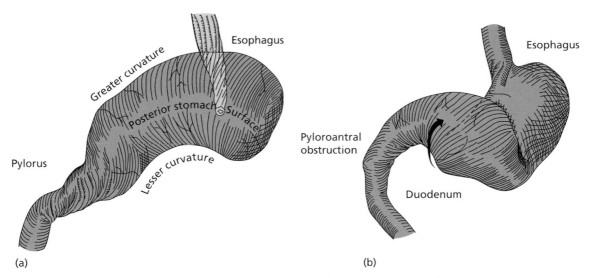

Figure 51.1 Illustration of (a) organoaxial and (b) mesenteroaxial gastric volvulus. In an organoaxial volvulus the stomach rotates horizontally on its pylorus and gastroesophageal junction axis. In a mesenteroaxial volvulus the stomach rotates vertically on an axis parallel to the gastrohepatic ligament.

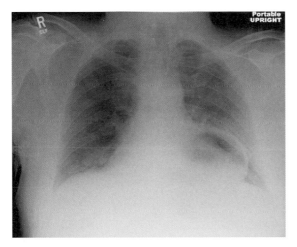

Figure 51.2 Chest X-ray of a large paraesophageal hernia demonstrating a retrocardiac air–fluid level in the upright anterior posterior projection.

gastroesophageal junction remains open allowing a NGT to be passed [8]. Chronic gastric volvulus, when symptomatic, causes vague, intermittent symptoms including abdominal pain, chest pain, vomiting, dysphagia, and early satiety [10].

Paraesophageal hiatal hernias may also present with anemia secondary to chronic gastrointestinal blood loss caused by gastric erosions (Cameron ulcers). These erosions result from venous engorgement of the stomach and its repetitive movement across the diaphragm [2,11]. In rare situations significant hematemesis can occur. Septic shock can ensue if ischemia or perforation has occurred. Strangulation of the arteries is a rare event due to the stomach's rich blood supply [8]. The more common cause of ischemia is venous obstruction and engorgement caused by gastric distension and hiatal obstruction of venous outflow.

Diagnosis

Case continued

Upon presentation to the ER, a chest X-ray and CT scan were done. Based on the findings, an UGI followed by an EGD was performed, confirming the diagnosis. The UGI showed that 70% of the stomach was intrathoracic with organoaxial rotation. It was a Type III hernia as the GEJ was located in the chest. The EGD was consistent with these findings and no evidence of ischemia (i.e., pneumatosis, bowel wall thickening, or enhancement) was visualized (Videos 23 and 24).

The diagnosis of hiatal hernia is highly dependent on radiographic and endoscopic findings as physical examination frequently provides little information. Type I hiatal hernias are typically diagnosed with esophagram and EGD. CT scan is not necessary. A paraesophageal hernia is diagnosed on chest X-ray when double air–fluid levels on an upright chest X-ray are seen. A retrocardiac air–fluid level on a lateral chest radiograph or an air-fluid level in the left chest is highly suggestive of a paraesophageal hernia.

Chest X-rays that are suggestive of gastric volvulus are typically followed with a CT scan and an UGI (considered the gold standard). The CT scan will show an "upside down stomach" in virtually all symptomatic patients with a paraesophageal hernia [3] (Figure 51.3).

An EGD should be attempted in hemodynamically stable patients with gastric volvulus to assess the distal esophagus and stomach and decompress the stomach by endoscopically gliding a NGT into it. Endoscopy may reveal an esophageal stricture or carcinoma in as high as 3% of this patient population [7]. Caution must be exercised not to over inflate the stomach, which may exacerbate the situation and cause perforation [2]. The stomach should always be completely deflated prior to removal of the scope.

Usually, esophageal pH monitoring is not helpful with Type II hernias and a complete esophageal motility study can be difficult to perform due to the distortion of the GEJ and distal esophagus [2]. On occasion it can be helpful to do a limited motility study to evaluate the amplitude of contraction in the distal esophageal body. If globally less than 20 mmHg a partial fundoplication should be considered. For Type I hernias, motility and pH monitoring provide invaluable information on the esophageal function as well as on the severity of the reflux, based on the DeMeester score [6].

Differential Diagnosis

The differential diagnosis of hiatal hernias and volvulus is broad and includes such common diseases as acute cholecystitis, biliary colic, and peptic ulcer disease [1]. Paraesophageal hernias commonly mimic a myocardial infarction or respiratory ailments such as pneumonia, asthma, and shortness of breath due to compression of the lung [5].

Therapeutics

Case continued

After the patient was adequately resuscitated, she was taken to the operating room for a laparoscopic repair of the paraesophageal hernia with reduction of the intrathoracic stomach and a Nissen fundoplication (Video 25).

Patients with Type I hernias and persistent GERD symptoms despite optimal medical treatment should be considered for an antireflux procedure, such as a Nissen

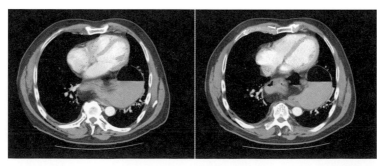

Figure 51.3 A CT scan of a patient with a large Type III hernia. Points of note include: (i) the gastroesophageal junction and the pylorus have both migrated into the chest cavity; (ii) the entire stomach has migrated into the chest, resulting in a so-called "intrathoracic stomach"; (iii) the stomach is volvulized by an organoaxial rotation resulting in a mechanical obstruction at the antrum as noted by the large amount of gastric contents in the stomach; and (iv) there is no CT evidence of gastric wall ischemia or perforation.

fundoplication. Further, patients with severe or recurrent complications of GERD, such as ulcers, strictures, bleeding, or repetitive aspiration also benefit from operative intervention. Laparoscopic Nissen fundoplication consists of a 360 degree fundoplication around the gastroesophageal junction with reduction of the hernia and closure of the diaphragmatic hiatus. It is the most common antireflux procedure performed today [6].

Operative therapy is the only treatment for types II–IV hiatal hernias. Conservative treatment of acute gastric volvulus with endoscopic reduction and percutaneous gastrostomy has been described in the literature. Currently, such an approach carries a high risk of perforation with further air insufflation and should be considered only in extremely poor surgical candidates [12,13].

Patients with acute gastric volvulus should be resuscitated by attempting to place a NGT. An emergent surgical consult should be obtained for laparotomy with reduction of the volvulus, sometimes via thoracotomy if it is a very large hernia or if there is suspicion of existing perforation [1,2]. If gastric necrosis is present a local excision, subtotal, or total gastrectomy needs to be performed [1]. To prevent hernia recurrence the stomach is brought below the diaphragm, a Nissen fundoplication is performed and one or two gastrostomies are placed to anchor the stomach to the anterior abdominal wall [14]. The diaphragmatic defect should be closed and buttressed with a biological mesh [1]. Most patients with acute or chronic gastric volvulus without peritonitis are repaired laparoscopically [15].

The treatment of asymptomatic patients with a paraesophageal hernia is controversial. Historically, prompt surgical repair was recommended for all patients regardless of symptoms based on a 1967 study that reported a mortality rate of 30% in patients with paraesophageal hernias [16]. More recent studies have shown that watchful waiting in high-risk patients is reasonable as the complication rate is currently thought to be significantly lower than previously reported. One study had no life-threatening complications after 78 months of follow-up of 23 asymptomatic patients with paraesophageal hernias [2]. Current recommendations are that symptomatic patients with evidence of esophageal mucosal damage (i.e., Barrett or esophagitis) or anemia, or asymptomatic patients who desire surgical intervention are surgical candidates and should undergo elective repair as outlined in Figure 51.4. Chronic gastric volvulus secondary to even-

trations of the diaphragm may be managed non-operatively as it is often intermittent and not likely to lead to strangulation [1].

Case continued

The patient underwent an UGI on postoperative day 1which revealed no leak and she was started on a clear liquid diet. Her diet was advanced and she was discharged on postoperative day 3.

Prognosis

A 10-year follow-up of patients who were symptomatic and underwent a Nissen fundoplication repair, shows 80% significant symptomatic improvement. When asked, 85% of patients would undergo the surgical therapy again [17]. Surgical therapy appears durable, with patients denying recurrence of their symptoms up to 4 years after surgery [2].

Sepsis secondary to strangulation is the leading cause of death from acute gastric volvulus, contributing to the historically reported 30–50% mortality rate [9]. Other complications of acute gastric volvulus include splenic rupture, pancreatic necrosis, omental avulsion, ulceration, perforation, and hemorrhage [8]. It is for this reason that surgery is usually recommended to patients with a paraesophageal hernia, as operative mortality rates in elective circumstances are less than 1% [5].

Take-home points

- Diaphragmatic hernias include traumatic, congenital, and hiatal hernias.
- Type I hiatal hernias (known as sliding hiatal hernias) constitute 90% of all hiatal hernias and are commonly associated with GERD.
- Diagnosis of a sliding hernias (Type I) require a video esophagram or EGD.
- In Type II hiatal hernias, known as paraesophageal hernias, the gastroesophageal junction is intra-abdominal with the gastric fundus and body herniating into the chest in a paraseophagel position.
- Type III hernias are a combination of Types I and II hernias and the gastroesophageal junction has slid intrathoracicly, but retains its relation to the gastric fundus as in the Type II hernias.

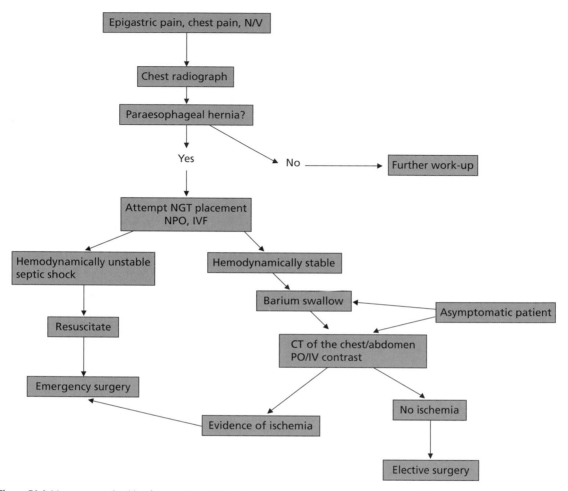

Figure 51.4 Management algorithm for a patient with a paraesophageal hernia and acute symptoms. N/V, nausea/vomiting; CXR, chest X-ray; NGT, nasogastric tube; NPO, nothing by mouth; IVF, intravenous fluids.

- Types II and III hernias can lead to gastric volvulus which, when acute, is a surgical emergency.
- Organoaxiol volvulus occurs in two-thirds of the patients with gastric volvulus and is recognized when the stomach rotates on its longitudinal axis (a line connecting the cardia to the pylorus).
- Acute gastric volvulus typically presents with Borchardt triad; epigastric pain, inability to vomit, and difficulty or inability to pass a NGT.
- A CT scan, video esophagram, and EGD confirm the diagnosis of gastric volvulus.
- The treatment of gastric volvulus is primarily surgical and includes reduction of the hernia, repair of the diaphragmatic defect, and fundoplication.

References

1 Yeo C, ed. *Shackelford's Surgery of the Alimentary Tract, 6th edn. Volvulus of the Stomach and Small Bowel*, White R, Jacobs D, eds, Vol. I. Philadelphia, PA: Saunders Elsevier, 2007: 1035–40.

2 Cameron J, ed. *Current Surgical Therapy*, 9th edn. Philadelphia, PA: Mosby Elsevier, 2008: 46–9.

3 Chau B, Dufel S. Gastric volvulus. *Emerg Med J* 2007; **24**: 446–7.

4 Murray JA, Demetriades D, Cornwell EE 3rd. Penetrating left thoracoabdominal trauma: the incidence and clinical presentation of diaphragm injuries. *J Trauma* 1997; **43**: 624–6.

5 Fischer J, ed. *Mastery of Surgery*, 4th edn. Philadelphia, PA: Lippincott, Williams, and Wilkins, 2007: 598–650.

6 Schwartz S, ed. *Principles of Surgery,* 8th edn. *Esophagus and Diaphragmatic Hernia*, Peters J, Demeester T, eds. Columbus: McGraw Hill, 2006: 835–73.

7 Landreneau RJ, Del Pino M, Santos R. Management of paraesophageal hernias. *Surg Clin North Am* 2005; **85**: 411–32.

8 Carter R, Brewer LA 3rd, Hinshaw DB. Acute gastric volvulus. A study of 25 cases. *Am J Surg* 1980; **140**: 99–106.

9 Wasselle JA, Norman J. Acute gastric volvulus: pathogenesis, diagnosis, and treatment. *Am J Gastroenterol* 1993; **88**: 1780–4.

10 Cozart JC, Clouse RE. Gastric volvulus as a cause of intermittent dysphagia. *Dig Dis Sci* 1998; **43**: 1057–60.

11 Weston AP. Hiatal hernia with cameron ulcers and erosions. *Gastrointest Endosc Clin North Am* 1996; **6**: 671–9.

12 Tabo T, *et al.* Balloon repositioning of intrathoracic upside-down stomach and fixation by percutaneous endoscopic gastrostomy. *J Am Coll Surg* 2003; **197**: 868–71.

13 Januschowski R. [Endoscopic repositioning of the upside-down stomach and its fixation by percutaneous endoscopic gastrostomy]. *Dtsch Med Wochenschr* 1996; **121**: 1261–4.

14 Gourgiotis S, *et al.* Acute gastric volvulus: diagnosis and management over 10 years. *Dig Surg* 2006; **23**: 169–72.

15 Teague WJ, *et al.* Changing patterns in the management of gastric volvulus over 14 years. *Br J Surg* 2000; **87**: 358–61.

16 Skinner DB, Belsey RH. Surgical management of esophageal reflux and hiatus hernia. Long-term results with 1,030 patients. *J Thorac Cardiovasc Surg* 1967; **53**: 33–54.

17 Cowgill SM, *et al.* Ten-year follow up after laparoscopic Nissen fundoplication for gastroesophageal reflux disease. *Am Surg* 2007; **73**: 748–52; discussion 752–3.

CHAPTER 52

Surgery for Peptic Ulcer Disease

Henry Lin[1] and Daniel B. Jones[2]

[1] National Naval Medical Center and Walter Reed Army Medical Center, Bethesda, MD, USA
[2] Section Minimally Invasive Surgery, Beth Israel Deaconess Medical Center, Boston, MA, USA

Summary

The number of operations for management of peptic ulcer disease (PUD) has decreased and the history of these key operations is briefly reviewed here. Treatment of PUD has shifted from the paradigm of acid hypersecretion to colonization by *H. pylori*. Treatment for perforation, bleeding, obstruction, or refractory disease depends on the status of the patient, co-morbidities, the *H. pylori* status, and the patient's dependence on ulcerogenic medication, for example NSAIDs and ASA. A perforated peptic ulcer should be closed, followed by consideration of definitive antiulcer surgery. Bleeding usually stops spontaneously or with endoscopic therapy, but some patients will require urgent surgery to control refractory bleeding. Refractory ulcers and obstruction due to ulcer disease are uncommon in the era of *H. pylori* eradication and proton pump inhibitor therapy. Laparoscopic approaches to traditional peptic ulcer surgery are becoming more popular. While surgery can cure PUD, there are often postoperative symptoms and complications which must be managed.

Case

A 73-year-old woman with arthritis and history of asthma presents with an acute onset of epigastric pain 2 h ago. She is afebrile with a heart rate of 96 and is normotensive. Medications include intermittent ibuprofen, ranitidine, and steroids for asthma exacerbations. On physical examination, there is significant epigastric tenderness with rebound tenderness. White blood cell count is $12 \times 10/mm^3$. Acute abdominal series demonstrates free air.

Epidemiology

There has been a paradigm shift in peptic ulcer disease (PUD) over the past two decades from a focus on acid hypersecretion to an emphasis on gastric *Helicobacter pylori* [1,2]. *H. pylori* is present in 80–100% of duodenal ulcers (DU). Approximately 50–60% of peptic ulcers are caused by non-steroid anti-inflammatory drugs (NSAIDs) or acetylsalicylic acid (ASA) in *H. pylori*-

negative patients [3]. In addition, NSAIDs and aspirin are associated with 32–60% of perforated PUD in *H. pylori*-negative patients [3]. Of the 10–15% PUD patients who are *H. pylori*-negative and not taking NSAIDs [3], hypersecretors and Zollinger–Ellison syndrome must be excluded by checking gastrin levels. Cocaine can cause gastric perforation, usually prepyloric, probably related to ischemia. Smoking is also a risk factor for perforation and refractory ulcers [2].

Pathophysiology

Peptic ulcer disease can manifest either as gastric or duodenal ulcers. Gastric ulcers are divided into five types, which are depicted in Figure 52.1, and may guide therapy. The complications of both gastric and duodenal ulcers include perforation, bleeding, and obstruction. Surgical therapy is reserved for ulcers that fail to respond to medical therapy and for complications of ulcer disease. Expected referrals to surgeons will be in only 5–10% of patients with chronic PUD, given the rapid expansion in use of antisecretory agents [4]. There is a growing consensus that vagotomy is rarely, if ever, needed [5].

Practical Gastroenterology and Hepatology: Esophagus and Stomach, 1st edition. Edited by Nicholas J. Talley, Kenneth R. DeVault and David E. Fleischer. © 2010 Blackwell Publishing Ltd.

Clinical Features

Patients present with epigastric pain which is typically burning, stabbing, or gnawing, and worse in the morning. Food and antacids promptly relieve symptoms [6]. Atypical presentations may include bleeding or perforation with or without the typical symptoms.

Bleeding PUD presents with hematemesis [7] and occasionally melena that is severe and sudden (see Chapter 47 for a treatment algorithm).

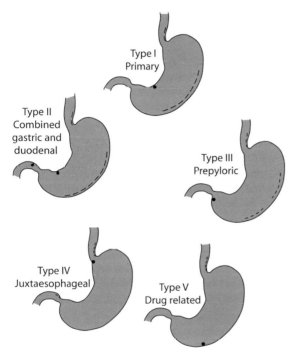

Figure 52.1 Traditional description of five types of gastric ulcers. Reproduced from Rege RV, Jones DB, Spechler SJ. Current role of surgery in peptic ulcer disease. In: *Sleisenger and Fordtran's Gastrointestinal and Liver Disease*, Vol. 1, Issue 1. Copyright Elsevier: Saunders, PA, 2002: 732–809, Fig. 42-9. With permission from Elsevier.

Perforated ulcer may cause sudden onset of severe upper abdominal pain which rapidly becomes generalized over hours [3] and can be unrelenting [1]. These patients may have a history of "dyspepsia," NSAIDs or aspirin abuse, and be *H. pylori* positive [3].

Perforation

Diagnosis (Table 52.1)

On plain film radiology, pneumoperitoneum is 92% sensitive for perforated peptic ulcer disease [3] and is usually subphrenic in location [1]. This pneumoperitoneum can be seen on either an upright portable chest X-ray or a left lateral decubitus abdominal plain film in which the patient has been in that position for at least 5 min. Typically, as little as 5 mL of pneumoperitoneum can be visualized. Ultrasound can demonstrate a "fisheye sign" when the anterior wall of the duodenum is perforated.

Computed tomography (CT) scan of the abdomen and pelvis can demonstrate the following changes: in 50% of patients, there are occasionally inflammatory changes in paraduodenal tissue and the tissues of the right subhepatic space; in 75% of patients, there is fluid in the right subhepatic space. CT is usually of little value until 6h or longer from symptom onset if no pneumoperitoneum is visualized on plain films or ultrasound.

Therapeutics

In general, if the patient is suspected of having a perforated ulcer [8], recommendations are to operate unless the patient is moribund or clinically improving with a sealed perforation. There are several potential operations to be considered in this situation. If there is a significant leak, then oversew of the ulcer and/or a Graham patch (Figure 52.2) is performed, but it is also usually reasonable to consider performing definitive surgery to improve

Table 52.1 Diagnosis of peptic ulcer.

Diagnosis	Symptoms	Physical exam findings	Diagnostic studies
Duodenal ulcer	Epigastric pain: burning, stabbing, gnawing	±Epigastric tenderness	±UGI or EGD
Perforated	Severe upper abdominal pain, sudden onset	Diffuse abdominal tenderness	Plain film: pneumoperitoneum
Bleeding	Hematemesis; occasionally severe melena	±Melena	±NGT lavage, EGD

EGD, esophagogastroduodenoscopy; UGI, upper gastrointestinal contrast study; NGT, nasogastric tube.

the odds of healing and to decrease the chance of recurrence. All patients with routine or complicated peptic ulcer disease should be tested and treated for *H. pylori* (see Chapter 44 for details).

Potential Ulcer Surgeries

• **Truncal vagotomy** and drainage with either pyloroplasty or antrectomy has traditionally been performed for acid reduction. A drainage procedure is required after vagotomy to compensate for delayed gastric emptying.

• **Pyloroplasty** (Figure 52.3) opens the pylorus longitudinally and closes the opening transversely to minimize narrowing. A pyloroplasty is preferred to antrectomy when the patient is critically ill or when inflammation associated with the ulcer precludes an antrectomy.

• **Antrectomy** (Figure 52.4) is a more definitive procedure (Table 52.2). After antrectomy, either a Bilroth I or Bilroth II reconstruction is performed.

• **Billroth I** reconstruction (Figure 52.5) fashions a gastroduodenostomy and is done when the pylorus and duodenum are easily mobile, e.g. after an early perforation before the onset of inflammation prevents mobilization.

• **Billroth II** reconstruction (Figure 52.6a,b) is a gastrojejunostomy that is performed when the severity of the disease or inflammation, such as in a delayed or chronic presentation, prevents mobilization, e.g., late perforation.

• **Highly selective vagotomy** (HSV) has been used to avoid the dumping syndrome (explosive diarrhea) that is associated with the more proximal truncal vagotomy [4]. Because HSV takes longer to perform, it can only be performed when the patient is otherwise stable. All branches of the vagal nerves to the stomach wall are divided except the "crow's foot" branches of nerve of Latarjet [5,9], that is the vagal innervation to the pylorus. Also preserved are the hepatic branch of anterior vagal trunk and the celiac branch of posterior vagal trunk. The criminal nerve of Grassi is taken to assure completion of the highly selective vagotomy. Recommendations for surgeons are to start the dissection proximal to crow's foot and dissect proximally [5].

• **Roux-en-Y gastrojejunostomy** (Figure 52.7) is used to resolve or prevent the problems of bile reflux associated with Bilroth II and does not require the mobility for the anatomy of the Bilroth I reconstruction.

The decision to perform the operation laparoscopically or via open technique will depend on individual surgeon's skill, whether the ulcer is causing significant bleeding, and the patient's condition. There are, however, a few relative contraindications to laparoscopic approach: pre-existing gastric outlet obstruction and greater than 1.5–2 cm perforation which prevents technically feasible closure. Of note, the laparoscopic technique does result in a higher re-operative rate. Not all but many experts argue that a parietal cell vagotomy should be considered for indications listed in Table 52.2.

Contraindications to definitive ulcer surgery include serious medical illness (myocardial infarction, congestive heart failure, uncontrolled diabetes, chronic obstructive pulmonary disease, renal failure) and shock or hemodynamic instability.

Bleeding

Upper GI bleeding may presents with hematemesis or acute onset of melena. Acute management begins with the Emergency Department physician or primary care manager, but should quickly include the gastroenterologist, radiologist, and surgeon (see also Chapter 47 for a treatment algorithm). Most patients undergo esophagogastroduodenoscopy (EGD) early in the course of significant bleeding and the findings from that endoscopy can be used to predict both rebleeding risk and mortality. The risk of rebleeding in a patient who is *H. pylori* positive, has a gastric ulcer, and has a low-risk endoscopic appearance is 1%/month. For a peptic ulcer with a visible vessel located on the posterior wall of the duodenum, there is a high risk of massive rebleeding secondary to the presence of the gastric duodenal artery in that location. For an observed, non-arterial hemorrhage from gastric ulcer, the rebleed rate ranges between 10 and 53%. Additionally, the rebleed event usually occurs before hospital day 4 and is associated with increased mortality.

Indications for surgical treatment of bleeding duodenal ulcer include:

1 Failed endoscopic treatments (dependent on presence of multiple co-morbidities, age >60, previous history of ulcer diathesis).

2 A second endoscopic treatment is controversial. Some data support a second attempt at endoscopic control and others have suggested a high likelihood of failure. The decision needs to be individualized and some patients should be taken urgently to the operating

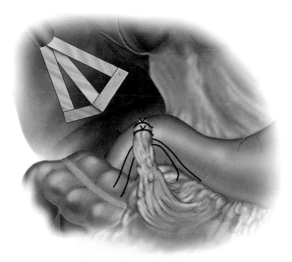

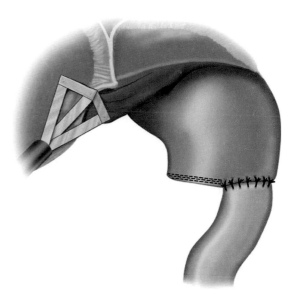

Figure 52.2 Graham (omental) patch. Reproduced from Jones DB, Maithel SK, Schneider BE. Laparoscopic management of peptic ulcer disease. In: *Atlas of Minimally Invasive Surgery.* Cine-Med, 2006: 217. Reprinted with permission from Cine-Med, Inc., 127 Main Street North, Woodbury, CT 06798. Copyright© Cine-Med, Inc.

Figure 52.4 Antrectomy. Reproduced from Jones DB, Maithel SK, Schneider BE,. Laparoscopic partial gastrectomy. In: *Atlas of Minimally Invasive Surgery.* Copyright Cine-Med, 2006: 183, Fig H. Reprinted with permission from Cine-Med, Inc., 127 Main Street North, Woodbury, CT 06798. Copyright© Cine-Med, Inc.

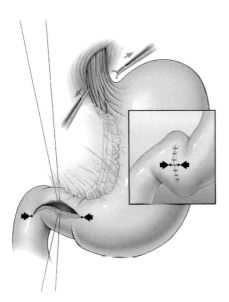

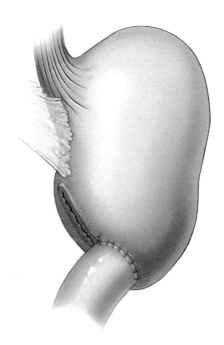

Figure 52.3 Pyloroplasty. Reproduced from Rege RV, Jones DB, Spechler SJ. Current role of surgery in peptic ulcer disease. In: Feldman M, Friedman LS, Sleisenger MH, eds. *Sleisenger and Fordtran's Gastrointestinal and Liver Disease*, Vol. 1, Issue 1. Copyright Elsevier: Saunders, PA, 2002: 732–809, Fig. 42–2. With permission from Elsevier.

Figure 52.5 Bilroth I (gastroduodenostomy). Reproduced from Rege RV, Jones DB, Spechler SJ. Current role of surgery in peptic ulcer disease. In: *Sleisenger and Fordtran's Gastrointestinal and Liver Disease*, Vol. 1, Issue 1. Copyright Elsevier: Saunders, PA, 2002: 732–809, Fig. 42–5. With permission from Elsevier.

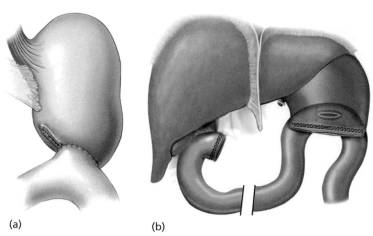

(a)   (b)

Figure 52.6 (a) Bilroth II (gastrojejunostomy). Reproduced from Rege RV, Jones DB, Spechler SJ. Current role of surgery in peptic ulcer disease. In: *Sleisenger and Fordtran's Gastrointestinal and Liver Disease*, Vol. 1, Issue 1. Copyright Elsevier: Saunders, PA, 2002: 732–809, Fig. 42–6. With permission from Elsevier. (b) Bilroth II, laparoscopic approach. Reproduced from Jones DB,

Maithel SK, Schneider BE. Laparoscopic partial gastrectomy. In: *Atlas of Minimally Invasive Surgery*. Copyright Cine-Med, 2006: 189, Fig. M-b. Reproduced with permission from Cine-Med, Inc., 127 Main Street North, Woodbury, CT 06798. Copyright© Cine-Med, Inc.

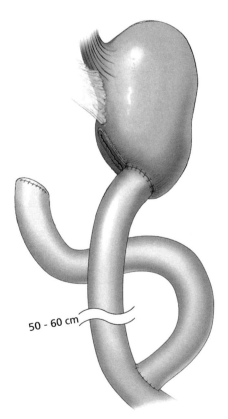

Figure 52.7 Roux-en-Y gastrojejunostomy. Reproduced from Rege RV, Jones DB, Spechler SJ. Current role of surgery in peptic ulcer disease. In: *Sleisenger and Fordtran's Gastrointestinal and Liver Disease*, Vol. 1, Issue 1. Copyright Elsevier: Saunders, PA, 2002: 732–809, Fig. 42-8. With permission from Elsevier.

Table 52.2 Treatment of peptic ulcer.

Indications for surgery [Ref.]	Additional factors	Treatment	Recurrence	
Perforation + chronic DU	*H. pylori* neg.	Graham patch ± PCV, or TV + P [10] w/ulcer excision [3]	15–20% recur	
Chronic bleeding [1]		TV + A → BI > BII	2% recur [1]	Highest mortality rate
Intractable [1]	Gastrinoma excluded	PCV	15–20% recur	
Gastric outlet obstruction [1]	GU or DU	TV + A → BI > BII > GJ [3,10]	2% recur [1]	Almost disappeared [1]
Perforated DU				
+Prior ulcer complications		Graham patch ± PCV [4], or TV + P w/ulcer excision	15–20% recur	
+Prior *H. pylori* treatment [4]	Tx failure [4] or known *H. pylori* neg.	Graham patch ± PCV, or TV + P w/ulcer excision	15–20% recur	
+Non-compliant [4]		Graham patch ± PCV, or TV + P w/ulcer excision	15–20% recur	
+NSAID-dependent [4], steroid-dependent [8]	±No toleration of PPIs or cytoprotective agents	Graham patch ± PCV, or TV + P w/ulcer excision	15–20% recur	
+age <40		Graham patch ± PCV, or TV + P w/ulcer excision	15–20% recur	
Perforated DU >2 cm [3,9]		TV + A [4] → BII		
+Bleeding		TV + P [4], resection of perforation, U-stitch bleeding		
+Pregnant		Plication only [11]		
Perforated GU [8]				
(>1–2 cm proximal to pyloric vein), HD stable		±TV + A → BI [3,10]		
HD stable + long h/o PUD		TV + A → BI [3,10]		
HD stable + failed TV + P		TV + A → BI [3,10]		
h/o ulcer + not good candidate for resection		±IV + P	5% recur	
H. pylori + untreated, not NSAID-dependent		(Lap) ulcer biopsy/ excision + omentoplasty		
Elderly or unstable or difficult location of perforation		Ulcer excision + 1° closure ± omentoplasty [10]		
Previous operation for DU	Prior vagotomy	Require 60–70% gastric resection → BI		
Previous operation for DU	Prior adequate gastrectomy	TV ± re-resection ± r/o ZE		
Bleeding DU				
Actively bleeding DU [1,7,9]	High risk, unstable	Suture bleeding vessel, TV + P	5% recur	
Actively bleeding DU [1,7,9]	High risk, unstable + no Previous med Tx	Suture bleeding vessel + Med Tx [7,9]		
Actively bleeding DU [7,9]	Young, HD stable, min. co-morbidities	Suture bleeding vessel, PCV + P	Recurrent bleed → mortality 30% [2]	
Bleeding GU				
Bleeding from GU [8]	Unstable, urease +	Ulcer excision + *H. pylori* treatment		
Bleeding from GU [8]	Unstable	Oversew ulcer [8,9] vs. wedge excision + TV + P [9]		

Table 52.2 (continued)

Indications for surgery [Ref.]	Additional factors	Treatment	Recurrence
Rebleeding controlled from GU [8,9], NSAID-dependent	Stable	Distal gastrectomy → BI [8,9]	
Rebleeding controlled from GU [8,9], NSAID-dependent	GU II	+(TV + A [6,9]) < PCV [6]	
Rebleeding controlled from GU [8,9], NSAID-dependent	GU III	+(TV + P [9]) < PCV [6]	
Rebleeding controlled from GU [8,9], NSAID-dependent	GI IV	Biopsy ulcer, oversew ulcer [+9], ligate left gastric artery vs. subtotal gastrectomy + RNY esophagogastrojejunostomy	
Dieulefoy ulceration		suture ligation	

DU, duodenal ulcers; PCV, parietal cell vagotomy; TV, truncal vagotomy; P, pyloroplasty; BI, Bilroth; GU, gastric ulcer; A, antrectomy; GJ, gastrojejunostomy; Tx, treatment; GI, gastrointestinal; PPIs, proton pump inhibitor; ZE, Zollinger–Ellison syndrome; r/o, rule out; h/o, history of; Med, medical.

room. Morbidity and mortality increase with delayed intervention.

3 Failure of interventional radiology embolization—interventional radiology embolization of the gastric duodenal artery is reserved for bleeds >1 mL/min, especially in the poor surgical risk patients and in patients with multiple previous operations that make access to duodenum difficult.

4 Three to 6 units or more of packed red blood cells transfused without indication of cessation of bleeding or this amount transfused within a 24-h period [7]—again, some centers would do another endoscopy at this point, while others would move directly on to surgery.

5 "Giant gastric ulcer" i.e., >3 cm—malignancy must be excluded in these cases since there is a 30% incidence [8] in this situation. Also, rebleeding and failure are typical for these giant ulcers. After biopsy, the mucosal surface is cauterized or oversewn and an omental patch may be overlaid.

6 Twelve weeks of persistent bleeding despite medical treatment.

Refractory PUD

Refractory peptic ulcers in the era of *H. pylori* eradication and acid-suppressing agents such as proton pump inhibi-

tors are relatively rare. If a patient has persistent symptoms and a non-healing ulcer, NSAID or aspirin use should be strongly suspected. Surgery may be considered if an ulcer persists and *H. pylori* has been eradicated, the patient has not taken NSAID or aspirin, and has been treated adequately with an acid blocker. Surgeries for refractory ulcer disease are the same as those listed in the section on perforation above.

PUD induced obstruction is also much less common than in the past. Ongoing NSAID use should always be considered in these patients. A vagotomy and gastric emptying procedure can be curative, but most patients will continue to have some symptoms after that surgery.

Complications of Surgery

Recurrent or marginal ulcers can occur. If the patient has already had a truncal vagotomy, a modified glucose feeding test should be performed to evaluate the completeness of vagotomy [1]. If the patient has had an antrectomy, an evaluation to exclude retained antrum should be performed. These patients need to be considered for the exclusion of gastrinoma or Zollinger–Ellison syndrome. Ongoing NSAID use should also be considered. Placing an ambulatory pH probe in the residual stomach is another method to access ongoing acid secretion.

Postoperative gastroparesis may be treated with prokinetic agents (although safe effective agents in this class are somewhat lacking). Afferent loop syndrome occurs when partial obstruction of the limb of jejunum between the ligament of Treitz and the anastomosis to the stomach causes intermittent distension of the duodenum and proximal jejunum. Bile (alkaline) reflux gastritis occurs in almost every patient but is only clinically significant in a subset of patients when severe epigastric pain and sometimes bilious emesis occurs with gastric mucosal damage. In some situations, revising the surgery to a Roux-en-Y is required to isolate the stomach from the refluxed bile.

Gastric adenocarcinoma is increased in patients with gastric ulcer, but not with duodenal ulcer, regardless of whether PUD surgery has been performed.

Postvagotomy diarrhea typically occurs 1 h postprandially [1] and usually resolves over 1 year with diet changes. Only 10% of these patients require medical intervention such as codeine and loperamide. Dumping syndrome is another postoperative symptom that may be treated with dietary changes and in some more severe situations with octreotide.

Case continued

The patient had a portable upright chest X-ray that showed a small amount of free air under the left hemidiaphragm. She otherwise looked unchanged. Over the next few hours her abdomen became more distended and she underwent an exploratory laparotomy. This demonstrated a confined perforation in the anterior portion of the proximal duodenum. The perforation was closed and a highly selective vagotomy was performed. Her symptoms improved and several weeks later she underwent an EGD that showed a well-healed duodenal ulcer. Follow-up *H. pylori* testing was negative. It was suggested she avoid NSAID type medications in the future.

Take-home points

- The number of operations for management of PUD has decreased.
- Treatment of PUD has shifted from the paradigm of acid hypersecretion to colonization by *H. pylori*.
- Treatment for perforation depends on the status of the patient, co-morbidities, the *H. pylori* status, and the patient's dependence on ulcerogenic medication, e.g. NSAIDs and ASA.
- Surgical therapy in general includes Graham patch or oversew the ulcer without vagotomy.
- The treating provider should follow-up with determination of the *H. pylori* status.

References

1 Mulholland MW, Kauffman Jr, GL, Conter RL. In: Greenfield L, ed. *Surgery: Scientific Principles and Practice*. J.B. Lippincott Company, PA, 1993: 674–701.

2 Stabile BE. Redefining the role of surgery for perforated duodenal ulcer in the Helicobacter pylori era. *Ann Surg* 2002; **31**: 159.

3 Baker RJ. The perforated duodenal ulcer. In: Fischer JE, *et al.*, eds. *Mastery of Surgery*. Lippincott Williams and Wilkins, 2007: 891–901.

4 Siewert JR, Bumm R. Distal gastrectomy with billroth I, billroth II, or roux-Y reconstruction. In: Fischer JE, *et al. Mastery of Surgery*. Lippincott Williams and Wilkins, 2007.

5 Yahchouchy E, Debet A, Fingerhut A. Crack cocaine-related prepyloric perforation treated laparoscopically. *Surg Endosc* 2001; **16**: 220.

6 Jones DB, Maithel S, Schneider B. *Atlas of Minimally Invasive Surgery*. Woodbury, CT: *Cine-Med*, 2006.

7 Schirmer BD. Bleeding duodenal ulcer. In: Fischer JE, *et al.*, eds. *Mastery of Surgery*. Lippincott Williams & Wilkins, PA, 2007: 882–91.

8 Schlinkert RT, Kelly K. Upper GI bleeding. In: *ACS Surgery: Principles and Practices*. WebMD Corporation, NY, 2002: 286–91.

9 Rotstein OD, Nathens AB. Approach to peritonitis and intra-abdominal abscess. In: *ACS Surgery: Principles and Practices*, 2002: 1244.

10 Howell HS. When repair is enough for perforated duodenal ulcer. *Contemp Surg* 2008; **64**: 521–4.

11 Mercer DW, Robinson EK. Stomach. In: Townsend CM, *et al.*, eds. *Sabiston Textbook of Surgery*, 18th edn. Saunders, 2007; online.

CHAPTER 53

Esophageal and Gastric Involvement in Systemic and Cutaneous Diseases

John M. Wo

Division of Gastroenterology/Hepatology, University of Louisville School of Medicine, Louisville, KY, USA

Summary

Esophageal and gastric manifestations in systemic and cutaneous diseases vary a great deal. Some patients have debilitating symptoms, while others may have minimal symptoms with impaired physiologic function. Some patients may be asymptomatic but at risk for developing cancer. In this chapter, the esophageal and gastric manifestations of the connective tissue, endocrine, inflammatory, neuromuscular, and cutaneous diseases are reviewed.

Case

A 47-year-old female developed Raynaud phenomenon 6 years ago. An evaluation for a cough 4 years led to the diagnosis of interstitial lung disease. Two years ago skin changes were found and the diagnosis of scleroderma was made. She was referred by the rheumatologist for a series of complaints that included dry mouth, dysphagia, heartburn, bloating, and constipation. Her salivation has decreased and the test for Sjögren is positive. At endoscopy there is a 4-cm area of salmon-colored mucosa in the distal esophagus and a stricture is found at the squamocolumnar junction. Duodenal aspirates reveal bacterial overgrowth. Gastric emptying study shows delayed emptying at 2 and 4 h. Biopsy of the distal esophagus shows intestinal metaplasia without dysplasia. The stricture is dilated. She is placed on a proton pump inhibitor and a prokinetic agent and treated for bacterial overgrowth. Her upper gastrointestinal symptoms abate although she still complains of constipation.

Connective Tissue Diseases

Systemic Sclerosis (Table 53.1)

Systemic sclerosis (SSc), also known as systemic sclero-derma, is a generalized disorder of the small arteries with

Practical Gastroenterology and Hepatology: Esophagus and Stomach, 1st edition. Edited by Nicholas J. Talley, Kenneth R. DeVault and David E. Fleischer. © 2010 Blackwell Publishing Ltd.

proliferation of fibrosis affecting the skin and multiple organs. The gastrointestinal (GI) tract is the third most common organ affected after skin thickening and Raynaud phenomenon. In the early stages of SSc, there are thickened capillary basement membrane, swollen endothelial cells, and arteriolosclerosis. In the later stages, there is extensive collagen infiltration in the lamina propria toward the muscularis mucosa in the esophagus and stomach. Unlike the renal, cardiac, and pulmonary manifestations of SSc, where the mortality is increased, esophageal involvement does not affect overall mortality [1]. Esophageal symptoms are common, occurring in 50 to 80% of the patients. Severity of gastro-esophageal reflux disease (GERD) is correlated with impairment of distal esophageal peristalsis (Figure 53.1b). Erosive esophagitis and interstitial lung disease has been associated with esophageal aperistalsis in patients with SSc [2]. The function of the proximal striated esophagus is preserved. The extent of the GI dysmotility can be severe and diffuse, causing esophageal aperistalsis, gastroparesis, and chronic intestinal pseudo-obstruction (CIP).

Inflammatory Myopathies (Table 53.1)

Inflammatory myopathies consist of a heterogeneous group of acquired disorders including polymyositis, dermatomyositis, and inclusion-body myositis. They are

Table 53.1 Connective tissue diseases affecting the esophagus and stomach.

Clinical features	Diagnostic testing	Therapeutics
Systemic sclerosis (scleroderma)		
Symptoms: heartburn, regurgitation, dysphagia, dyspepsia, nausea, vomiting, early satiety, weight loss, GI bleeding Manifestations: GERD, gastroparesis, gastric telangiectasia, iron deficiency anemia	EGD: esophagitis, reflux stricture, Barrett esophagus uncommon, "watermelon" stomach Esophageal manometry and MII: low LES pressure, impaired acid and bolus clearance, impaired distal esophageal contraction, aperistalsis (Figure 53.1b) pH & impedance monitoring: acid and non-acid reflux, especially at night Others: delayed gastric emptying, abnormal slow waves and diminished postprandial power by EGG	Avoid eating late before bed High-dose PPI for GERD Prokinetics for gastroparesis, avoid indigestible solids Avoid antireflux surgery Endoscopic therapy for "watermelon" stomach
Inflammatory myopathies (polymyositis and dermatomyositis)		
Symptoms: oropharyngeal dysphagia, choking, dysphonia, aspiration, heartburn, regurgitation, nausea, vomiting, early satiety Manifestations: oropharyngeal dysfunction, GERD, gastroparesis	EGD: esophagitis Videofluoroscopy: oropharyngeal dysfunction, poor relaxation of UES Esophageal manometry: poor UES relaxation by solid state manometry, diminished proximal and distal pressures Others: delayed gastric emptying	PPI for GERD Prokinetics for gastroparesis Swallowing therapies Treatment for inflammatory myopathy (steroids, others) Look for paraneoplastic disease in dermatomyositis
Mixed connective tissue diseases		
Symptoms and manifestations: similar to scleroderma and inflammatory myopathies	Similar to scleroderma and inflammatory myopathies	Similar to scleroderma and inflammatory myopathies
Sjögren syndrome		
Symptoms: dysphagia, heartburn, dyspepsia, nausea Manifestations: chronic atrophic gastritis is common, mucosa-associated lymphoid tissue lymphoma	Esophageal manometry: variable but usually normal, simultaneous contractions, aperistalsis rare	Correct lack of saliva: chew sugarless gum, mucous-containing lozenges, cholinergic agonists Increase fluid intake
Systemic lupus erythematosus		
Symptoms: heartburn, regurgitation, chest pain, anorexia, nausea, vomiting, epigastric pain Manifestations: GERD, gastroparesis, gastric ulcers from vasculitis	Esophageal manometry: variable, low LES pressure, impaired distal esophageal peristalsis, aperistalsis rare Others: delayed gastric emptying	PPI for GERD Prokinetics for gastroparesis

EGG, electrogastrography; LES, lower esophageal sphincter; MII, multichannel intraluminal impedance; PPI, proton pump inhibitors; UES, upper esophageal sphincter; GERD, gastroesophageal reflux disease; EGD, esophagogastroduodenoscopy.

characterized by proximal muscle weakness with difficulty lifting the arms, climbing steps, and arising from chairs. The diagnosis of inflammatory myopathy is based on elevated muscle enzymes, electromyography, and muscle biopsy. Dermatomyositis is recognized by the characteristic heliotrope rash, periorbital edema, and papular scaly lesions over the knuckles (Gottren signs)

(Figure 53.2). There is a threefold increase in risk of cancer after making a diagnosis of dermatomyositis, especially for ovarian, lung, pancreatic, stomach, and colorectal cancers, and non-Hodgkin lymphoma. Inclusion body myositis causes a slowly progressive weakness of proximal and distal muscles in older patients. Weak pharyngeal striated muscles and uncoordinated

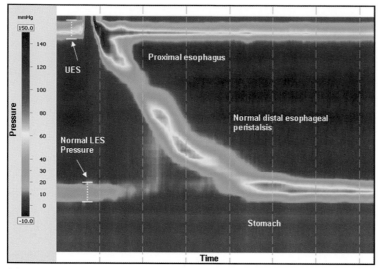

(a)

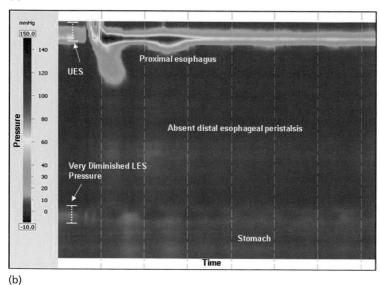

(b)

Figure 53.1 Pressure topography from high-resolution esophageal manometry in an asymptomatic individual with normal esophageal peristalsis (a) and in a patient with systemic scleroderma who has diminished lower esophageal sphincter (LES) pressure and absent esophageal peristalsis (b). Note that the pressures of the upper esophageal sphincter (UES) and proximal esophagus are preserved in scleroderma.

swallowing may cause oropharyngeal dysfunction, which may be the presenting complaint rather than the proximal skeletal muscle weakness [3]. Reflux symptoms are less common than in SSc, but severe upper GI dysmotility has been reported. Cricopharyngeal myotomy has been advocated in patients with poor upper esophageal sphincter relaxation, but the presence of severe GERD and gastroparesis should be excluded to prevent regurgitation to the throat and aspiration after surgery.

Mixed Connective Tissue Disease (Table 53.1)

Mixed connective tissue disease (MCTD) is a syndrome characterized by overlapping features of SSc, systemic lupus erythematosus (SLE), inflammatory myopathies, and rheumatoid arthritis. The systemic features of MCTD are Raynaud phenomenon, polyarthritis, swelling of the hands, myalgia, and esophageal dysfunction. The upper GI manifestations of MCTD are also an overlap of the

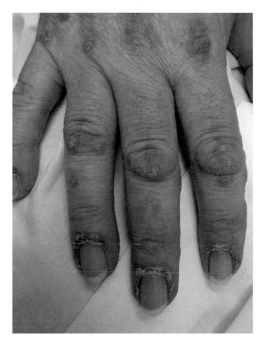

Figure 53.2 Papular scaly lesions over the knuckles (Gottren signs) in a patient with dermatomyositis. (Illustration courtesy of Dr Jeff Callen, University of Louisville, Louisville, KY.)

neural dysfunction and smooth muscle atrophy of SSc and striated muscle weakness of polymyositis. Heartburn and regurgitation are common, occurring up to half of patients with MCTD [4].

Sjögren Syndrome (Table 53.1)

Sjögren syndrome is a chronic autoimmune disorder associated with the destruction of salivary and lacrimal glands. It can present as a primary disorder or associated with other connective tissue disorders. It is believed that the absence of saliva, acting as a lubricant, may lead to impaired solid bolus transit through the esophagus. Most patients localize the dysphagia sensation to the pharyngeal region [5]. Chronic atrophic gastritis and secondary hypergastrinemia are common. Sjögren syndrome has been associated with mucosal associated lymphoid tissue (MALT) lymphoma, a form of non-Hodgkin B-cell lymphoma, of the salivary glands and other mucosal extranodal sites including the stomach. Gastric MALT lymphomas are usually less responsive to *H. pylori* therapy.

Systemic Lupus Erythematosus (Table 53.1)

Anorexia, nausea, vomiting, and abdominal pain are common complaints in patients with systemic lupus erythematosus (SLE). The precise cause of anorexia and abdominal pain are difficult to identify. Some patients with SLE have overlapping features of SSc, polymyositis, and MCTD, which all can affect the esophagus. Salivary gland dysfunction may contribute to symptoms of dysphagia or impaired acid clearance. Esophageal aperistalsis, gastroparesis, and CIP have been reported in some cases of SLE.

Endocrine and Metabolic Diseases

Diabetes Mellitus (Table 53.2)

Diabetes affects multiple levels in the neuromuscular control of esophagus and stomach. The pathology of diabetic gastroparesis consists of demyelination of the vagus nerve, loss of parasympathetic and sympathetic fibers, and degeneration of the interstitial cells of Cajal in the enteric nervous system. Diabetic patients have a higher perception threshold in the esophagus. Reflux symptoms in diabetics are unreliable predictors for the presence of GERD. In studies of unselected diabetics, delayed gastric emptying of solids was present in 40 to 50% of the patients. Many of these diabetics have no gastric symptoms. Hence, a patient's symptoms should be clinically correlated with delayed gastric emptying before make a diagnosis of diabetic gastroparesis. Evaluation and treatment of diabetic gastroparesis is described in details in Chapter 46.

Hypothyroidism (Table 53.2)

Oropharyngeal dysphagia has been reported in patients with myxedma associated with edematous facies and periorbital edema. Dysphagia responds well with thyroid replacement therapy, and the manometric abnormalities are reversible. Hypothyroidism is a known cause of hypomotility of the GI tract causing constipation and small bowel ileus, but cases are now rare because hypothyroidism is easily detected and treated. The underlying histology in myxedema small bowel ileus is the infiltration of the stroma, muscle fibers, and myenteric plexus by mucinous protein complexes.

Table 53.2 Endocrine and metabolic diseases affecting the esophagus and stomach.

Clinical features	Diagnostic testing	Therapeutics
Diabetes mellitus		
Symptoms: heartburn, regurgitation, dysphagia, chest pain, nausea, retching, vomiting, early satiety, effortless regurgitation of undigested foods, weight loss Manifestations: GERD, "silent" reflux is common, gastroparesis, impaired gastric accommodation	Esophageal manometry: variable, low LES pressure, impaired peristalsis, simultaneous contractions Gastric scintigraphy and breath test: delayed gastric emptying Others: abnormal slow wave frequency and diminished postprandial power by EGG, abnormal gastric barostat	Antiemetics for nausea and vomiting Treat hyperglycemia PPI for GERD Prokinetics for gastroparesis Gastric electrical stimulation for severe vomiting-predominant gastroparesis
Hypothyroidism		
Symptoms: oropharyngeal dysphagia Manifestations: oropharyngeal dysfunction, esophageal aperistalsis	Videofluoroscopy: oropharyngeal dysfunction, poor UES relaxation Esophageal manometry: reduced LES pressure, low amplitude, aperistalsis rare	Thyroid hormone replacement
Hyperthyroidism		
Symptoms: oropharyngeal dysphagia, dysphonia, nasal regurgitation, choking, weight loss, muscle wasting Manifestations: oropharyngeal dysfunction	Videofluoroscopy: oropharyngeal dysfunction Others: delayed gastric emptying, abnormal EGG	Treat hyperthyroidism Identify and treat underlying cause
Hypercalcemia		
Symptoms: dysphagia, anorexia, nausea, vomiting Manifestations: gastroparesis	Esophageal manometry: usually normal, diminished LES pressure Others: delayed gastric emptying, abnormal EGG	Treat hypercalcemia Identify and treat underlying cause

EGG, electrogastrography; LES, lower esophageal sphincter; PPI, proton pump inhibitors, GERD, gastroesophageal reflux disease.

Hyperthyroidism (Table 53.2)

Hyperthyroidism can cause a variety of neurologic manifestations, such as thyrotoxic myopathy and periodic paralysis. The precise cause of oropharyngeal dysphagia may be difficult to determine because myasthenia gravis, hypercalcemia, and hypokalemia may coexist in thyrotoxicosis. Patients with dysphagia most likely have marked weight loss and muscle wasting associated with severe hyperthyroidism. Abnormal vagal autonomic function, gastric myoelectrical activity, and delayed of gastric emptying has been described in patients with hyperthyroidism [6].

Hypercalcemia (Table 53.2)

Hypercalcemia is a common manifestation of many disorders, such as hyperparathyroidism, paraneoplastic syndrome, and disorders of increased bone turnover. Chronic hypercalcemia results in the depression of the nervous system because the neuronal membrane becomes impermeable to sodium ions, thus it is unable to generate action potentials. Striated and smooth muscle contractility is reduced. Dysphagia to solids has been reported in patients with hypercalcemia associated with a paraneoplastic syndrome. Dysphagia improves after the correction of hypercalcemia.

Inflammatory Diseases

Crohn Disease (Table 53.3)

Crohn disease is a systemic inflammatory disorder affecting the entire GI tract. Esophageal and gastric involvement is rare, and it is always associated with ileocolonic Crohn disease. The esophageal inflammation can be transmural causing extensive fibrosis and fistula formation to the bronchopulmonary tree, mediastinum, and pleura. Dysphagia can be severe with weight loss in a patient with a long narrowed esophageal stricture.

Table 53.3 Inflammatory diseases affecting the esophagus and stomach.

Clinical features	Diagnostic testing	Therapeutics
Crohn disease Symptoms: dysphagia, odynophagia, chest pain, epigastric pain, hematemesis, weight loss Manifestations: esophageal ulcers, long esophageal stricture, fistula, isolated esophageal or gastric Crohn is rare	Barium esophagram: shallow ulcers, irregular mucosa, stricture, fistula EGD: esophageal erosions and ulcers, cobblestone mucosa, prominent scarring (Figure 53.3a,b) Biopsy: chronic non-specific lymphohistocytic inflammation, non-caseating granuloma uncommon	Treat underlying Crohn Esophageal dilation Surgery may be needed if fistula refractory to treatment for Crohn
Behçet disease Symptoms: oral pain, chest pain, dysphagia, odynophagia, epigastric pain, hematemesis Manifestations: oral and esophageal apthous ulcers, esophageal stricture, fistula, esophageal varices from superior vena cava thrombosis	Similar to Crohn disease Biopsies: non-specific ulcerations with neutrophilic inflammatory infiltrate	Corticosteroids may be helpful Esophageal dilation
Sarcoidosis Symptoms: dysphagia, early satiety, epigastric pain, nausea, vomiting, weight loss, hematemesis Manifestations: extrinsic compression of esophagus, infiltration of esophagus and stomach, involvement of enteric nervous system, laryngeal involvement (Figure 53.4), subglottic stenosis	Barium esophagram: narrowing at level of carina, mimic achalasia EGD: esophageal stricture, extrinsic esophageal compression, gastric mucosal nodularity, gastric ulcerations Biopsy: non-caseating, giant-cell granuloma, mononuclear infiltrates Esophageal manometry: variable, impaired LES relaxation, reduced amplitude, aperistalsis Others: CXR/CT scan shows hilar and mediastinal lymphadenopathy	Treat underlying sarcoidosis Treat impaired LES relaxation with botulinum toxin injection

LES, lower esophageal sphincter, EGD, esophagogastroduodenoscopy; CXR, chest X-ray.

Barium esophagram is helpful to determine the length of esophageal stricture and the presence of fistula. Endoscopic findings are variable. They may consist of prominent esophageal scarring with or without active ulcerations (Figures 53.3a,b). There is no randomized controlled trial to assess the treatment of esophageal and gastric Crohn disease. Upper GI Crohn is a complicated problem in adults, and many patients may require surgical intervention [7].

Behçet Disease (Table 53.3)

Behçet disease is an idiopathic systemic vasculitis with chronic relapsing symptoms. Systemic vasculitis, hyperfunction of neutrophils, and autoimmune inflammatory response are the predominant features. Patients with Behçet disease cluster along the ancient Silk Road from eastern Asia to the Mediterranean basin, especially in Turkey, Japan, Korea, China, Iran, and Saudi Arabia. Major clinical features of Behçet disease are recurrent oral ulcers, genital ulcers, uveitis, erythema nodosum, and papulopustular skin lesions. The prevalence of GI involvement varies among countries, the highest being in Japan (50 to 60%). Behçet disease may affect the GI tract as small blood vessel disease with mucosal inflammation causing ulceration or as large blood vessel disease resulting in intestinal ischemia and infarction. Many aspects are similar to Crohn disease. Penetrating ulcers can develop into fistulae. Esophageal ulcers usually parallel oral ulcers in Behçet disease. There are no sign, laboratory test, or histology specific for Behçet disease.

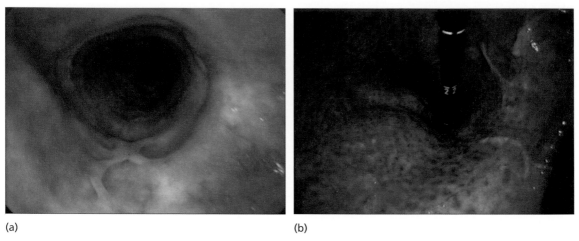

(a)   (b)

Figure 53.3 Endoscopic findings in a patient with Crohn disease complaining of dysphagia. There were prominent scaring without active ulceration in the mid-esophagus (a) and diffuse, non-specific granularity in the stomach (b). (Illustration courtesy of Dr Gerald Dryden, University of Louisville, Louisville, KY.)

Sarcoidosis (Table 53.3)

Sarcoidosis is a systemic disorder of unknown etiology characterized by accumulation of T lymphocytes, macrophages, and non-caseating epithelial granuloma. It affects nearly all ages, ethnicities, and geographical regions. It affects the lungs in 90% of the patients, less frequently affecting the lymph nodes, skin, eyes, nasopharynx (Figure 53.4), and liver. Direct granulomatous infiltration of the esophagus can result in a markedly thickened esophagus with extensive demyelinization and axonal loss of the myenteric plexus. The stomach is the most common site of GI involvement, and it may present as a subclinical, ulcerative, or infiltrative process. Endoscopic biopsy may reveal the typical non-caseating, granulomatous inflammation, but special stains are needed to exclude tuberculosis and histoplasmosis. If bronchoscopy is non-diagnostic, endoscopic ultrasound-guided fine-needle aspiration can obtain adequate tissue to diagnose sarcoidosis [8]. In rare cases of secondary achalasia, botulinum toxin injection and Heller myotomy may improve dysphagia, but symptoms usually persist.

Neuromuscular Diseases

Neuromuscular diseases represent a category of acquired and primary disorders affecting the motor neurons,

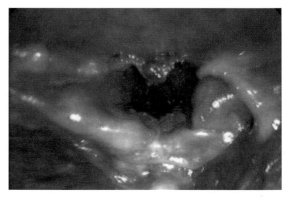

Figure 53.4 Sarcoid inflammatory infiltration of the larynx, identified during esophagogastroduodenoscopy.

peripheral nerves, neuromuscular junctions, and muscles. Abnormalities involving the parasympathetic, sympathetic, and enteric nervous systems can potentially affect the esophagus and stomach.

American Trypanosomiasis (Chagas Disease) (Table 53.4)

A Brazilian, Carlos Chagas, first described the tropical protozoan parasitic infection caused by *Trypanosoma cruzi*, which is an endemic disease in rural Central and South America. Transmission to humans occurs when

Table 53.4 Neuromuscular diseases affecting the esophagus and stomach.

Clinical features	Diagnostic testing	Therapeutics
American trypanosomiasis (Chagas disease)		
Symptoms: dysphagia, odynophagia, chest pain, regurgitation, aspiration, weight loss Manifestations: esophageal aperistalsis, megaesophagus	Barium esophagram: dysrhythmic contractions, dilated esophagus, mimic esophagus Esophageal manometry: variable, diminished LES pressure, impaired LES relaxation, multipeaked waves, low peristaltic amplitude, aperistalsis Others: abnormal EGG, impaired gastric accommodation, rapid gastric emptying	Benznidazole, nifurtimox for *T. cruzi* but not effective in chronic disease Similar to achalasia: pneumatic esophageal dilation, botulinum toxin injection to LES, surgical myotomy, esophageal resection for megaesophagus
Amyloidosis		
Symptoms: hoarseness, dysarthria, heartburn, dysphagia, nausea, vomiting, weight loss, hematemesis Manifestations: oropharyngeal dysfunction, infiltration of oropharynx and thyroid, mimic achalasia, gastric lymphoma, gastric outlet obstruction	Barium esophagram: mimic achalasia Esophageal manometry: variable findings, diminished peristalsis, aperistalsis, impaired LES relaxation EGD: esophageal and gastric mucosal granularity, erosions, ulcers, gastric polyps, large gastric folds Biopsy: biopsy from rectum, abdominal fat pad, bone marrow, or sural nerve may reveal the amorphous protein deposit staining pink by H&E (Figure 53.5a,b) or apple-green appearance by Congo red staining under polarized light	Identify and treat underlying cause Prokinetics for gastroparesis
Paraneoplastic syndromes		
Symptoms: dysphagia, regurgitation, weight loss, early satiety, nausea, vomiting Manifestations: esophageal aperistalsis, gastroparesis	Esophageal manometry: impaired LES relaxation, simultaneous contractions, aperistalsis, EGD: usually normal Serum: paraneoplastic autoantibodies Others: imaging to look for underlying cancer	Identify and treat underlying cancer are essential Prokinetics for gastroparesis

EGG, electrogastrography; EGD, esophagogastroduodenoscopy; LES, lower esophageal sphincter.

the feces of reduviid insects containing *T. cruzi* contaminate a bite, mucosal surface, or the conjunctiva. Infection can also be transmitted from the mother to her fetus, through blood transfusion, organ donation, and accidental exposure in laboratory workers. The parasite then spreads hematogeneously to internal organs. Acute Chagas disease consists of 4 to 6 weeks of fever, malaise, and generalized lymphadenopathy. During the indeterminate phase, infected individuals are asymptomatic with low-grade parasitemia and detectable *T. cruzi* antibodies. Most individuals remain in the indeterminate phase, but 10 to 30% progress to chronic Chagas disease. The cause of chronic Chagas disease is likely infection-induced, immune-mediated tissue damage. Denervation of inhibitory and excitatory myenteric neurons has been described followed by the replacement of neural structures by fibrosis.

The esophagus is affected in 7 to 10% of the chronic *T. cruzi* infected individuals in the endemic areas. Dysphagia is mostly intermittent and mild in early disease when the esophagus is not dilated. In the late stages, dysphagia becomes persistent with regurgitation, aspiration, and weight loss. Aperistalsis is a universal finding in patients with a megaesophagus. Chronic infection can be detected by serum antibodies, but false-positive reactions may occur in connective tissue diseases, leishmaniasis, malaria, and syphilis. Medical treatment with benznidazole and nifurtimox eradicates *T. cruzi* in only less than 50% of the patients and the chronic clinical course is not affected. In end-stage megaesophagus, surgical resection may be required, but perioperative mortality is significant [9]. Laparoscopic transhiatal subtotal esophagectomy through a left cervicotomy is a feasible approach, but surgical expertise is required [10].

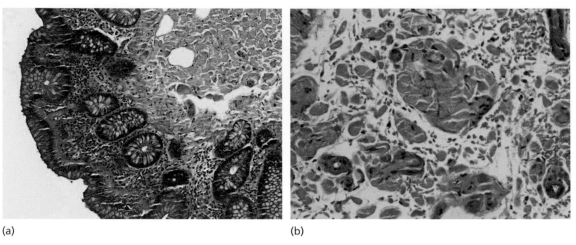

(a)   (b)

Figure 53.5 Rectal biopsy in a patient with amyloidosis. Low power (a) and high power fields (b) of light microscopy show the pink, homogeneous protein deposit in the submucosa using routine hematoxylin and eosin staining. (Illustration courtesy of Dr Walter Jones, Floyd Memorial Hospital, New Albany, IN.)

Amyloidosis (Table 53.4)

Amyloidosis is a group of disorders caused by the deposition of insoluble fibril proteins that are resistant to proteolysis. The most common subtype is AL (light chain) from primary idiopathic amyloidosis or multiple myeloma. Secondary amyloidosis has been associated with various chronic inflammatory, infectious, and neoplastic diseases. The amyloid protein has been found in the esophagus and stomach within the mucosa, submucosa, and smooth muscle. The myenteric plexus itself usually remains intact. The most common site of GI involvement is the rectum, followed by the colon, small intestine, esophagus, and stomach. Only 8% of patients with primary amyloidosis have GI involvement, and only 1% had symptomatic gastric amyloidosis [11]. Congo red staining of the endoscopic biopsies is often diagnostic, showing the characteristic apple-green birefringence under polarized light. Rectal biopsy and abdominal fat pad aspirate can be obtained if needed (Figure 53.5a,b). Treatment of amyloidosis should be directed toward the primary cause, although effective treatment is not available.

Paraneoplastic Syndromes (Table 53.4)

Paraneoplastic syndromes refer to the remote effects of malignancy on various organ systems. Cancer cells express antigens mimicking neuronal tissues, thus producing an autoimmune response. Small cell lung cancer

accounts for approximately 80% of the paraneoplastic syndromes, followed by breast, ovarian, and Hodgkin lymphoma. The myenteric plexus is infiltrated with lymphocytes and plasma cells associated with neuronal degeneration. The GI manifestations are very variable and often present before the cancer can be detected. Many patients may be misdiagnosed with primary achalasia or idiopathic gastroparesis. Paraneoplastic syndrome should be considered in patients with new onset of severe GI dysmotility of unclear etiology, especially in older individuals with weight loss and in patients at risk for lung and breast cancers. A diagnostic panel of serum antineuronal antibodies has been advocated [12].

Cutaneous Syndromes

Many acquired and inherited cutaneous diseases may affect the oropharynx and the proximal esophagus, since they share a similar stratified squamous epithelium. The aim of this section is not to diagnose each of these dermatologic diseases, but to recognize the GI manifestations and to provide appropriate management and referral. Cutaneous diseases should be considered in patients with proximal esophageal ulcers and strictures. Underlying causes should be identified in the acquired

Table 53.5 Cutaneous autoimmune diseases affecting the oropharynx and esophagus.

Clinical features	Diagnostic testing	Therapeutics
Pemphigus (pemphigus vulgaris, paraneoplastic, drug-induced)		
Symptoms: oral and buccal burning, dysphagia, odynophagia, hematemesis, weight loss Manifestations: blistering skin lesions, buccal mucositis (Figure 53.6), esophagitis dissecans superficialis, esophageal strictures, subglottic stenosis	EGD: proximal esophageal bullae, erosions, ulcers, webs, proximal stricture, linear furrows, white pseudomembrane, exfoliated mucosa sloughing Biopsy: suprabasilar acantholysis, clumps of acantholytic cells within blister (Tzank cells), intraepithelial mononuclear inflammation, intraepithelial deposits of IgG and C3 in intercellular space by immunofluorescence Serum: ELISA for anti-Dsg3 and anti-Dsg1 antibodies	Identify and treat underlying cause, such as paraneoplastic, drugs (penicillamine, ACE-inhibitors, rifampin, fludarabine) Treatment for pemphigus (steroid, immunomodulating agents) Endoscopic dilation Maintain nutrition
Pemphigoid (bullous pemphigoid, mucous membrane pemphigoid, paraneoplastic, drug-induced)		
Symptoms: similar to pemphigus Manifestations: similar to pemphigus except more prominent oral ulcers, desquamative gingivitis, conjunctivitis, eruptions may be generalized	EGD: similar to pemphigus Biopsy: subepithelial mononuclear inflammation, subepithelial deposits of IgG, IgA and C3 along basement membrane zone by immunofluorescence Serum: bullous pemphigoid antigen-2 antibodies	Identify and treat underlying cause, such as paraneoplastic, drugs (penicillamine, ACE-inhibitors, rifampin, fludarabine) Treatment for pemphigoid (steroid, dapsone, others)
Epidermolysis bullosa (acquired, inherited)		
Symptoms: similar to pemphigus Manifestations: similar to pemphigus, mechanical or trauma-induced skin and mucosal blisters with scaring	EGD: similar to pemphigus, endoscope may cause further mucosa damage Biopsy: similar to pemphigus Serum: antibodies for basement membrane zone antibody	Identify and treat underlying cause, such as amyloidosis, multiple myeloma, inflammatory bowel disease Dilation may induced mucosal bullae
Lichen planus		
Symptoms: oral pain, dysphagia, odynophagia, weight loss Manifestations: non-blistering skin lesions, similar to pemphigus but always associated with oral lichen planus	EGD: proximal esophageal lacy white papules, pinpoint erosions, desquamation, pseudomembrane, stricture of proximal esophagus Biopsy: histiocytic infiltration within epithelium, negative immunofluorescent stain for IgG, IgA and IgM.	Identify and treat underlying cause, such as hepatitis C, drugs (chloroquine, methyldopa, penicillamine), secondary syphilis, graft-versus-host syndrome)

EGD, esophagogastroduodenoscopy; ACE, angiotensin-converting enzyme; ELISA, enzyme-linked immunosorbent assay test.

syndromes. The risk of oropharyngeal and GI cancers should be recognized.

Pemphigus (Table 53.5)

Pemphigus is a group of autoimmune intraepithelial blistering diseases involving the skin and mucous membrane. It is the result of the interaction between the genetically predisposed individuals and exogenous factor. Ethnic groups from the Mediterranean and South Asia are at increased risk. The autoantibodies of pemphigus disrupt the cell-to-cell adhesion to the epithelium, causing the characteristic skin blisters that may be several centimeters in size. Pemphigus vulgaris is the most common form with painful oropharyngeal erosions, which may precede the skin blisters by weeks or months (Figure 53.6). Paraneoplastic pemphigus has been described in lymphoproliferative disorders, melanoma, carcinoid, gastric, lung, and ovarian cancers. Pemphigus

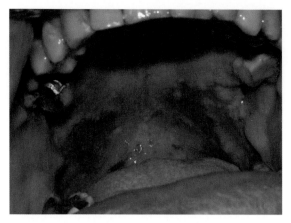

Figure 53.6 Oral ulceration and buccal mucositis in a patient with pemphigus vulgaris. (Illustration courtesy of Dr Jeff Callen, University of Louisville, Louisville, KY.)

may also affect the larynx, nasal mucosa, cervix, and anal canal. Esophageal biopsy, using a "rocking" forcep to maximize the mucosal contact and the depth of the biopsy specimen, can identify the suprabasilar acanthosis by histology and intraepithelial immune complexes by immunofluorescence to diagnose pemphigus [13]. Indirect immunohistochemical staining can be performed from a paraffin block of past specimens.

Pemphigoid (Table 53.5)

Pemphigoid is a group of autoimmune subepithelial blistering diseases with autoantibodies disrupting the adhesion of the epithelium to the basement membrane, resulting in dermal–epidermal separation and skin blisters. Bullous pemphigoid affects older patients and is the most common type, but mucosal involvement is rare. Mucous membrane pemphigoid (cicatricial pemphigoid) has a 2:1 predilection for women. Paraneoplastic pemphigoid has also been reported with lymphoma, gastric and renal cancers. Esophageal manifestations of pemphigoid have been reported in case reports and are similar to pemphigus. Desquamative gingivitis and conjunctivitis are common in mucous membrane pemphigoid. Cutaneous and mucosal scaring is more prominent. Esophageal biopsies can identify the subepithelial immune complexes of pemphigoid by immunohistology, in contrast to the intraepithelial deposits of pemphigus.

Acquired and Inherited Epidermolysis Bullosa (Table 53.5)

Epidermolysis bullosa acquisita is an acquired mucocutaneous syndrome characterized by skin fragility and spontaneous and trauma-induced mucocutaneous blisters (Table 53.5). It is associated with autoimmunity to type VII collagen, the anchoring protein for attaching the epidermis to the dermis layer. Tense blisters tend to occur on trauma-prone areas, such as the palms, soles, elbows, and knees. Esophageal mucosa may be damaged by the endoscope itself. Epidermolysis bullosa is also a group of rare inherited syndromes with very similar manifestations as the acquired form. The clinical and immunohistological findings of epidermolysis bullosa mimic mucous membrane pemphigoid, because they both cause subepithelial blisters.

Lichen Planus (Table 53.5)

Lichen planus is a chronic, relapsing inflammatory disorder of the skin, nails, and mucous membrane. It causes mucocutaneous ulceration without blistering by a lymphocytic cell-mediated response against the basal epithelium. The mean age of onset is 40 to 50 years old. The skin findings consist of the five P's of lichen planus: pruritic, planar (flat), polyangular, and purple papules. There are various forms of lichen planus, from a few localized lesions to a more generalized eruption. Esophageal lichen planus is rare, occurs in only 1% of patients with oral lichen planus, and almost exclusively in women [14]. Histology may show a dense lymphocytic infiltrate at the junction of the squamous mucosa and lamina propria. Immunohistochemical stain may reveal a mixture of CD8 and CD4 T-lymphocytes with negative staining for IgG, IgA and IgM. Oral and esophageal squamous carcinomas may develop in patients with mucosal lichen planus.

Cutaneous Hyperkeratosis Syndromes (Table 53.6)

Cutaneous hyperkeratosis syndromes are rare inherited or acquired disorders with a thickening of the skin and squamous mucosa with or without hyperpigmentation. The reader is referred to Table 53.6 for a summary of the manifestations, diagnostic testing, and therapy. Endoscopy may be the first sign of the syndrome by finding esophageal and gastric benign or malignant lesions. It is important to recognize these syndromes,

Table 53.6 Cutaneous hyperkeratosis syndromes involving the esophagus and stomach.

Summary	Clinical features	Diagnostic testing	Therapeutics
Hyperkeratosis plantaris and palmaris (tylosis)			
Rare, autosomal dominant inherited mucocutaneous syndrome Tylosis-esophageal cancer gene on chromosome 17q25 locus, but mutation is unknown Lifetime risk for esophageal squamous carcinoma is very high in affected family members [15]	Symptoms: may be asymptomatic, dysphagia, weight loss Manifestations: symmetric focal or diffuse hyperkeratosis of palms and soles, pruritic and painful dermal fissures, esophageal and oral cancers	EGD: esophageal papillomatosis, esophageal cancer	Surveillance for esophageal cancer for at-risk family members Genetic testing not available Genetic counseling
Acanthosis nigricans			
Rare acquired syndrome with or without hyperpigmentation Multiple subtypes Paraneoplastic is common (gastric adenocarcinoma, uterine, liver, intestinal, ovarian, renal, breast, and lung cancer); cancer secretes tumor growth factors to mimic epidermal growth factor Mucosal lesions may progress to oral and esophageal squamous cancers	Symptoms: may be asymptomatic, dysphagia, weight loss Manifestations: multiple small hyperpigmented raised plaques of flexor surfaces (palm, neck, arms, axilla), esophageal papillomas, esophageal squamous cancer	EGD: similar to tylosis, esophageal papillomatosis, esophageal cancer Biopsy: papilloma, no significant inflammation	Identify and treat underlying cause (scleroderma, dermatomyositis, lupus, paraneoplastic from gastric cancer)
Multiple hamartoma syndrome (Cowden syndrome)			
Autosomal dominant inherited syndrome, mutation of *PTEN* tumor-suppressor gene on chromosome 10q23 Increased risk for breast, thyroid, endometrial cancers	Symptoms: may be asymptomatic, dysphagia, epigastric pain, GI bleeding Manifestations: hyperkeratosis of soles and palms, oropharyngeal papillomas, hamartomatous polyposis (GI tract, breast, thyroid, skin and uterus)	EGD: esophageal and gastric polyposis Biopsy: epithelial hyperplasia, hamartomas, esophageal glycogen acanthosis	Identify and screen for cancers Genetic testing available Genetic counseling for patient and family
Dyskeratosis congenita			
Group of congenital syndromes with variable inheritance Telomerase deficiency resulting in accelerated cell loss (skin, mucosal lining) Increase risk for bone marrow failure and cancer	Symptoms: dysphagia, fatigue Manifestations: abnormal skin pigmentation, nail dystrophy, oral leucoplakia, premature graying and hair loss, esophageal strictures	EGD: proximal esophageal webs	Endoscopic dilation Genetic counseling for patient and family
Acrokeratosis paraneoplastica (Bazex syndrome)			
Rare, acquired paraneoplastic cutaneous syndrome Skin lesion may precede aerodigestive tract cancer (oral cavity, larynx, pharynx, lung, esophagus) [16] Affect mostly men Etiology unclear	Symptoms: asymptomatic, dysphagia Manifestations: scaly, psoriasis-like skin lesions of the ears, nose, hands, feet, nails; hyperkeratosis of plaques of palms, soles	EGD: primary esophageal cancer	Identify and treat underlying cancer Skin lesions improved with cancer treatment

EGD, esophagogastroduodenoscopy.

since the patients are at risk for developing GI and other systemic cancers. Management depends on making the right diagnosis, identify the underlying cause, providing proper surveillance, and genetic counseling for the family.

Take-home points

- The gastrointestinal tract is the third most common organ involved in systemic sclerosis after skin thickening and Raynaud phenomenon.

- There is a threefold increase in the risk of cancer in patients with dermatomyositis, especially for ovarian, lung, pancreatic, stomach, colorectal cancers, and non-Hodgkin lymphomas.

- Mixed connective tissue disease is a syndrome characterized by overlapping features of systemic sclerosis, systemic lupus erythematosus, inflammatory myopathies, and rheumatoid arthritis.

- In studies of unselected diabetics delayed gastric emptying of solids were seen in 40–50% of patients. Many of these diabetics have no gastric symptoms.

- Esophageal and gastric involvement in Crohn disease is rare and always associated with ileocolonic Crohn disease.

- The stomach is the most common site of GI involvement in sarcoidosis.

- The esophagus is affected in 7–10% of patients of chronic *T. cruzi* infected individuals in endemic areas with Chagas disease.

- Paraneoplastic syndrome should be considered in patients with new onset of severe GI dysmotility of unclear cause especially in older individuals with weight loss and in patients at risk for lung and breast cancer.

- Esophageal lichen planus is rare and it occurs in only 1% of patients with oral lichen planus and this is almost exclusively in women.

References

1 Ioannidis JP, Vlachoyiannopoulos PG, Haidich AB, *et al.* Mortality in systemic sclerosis: an international meta-analysis of individual patient data. *Am J Med* 2005; **118**: 2–10.

2 Marie I, Ducrotte P, Denis P, *et al.* Oesophageal mucosal involvement in patients with systemic sclerosis receiving proton pump inhibitor therapy. *Aliment Pharmacol Ther* 2006; **24**: 1593–601.

3 Oh TH, Brumfield KA, Hoskin TL, *et al.* Dysphagia in inflammatory myopathy: clinical characteristics, treatment strategies, and outcome in 62 patients. *Mayo Clin Proc* 2007; **82**: 441–7.

4 Marshall JB, Kretschmar JM, Gerhardt DC, *et al.* Gastrointestinal manifestations of mixed connective tissue disease. *Gastroenterol* 1990; **98**: 1232–8.

5 Mandl T, Ekberg O, Wollmer P, *et al.* Dysphagia and dysmotility of the pharynx and oesophagus in patients with primary Sjogren's syndrome. *Scand J Rheumatol* 2007; **36**: 394–401.

6 Barczynski M, Thor P. Reversible autonomic dysfunction in hyperthyroid patients affects gastric myoelectrical activity and emptying. *Clin Auton Res* 2001; **11**: 243–9.

7 Yamamoto T, Allan RN, Keighley MR. An audit of gastroduodenal Crohn disease: clinicopathologic features and management. *Scand J Gastroenterol* 1999; **34**: 1019–24.

8 Annema JT, Veselic M, Rabe KF. Endoscopic ultrasound-guided fine-needle aspiration for the diagnosis of sarcoidosis. *Eur Respir J* 2005; **25**: 405–9.

9 Pinotti HW, Felix VN, Zilberstein B, *et al.* Surgical complications of Chagas' disease: megaesophagus, achalasia of the pylorus, and cholelithiasis. *World J Surg* 1991; **15**: 198–204.

10 Crema E, Ribeiro LB, Terra JA, Jr, *et al.* Laparoscopic transhiatal subtotal esophagectomy for the treatment of advanced megaesophagus. *Ann Thorac Surg* 2005; **80**: 1196–201.

11 Menke DM, Kyle RA, Fleming CR, *et al.* Symptomatic gastric amyloidosis in patients with primary systemic amyloidosis. *Mayo Clin Proc* 1993; **68**: 763–7.

12 Pittock SJ, Kryzer TJ, Lennon VA. Paraneoplastic antibodies coexist and predict cancer, not neurological syndrome. *Ann Neurol* 2004; **56**: 715–19.

13 Galloro G, Diamantis G, Magno L, *et al.* Technical aspects in endoscopic biopsy of lesions in esophageal pemphigus vulgaris. *Dig Liver Dis* 2007; **39**: 363–7.

14 Eisen D. The evaluation of cutaneous, genital, scalp, nail, esophageal, and ocular involvement in patients with oral lichen planus. *Oral Surg Oral Med Oral Pathol* 1999; **88**: 431–6.

15 Ellis A, Field JK, Field EA, *et al.* Tylosis associated with carcinoma of the oesophagus and oral leukoplakia in a large Liverpool family—a review of six generations. *Eur J Cancer B Oral Oncol* 1994; **30B**: 102–12.

16 Bolognia JL. Bazex syndrome: acrokeratosis paraneoplastica. *Semin Dermatol* 1995; **14**: 84–9.

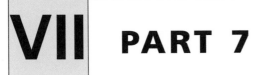

PART 7

Functional Disease

54

CHAPTER 54
Functional Esophageal Disorders

Sami R. Achem and Kenneth R. DeVault

Division of Gastroenterology and Hepatology, Mayo Clinic, Jacksonville, FL, USA

Summary

The functional esophageal disorders (FED) represent chronic symptoms suggestive of esophageal disease without identifiable structural or mucosal abnormalities. Up to 42% of the US population suffers from FED. Functional heartburn has recently been defined by the Rome III consensus as patients with heartburn and regurgitation, normal endoscopy, normal acid contact time on pH testing, and negative symptom index correlation. Functional dysphagia is defined as an abnormal sensation of bolus transit through the esophagus body in the absence of gastroesophageal reflux disease, structural lesions, and motility disorders. The etiology and pathogenesis of these two conditions is poorly understood and probably multifactorial. Increased visceral sensitivity to acid or other stimuli is considered to account for patient's symptoms. More research is needed to identify the mechanism(s) triggering symptoms that will lead to effective targeted therapies. This chapter reviews our current understanding regarding evaluation, pathogenesis, and management of these challenging conditions.

Case

A 49-year-old female pharmacist presents for evaluation of frequent and persistent retrosternal heartburn and regurgitation for more than 9 months. She was initially treated with omeprazole 20 mg daily 40 min prior to breakfast for 8 weeks. Since she did not respond, her physician increased omeprazole to 20 mg twice daily (40 min before breakfast and dinner). After additional 8 weeks of therapy, she seeks consultation for unabated symptoms. An esophagogastroduodenoscopy (EGD) is performed and shows normal results. Esophageal biopsies were negative for eosinophilic esophagitis. A pH impedance test reveals excellent acid inhibition on double-dose proton pump inhibitor (PPI) therapy, no evidence of non-acid reflux, and multiple symptomatic episodes, none correlating with acid or non-acid reflux. An esophageal motility test and a gastric emptying study at 4 h are normal.

Introduction

Functional esophageal disorders (FED) represent chronic symptoms suggestive of esophageal disease that have no

Practical Gastroenterology and Hepatology: Esophagus and Stomach, 1st edition. Edited by Nicholas J. Talley, Kenneth R. DeVault and David E. Fleischer. © 2010 Blackwell Publishing Ltd.

readily identified structural or metabolic basis [1]. FED affects a large proportion of the US population. In a national survey (n = 5430), up to 69% of the population reported suffering from at least one of 20 possible functional digestive symptoms, 42% specifically complained of functional esophageal symptoms (functional heartburn (FH) in 32.6% and functional dysphagia (FD) in 7.5%) [2]. Patients with FED represent a major clinical challenge. This is due to the poorly understood and likely multifactorial source of their symptoms. No single agent or intervention has resulted in complete symptom relief. The purpose of this chapter is to focus on our current understanding of FH and FD.

Functional Heartburn

Current Concepts: Gastroesophageal Reflux Disease, Non-erosive Reflux Disease, Erosive Esophagitis, and Functional Heartburn

The recently convened consensus meeting in Montreal defined gastroesophageal reflux disease (GERD) as when reflux of stomach contents produces troublesome symptoms and/or complications [3]. The most commonly recognized symptoms of GERD are heartburn and regurgitation. While GERD has been reported to occur weekly in 20% of the population, esophageal mucosal injury does not occur universally and, in fact, most patients with GERD have non-erosive reflux disease (NERD).

Symptomatic GERD can be further classified on the basis of endoscopic findings as: normal endoscopy, erosive esophagitis (EE), and Barrett esophagus (BE). Patients with normal mucosal appearance not only represent the majority of the GERD population but, based on the recently reported Rome III criteria [1] and using pH testing, they can be further stratified into three categories: (i) NERD with abnormal acid contact time, (ii) NERD with normal acid contact time, but positive symptom index (SI), and (iii) functional heartburn (FH), those with normal acid contact time and negative SI.

Epidemiology

The epidemiology of FH remains insufficiently studied. A Swedish study reported data from two adult populations who responded to a GERD questionnaire and underwent EGD; 3000 subjects were studied, 1000 eventually undergoing EGD; 400 of these patients had GERD symptoms with a normal endoscopy in 67.8% [4]. Similar figures were found in a large Japanese population study where NERD occurred in 61–86% [5]. Since pH testing was not done in either study it is not possible to determine the actual prevalence rates of NERD versus FH.

Pathogenesis

A number of differences [6] have been identified between EE and NERD and are summarized in Table 54.1. The exact mechanism(s) explaining symptoms in patients with NERD or FH remain unclear. However, the abnormalities listed in Table 54.1 suggest that while defective esophageal clearance may be more commonly present in EE (hiatal hernia and motility disorders), patients with NERD may have defects in sensory perception (visceral hypersensitivity). Acid may disrupt the intercellular connections of the squamous esophageal mucosa exposing nociceptive nerve fibers to normal or modest acid quantities, and so generating symptoms.

On the other hand, factors other than acid may also trigger symptoms. For instance, it has been shown that stress may increase the intercellular connections of the squamous esophageal mucosa exposing sensory nerve fibers to injurious substances (acid, bile, etc.). This information may explain the potential role of psychological factors in the causation of symptoms. Other investigators have also found that longitudinal muscle contraction of the esophagus, detected by intraluminal ultrasound but not by conventional esophageal motility tests, produces the sensation of heartburn. Heartburn can also result from increased perception of normal peripheral stimuli at the central level [7].

The recent introduction of pH impedance suggests that in patients with GERD failing PPI therapy, symptoms may be due to acid reflux in only 11%. By contrast, non-acid reflux potentially explained symptoms in 31%, and 58% had neither acid nor non-acid reflux [8]. Taken together, these observations underscore the role of mechanisms other than acid or non-acid reflux in the cause of symptoms in NERD and explain the heterogeneous response of patients with NERD to acid-suppressive therapy.

Table 54.1 Differences between erosive esophagitis (EE) and non-erosive reflux disease (NERD).

Parameter	EE	NERD
Hiatal hernia	Common	Rare
Esophageal motility disorder	Common	Rare
Abnormal acid contact time	More commonly abnormal	Less likely abnormal or normal
Proximal migration of GERD events on pH and impedance testing	Significant less proximal esophageal migration of acid reflux events	Events more likely to extend more proximally and more homogeneous esophageal acid exposure
Sensitivity response to esophageal acid infusion proximal esophagus	Mildly increased	Significantly increased, particularly in functional heartburn (more sensitive than NERD)
Bile reflux	More common	Less likely

GERD, gastroesophageal reflux disease.

Clinical Features

Clinical symptoms do not distinguish EE from NERD. Phenotypically, EE patients tend to be older and more commonly males than NERD subjects. A number of population-based studies have found unique features in patients with GERD in relation to control subjects, such as a higher than expected prevalence of irritable bowel syndrome, anxiety, depression, and low socioeconomic status [9,10,11]. However, there are no data indicating whether these differences apply to patients with EE, NERD, or FH.

One of the few studies grouping patients according to phenotype (EE, NERD, or FH) found that patients with FH had acid reflux on pH impedance that reached significantly higher levels of the esophagus than the observed in patients with EE or NERD. Studies are needed to determine if there are specific markers that can help predict which patient is more likely to have NERD, specifically FH. Until such data become available, endoscopy and pH testing need to be done to lead to objective classification of symptomatic patients. This is important since therapeutic outcomes vary based on phenotypic distribution. Despite the fact that patients with NERD have apparently normal mucosa, their quality of life is as impaired as those with EE and they appear more difficult to treat.

Natural History

Whether NERD evolves into EE or BE is not well known, but appears unlikely. Few studies are available addressing the long-term course of NERD patients and those available fail to standardize diagnostic groups (EE, NERD, or FH) or treatment criteria. In a prospective study of patients with NERD (n = 1717), follow up after 2 years showed that 25% progressed to EE Los Angeles (LA) A/B, and 0.6% to LA C/D. BE developed in only 0.5% [12]. Again, it is not possible to separate NERD patients from FH in this study since pH testing was not done. The reason(s) some patients develop EE while others have NERD is not well understood. In the previously cited study, men and patients with LA grade A/B were more likely to develop EE [12]. Interesting data from a long-term, prospective study of GERD patients were recently reported. In this preliminary report [13], 2000 patients with varying severity of GERD were followed for 5 years and were treated at the discretion of their health-care providers (usually symptom-driven therapy). The initial

impairment of quality of life improved after initial diagnosis, regardless of subsequent therapy, and this improvement tended to persist. The major determinant of persistently impaired quality of life was ongoing night-time symptoms.

Treatment

Treatment of FH remains insufficiently studied. Most publications reporting data on NERD patients precede the Rome III criteria and so do not distinguish between NERD and FH. Thus, the following summary regarding therapy needs to be put into perspective given this limitation (Table 54.2).

Dean *et al.* performed a systematic review of the literature regarding the effectiveness of PPI therapy in NERD using Medline articles from 1980 to 2002 [14]. Patients with NERD were included and end points were complete heartburn resolution (no heartburn in the preceding 7 days) or "sufficient" heartburn resolution (less than 1 day of moderate heartburn in the preceding 7 days). pH testing was not required for study inclusion, therefore it is not possible to determine outcome differences between GERD, NERD, and FH subjects. Seven placebo-controlled trials were ultimately identified. PPIs and dose used in those studies were: omeprazole 10, 20 mg; rabeprazole 10, 20 mg; esomeprazole 20, 40 mg. The major findings were that therapeutic gains for PPI therapy over placebo ranged from 25 to 30% for complete heartburn resolution and 30 to 35% for sufficient heartburn resolution. Pooled response rates showed a significantly higher

Table 54.2 Functional heartburn concepts.

1 Compared to placebo, PPI therapy in NERD provides clinical improvement

2 Patients with EE treated with PPI have an overall better response than NERD patients [18]

3 A time lag of progressive improvement from 2 to 4 weeks in NERD suggests that longer therapeutic trials may afford better symptom resolution

4 Most therapeutic studies to date have not addressed therapeutic efficacy in FH as defined by Rome III but instead have focused on NERD

5 Although many investigators recommend the use of visceral analgesic agents for FH not responding to PPI therapy, there are no available clinical trials proving the efficacy of this approach

PPI, proton pump inhibitor; NERD, non-erosive reflux disease; EE, erosive esophagitis; FH, functional heartburn.

improvement in EE than in NERD (56 versus 37%). An important finding was the gradual improvement from 2 to 4 weeks in NERD. This observation suggests that longer therapeutic trials may afford better symptom resolution.

A large multicenter, multinational, controlled trial compared daily AM doses of esomeprazole 40 mg to esomeprazole 20 mg or omeprazole 20 mg for 4 weeks in NERD patients. The main efficacy point was complete heartburn resolution at 4 weeks (no days with heartburn episodes during the last 7 days before visit 3). At 4 weeks, complete symptom resolution was achieved by 56.7 to 70.3% of the patients with no statistical differences among the various PPI types or doses, although, numerically esomeprazole 40 mg treated subjects obtained the highest improvement (70.3%). This study also showed considerable therapeutic gain from 2 to 4 weeks [15].

In a study from Sweden, 509 NERD patients were randomized to omeprazole 20 mg, 10 mg daily, or placebo for 4 weeks. This study showed that complete absence of heartburn for the different regimens was 46, 31, and 13%, respectively. During an open-treatment phase of non-responsive placebo patients, resolution of heartburn was reached with omeprazole in more than 85% of patients. This study was unique in that pH testing was done prior to entry and showed that subjects with higher acid contact time obtained better response, although no data were provided regarding SI and consequently FH [16].

The predictive value of PPI response in NERD at 1 week was evaluated during a recent trial. This study showed that patients with NERD who had complete resolution of their heartburn by days 5–7 of PPI use had an 85% probability of complete resolution of heartburn after 4 weeks. In contrast, those with persistent heartburn on days 5–7 of acid suppression therapy had a 22% probability of complete resolution of heartburn after 4 weeks [17].

Diagnostic Evaluation

Most patients with typical heartburn and regurgitation symptoms do not undergo endoscopy, unless they report alarming symptoms (dysphagia, weight loss, bleeding). Symptomatic patients without alarming symptoms will likely be treated with a 4 to 8-week trial of a PPI. Approximately 25–42% of these patients fail to respond to this approach [19]. Diagnostic possibilities at this stage include: (i) inappropriate PPI intake (not taken 30–60 min before breakfast meal) or (ii) non-compliance. If neither possibility is identified, patients may be switched to a single dose of second-generation PPI (esomeprazole 40 mg 30–60 min before breakfast) for 8 weeks, or they may increase the original PPI to twice daily (again, to be taken 30–60 min before breakfast and dinner).

For patients not responding to the above program, an EGD will help classify patients into EE or NERD. For patients whose endoscopic evaluation shows no evidence of EE, pH testing while on double-dose PPI or second-generation PPI can help determine if they have persistent GERD. This evaluation may be done with pH impedance or a wireless pH capsule, Bravo (Medtronics, Minneapolis, MN); pH impedance offers the advantage that, in addition to establishing whether sufficient acid inhibition is taking place, it may uncover non-acid reflux. However, we lack sufficient information regarding outcomes for patients with non-acid reflux (i.e., what is the best approach to therapy). For patients with negative pH testing (no evidence of acid reflux or non-acid reflux), an esophageal motility test and gastric emptying will help exclude the possibility of a motility disorder.

Patients refractory to PPI therapy without evidence of motility disorders and negative pH test (both acid contact time and SI association) have FH. Since these patients failed a double-dose PPI program for 8 weeks, do not have evidence of abnormal contact time or non-acid reflux on pH testing, and have a negative SI, it is speculated that visceral hyperalgesia may be the cause of their symptoms. A low-dose tricycle antidepressant (TCA) or a selective serotonin receptor antagonist (SSRI) is suggested as next treatment choice. However, to date, there are no clinical controlled trials showing the benefits of this approach.

Functional Dysphagia

This disorder is defined by the Rome III consensus as "an abnormal sensation of bolus transit through the esophagus body in the absence of GERD, structural lesions and histopathology-based esophageal motor disorders" [1]. The criteria should have a minimum duration of 3 months and onset of symptoms of at least 6 months. In contrast to FH, FD has received less attention in the literature and remains incompletely studied.

Epidemiology

Few studies are available that shed light into the epidemiology of FD. In the previously mentioned house-hold study of the US population, 7.5% reported FD [2]. There are no epidemiological data available using current Rome III criteria definition.

Clinical Features

The evaluation of patients with recurrent dysphagia should include esophageal tests to exclude mechanical sources of dysphagia, motility disorders, and GERD. These patients should have a barium swallow with a radio-opaque bolus challenge, endoscopy, and esophageal biopsies to exclude eosinophilic esophagitis. If those studies are non-diagnostic, esophageal motility tests should be considered. The value of esophageal motility testing in patients with non-obstructive dysphagia has been described by Chen and Orr [20]. These investigators grouped patients with non-obstructive dysphagia into those with solid and liquid dysphagia and solid-food dysphagia only. The most common finding in both groups was a normal study (NS) (55 vs. 63% NS; solid and liquid dysphagia vs. solid dysphagia, respectively), followed by non-specific esophageal motility disorder (26 vs. 25% NS), and achalasia (12 vs. 3% NS). Diffuse esophageal spasm and nutcracker esophagus were seen in less than 10%. GERD should also be excluded with a pH test, although some authorities regard a double-dose PPI trial for at least 8 weeks as reasonable diagnostic/therapeutic alternative. In the study mentioned above [20], pH testing was abnormal in 58% of patients with solid-food dysphagia versus 29% of patients with solids and liquid-food dysphagia (p = .02). Medication-induced dysphagia should be considered in the differential diagnosis of unexplained dysphagia. A recent study of 153 adults discovered that 5.4% were taking medications potentially associated with dysphagia and 31.7% with drugs that can result in dry mouth or other oral-stage-related side effects [21].

Pathogenesis

The mechanism underlying FD is insufficiently understood. Intraesophageal balloon distension studies have shown an increased threshold perception consistent with a defect in visceral sensitivity [22]. Other studies also using balloon distension techniques have shown both reproduction of dysphagia and generation of abnormal motility patterns, suggesting a defect in the neural circuit of the esophagus [23]. A number of investigators have reproduced patient's dysphagia and identified an abnormal esophageal motor response during food-provoked but not water-provoked swallows [24]. In addition, patients with non-obstructive dysphagia show a defect in the triggering of secondary peristalsis and functional clearance by impedance manometry [25,26]. Increased stress can also induce abnormal esophageal motility responses [27] although there are no data that stress can be linked directly to FD.

Treatment

There are no randomized controlled trials for the management of patients with FD. Treatment remains uncontrolled and anecdotal. In the absence of data, strategies have included reassurance, careful food mastication, and preventing any precipitating factors (psychological or alimentary). Other treatment programs have included empiric esophageal dilation, visceral analgesics, esophageal muscle relaxants, and botulinum toxin. The risk–benefit ratio of these approaches should be carefully considered in treating FD since there are no outcome studies supporting the use of any one particular approach.

Case continued

The patient had a negative work-up for esophageal obstruction, mucosal disease (including eosinophilic esophagitis), esophageal and gastric dysmotility, and refractory (acid or non-acid) reflux. The most likely diagnosis at this point is functional heartburn. The patient has also failed a twice daily PPI trial and combination of a negative pH test and lack of response suggests that reflux is unlikely to be the cause of these symptoms. While there are no trials to confirm this approach, a trial of a low-dose TCA or SSRI would be reasonable. Reassurance, psychological based therapy, and swallowing therapy would be reasonable alternatives as well.

Take-home points

Functional heartburn:
• Functional Heartburn (FH) is a recently identified concept defined as symptoms of heartburn and/or regurgitation, normal endoscopy (non-erosive reflux disease or NERD), and pH testing demonstrating normal acid contact time and negative symptom index (SI) correlation.

- Since the criteria for FH has only recently been redefined (Rome III consensus 2006), previous studies reporting FH were likely contaminated with NERD patients (they did not include pH testing and or SI information).

- The etiology of FH is unknown. Proposed causes include: increased susceptibility of the esophageal mucosa to reflux-mediated injury, and an enhanced recognition of perception stimuli by esophageal nerve fibers at the esophageal or central nervous system levels.

- It is unknown why some patients develop NERD or FH while others evolve into erosive disease. Most patients with NERD, however, do not seem to progress to erosive disease or Barrett esophagus (BE).

- Present data regarding treatment of FH are primarily derived from therapeutic trials in NERD since there are no treatment trials of patients with FH as recently defined by Rome III.

- Based on current available treatment information (mostly from NERD populations), proton pump inhibitor (PPI) therapy provides between 29 and 70% response rates. Patients with erosive esophagitis (EE) treated with PPI have an overall better response than NERD patients. Visceral analgesic agents are recommended for FH not responding to PPI therapy despite lack of controlled trials to validate their use.

- Patients with FH have no evidence of endoscopic mucosal damage, but their quality of life is as impaired as those with erosive disease and they are more resistant to acid-suppressive therapy.

Functional dysphagia:

- Functional dysphagia (FD) is defined as an abnormal sensation of bolus transit through the esophagus body in the absence of reflux, structural lesions, abnormal histology, or esophageal motor disorders.

- The cause of FD is not understood. Abnormal sensitivity to visceral stimulation, psychological disturbances, and defects of the esophageal neural circuit have been proposed as possible causes.

- The treatment of FD remains anecdotal and uncontrolled. Therapies used include: reassurance, empirical esophageal dilation, smooth muscle relaxants, visceral analgesics, botulinum toxin, acid inhibition, and psychological interventions.

References

1 Galmiche JP, Clouse RE, Balint A, *et al.* Functional esophageal disorders. *Gastroenterology* 2006; **130**: 1459–65.

2 Drossman DA, Li Z, Andruzzi E, Temple RD, *et al.* U.S. householder survey of functional gastrointestinal disorders. Prevalence, sociodemography, and health impact. *Dig Dis Sci* 1993; **38**: 1569–80.

3 Vakil N, van Zanten SV, Kahrilas P, *et al.* The Montreal definition and classification of gastroesophageal reflux disease: a global evidence-based consensus. *Am J Gastroenterol* 2006; **101**: 1900–20.

4 Ronkainen J, Aro P, Storskrubb T, *et al.* High prevalence of gastroesophageal reflux symptoms and esophagitis with or without symptoms in the general adult Swedish population: a Kalixanda study report. *Scand J Gastroenterol* 2005; **40**: 275–85.

5 Mishima I, Adachi K, Aridima N, *et al.* Prevalence of endoscopically negative and positive gastroesophageal reflux disease in the Japanese. *Scand J Gastroenterol* 2005; **40**: 1005–9.

6 Thoua NM, Khoo D, Kalantzis C, *et al.* Acid-related oesophageal sensitivity, not dysmotility, differentiates subgroups of patients with non-erosive reflux disease. *Aliment Pharmacol Ther* 2008; **27**: 396–403.

7 Fass R, Naliboff B, Higa L, *et al.* Differential effect of long-term acid exposure on mechanosensitivity and chemosensitivity in humans. *Gastroenterology* 1998; **115**: 1363–73.

8 Mainie I, Tutuian R, Shay S, *et al.* Acid and non-acid reflux in patients with persistent symptoms despite acid suppressive therapy: a multicentre study using combined ambulatory impedance-pH monitoring. *Gut* 2006; **55**: 1398–402.

9 Pimentel M, Rossi F, Chow EJ, *et al.* Increased prevalence of irritable bowel syndrome in patients with gastroesophageal reflux. *J Clin Gastroenterol* 2002; **34**: 221–4.

10 Jansson C, Nordenstedt H, Wallander MA, *et al.* Severe gastro-oesophageal reflux symptoms in relation to anxiety, depression and coping in a population-based study. *Aliment Pharmacol Ther* 2007; **26**: 683–91.

11 Jansson C, Nordenstedt H, Johansson S, *et al.* Relation between gastroesophageal reflux symptoms and socioeconomic factors: a population-based study (the HUNT Study). *Clin Gastroenterol Hepatol* 2007; **5**: 1029–34.

12 Labenz J, Nocon M, Lind T, *et al.* Prospective follow-up data from the ProGERD study suggest that GERD is not a categorical disease. *Am J Gastroenterol* 2006; **101**: 2457–62.

13 Nocon M, Leodolter A, Labenz J, *et al.* Health-related quality of life in patients with gastroesophageal reflux disease under routing care. A 5-year follow-up from the Progerd study. *Gastroenterology* 2009; **135**: A-80.

14 Dean BB, Gano AD Jr, Knight K, *et al.* Effectiveness of proton pump inhibitors in nonerosive reflux disease. *Clin Gastroenterol Hepatol* 2004; **2** : 656–64.

15 Armstrong D, Talley NJ, Lauritsen K, *et al.* The role of acid suppression in patients with endoscopy-negative reflux

disease: the effect of treatment with esomeprazole or omeprazole. *Aliment Pharmacol Ther* 2004; **20**: 413–21.

16 Lind T, Havelund T, Carlsson R, *et al.* Heartburn without oesophagitis: efficacy of omeprazole therapy and features determining therapeutic response. *Scand J Gastroenterol* 1997; **32**: 974–9.

17 Talley NJ, Armstrong D, Junghard O, *et al.* Predictors of treatment response in patients with non-erosive reflux disease. On demand therapy with omeprazole after initial improvement, resulted in remission rates of 83% in NERD (omeprazole 20 mg) or 69% (omeprazole 10 mg) versus 56% in the placebo arm for 6 months. *Aliment Pharmacol Ther* 2006; **24**: 371–6.

18 Carlson R, Dent J, Watts R, *et al.* Gastro-esophageal reflux disease in primary care: an international study of different treatment strategies with omeprazole. *Eur J Gastroenterol Hepatol* 1998; **10**: 119–24.

19 Richter JE. How to manage refractory GERD. *Nat Clin Pract Gastroenterol Hepatol* 2007; **4**: 658–64.

20 Chen CL, Orr WC Comparison of esophageal motility in patients with solid dysphagia and mixed dysphagia. *Dysphagia* 2005; **20**: 261–5.

21 Gallagher L, Naidoo P. Prescription drugs and their effects on swallowing. *Dysphagia* 2008; **24**: 159–66.

22 Bohn B, Bonaz B, Gueddah N, *et al.* Oesophageal motor and sensitivity abnormalities in non-obstructive dysphagia. *Eur J Gastroenterol Hepatol* 2002; **14**: 271–7.

23 Deschner WK, Maher KA, Cattau EL Jr, *et al.* Manometric responses to balloon distention in patients with nonobstructive dysphagia. *Gastroenterology* 1989; **97**: 1181–5.

24 Cordier L, Bohn B, Bonaz B, *et al.* [Evaluation of esophageal motility disorders triggered by ingestion of solids in the case of non-obstructive dysphagia]. *Gastroenterologie Clinique Biologique* 1999; **23**: 200–6.

25 Schoeman MN, Holloway RH. Secondary oesophageal peristalsis in patients with non-obstructive dysphagia. *Gut* 1994; **35**: 1523–8.

26 Chen CL, Szczesniak MM, Cook IJ. Identification of impaired oesophageal bolus transit and clearance by secondary peristalsis in patients with non-obstructive dysphagia. *Neurogastroenterol Motil* 2008; **20**: 980–8.

27 Valori RM. Nutcracker, neurosis, or sampling bias? *Gut* 1990; **31**: 736–7.

CHAPTER 55

Functional Gastroduodenal Disorders

Gerald Holtmann

University Hospital Essen, Essen, Germany *and* Faculty of Health Sciences, University of Adelaide, Adelaide, SA, Australia

Summary

Functional disorders of the stomach present with chronic or relapsing symptoms, which include (epigastric) fullness, early satiety, bloating, discomfort, and nausea. After exclusion of structural or biochemical abnormalities that may cause these symptoms, altered gastric (or gastroduodenal) function is assumed as the cause of symptoms. Patients in this category are frequently labeled as having functional dyspepsia, a condition that is included into the Rome III definitions. For research purposes two entities are now recognized: the postprandial distress syndrome (PDS) with predominant meal-related symptoms and the epigastric pain syndrome (EPS) with pain in the epigastric area as the main feature. A proper clinical assessment with a thorough history is key to the diagnosis. Routine laboratory studies, ultrasound of the gall bladder and pancreas, and esophagogastroduodenoscopy (EGD) will exclude the majority of conditions that cause (organic) dyspepsia. The etiology of functional disorders of the stomach is still poorly understood and most likely many factors, including genetic susceptibility and environmental factors such as stress, may play a role.

There are limited treatment options. For PDS, dietary counseling and gastroprokinetic agents such as metoclopramide might be used. Smooth muscle relaxants may help. For EPS, acid-suppressing drugs are first-line therapy. For non-responders low doses of psychotropic drugs (preferably tricyclic antidepressants) might be advisable.

Case

A 37-year-old female high school teacher is referred for assessment of chronic, relapsing upper abdominal discomfort. Symptoms manifested 5 years ago. She had just returned from a holiday trip to Indonesia where she had acquired traveler's diarrhea. After treatment by a local doctor, her symptoms quickly settled. One week after her return, she experienced severe nausea without vomiting and since then she suffered from episodes of moderately severe upper abdominal discomfort. Symptoms are localized between the navel and the lower part of the sternum. She is frequently unable to finish a normal meal because of early satiety and fullness. Fullness is bothering her even after hours of fasting. Her body weight initially decreased by 2.5 kg (5 lb) but has remained stable throughout the last 3 years. She initially was managed by a wide array of

treatments including prokinetics, antacids, and antisecretory drugs. Since there was no long-lasting improvement, she had a diagnostic work-up. Routine laboratory tests including blood glucose were normal. EGD did not reveal structural abnormalities. Histology was negative for *H. pylori*.

Introduction

Disorders of the gastric and duodenal function present with a variety of symptoms. Patients may complain of pain, burning sensations, discomfort, early satiety, regurgitation, rumination, or other symptoms or combinations of symptoms. While in patients with these symptoms a structural abnormality needs to be considered, a large proportion will not have identifiable structural abnormalities as the cause of symptoms. In a recent study [1], most patients with upper abdominal symp-

Practical Gastroenterology and Hepatology: Esophagus and Stomach, 1st edition. Edited by Nicholas J. Talley, Kenneth R. DeVault and David E. Fleischer. © 2010 Blackwell Publishing Ltd.

toms referred for endoscopy did not have an underlying structural abnormality (e.g., no peptic ulcer, no cancer, no relevant mucosal inflammation). It is also common clinical experience that patients with severe structural lesions (e.g., large bleeding ulcers) have no or very little symptoms prior to the manifestation of the complication.

In the absence of structural (or biochemical) abnormalities explaining the symptoms, a functional disorder is believed to cause the symptoms [2]. While this may imply a distinct dichotomy, organic versus functional causes of symptoms, it needs to be recognized that the absence of structural or biochemical abnormalities explaining symptoms refers only to well-recognized structural abnormalities such as peptic ulcer disease. Considering the prevalence of functional disorders it is possible—if not highly likely—that distinct causes for these functional disorders will be identified eventually. For example, there is now emerging evidence, that functional GI disorders are associated with specific genetic risk factors [3,4] and at least in patients with irritable bowel syndrome (IBS), a condition that frequently overlaps with functional dyspepsia, activated immune function is observed [5]. Indeed, functional disorders of the gastroduodenal region with dyspeptic symptoms and symptoms of IBS frequently overlap.

Epidemiology

Various studies have demonstrated prevalence rates of uninvestigated dyspepsia (UD) ranging from 7 to 45%. Most likely this reflects different definitions rather than true differences in the epidemiology. Prevalence rates of functional dyspepsia range from 11 to 29%. However, not all "subjects" with dyspeptic symptoms become patients and a considerable proportion of dyspeptics will never seek medical attention simply because symptoms are not bothersome. On the other hand, some people might be concerned about very minimal symptoms and thus seek medical attention. In these patients limited diagnostic work-up and reassurance might be sufficient. Interestingly, risk factors for functional dyspepsia (FD) include female gender, psychological disturbances, and in some studies lower socioeconomic status, smoking, and increased caffeine intake [6,7].

Categorization of Functional Disorders of the Stomach and Gastroduodenal Region

Dyspepsia is believed to be the key symptom complex caused by disordered function of the gastroduodenal region. This term dyspepsia is actually derived from the Greek words dys ("bad") and peptein ("digestion"). Dyspepsia refers to several symptoms such as epigastric pain, nausea, and early satiety (Table 55.1). If these symptoms are of chronic or relapsing nature, and if there are no structural lesions or biochemical abnormalities that can explain the symptoms, a functional abnormality is believed to cause the symptoms.

While dyspepsia and functional dyspepsia have been the key concepts for many years [8], more recently functional dyspepsia and other conditions referred to the gastroduodenal region were redefined and recategorized by Rome III [9]. Based upon this, there are four categories of functional gastroduodenal disorders. The first category includes what formerly was referred to as functional dyspepsia. The second category refers to belching disorders, the third to nausea and vomiting disorders, and the forth to rumination syndromes in adult. The various categories are summarized in Table 55.2.

Functional Dyspepsia

Dyspepsia is defined by Rome III to comprise the presence of one or more of the following symptoms only: postprandial fullness, early satiety, and epigastric burning or epigastric pain. Unexplained nausea and vomiting, and heartburn, were included in other categories.

While the term functional dyspepsia is used clinically as an overarching umbrella, the most recent categorization, however, suggests (at least for research purposes) that there are two distinct entities: the epigastric pain syndrome (EPS) and the postprandial distress syndrome (PDS). PDS is characterized by meal-induced dyspeptic symptoms (bothersome postprandial fullness during or after a normal sized meal) or early satiation that prevents the finishing of a regular sized meal. Based on Rome III, one or both of these must have been present for at least the last 3 months with an onset of symptoms at least 6 months prior to diagnosis. Symptoms of upper abdominal bloating, postprandial nausea, and epigastric pain may frequently coexist.

Table 55.1 Definition of symptoms potentially originating from the gastroduodenal region.

Dyspepsia	Derived from the Greek word "δυς-" (Dys-) and "πέψη" (Pepse); indigestion, difficult digestion
Epigastric pain	Subjective and unpleasant feeling, might be described as a feeling of tissue being damaged, otherwise difficult to define. This sensation is localized between the umbilicus and lower end of sternum, between the midclavicular lines.
Epigastric burning	Pain located in the epigastrium that has a burning quality without radiation to the chest
Discomfort	Subjective, negative feeling in the upper abdomen that does not reach the level of pain, may occur in relationship to meals (early satiety, postprandial fullness)
Nausea	From the Greek word Ναυτεία, sensation of unease and discomfort in the stomach with an urge to vomit
Heartburn	Painful burning sensation behind the sternum; usually associated with regurgitation of gastric acid
Belching, burping	Release of gas from the digestive tract via the esophagus through the mouth
Postprandial fullness	Unpleasant sensation like prolonged persistence of food in the stomach
Early satiation	Feeling that the stomach is inappropriately (in relation to the ingested meal) overfilled soon after starting to eat; patient is frequently unable to finish a normal meal

Table 55.2 Rome III classification of functional gastroduodenal disorders.

B	Functional gastroduodenal disorders
B1	Functional dyspepsia (for application in clinical practice but not otherwise useful)
B1a	Postprandial distress syndrome
B1b	Epigastric pain syndrome
B2	Belching disorders
B2a	Aerophagia
B2b	Unspecified excessive belching
B3	Nausea and vomiting disorders
B3a	Chronic idiopathic nausea
B3b	Functional vomiting
B3c	Cyclic vomiting syndrome
B4	Rumination syndrome in adults

In contrast, EPS refers to pain or burning localized to the epigastrium of at least moderate severity that occurs at least once per week. The pain must be intermittent in nature though not relieved by defecation or passage of flatus. In patients with suspected EPS, it is important that symptoms must not fulfill the criteria of gall bladder or sphincter of Oddi disorders. Symptoms should not be relieved or triggered by meals. While the two disorders are believed to represent two distinct entities, it needs to be emphasized that, in the clinical reality, overlap often occurs.

Belching Disorders

Belching disorders include the subcategories of aerophagia and unspecified excessive belching. Belching typically results from swallowing air (aerophagia). While belching is a complaint frequently reported by patients, there are very few data from large cohorts.

Nausea and Vomiting

The third category comprises: a chronic idiopathic nausea (frequent bothersome nausea without vomiting); functional vomiting (recurrent vomiting in the absence of self-induced vomiting, or underlying eating disorders, metabolic disorders, drug intake, or psychiatric or central nervous system disorders); and cyclic vomiting syndrome (stereotypical episodes of vomiting with vomiting-free intervals).

Rumination in Adults

Rumination is a syndrome characterized by repetitive regurgitation of small amounts of food from the stomach. The food is then partially or completely rechewed, reswallowed, or expelled. Patients with rumination syndrome are frequently misdiagnosed as having vomiting due to gastroparesis, or gastroesophageal reflux. Thus this syndrome needs to be taken into consideration in the differential diagnosis of any patient with regurgitation, self-reported vomiting (especially postprandial), and weight loss. There is as yet no specifically targeted therapy, but explanation, reassurance, and behavioral therapy are the treatment options in adults.

Pathogenesis

The precise pathophysiology of functional disorders of the gastroduodenal region remains poorly understood. While a number of abnormalities of gastric motor and sensory function (e.g., delayed gastric emptying, impaired postprandial fundic relaxation, heightened sensory function) have been identified, these abnormalities only at best partly explain the symptom pattern. Thus patients with heightened visceral sensory function may not have a specific symptom pattern [10]. As a consequence, it might be speculated that this pathophysiologic mechanism may simply represent markers of an underlying functional abnormality but does not represent the mechanism that needs to be targeted to improve symptoms or cure these disorders.

It is important to conceptionally categorize factors that are associated with the clinical manifestation of functional disorders of and pathomechanisms that can be targeted to alter the natural history of the disease. So far, there are only pathomechanisms that appear to be associated with the manifestation of the condition, but evidence that targeting these mechanisms changes the course of disease or even cures them are lacking. More recently, genetic risk factors such as *GNB3* have been identified [3] and activation of specific immune cells has been observed [11]. Mild duodenal eosinophilia in functional dyspepsia has also been observed [12]. However, the associated risk is small. This may suggest that the pathophysiology is multifactorial.

In the absence of structural abnormalities, a central nervous system abnormality might be suspected. Indeed, patients with these conditions have a high prevalence of psychiatric co-morbidities. Individuals with functional dyspepsia have been shown to be more psychologically disturbed, in terms of being more anxious and depressed [13–18].

Diabetes mellitus with underlying autonomic neuropathy may cause postprandial fullness, early satiety, nausea, and vomiting, but symptoms correlate poorly with gastroparesis. Poor glycemic control may contribute [19]. Other metabolic disturbances (e.g., hypothyroidism, hypercalcemia) also can produce upper GI symptoms.

Management

In patients with typical symptoms (see above) the targets of treatment are: (i) to identify all patients with potentially curable or life-threatening conditions; (ii) to minimize risks and complications of diagnostic measures and treatments; and (iii) to alleviate the most bothersome symptoms. While it would be simple to do a comprehensive diagnostic work-up in all patients, functional gastrointestinal disorders are highly prevalent. Thus strategies need to be developed and implemented to optimize the utilization of diagnostic measures. The diagnostic algorithms for dyspepsia will be addressed elsewhere and are well described in the literature [20]. However, it needs to be emphasized that the risk of structural lesions as a cause of symptoms is low in younger patients in regions with a low *H. pylori* prevalence and in the absence of nonsteroidal anti-inflammatory drug intake. While functional disorders of the gastroduodenal region are of a chronic nature, it is important that patients have realistic expectations regarding their long-term perspective. Thus patient expectations need to be explored, the management tailored accordingly, and if necessary expectations modified towards a more realistic view by careful explanation and education of the patient.

Diagnostic Approach and Treatment

While a diagnostic test may not only guide the physician towards the diagnosis of a functional gastroduodenal disorders by ruling out relevant structural abnormalities, it may also reassure the patient. Convincing the patient that the necessary tests have been done to sufficiently rule out relevant structural lesions is important in addressing the patient's concerns and may represent an important step of therapy.

On the other hand, the comprehensive diagnostic work-up in all patients, or even worse the frequent repetition of readily available diagnostic measures, is unlikely to result in any improvement of outcomes. Careful assessment of history (and review of available results of diagnostic tests) followed by a careful explanation of the underlying causes of the symptoms and the nature of the condition followed, if required, by an empirical treatment might be completely sufficient for a large proportion of patients. While disordered function is believed to play a role in the manifestation of symptoms, testing for specific disturbances such as delayed gastric emptying or impaired sensory function cannot be recommended as a routine diagnostic measure. The diagnostic measures are listed in Table 55.3.

With regard to the various management options in uninvestigated dyspepsia, a large number of studies have compared various first-line management strategies, namely empirical acid suppression, test and treat for *Helicobacter pylori*, initial endoscopy, acid suppression then endoscopy, test and treat then proton pump inhibitor (PPI) then endoscopy. At all ages, endoscopy was less cost effective than other strategies. PPI therapy was the most cost-effective strategy in 30 year olds with a low prevalence of *H. pylori*. In 60 year olds, *H. pylori* test and treatment was the most cost-effective option. Acid suppression alone was more cost-effective than either endoscopy or *H.*

Table 55.3 Diagnostic studies to be considered in the patient with suspected functional gastroduodenal disorders.

Useful

  Clinical examination and review of available test results
  If not done before, EGD during a symptomatic period off acid
    suppression
  Helicobacter pylori testing

Optional
  Routine hematologic and biochemical tests (full blood count,
    ESR or CRP, serum glucose measurement, liver function tests,
    electrolytes and creatinine, calcium, thyroid function)
  Ultrasonography of the gall bladder, liver, and pancreas (low
    yield of relevant pathology; incidental gall stones may be
    found)
  24- or 48-h esophageal pH testing to rule out non-erosive reflux
    disease (if responsive to PPI)

Uncertain clinical value
  Gastric-emptying study
  Fundic relaxation (e.g., using barostat, SPECT, ultrasound, or
    MRI)
  Water or nutrient load test (global gastric function test)
  Electrogastrography
  Gastroduodenal manometry

CRP, C-reactive protein; ESR, erythrocyte sedimentation rate; SPECT, single photon emission computed tomography; MRI, magnetic resonance imaging; EGD, esophagogastroduodenoscopy.

pylori tests and treatments in younger dyspepsia patients with a low prevalence of infection [21]. Thus with regard to clinical outcomes and cost efficacy, most guidelines recommend empiric acid inhibition as the first line of therapy if alarm feature are missing [20].

In the literature there are many clinical trials focusing on the treatment of patients with non-ulcer dyspepsia (NUD), functional dyspepsia, idiopathic dyspepsia, and similar entities that all fall into the same category of symptoms referred to the upper gut in the absence of relevant structural lesions. For all trials there is a remarkable placebo response that ranges from 20 to 60%. This placebo response most likely is mainly due to the fluctuating course of symptoms and not due to true psychological effects. Nevertheless, antisecretory therapy with histamin-2-receptor antagonists (H_2RA) and PPIs appeared to be significantly more effective in this condition than placebo. A recent meta-analysis also concluded that the trials evaluating prokinetic therapy were difficult to interpret. While they demonstrated a significant effect, they were usually based on a small sample size and there was clear evidence for publication bias [22]. On the other hand, some large well controlled studies demonstrated efficacy of prokinetic therapy [23].

Colonization of the stomach with *H. pylori* is a risk factor for peptic ulcer disease. In undiagnosed dyspepsia, a test and treat strategy might be an option to avoid endoscopies in patients presenting with dyspepsia. Based on clinical studies, the *H. pylori* test and treat strategy for (previously undiagnosed) dyspeptic patients younger than 55 years appears to be safe and may result in lower costs than initial endoscopy with similar clinical outcomes [24]. Other decision analysis data suggest that if *H. pylori* eradication fails to relieve symptoms, PPI empiric therapy is more cost effective than endoscopy [25]. On the other hand, *H. pylori* eradication is very unlikely to improve symptoms in the long term, if peptic ulcer disease is ruled out and it is possible that the small effect in favor of *H. pylori* eradication therapy is simply due to undiagnosed peptic ulcer disease.

Acupuncture and acupressure can reduce chemotherapy-induced and postoperative nausea and vomiting but have not been tested in functional dyspepsia [26]. The value of gastric pacing in functional dyspepsia is also unclear [26].

Antidepressants are of uncertain benefit. Amitriptyline may be superior to placebo but data are very limited [27];

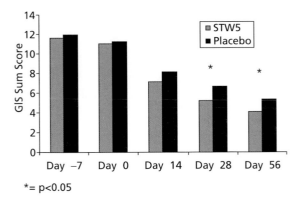

*= p<0.05

Figure 55.1 Course of Gastrointestinal Symptom Score (GIS Sum Score), ITT-population during 8 weeks of treatment with STW 5 (a novel prokinetic agent) or placebo. (From von Arnim U et al. [30]).

venlafaxine was no better than placebo in a larger trial [28].

Few controlled trials have evaluated the efficacy of psychological therapies in functional dyspepsia. In small trials greater improvement of symptoms in patients treated with cognitive psychotherapy than in a control group that received no specific treatment was seen. In patients with refractory symptoms, cognitive behavioral therapy was effective for the control of concomitant anxiety and depression [29]. Some herbal preparations also might be of value if efficacy is proven in placebo controlled clinical trials (Figure 55.1) [30]. The therapeutic measures are summarized in Table 55.4.

Case continued

A careful history is obtained and the available test results reviewed. In addition, the expectations of the patient were explored. The patient was concerned about the symptoms and the severity of them impairing her quality of life and thus she sought relief of her symptoms. Medication she had received before (acid-suppressing drugs and metoclopramide) had only temporarily relieved the symptoms. The patient appeared slightly depressed and concerned about potentially underlying, life-threatening disorders. Her sleep was disturbed with the inability to fall asleep. While the patient was without alarm features and was in a low-risk age group, she already had undergone a comprehensive diagnostic work-up including endoscopy, which had excluded *H. pylori* infection and sprue. Based on the long history of relapsing symptoms, and previous testing, the diagnosis of functional dyspepsia could be established. A low dose of tricyclic antidepressant was prescribed and her symptoms greatly improved.

Table 55.4 Treatments for functional gastroduodenal disorders.

First line
   Standard prokinetics (metoclopramide, domperidone, tegaserod)
   Anti–*Helicobacter pylori* therapy (unlikely to improve symptoms
      but minimizes risk of peptic ulcer disease)

Second line
   Tricyclic antidepressants (low dose)
   5-HT$_1$ agonists (e.g., buspirone, sumatriptan)
   Simethicone
   Sucralfate

Uncertain or unknown efficacy
   Promising new visceral analgesics
   Serotonin type 3 (e.g., ondansetron, alosetron)
   Gonadotropin-releasing hormone analogs
   Somatostatin analogs

Unlikely to be beneficial
   Antacids
   Prostaglandin analogs
   Motilinomimetics
   Anticholinergics/antispasmodics
   Nitrates

Take-home points

- Functional disorders of the stomach are characterized by symptoms referred to the upper abdomen that occur in the absence of known structural or biochemical abnormalities that can be detected utilizing routine diagnostic tests.

- Functional dyspepsia (which is the clinical manifestation of functional stomach disorders and is defined by the Rome III consensus) includes two entities: postprandial distress syndrome (PDS) with predominant meal-related symptoms and the epigastric pain syndrome (EPS).

- The precise causes of functional stomach disorders are as yet unknown.

- Defined abnormalities of stomach function are only present in a proportion of patients and may not be associated with the severity of symptoms.

- The diagnosis of a functional gastroduodenal diagnosis does *not* require evidence of disordered stomach function (e.g., delayed gastric emptying).

- The key to management is reassurance that no life-threatening disease is the cause of the symptoms. Dietary interventions and prokinetic as a trial of antisecretory medication (in patients with pain as the main symptom) may be considered. In treatment failures with severe symptoms, low-doses of tricyclic antidepressants are an option. Herbal therapy is another feasible approach, provided that there is sufficient clinical data (clinical trials) and safety data for a given preparation.

References

1 Vakil N, Talley N, van Zanten SV, *et al.* Cost of detecting malignant lesions by endoscopy in 2741 primary care dyspeptic patients without alarm symptoms. *Clin Gastroenterol Hepatol* 2009; **7**: 756–61.

2 Drossman DA. The functional gastrointestinal disorders and the Rome III process. *Gastroenterology* 2006; **130**: 1377–90.

3 Holtmann G, Siffert W, Haag S, *et al.* G-protein beta 3 subunit 825 CC genotype is associated with unexplained (functional) dyspepsia. *Gastroenterology* 2004; **126**: 971–9.

4 Camilleri CE, Carlson PJ, Camilleri M, *et al.* A study of candidate genotypes associated with dyspepsia in a U.S. community. *Am J Gastroenterol* 2006; **101**: 581–92.

5 Doring B, Pfitzer G, Adam B, *et al.* Ablation of connexin43 in smooth muscle cells of the mouse intestine: functional insights into physiology and morphology. *Cell Tissue Res* 2007; **327**: 333–42.

6 Mahadeva S, Goh KL. Epidemiology of functional dyspepsia: a global perspective. *World J Gastroenterol* 2006; **12**: 2661–6.

7 Gschossmann JM, Holtmann G, Mayer EA. [Epidemiology and clinical phenomenology of visceral pain]. *Schmerz* 2002; **16**: 447–51.

8 Talley NJ, Stanghellini V, Heading RC, *et al.* Functional gastroduodenal disorders. *Gut* 1999; **45** (Suppl. 2): II37–42.

9 Tack J, Talley NJ, Camilleri M, *et al.* Functional gastroduodenal disorders. *Gastroenterology* 2006; **130**: 1466–79.

10 Haag S, Talley NJ, Holtmann G. Symptom patterns in functional dyspepsia and irritable bowel syndrome: relationship to disturbances in gastric emptying and response to a nutrient challenge in consulters and non-consulters. *Gut* 2004; **53**: 1445–51.

11 Walker MM, Talley NJ, Prabhakar M, *et al.* Duodenal mastocytosis, eosinophilia and intraepithelial lymphocytosis as possible disease markers in the irritable bowel syndrome and functional dyspepsia. *Aliment Pharmacol Ther* 2009; **29**: 765–73.

12 Talley NJ, Walker MM, Aro P, *et al.* Non-ulcer dyspepsia and duodenal eosinophilia: an adult endoscopic population-based case-control study. *Clin Gastroenterol Hepatol* 2007; **5**: 1175–83.

13 Langeluddecke P, Goulston K, Tennant C. Psychological factors in dyspepsia of unknown cause: a comparison with peptic ulcer disease. *J Psychosom Res* 1990; **34**: 215–22.

14 Talley NJ, Fung LH, Gilligan IJ, *et al.* Association of anxiety, neuroticism, and depression with dyspepsia of unknown cause. A case-control study. *Gastroenterology* 1986; **90**: 886–92.

15 Talley NJ, Phillips SF, Bruce B, *et al.* Relation among personality and symptoms in non-ulcer dyspepsia and the irritable bowel syndrome. *Gastroenterology* 1990; **99**: 327–33.

16 Talley NJ, Jones M, Piper DW. Psychosocial and childhood factors in essential dyspepsia. A case-control study. *Scand J Gastroenterol* 1988; **23**: 341–6.

17 Drossman DA, Creed FH, Fava GA, *et al.* Psychosocial aspects of the functional gastrointestinal disorders. *Gastroenterol Int* 1995; **8**: 47.

18 Walker EA, Gelfand AN, Gelfand MD, Katon WJ. Psychiatric diagnoses, sexual and physical victimization, and disability in patients with irritable bowel syndrome or inflammatory bowel disease. *Psychol Med* 1995; **25**: 1259–67.

19 Bytzer P, Talley NJ, Leemon M, *et al.* Prevalence of gastrointestinal symptoms associated with diabetes mellitus: a population-based survey of 15,000 adults. *Arch Intern Med* 2001; **161**: 1989–96.

20 Talley NJ, Vakil NB, Moayyedi P. American gastroenterological association technical review on the evaluation of dyspepsia. *Gastroenterology* 2005; **129**: 1756–80.

21 Barton PM, Moayyedi P, Talley NJ, *et al.* A second-order simulation model of the cost-effectiveness of managing dyspepsia in the United States. *Med Decis Making* 2008; **28**: 44–55.

22 Moayyedi P, Delaney BC, Vakil N, *et al.* The efficacy of proton pump inhibitors in nonulcer dyspepsia: a systematic review and economic analysis. *Gastroenterology* 2004; **127**: 1329–37.

23 Holtmann G, Talley NJ, Liebregts T, *et al.* A placebo-controlled trial of itopride in functional dyspepsia. *N Engl J Med* 2006; **354**: 832–40.

24 Delaney BC, Innes MA, Deeks J, *et al.* Initial management strategies for dyspepsia. *Cochrane Database Syst* 2000; **2**: CD001961.

25 Spiegel BM, Vakil NB, Ofman JJ. Dyspepsia management in primary care: a decision analysis of competing strategies. *Gastroenterology* 2002; **122**: 1270–85.

26 Drossman DA, Corrazziari E, Talley NJ, *et al. The Functional Gastrointestinal Disorders. Diagnosis, Pathophysiology, and Treatment: a Multinational Consensus.* Degnon Associates, 2000.

27 Passos Mdo C, Duro D, Fregni F. CNS or classic drugs for the treatment of pain in functional dyspepsia? A systematic review and meta-analysis of the literature. *Pain Physician* 2008; **11**: 597–609.

28 van Kerkhoven LA, Laheij RJ, Aparicio N, *et al.* Effect of the antidepressant venlafaxine in functional dyspepsia: a randomized, double-blind, placebo-controlled trial. *Clin Gastroenterol Hepatol* 2008; **6**: 746–52.

29 Haag S, Senf W, Tagay S, *et al.* Is there a benefit from intensified medical and psychological interventions in patients with functional dyspepsia not responding to conventional therapy? *Aliment Pharmacol Ther* 2007; **25**: 973–86.

30 von Arnim U, Peitz U, Vinson B, *et al.* STW 5, a phytopharmacon for patients with functional dyspepsia: results of a multicenter, placebo-controlled double-blind study. *Am J Gastroenterol* 2007; **102**: 1268–75.

Index

Page numbers in *italic* refer to figures and tables.